www.harcourt-international.com

Bringing you products from all Harcourt Health Sciences companies including Baillière Tindall, Churchill Livingstone, Mosby and W.B. Saunders

- ▶ **Browse** for latest information on new books, journals and electronic products

- ▶ **Search** for information on over 20 000 published titles with full product information including tables of contents and sample chapters

- ▶ **Keep up to date** with our extensive publishing programme in your field by registering with **eAlert** or requesting postal updates

- ▶ **Secure online ordering** with prompt delivery, as well as full contact details to order by phone, fax or post

- ▶ **News** of special features and promotions

If you are based in the following countries, please visit the country-specific site to receive full details of product availability and local ordering information

USA: www.harcourthealth.com

Canada: www.harcourtcanada.com

Australia: www.harcourt.com.au

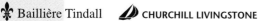 Baillière Tindall   CHURCHILL LIVINGSTONE   Mosby   W.B. SAUNDERS

HUTCHISON'S
CLINICAL METHODS

Commissioning Editor: Laurence Hunter
Project Development Manager: Sarah Keer-Keer
Project Controller: Nancy Arnott
Design direction: Judith Wright, George Ajayi

HUTCHISON'S
CLINICAL
METHODS

EDITED BY

MICHAEL SWASH MD FRCP FRCPath
Consultant Physician, The Royal London Hospital, London UK
Professor of Neurology
Barts and the London, Queen Mary's School of Medicine and Dentistry
London
UK

TWENTY-FIRST EDITION

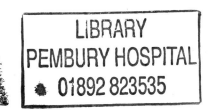

 W.B. SAUNDERS

EDINBURGH   LONDON   NEW YORK   PHILADELPHIA   ST LOUIS   SYDNEY   TORONTO   2002

W. B. Saunders
An imprint of Harcourt Publishers Limited

© Harcourt Publishers Limited 2002

▣ is a registered trademark of Harcourt Publishers Limited

First published 1897
Twenty first edition published 2002

Main edition
ISBN 0702025305

International edition
ISBN 0702025313

British Library Cataloguing in Publication Data
A catalogue record for this book is available from the British Library

Library of Congress Cataloging in Publication Data
A catalog record for this book is available from the Library of Congress

Note
Medical knowledge is constantly changing. As new information becomes available, changes in treatment, procedures, equipment and the use of drugs become necessary. The editors/authors/contributors and the publishers have, as far as it is possible, taken care to ensure that the information given in this text is accurate and up to date. However, readers are strongly advised to confirm that the information, especially with regard to drug usage, complies with the latest legislation and standards of practice.

The publisher's policy is to use **paper manufactured from sustainable forests**

Printed in India

PREFACE TO THE TWENTY-FIRST EDITION

The scope and technology of medicine continues to evolve, and clinical methods consequently evolve and require new techniques and approaches. Nonetheless, the core skills of communication, clinical examination, objective assessment, and planning relevant investigation and management, are as important to clinical practice as ever. Only learning and experience can develop these skills. Medicine is a profession: there is a relationship of trust between patient and doctor, and the doctor is recognised to have acquired knowledge and skills relevant to the practice of medicine. In addition, a code of ethics binds the doctor to certain modes of conduct in the clinical relationship with a patient and in relations with colleagues. All these matters are part of clinical methods in the modern world. Understanding established and new clinical methods and how they inter-relate is essential. *Hutchison's Clinical Methods* seeks to teach an integrated approach to clinical practice, so that new methods and investigations are merged into established patterns. Therefore, it continues to be a book for students of all ages.

We all find new things to learn every day, and the more alert we are the more we find there is to learn. In order to learn it is necessary to understand what we know. Knowledge and understanding are the keys to good practice.

With the advent of the Internet, and the easy availability of information, people are generally better informed than in the past. The modern doctor needs to be aware of this and to develop particular skills in dealing with the informed patient and their family. A firm foundation in clinical methods is essential to this process.

The text of this 21st edition reflects the need for an integrated approach to medicine. It is organized into both body system-related and problem-oriented chapters. The basic methods of cardiology, neurology and other specialties are described in chapters devoted to these topics. The special skills required in obstetrics and gynaecology, children, the elderly, or in the unconscious patient, for example, are discussed in separate chapters. There has been much re-writing and readers familiar with earlier editions will notice many changes, and much new material. The organization of the book, however, continues to follow the outline used by Hutchison, in the first edition, published in 1897.

In this new edition, there are many new illustrations and diagrams. Colour has been used whenever possible to enhance clarity. All the existing chapters have been substantially revised and brought up-to-date, and a number of entirely new chapters added, for example in oncology and traumatic injury. The book covers much new ground and reflects recent developments in clinical practice. Because of the importance of diagnostic imaging in contemporary clinical practice, a new chapter is devoted to this topic, with a panel of illustrations reflecting its scope within the modern hospital. In addition, appropriate images are used in each chapter. The chapter on ethics in medical practice, an issue of increasing importance in everyday practice, is updated. The introductory chapters have been shortened to avoid duplication with material that appears later. Quantitative methods have been introduced whenever relevant.

There are several new contributors, who are members of the consultant staff of the Royal London Hospital or of St Bartholomew's Hospital; these two venerable London teaching hospitals, and the Royal London Chest Hospital, merged in 1995. The new contributors to Hutchison's Clinical Methods from 'Barts' are most warmly welcomed. All the contributors to the book are accustomed to working closely together, and the book reflects these close professional relationships.

Throughout the book, the relevance of abnormal findings is explained in the context of diagnosis and management, and the book can therefore be used as an adjunct to a standard textbook of medicine, surgery or specialty. It may be read cover to cover or used section by section as seems appropriate. Readers' comments, as always, are welcomed.

Michael Swash
The Royal London Hospital

SIR ROBERT HUTCHISON MD FRCP (1871–1960)

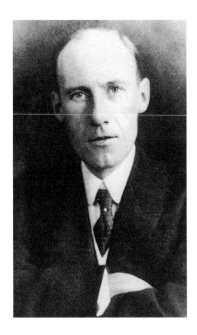

CLINICAL METHODS

A GUIDE TO THE PRACTICAL STUDY
OF MEDICINE

BY

ROBERT HUTCHISON, M.D., M.R.C.P.
DEMONSTRATOR IN PHYSIOLOGY, LONDON HOSPITAL MEDICAL COLLEGE

AND

HARRY RAINY, M.A., F.R.C.P.Ed., F.R.S.E.
UNIVERSITY TUTOR IN CLINICAL MEDICINE, ROYAL INFIRMARY, EDINBURGH

WITH 137 ILLUSTRATIONS AND 8 COLOURED PLATES

CASSELL AND COMPANY, LIMITED
LONDON, PARIS & MELBOURNE
1897
ALL RIGHTS RESERVED

Clinical Methods began in 1897, three years after Robert Hutchison was appointed Assistant Physician to The London Hospital. He was appointed full physician to The London and to the Hospital for Sick Children, Great Ormond Street, in 1900. He steered *Clinical Methods* through no less than 13 editions, at first with the assistance of Dr H. Rainy and then, from the 9th edition, published in 1929, with the help of Dr Donald Hunter. Although Hutchison retired from hospital practice in 1934 he continued to direct new editions of the book with Donald Hunter, and from 1949 with the assistance also of Dr Richard Bomford. The 13th edition, the first produced without Hutchison's guiding hand, was published in 1956 under the direction of Donald Hunter and Richard Bomford. Dr A. Stuart Mason and the present author joined Richard Bomford on Donald Hunter's retirement to produce the 16th edition, published in 1975, and following Richard Bomford's retirement prepared the 17th, 18th and 19th editions. Each of these editions was revised with the help of colleagues at The Royal London Hospital, in keeping with the tradition that lies behind the book.

During the many years of its continuous publication *Clinical Methods* has been translated into many languages. Indeed it is one of the great pleasures of association with the book to receive letters from far parts of the world, offering friendly advice, criticism and correction. Students have often noted errors that have escaped the eye of the editors.

Sir Robert Hutchison died in 1960 in his 90th year. It is evident from the memoirs of his contemporaries that he had a remarkable personality. Many of his clinical sayings became, in their day, aphorisms to be remembered and passed on to future generations of students. Of these the best known is his petition, written in his 82nd year:

'From inability to let well alone;
from too much zeal for the new and contempt for what is old;
from putting knowledge before wisdom, science before art, and cleverness before common sense;
from treating patients as cases;
and from making the cure of the disease more grievous than the endurance of the same, Good Lord, deliver us.'

Michael Swash
The Royal London Hospital

CONTRIBUTORS

Mr Trevor Beedham
Consultant Gnynaecologist
The Royal London Hospital
London

Professor Gerry Bennett
Consultant Geriatrician
The Royal London Hospital
and Professor of Healthcare of the Elderly,
Barts and the London, Queen Mary School of
Medicine and Dentistry
London

Dr Jamie Cavenagh
Honorary Consultant in Haematology
The Royal London Hospital
and Senior Lecturer in Haematology,
Barts and the London, Queen Mary School of
Medicine and Dentistry
London

Dr Rino Cerio
Consultant Dermatologist
The Royal London Hospital
London

Dr Otto Chan
Consultant Radiologist
Department of Medical Imaging
The Royal London Hospital
London

Dr Gordon Cook
Trust Centre Wellcome for History of Medicine
and Honorary Lecturer in Clinical Pathology
Barts and the London, Queen Mary School of
Medicine and Dentistry
London

Mr Frank Cross
Consultant Surgeon
The Royal London Hospital
London

Dr John Cunningham
Consultant Physician
The Royal London Hospital
London

Dr David D'Cruz
Consultant Physician
Louise Cotte Lupus Unit
St Thomas's Hospital
London

Dr Chris Gallagher
Consultant Oncologist
Department of Medical Oncology
St Bartholomew's Hospital
London

Dr Beng Goh
Consultant in GU Medicine
Ambrose King Centre
The Royal London Hospital
London

Dr Roger Harris
Consultant Paediatrician
The Royal London Hospital
and Senior Lecturer in Paediatrics,
Barts and the London, Queen Mary School of
Medicine and Dentistry
London

Dr Gary John
Consulant Clinical Biochemist
The Royal London Hospital
London

Mr Guy Kenyon
Consultant Otolaryngologist
The London Independant Hospital
London

Mr Ivor Levy
Consultant Ophthalmic Surgeon
75 Harley Street
London
and Consultant Opthalmic Surgeon
The Royal London Hospital
London

Dr Peter Mills
Consultant Cardiologist
The London Chest Hospital
London

Professor John Monson
Consultant Endocrinologist
St Bartholomew's Hospital
and Professor of Endocrinology
Barts and the London, Queen Mary School of
Medicine and Dentistry
London

Dr John Moore-Gillon
Consultant Physician
Department of Respiratory Medicine
St Bartholomew's Hospital
London

Dr Howard Ring
Consultant Psychiatrist and Senior Lecturer in
Psychiatry
Barts and the London, Queen Mary School of
Medicine and Dentistry
London

Professor Paul Swain
Consultant Gastroenterologist
Royal London Hospital
and Professor of Gastroenterology
Barts and the London, Queen Mary School of
Medicine and Dentistry
London

Professor Michael Swash
Consultant Physician
The Royal London Hospital
& Professor of Neurology
Barts and the London, Queen Mary School of
Medicine and Dentistry
London

Dr Adam Timmis
Consultant Cardiologist
London Chest Hospital
London

CONTENTS

1
PATIENT AND DOCTOR

INTRODUCTION

The word 'patient' is derived from the Latin *patiens*, a word meaning sufferance or forbearance. The purpose of medical practice is to relieve suffering. In order to achieve this purpose, it is important to make a diagnosis, to know how to approach treatment and to design an appropriate scheme of management for each patient. It is therefore essential to understand each person as fully as possible, whatever their social class, income or ethnic and cultural background. The wise doctor must not only elucidate the problems posed by disease but also apply his or her skill to advise patients and families how to manage these problems. The distinction between cure of disease and relief of symptoms remains as valid today as in the past. No patient should leave a medical consultation feeling that they will 'just have to live with it', even when the disease is incurable.

Clinical methods, the skills doctors use to achieve this aim of excellence in clinical practice, are acquired during a lifetime of practice. Indeed, they evolve and change as new techniques and new concepts arise. There is always something new to learn. Clinical methods are learned by a combination of study and experience.

The initial aims of any first consultation are diagnosis and understanding the nature of the patient's perception of the problem. This double aim requires knowledge of disease and its patterns of presentation, together with an ability to interpret a patient's symptoms and signs. Appropriate skills are needed to elicit the symptoms from the patient's description and conversation, and the signs by observation and by physical examination. Difficulties posed by differences in educational level or by the variety of cultural and ethnic backgrounds found in modern life must be accepted and factored into the interpretation of the data acquired during the consultation. This requires not only experience and considerable knowledge of people, in general, but also confidence in one's ability to strike up a relationship with very different individuals.

It is often worthwhile asking what the patient (and the family) expect to gain or learn from the consultation. Sometimes the answer is surprising; the aim may be to check another physician's diagnosis, or to obtain verification of inability to work, or to seek an opinion useful in relation to some legal matter or in the pursuit of compensation following injury, rather than to seek cure of a disease. Sometimes people come because their families have insisted, and not from any personal desire to seek a medical opinion. All these reasons are nonetheless valid; every consultation should be taken seriously, and every patient should be evaluated thoroughly. If a patient indicates that he or she does not wish to discuss certain topics, or to be examined fully, this wish must be respected, even though it may make the consultation incomplete and cause difficulties in advising on further investigations or therapy.

There are two main steps in making a diagnosis:

- The first is to establish the clinical features by history and examination—this represents the clinical database
- The second is to interpret the clinical database in terms of disordered function and potential causative pathologies, whether physical, mental, social, or a combination of these.

This book is about this process.

SETTING THE SCENE

Most medical encounters or consultations occur in the out-patient setting. Here there is opportunity for introducing a stereotyped situation. The consultation room and the waiting area, together with the registration procedure, are always the same, and the same nurses, clerks and other employees will work there. Every patient can therefore be assessed against this constant background. The degree of confidence, fear or concern, the personality and the social skills of each patient can be rapidly assessed by the staff and by the doctor. This can be important in understanding the nature of the problem presented by any individual.

Either go yourself to fetch the patient from the waiting room or have the patient brought into the consulting room by a nurse or receptionist. Introduce yourself and offer a greeting. Observe the response unobtrusively, but with care. Does the patient smile, or appear furtive or anxious? Does the patient make good eye contact with you? Is he or she frightened? Or depressed? Are posture and stance normal? Is the patient short of breath, or wheezing? In some conditions (e.g. congestive heart failure, uraemia, Parkinson's disease, stroke, severe anaemia, jaundice) the nature of the problem will be immediately obvious.

Pleasant surroundings are very important. It is essential that both patient and doctor feel at ease, and especially that neither feels threatened by the encounter. Avoid having patients full-face in front of you. You will wish to take some notes during consultations and yet you will need to be able to see your patients and establish eye contact, and to show sympathy and awareness of their needs during the discussion of symptoms, much of which may be distressing or even embarrassing. If patients sit to your left, at an angle to your desk, the situation is less formal, and clues such as agitated foot and hand

movements are more evident. This is also a good position for someone in a wheelchair, who is otherwise likely to be at some distance because the foot pieces of the chair project forward. Other people present can arrange themselves beside the patient, or further round to your left, or in front of you. This disposition of seating arrangements also makes it clear that it is the patient who is the centre of attention, rather than any other of those present.

ACCOMPANYING PERSONS

Some people come to consultations alone, others with one or more friends or family members. Always spend time during the initial exchange of greetings to identify who is present and to get some idea of the group dynamics. Who is the senior person present? What are the expectations of this consultation? What is the educational level of the people present? Have they perhaps seen many other doctors previously for the same problem? Ask patients whether they came alone, or whether there is someone waiting outside. Consider whether these people should also be interviewed, either with your patient or separately, perhaps while the patient is getting ready to be examined and there is an opportunity to talk with the accompanying person alone.

There is always a reason why people come accompanied. If there appear to be too many people present, or if you feel that the presence of others threatens your relationship with the patient at any time in the consultation, it is appropriate to consider asking the others to leave, if only briefly. Suggesting this may uncover dissension, so be prepared for this. It is reasonable, if in doubt, to ascertain *why* others wish to be present, and, certainly, whether this is also the patient's wish.

In certain ethnic groups, however—including, for example, many Asian and Muslim people—it is normal for the patient to be accompanied. A male patient will often be accompanied by his wife or by one or more male relatives, and a female patient may come with several other family members. An Asian woman will never come alone unless she is second or third generation in the UK, or otherwise acculturated to Western ways. Often the accompanying family members, especially male elders, will take on the task of describing the patient's symptoms, and may dictate how much questioning can be undertaken, and how intimate an examination will be allowed, particularly when the patient is female and the doctor is male. Sometimes, discussion is necessary in order to allow a reasonably complete examination to be accomplished.

COMMUNICATION

Rather than asking the patient immediately to start to describe the problem, it is better to engage in certain preliminaries. These will set the patient at ease and give an opportunity for both you and the patient, and any others present, to become sufficiently familiar with each other to proceed with confidence. Doctors may appear quite formidable and frightening to the patient. Try to avoid this, without losing a slight sense of formality and neutrality in the relationship.

First, check that you have the right patient—there may be several Mrs Smiths or Mr Patels waiting to see you. Check the address and the date of birth as well as the name. Look at the documentation, if any, but do not rely excessively on this until you have heard what the patient has to say; always prefer primary information to hearsay or someone else's opinion—even that of another doctor. Make it clear that, first and foremost, you want to hear what the patient has to say; you will inspire confidence by this.

There are two ways of beginning the history: either ask patients to describe their symptoms, or get the background information first. The latter is in many ways preferable, since the personal, social and medical history is then obtained without bias for the current complaints, and its true significance can thus be considered. It is a good idea to get at least some of this information at the beginning, particularly basic demographic information such as marital status and employment, basic family history and the main features of the past medical history (see Box 1.1). The details can be filled in later. If you know something about the person sitting with you at your desk you will be in a far better position to discuss symptoms and problems than if you know nothing about them. If you have any experiences in common—for example, you both know the place in which the patient lives or was brought up—then the relationship is easier to develop.

Remember that communication is a two-way process. It is the beginning of the doctor–patient relationship. Any fear or nervousness must be dispersed by bringing it out into the open. The doctor should be confident, attentive, dispassionate and friendly. It is not always easy to be all these things, but it is important. Any other worries the doctor may have should be put aside for the day.

THE HISTORY

Getting patients to start talking is a conversational skill. There are a number of possible approaches; it

BOX 1.1   Headings used in history-taking.

- Age and address
- Marital status
- Social and occupational history
- History of previous illness
- Family history
- Presenting complaint
- History of present illness
- Treatment history

is important to remain flexible and to be prepared to change your approach if it seems that a new start is needed. Try asking what the problem is or use the referral letter, if there is one, to ask a direct but open question to encourage a patient to talk, for example, 'What is the problem—can you describe it?' Ask for a description of what has happened. Encourage patients either to start at the beginning, or to describe the particular problem that worries them the most. Set up the relationship so that you start with an open situation. Expect patients to be open with you and be clear that you will be open with them. Avoid suspicion. Sometimes there is a background of a failed relationship between a patient and another doctor; sometimes patients are suspicious that you may exert some statutory power that will disadvantage them. If you feel there is a cloud developing in your relationship with a particular patient, try gently to find out why this is.

OBSERVE YOUR PATIENT
During the communication process make judgements about the patient's general demeanour. Is the person well-presented, clean, well-spoken, intelligent? Is there any sign of disability, whether mental or physical? What clues does the gestural language convey? Is the patient confident, knowledgeable, or perhaps depressed and miserable? Does he or she keep to the subject or ramble inconsequentially, or with suspicion of others? Is there embarrassment about something that is not spoken of? Is the patient talking about the things that really bother them? Look at the patient's clothes and belongings. Have they just been shopping? Are they reading anything and what is it? This will tell you a lot about your patient's language, interests and educational level.

TRUST YOUR PATIENT
Make it clear to your patients that you expect them to speak freely and give their own account of the problem. Avoid suggesting symptoms until the patient has finished this description, when you may wish to obtain more detail or to enquire specifically about certain symptoms not so far mentioned. If there are points that are not fully described, or which you think are important, do not be afraid to ask directly for more information. However, recognize that this will interrupt the patient's flow of recall, and that you will then need to restart the spontaneous description that you interrupted.

CATEGORIZING THE MAIN SYMPTOM
It is conventional to seek to identify the patient's main or presenting complaint. In practice this may not be relevant, since the problem may take the form of the progressive development of a sequence of symptoms and deficits rather than a simple symptom such as 'breathlessness'. Indeed, modern patients may already have had recourse to the internet and found informa-

tion about their symptoms and difficulties, and have found a reasonable diagnosis. Never feel threatened by the informed patient. Knowledge is itself a source of power and influence, and knowledgeable patients will have a much clearer concept of the options available and of the direction they would like management of their illness to take. This knowledge is also useful to you, as the physician. It is not a threat.

The internet is only one of several sources of information available to patients. All such sources are uncensored, and many are unconventional and provide information of dubious value. Nonetheless, all information has some value, and it should always be taken seriously and discussed in detail. An informed patient is generally an understanding and compliant patient.

NOTE-TAKING

When making notes, try to keep eye contact with the patient. Try also not to make notes only at times that might suggest what items of information you regard as important; listen, make up your mind what is being said and record enough to help you remember the important points. Later, you can write up a fuller account or, as many physicians do, dictate a full letter indicating the history, the weight placed on various items and, most importantly, what the patient actually said. What patients say, word for word, is often as important as any later reconstruction of the history.

DIRECT QUESTIONS

There is a time and place for direct questions in history-taking. Indeed, direct relevant questions are an essential component of sensitive history-taking. It is often best to store up direct questions until the patient has finished talking—you may well need to make notes to make sure you have not forgotten these points. Sometimes the patient or family will themselves embellish the history at the end of the initial account with more detail, and a little extra questioning in this context is often very valuable. If you are not sure of something, ask for more detail. If you have noticed an abnormality not mentioned by the patient (for example a rash, an abnormal posture, pallor, an injury or scar), ask about it directly. Often such abnormalities are discovered during the examination, and a further series of questions is necessary to establish whether this observation is relevant to the presenting problem, or has an unrelated and irrelevant basis. Useful subjects are listed in Box 1.2. Clearly, it is not appropriate to ask all these questions; select the most relevant or those than provide the best screening information.

When you think you have a clear understanding of the patient's story, you should take each main symptom in turn and examine it in detail. The first step is to make sure that you and the patient are talking about the same thing. Ask the patient to

BOX 1.2   Common symptoms in various bodily systems: the system review. This should be tailored to the clinical situation.

General features
- Weight
- Sleep
- Energy

Gastrointestinal system, abdomen and pelvis
Upper alimentary tract
- Pain
- Appetite
- Vomiting
- General characteristics of vomited matter
- Flatulence
- Water-brash
- Heartburn
- Dysphagia

Lower alimentary tract
- Diarrhoea
- Constipation
- Pain
- Liver and gallbladder
- Jaundice
- Pain

Genital system

Cardiovascular system
- Dyspnoea
- Pain or tightness
- Palpitation
- Cough
- Oedema

The blood
- Lassitude, dyspnoea and awareness
- Infections
- Blood loss
- Skin problems
- Diet
- Past history
- Drug history
- Occupational history
- Glandular enlargement

Respiratory system
- Cough
- Sputum
- Breathing
- Wheeze
- Chest pain

Urinary system
- Symptoms suggestive of renal failure
- Urine

BOX 1.2   (continued)

Nervous system
- Stroke
- Seizures
- Headache
- Other neurological symptoms

Locomotor system

Infants and children
- Special questions where relevant

rephrase any part of the story if the original description was unclear to you. Sometimes the history has to be elaborated before it can be understood. A patient may, for instance, complain of wind or flatulence. Since flatus is considered in Western culture to be an indelicate subject, it might be assumed that this means bringing up wind, whereas the patient may well mean passing wind by the back passage, or perhaps a feeling of wanting to get rid of wind but being unable to do so. Therefore enquire directly: 'Do you mean that you bring the wind up or that you pass it down or that you feel that you want to get rid of it but can't?' Although one should avoid, as far as possible, leading questions which themselves suggest an answer, other direct questions, such as 'Have you ever coughed blood?', may be essential. With experience, certain suggestions lend themselves to a rather stereotyped pattern of analysis. Remember that symptom analysis can be achieved only when the database is complete. Completion of the database is itself a function of the success of communication between doctor and patient.

CONTEXT
Try to relate the history as given to what you know from the preliminary information you have obtained about the patient's occupation, past medical history and family history. Consider whether there is more you need to know about this background. Look again at the referring letter (if there is one) and consider whether there are any unexplored clues there. The family history is often especially important. People with a family history of premature vascular disease have increased susceptibility, and there is a genetic influence in a large number of diseases, including psychiatric problems. A particularly informative question at this stage is 'What made you come to see me today (at this time)?' The answer may be 'My wife made me come—she's fed up with me complaining', or 'My friend at the club has just been diagnosed with cancer', or 'I have had enough at work and I want to get a letter for medical retirement'.

NON-VERBAL CLUES
When trying to establish the significance of a symptom, or when asking a potentially emotionally

laden question, it is essential to take account of non-verbal clues to the importance attached by the patient to the issue. Does the patient catch his or her breath, change breathing pattern, become pale or flushed, look agitated, show restless limb or body movements, become upset, or change eye contact? All these are well recognized and important signs of stress. Be careful to maintain cooperation if these features become evident. You will need to avoid antagonizing the patient; to continue to explore difficult issues requires tact and trust. Try putting down your pen and looking at the patient with interest and with direct eye contact.

VOCABULARY
Be careful to use words that the patient can understand. Your preliminary enquiries should have roughly established the intellectual and educational level of the patient. Talk about passing urine rather than micturition, or opening the bowels rather than defaecation. Discuss eating and swallowing in the domestic context. Introduce a discussion about travelling to work or about sports and hobbies in order to find out about mobility and exercise tolerance. Ask about washing, dressing, getting up, cooking and shopping. Very simple, everyday tasks are important. Can the dizzy man stand on one leg while putting on his trousers, or does he have to sit down? What did the patient watch on TV last night? What is in the news these days? Do the patient's clothes fit just as they used to, or have they become too small or too large?

SOCIAL ISSUES
Social circumstances are relevant in many issues, particularly in 'functional disorder', in which there are severe and disabling symptoms but few or no signs on examination. Common examples include headache, certain recurrent abdominal pains, non-specific chest pain, muscle and joint pain and some menstrual disorders. Relating these complaints to a social or personal conflict requires independent verification of the conflict and attachment of the symptom to the conflict. This is easy to suggest but more difficult to establish, and sometimes even more difficult to explain to the patient and the family. Organically based disorders must always be properly excluded by appropriate clinical assessment and investigation. The persistence of disabling symptoms in the absence of demonstrated organic disease should raise this issue.

The symptom or symptoms thus displayed can be seen as a call for help: these patients present physical symptoms acceptable to themselves, to their families and friends and to others such as employers or physicians as a complaint justifying medical assessment and sympathy. Some people are particularly likely to develop physical symptoms in relation to emotional, situational or personal stresses, and these may constitute a 'somatization disorder' in psychiatric terminology. Sometimes the situation is more complex, the symptom developing unconsciously as a conversion reaction in an hysterical illness. Sexual themes often dominate such illnesses.

EXAGGERATION

More commonly, however, the patient simply exaggerates: the headache is present 'all the time'; the patient has 'not slept for a moment for weeks'; the abdominal discomfort has been present without interruption 'for days and days'; the pain in the knee or back is 'agony', but the patient is too busy doing something else to come for an appointment when asked. Nevertheless, despite the exaggeration, the symptom is real, and with a sympathetic approach its underlying characteristics can be analysed.

In some cultures it is normal behaviour stoically to bear pain without complaint, whereas in others the converse pertains—the patient will describe pain 'all over the body' that is present 'all the time' and is 'too much' to bear. The pain is the same, but the person's attitude towards it is different.

DIFFICULT PATIENTS

While it is true that the doctor's role is always to establish a relationship with the patient, this cannot always be successfully accomplished. There are always reasons for this and the reasons are always important. If you find that you are not getting on with a patient, pause and think why this might be. Try a different approach. Say that you are not clear what the main problem is and try to start again. Get the patient to describe the problem again from the beginning. Ask if there is some matter that has not yet been discussed—'Is there anything else I should know about?' In the event that there is persistent failure in the relationship, consider the following issues.

ANGRY PATIENTS

Anger arises from resentment, sometimes from unspoken distress, and from perceived insults, usually in the medical context a belief that the patient is not believed by the doctor. This most easily results when the doctor rapidly concludes that a symptom is not of organic origin in the context of the patient's fear of a serious underlying condition. The woman with persistent tension headache is convinced that she has a brain tumour; her reaction to the diagnosis may be overt anger, since the symptom is important to her in exerting control over the domestic stresses in her life. The headache allows her to retire from the unwanted advances of her husband, or to compensate for the near criminal behaviour of her son. Abdominal pain and diarrhoea may prevent a patient from going out to meet others; backache may prevent work and allow disability payments. Uncovering the non-organic

nature of these complaints is threatening and may provoke anger.

Anger can also arise from other factors. The patient may have been kept waiting without explanation, or there may be another work-related appointment for which he or she is late. There may have been a row with someone at home or at work that day, and you may be caught in the residual distress. The patient may have a grievance against you, against a colleague of yours, or against the hospital or practice itself. These grievances are often more perceived than real, but they are real enough to the patient, and the only way to resolve them is to get the patient to say what the trouble is, and then to talk it through. When the grievance is about an institution, this may be difficult since there is no one immediately responsible with whom the matter can be discussed directly, and the only recourse may be to offer an apology and try to start again. Try saying 'I am sorry to see you upset—can you tell me what it is that is causing you this problem?' and 'Can I help to put things right for you?'

CONTROLLING THE CONSULTATION

Always stop yourself from showing an angry reaction in response—although this may be difficult, it is important in order that you can remain in charge of the situation. *Violence* is sometimes experienced, especially in Emergency Room practice when some patients may be under the influence of alcohol or other substances. At the slightest hint of violence, seek help. If it is reasonably likely that a patient will be violent, undertake the examination with another person, preferably a bulky male assistant. Adopt a soothing attitude, and keep talking quietly and reassuringly. Take precautions to protect yourself from potential assault—fortunately this is rare.

If a patient is so angry that this dominates the consultation, it is wise to *close the consultation*, to offer another consultation on another occasion, or to offer to arrange consultation with another doctor, even at another hospital. To attempt to pursue the matter will sometimes simply raise the level of anger. No benefit will result to the patient or to you.

DISTRESS

The anxious patient is often distressed. This is due to worry, concern, fear or unresolved personal problems or conflicts. Seek opportunities for the patient to discuss any underlying issues so that the distress can be assuaged. Be sympathetic but firm in your approach, as well as strictly neutral and non-judgmental. Often the most marked distress is a result of apparently trivial problems that have become magnified by rumination and rehearsal—once discussed these can be resolved.

TEARFULNESS

This may indicate overwhelming distress or, more commonly, relief that the doctor has begun to understand a problem that no one else has listened to. Sometimes an emotionally distressing topic may be inadvertently touched on, and the patient starts to weep. Clearly, this is an important moment in the history, and care should be taken to skirt around it and then come back to it, or even to ask the patient to discuss it further at the time. It is usually best to resolve the concern as soon as possible.

The commonest cause of distress and tearfulness is grief—bereavement distress may persist for many months or even years when it is not discussed, and the mourning process brought out in public. Grief is a normal reaction, and should be discussed in this context. Occasionally, counselling from a priest or other religious adviser (or even a psychologist in the case of inappropriately prolonged grief) will be helpful.

The term 'catastrophic reaction' was introduced by the German neuropsychologist Goldstein, from his experience of soldiers in the First World War, to describe the sudden flood of distress and weeping that can occur in a conversation when an emotionally charged event is touched upon. The reaction may be so overwhelming that no further conversation is possible, and the consultation should be resumed on another occasion. The patient may require tea and sympathy to recover some equanimity. In people with brain injury, this catastrophic reaction is released and more prominent, and indeed may hamper communication and rehabilitation.

CONFUSION
The muddled patient is ill. There may be a progressive dementia, or drug abuse, a toxic confusional state, or a metabolic encephalopathy. Always remember the possibility of a focal brain disorder, especially aphasia, and also previous head injury. Test the mental status using the short-form mental state test—you can interpolate this into the history by saying 'I just want to ask you some simple questions', before continuing to try to get the patient to tell you about the symptoms and problems. Find a member of the family, or a close friend, and talk to them. Confused patients are often garrulous and circumlocutory, switching from one topic to another without ever getting to detail. The conversation is always superficial, sometimes amusing, but devoid of content or fact.

UNRELATED INFORMATION
A problem to those physicians wishing to take the history in chronological order—'Start at the beginning and tell me all about it'—is that people usually start with the part of the problem that they regard as the most important. This is, of course, entirely relevant from the patient's viewpoint, and it is also important to the doctor, since the issue that most bothers the patient is then brought to attention. Patients want their symptoms relieved, and the disease cured. The latter may not always be possible,

so it is important to be aware of the important symptoms since, for example, pain may be relieved even though the underlying cause of the pain is still present.

Unrelated information, introduced more or less without context into the consultation, is often of particular importance. When presented with another, apparently disparate point, note it carefully and come back to it later. It may fall naturally into place but it may also be a clue to the nature of the underlying disorder. For example, the patient with fatigue may describe a fleeting rash or joint pain that suggests systemic lupus erythematosus as the underlying cause.

INTERPRETERS
Any information taken through a third party is liable to distortion. This is most likely to occur if the interpreter is a close family member, for example a husband translating for his wife when the marital relationship may itself be part of the underlying problem. Trained independent interpreters are available in many hospitals, and may be invaluable in obtaining the history. Information obtained in this way is, however, never as good as first hand information, and it is often wise to make an attempt to communicate in broken English, or your own smattering of the patient's language in order to try to get a direct feel for the problem. Your relationship needs to be with the patient rather than with the third party.

A particular problem with interpreted histories is that the interpreter may simply summarize the patient's complaint, describing it as 'pain in the chest' rather than giving the detail that you may suspect was available from the conversation between interpreter and patient, and that you know you require. Ask for this detail.

SPEAKING TO RELATIVES AND OTHERS
If others have come to the consultation it is reasonable to suppose they have done so with the agreement of the patient. It is wise to check this however, perhaps while you are examining the patient, when the accompanying people will usually not be present.

Information obtained from a concerned and observant relative is often particularly valuable. There may be an objective account of the symptoms, indicating their relative severity and their duration with some accuracy. Other features may have been noticed. The onset may be more precisely recognized. A link with other personal or medical events may be apparent. The patient's non-compliance with prescribed medication may be brought to light. Hitherto undisclosed stresses at work, at home, or with others may be described.

SYMPTOM ANALYSIS

The objective of the history is to identify the disturbance of function and structure responsible for the patient's symptoms. Symptoms always have a *physiological* or *anatomical* basis. Thirst is an example of a physiological symptom.

Thirst must first be distinguished from the dry mouth of oral infections or of defective salivary secretion. Compulsive water drinkers complain of severe thirst but are seldom woken up by it. Thirst, however, is most commonly the prime symptom of loss of body water (with or without loss of salt). The main causes of reduced body water content are reduced water intake or excessive loss of body water, for example from vomiting, diarrhoea, increased sweating (with fever or exposure to heat), increased output of urine and severe haemorrhage. Simple questions or observations will reveal the immediate disorder of function or functions that are responsible for the symptom, but further questions and investigations may be necessary to explain it in terms of pathology.

Thirst associated with loss of body water due to increased urinary output should suggest diabetes mellitus. In this disorder the urine contains glucose and is of high specific gravity. In diabetes insipidus, on the other hand, the urine is of low specific gravity (< 1.010). The passage of large amounts of urine with a specific gravity of 1.010 (isotonic with plasma) in renal failure may be sufficient to cause a thirst that persists both by day and night. Hypercalcaemia, by diminishing the action of antidiuretic hormone and so increasing water loss, may produce thirst. Finally, the administration of diuretics (including excessive tea or coffee drinking and alcohol) may promote salt and water loss with increased urine volume and so cause thirst.

ANALYSIS OF PAIN

Perhaps the commonest complaint which brings a patient to a doctor is pain. Systematic analysis of this symptom is important, and illustrates the way in which the nature of a symptom can be further explored (see Box 1.3). A standardized approach is essential:

Site
Where is it? Note whether the patient points with a finger to one spot or with the hands to an area on the affected part of the body.

> **BOX 1.3   Analysis of pain as a symptom.**
>
> - Site
> - Radiation
> - Severity
> - Timing and duration
> - Character
> - Occurrence or aggravation
> - Relief

Radiation
Does it stay in one place, or does it move or spread? It may gradually extend, or shoot along the distribution of a peripheral nerve or nerve root.

Severity
Does it interfere with daily activities or keep the patient awake at night? If the answer to these questions is 'Never', the pain is unlikely to be severe; however, some people are quite stoic in enduring severe pain. Patients who use exaggerated terms such as 'continual agony' are usually seeking sympathy and one should try to discover the real reason for their distress, which is more often social or psychological than the result of serious physical illness. Headache that never lets up, day or night, and that apparently prevents sleep—'I can't sleep at all with it, doctor'—is strongly suggestive of anxiety and depressive symptoms.

Timing and duration
When did it start? When does it come and when does it go? Has it changed since it began?

Character
What is it like? Descriptions of the character of a pain (e.g. stabbing, burning, pricking, gnawing) may be helpful, although it is very difficult for anyone to describe a pain in words. The distinction between an abdominal colic, which waxes and wanes and may cause a patient to roll about, and a steady pain like that of peritonitis, which causes the patient to try to avoid all movement, is very important in diagnosis.

Occurrence or aggravation
What brings it on? What makes it worse? Pain in the centre of the chest which always comes on after a certain amount of exertion, or is made worse by exertion, is probably due to ischaemia of the heart (angina). A very similar pain which comes on a short time after eating is probably oesophageal.

Relief
What makes it better? Pains may be relieved by simple measures. Pain arising in the musculoskeletal system, for instance, may be relieved by a change of position. Upper gastrointestinal pains (e.g. duodenal ulcers) are usually promptly relieved by eating. Lower gastrointestinal pains may be relieved by defaecation or the passage of wind. Cardiac pain, brought on by exertion, is relieved by rest. The discomfort of oesophageal reflux is often relieved by belching. Any definite relief by simple responses or manoeuvres may be a valuable clue to the disturbance of function or structure involved.

The effect of drugs is also important. Ischaemic cardiac pain is usually promptly relieved by trinitrites. Musculoskeletal pains are usually relieved by simple analgesics such as aspirin, while discomforts associated with stress and tension are not.

CHRONOLOGY

The time course of the development of individual symptoms, and the timing of the onset of new symptoms, is important in understanding the development of the illness. This information tells much about the nature of the pathological process. Vascular disorders often have a sudden onset, as in stroke or myocardial infarction, or produce symptoms in relation to exertion of a certain degree, as in intermittent claudication of the legs from vascular insufficiency in the femoral circulation, or angina in coronary artery disease. Cancer presents as an enlarging lump, as a haemorrhage (e.g. haemoptysis or melaena), or with progressive symptoms due to organ failure. Degenerative diseases such as Parkinson's disease cause slowly progressive deficits. Inflammatory diseases cause fever, pain and restriction of movement (e.g. abdominal inflammation or inflammatory joint disease). Infections are usually characterized by local symptoms from the organ affected (e.g. breathlessness in pneumonia), together with fever and other systemic inflammatory symptoms. In all of these examples the local features, the general features, and the chronology of the development of these features are all important in making the diagnosis.

Often the diagnosis can be suggested from the history alone. It is worth remembering that in the history the patient is telling you about the symptoms resulting from disordered physiology and/or anatomy, and also how the illness developed. The examination can only give a snapshot of the abnormalities detectable at that particular time. The history is therefore almost always more important than the physical examination. Often the examination simply confirms what the patient has already told the doctor.

LIMITATIONS IN HISTORY-TAKING

Apart from the obvious limitations caused by language difficulties, or by mental and psychological disorders, there is an inevitable limitation in that patients are often describing abnormalities in their sense of well-being of which they have had no previous personal experience. This lack of experience limits the person's ability to give a coherent account. When the mind itself is disordered, as in psychiatric and many neurological disorders, there are further difficulties. Have sympathy for patients who struggle to find words and phrases to describe their symptoms; give them time to express themselves; indicate that you understand the difficulties they are experiencing. Never show impatience, even if you are short of time, since this will make the process more difficult. If you really have not got time, come back later when you are less pressed. Every patient deserves to have your unbroken attention during the time you are talking with them. Always talk *with* a patient, never at them or to them. Try to be on the patient's level at all times.

PREVIOUS ILLNESSES

It is often important to revisit the past history when current problems have been discussed in detail or, if you did not ask about this at the beginning, to introduce the subject at the end of the enquiry into current symptoms. Be clear that the patient's description of the diagnosis of an earlier illness is consistent and likely to be correct. If it seems important, ask where the previous illness was treated, and consider requesting information from the other doctor or hospital. Check whether the patient is taking medication, and do not forget to enquire about non-prescription proprietary treatments (for example used for pain relief) and also about alternative or herbal remedies—some of the latter can be powerful and may produce serious unwanted effects, including, for example, renal failure. If it seems relevant, ask simply and without coyness about sexual orientation and consider then asking about HIV exposure. Consider also asking about substance abuse if there are any clues that suggest this could be important (e.g. sleeping rough, an unconventional lifestyle, work in susceptible occupations such as the popular music industry or, if a European, residence in high incidence areas such as the Far East).

SPECIAL QUESTIONS FOR WOMEN

It may be relevant to ask if a woman is taking an oral contraceptive, whether the menstrual periods are regular, and about the cycle, and whether there are menopausal symptoms (e.g. hot flushes and irregular periods). The obstetric history may also be important, for example in a woman presenting with urinary or faecal incontinence. Migraine may be triggered by menstruation, and heart failure by pregnancy. Many women work long hours. They may have a full-time job, with commuting. When they get home there may be a child who is looked after by a child-minder in the working day, but requires time with its mother as well, and then there is cooking and housework to be done. All this is difficult to contain or cope with.

OCCUPATIONAL HISTORY

This is sometimes important (see Box 1.4 for some suggested questions). The classic industrial illnesses, such as lead poisoning and other toxic exposures are now extremely rare in developed industrial countries, but accidental exposure continues to occur, usually in relation to domestic usage. Other problems such as asbestos exposure or silicosis produce effects many years after exposure, and a careful chronological occupational history may be required to elucidate the exposure.

The work experience is also very important. Work is often a highly pressured environment in the West,

- Is the job dusty, and if so what tools make the dust?
- Are there fumes or vapours, and if so what are the chemical substances involved? (Most of the toxic substances encountered in dangerous trades enter the body by inhalation, although some solvents penetrate the skin.)
- Is a hood installed over the bench, and is it connected to a suction system?
- Is protective clothing provided?
- Is a special suit and goggles required, and why?
- Has any similar illness affected a fellow employee? (Certain occupational hazards are associated with office work, for example repetitive strain injury and migraine induced by stress or inappropriate lighting.)

with expectations of long or irregular hours, especially in work in financial services in big cities. The hours of other less skilled workers are generally more regulated, but many people work extra hours, or have anther job in addition to their main occupation, and personal life may therefore be restricted, leading to social problems that need to be addressed as part of the process of management.

GENETIC HISTORY

In many diseases there is a genetic background to onset and causation. Some diseases (e.g. Friedreich's ataxia, Huntington's disease, cystic fibrosis, muscular dystrophies and cardiomyopathies) are inherited with dominant, recessive or sex-linked patterns of transmission. Mitochondrial inheritance is also now well understood, especially in certain brain and muscle diseases, but also in renal and gastrointestinal disease. A new era of understanding of genetic factors in the presentation and development of disease is beginning, and this will have profound effects on medical practice. The genetic history has therefore become important.

Inherited disorders are generally more common in populations in which first cousin marriages are common, as happens in isolated communities, and in certain religious groups, especially some Muslim communities. Careful enquiry about the family history, with a family tree drawn to show all family members on both paternal and maternal sides of the family, together with the causes and ages of death, will usually demonstrate any inherited disorders. Diabetes and coronary artery disease also show inherited factors in their causation, although there are major interacting environmental factors, such as dietary factors. Some Mendelian disorders can be tested for preclinically by DNA analysis. When families request this testing, genetic counselling is required in order that the full implications are under-stood. Generally, children should be excluded unless there is the possibility of therapy that will prevent the onset of the disorder.

NEGATIVE DATA

It is sometimes as important to record that a symptom was *not* present as to record that it was present. Under each system therefore (See Box 1.2), the absence of the most important symptoms (e.g. breathlessness and cough in the case of the respiratory system, breathlessness on exertion or cardiac pain in the case of the cardiovascular system, and paralysis, headaches or fits in the case of the nervous system) should be recorded, if relevant.

THE PHYSICAL EXAMINATION

The techniques for examination of the different bodily systems are described in the system-specific chapters of this book. It is important to develop a routine of physical examination which combines speed with thoroughness, sensitivity and alertness, but which disturbs the patient no more than necessary. It need hardly be said that the examination must be carried out as gently as possible, without tiring the patient needlessly. In severely ill patients it may be necessary to postpone a routine examination and to perform only the examination required for provisional diagnosis and treatment. Very ill patients must obviously be treated with special care and consideration.

Different doctors have different routines for examining patients in different circumstances. Always plan the examination. Does the information obtained from the history suggest that particular abnormal features will be found on examination? What else should be looked for? For example, if the patient has vomited blood and has a history of heavy alcohol ingestion, the liver may be found to be enlarged, there may be signs of hepatic failure and there could also be neurological abnormalities.

Start the examination in a manner that is relevant to the patient's symptoms. For example, if the presenting symptom is sciatica, start with the legs and the spine. However, a systematic approach to each functional system is essential in order to gain information that is both *complete* and *relevant*. This routine serves to remind the clinician of any omissions. Always try to be thorough. With experience you will become more confident in looking directly for certain signs suggested by the history, and then conducting a systematic examination in this context.

GENERAL APPROACH

A physical examination requires a cooperative patient and a quiet, warm and well-lit room equipped with a couch, a chair and some steps to help disabled people get onto the couch. Daylight is better than artificial light, which may mask changes in skin colour, for example the faint yellow tinge of slight jaundice. A fairly complete examination can be carried out with a patient sitting in a chair, or in a wheelchair, but this is difficult and likely to be limited. Although in practice a physical examination may have to be made under all sorts of circumstances, every attempt should be made to reassure and relax the patient.

For a complete examination the patient should be asked to undress completely, or at least to under-clothes, and to lie on the couch or bed covered with a sheet or dressing-gown. Patients are often examined while wearing underpants, but it is essential to remember to examine the buttocks and genitalia. Ideally a chaperone should be present when a male doctor is examining a female patient, and always during rectal and vaginal examinations, both to reassure the patient and to protect the doctor from subsequent accusations of improper conduct.

In considering the general appearance, it is important to make a rapid assessment of the degree of illness. This is not making a diagnosis. One has simply to answer the question: 'Does this patient look well, mildly ill, or severely ill and therefore in need of urgent attention?' Experienced nurses are often highly skilled in this kind of assessment and their opinion should never be ignored. Some severely ill patients complain little; and occasionally one meets a patient whose appearance of excellent health belies protestations of unbearable agony.

Every moment of the consultation is important. Abnormalities will be recognized as soon as you meet the patient, and you may well notice things about the patient during history-taking. Watching the patient getting undressed or dressed is often especially revealing of neurological and rheumatological disorders, and may reveal the degree of pain. It has been said that the experienced doctor 'begins the examination on meeting the patient, and continues taking the history until the consultation ends'. An abnormal finding on examination may indicate the need for further questions. Although the examination may provide information about organs and functions, in physical examination as well as in history-taking it is important to try to view the patient as a whole person, recognizing the patient's reaction to his or her illness as an important component in understanding the symptoms. Box 1.5 shows a summary plan for the physical examination.

THE MENTAL AND EMOTIONAL STATE

Try to make some initial assessment of the patient's intelligence and mental and emotional state, but recognize that this initial impression may be inaccurate. Vocabulary and command of language are generally a good guide. Sometimes a book or magazine carried

---

> **BOX 1.5   The physical examination: summary of plan.**
>
> - Mental and emotional state
> - Physical attitude
> - Gait
> - Physique
> - Face
> - Skin
> - Hands
> - Feet
> - Neck
>   - lymphatic and salivary glands
>   - thyroid gland
>   - pulsation
> - Breasts
> - Axillae
> - Temperature
> - Pulse
> - Respiration
> - Odours

---

by the patient may provide a reliable clue. Observation, as well as the history, assist in the assessment of the emotional state. Thus an anxious person may be restless, with wide palpebral fissures and sweating palms. Is the anxiety reasonable in the circumstances or is the patient overanxious? In depression, the lowered mood, inability to concentrate or make decisions, mental retardation, apathy or even obvious misery may be clearly evident; however, these features may not be obvious, although important and leading to physical symptoms. Apparently severe disability, without appropriate concern or anxiety, should suggest a non-organic disorder, or even hysteria (*la belle indifférence*).

THE PHYSICAL ATTITUDE

The patient's posture may give valuable information. Severely ill patients slip down the bed or chair into uncomfortable attitudes which they are unable to correct. Patients with heart failure sit up because they may become dyspnoeic if they lie flat (*orthopnoea*). Patients with abdominal pain due to peritonitis lie still, while patients with colic are restless or may even roll about in futile attempts to find relief. People with painful joint diseases often have an attitude of helplessness. Various neurological disorders produce characteristic postures (Ch. 11). In the severest cases of meningitis the neck may be bent backwards so that the head appears to bore into the pillow (*neck retraction*).

THE GAIT

The gait should always be observed in patients able to walk. Important abnormalities of gait are described in Chapters 10 and 11, but remember that simple things like a painful corn, an ill-fitting shoe or a strained muscle may produce a temporary limp. The gait is best observed as the patient walks into the consulting room, or to the couch prior to the formal examination, since this represents the patient's natural gait. Under formal examination the gait may appear more abnormal as the patient may then try to demonstrate certain subjective abnormalities to the physician. Much can be learned by observing the unconscious signals of confidence, distress, anxiety, depression and other moods and emotions. An attempt should always be made to encourage a patient examined in bed to try to sit up, stand and walk. It may even be helpful to ask the patient to jump, hop or walk an imaginary narrow line.

PHYSIQUE

Much can be learned from a general inspection of the patient's physique. Is the appearance consistent with the patient's chronological age? Is he or she tall, short, fat, thin, muscular or asthenic? Are there any obvious deformities and is the body proportionate? Height should be roughly equal to the fingertip-to-fingertip measurement of outstretched arms and twice the leg length from pubis to heel. Dwarfism, with a stocky body and very short legs, is characteristic of achondroplasia. Hypopituitarism arising in childhood produces a proportionate but dwarfed adult with an unusually youthful appearance. In acromegaly the features are coarsened and the jaw, hands and feet are large. Young people with acromegaly may continue to gain height.

'Ideal' weights (as used in life insurance) are listed in Tables 1.1 and 1.2 Obesity is mostly a problem of developed countries. In some parts of the world signs of malnutrition such as wasting, apathy, anaemia and skin changes may be encountered; they should also be looked for in neglected elderly patients in developed countries such as Britain. A history of weight gain or loss can be checked by observation, remembering that fluid retention (*oedema*) will increase weight. Obvious weight loss, even when food intake has increased, is a feature of thyrotoxicosis and diabetes mellitus. Psychogenic loss of appetite in girls (*anorexia nervosa*) causes extreme emaciation while physical activity remains unimpaired. Vegetarians may be unusually thin, or may develop obesity if the diet contains much fat and carbohydrate.

THE FACE

Observe the patient's face. The expression, and particularly the eyes, indicate real feelings better than words. Some diseases, for example Parkinson's disease, depression, hypothyroidism, thyrotoxicosis, acromegaly, third and seventh cranial nerve palsies and paralysis of the cervical sympathetic nerve (Horner's syndrome, Fig. 12–16), produce characteristic facial appearances.

Parotid swellings are obvious on inspection of the face. The tender bilateral parotid swelling of mumps or the unilateral swelling with reddening of the skin from acute parotitis can be contrasted with the nonbilateral persistent enlargement, accompanied by dry, tearless eyes of Sjögren's syndrome, or the more

TABLE 1.1   Ideal weights for men aged 25 and over.

Height			Small frame		Medium frame		Large frame	
ft	in	cm	lb	kg	lb	kg	lb	kg
5	2	157.5	112–120	50.8–54.4	118–129	53.8–58.5	126–141	57.2–64.0
5	3	160.0	115–123	52.2–55.8	121–133	54.9–60.3	129–144	58.5–65.3
5	4	162.6	118–126	53.5–57.2	124–136	56.2–61.7	132–148	59.9–67.1
5	5	165.1	121–129	54.9–58.5	127–139	57.6–63.0	135–152	61.2–68.9
5	6	167.6	124–133	56.2–60.3	130–143	59.0–64.9	138–156	62.8–70.8
5	7	170.2	128–137	58.1–62.1	134–147	60.8–66.7	142–161	64.4–73.0
5	8	172.7	132–141	59.9–64.0	138–152	62.6–68.9	147–166	66.7–75.3
5	9	175.3	138–145	61.7–65.8	142–156	64.4–70.8	151–170	68.5–77.1
5	10	177.8	140–150	63.5–68.0	146–160	66.2–72.6	155–174	70.3–78.9
5	11	180.3	144–154	65.3–69.9	150–165	68.0–74.8	159–179	72.1–81.2
6	0	182.9	148–158	67.1–71.7	154–170	69.9–77.1	164–184	74.4–83.5
6	1	185.4	152–162	68.9–73.5	158–175	71.7–79.4	168–189	76.2–85.7
6	2	188.0	156–167	70.8–75.7	162–180	73.5–81.6	173–194	78.5–88.0
6	3	190.5	160–171	72.6–77.6	167–185	75.7–83.5	178–199	80.7–90.3
6	4	193.0	164–175	74.4–79.4	172–190	78.1–86.2	182–204	82.7–92.5

Heights are measured wearing ordinary shoes and weights in ordinary indoor clothing.
Notice that tables of this kind make no allowance for 'middle-aged spread'.

TABLE 1.2   Ideal weights for women aged 25 and over.

Height			Small frame		Medium frame		Large frame	
ft	in	cm	lb	kg	lb	kg	lb	kg
4	10	147.3	92–98	41.7–44.5	96–107	43.5–48.5	104–119	47.2–54.0
4	11	149.9	94–101	42.6–45.8	98–110	44.5–49.9	106–122	48.1–55.3
5	0	152.4	96–104	43.5–47.2	101–113	45.8–51.3	109–125	49.4–56.7
5	1	154.9	99–107	44.9–48.5	104–116	47.2–52.8	112–128	50.8–58.1
5	2	157.5	102–110	46.3–49.9	107–119	48.5–54.9	115–131	52.2–59.4
5	3	160.0	105–113	47.6–51.3	110–122	49.9–55.3	118–134	53.5–60.8
5	4	162.6	108–116	49.0–52.6	113–126	51.3–57.2	121–138	54.9–62.6
5	5	165.1	111–119	50.3–54.0	116–130	52.6–59.0	125–142	56.7–64.0
5	6	167.6	114–123	51.7–55.8	120–135	54.4–61.2	129–146	59.5–66.2
5	7	170.2	116–127	53.5–57.6	124–139	56.2–63.0	133–150	60.3–68.0
5	8	172.7	122–131	55.3–59.4	128–143	58.1–64.9	137–154	62.1–69.9
5	9	175.3	126–135	57.2–61.2	132–147	59.9–66.7	141–158	64.0–71.7
5	10	177.8	130–140	59.0–63.5	136–151	61.7–68.5	145–163	65.8–73.9
5	11	180.3	134–144	60.8–65.3	140–155	63.5–70.3	149–168	67.6–76.2
6	0	182.9	138–148	62.6–67.1	144–159	65.3–72.1	153–173	69.4–78.5

Heights are measured wearing ordinary shoes and weights in ordinary indoor clothing.
Notice that tables of this kind make no allowance for 'middle-aged spread'.

irregular unilateral painless lump of a mixed parotid tumour.

The cheeks give information regarding the patient's health: in anaemia and hypopituitarism they are pale; in the nephrotic syndrome they are pale and puffy; in cases of mitral stenosis there is sometimes a bright circumscribed flush over the malar bones; in many persons who lead an open-air life they are red and high-coloured; in congestive heart failure they may also be high-coloured, but the colour is of a bluish tint which cannot be mistaken for the red cheeks of weather-beaten people. In some cases of systemic lupus erythematosus there is a red raised eruption on the bridge of the nose extending on to the cheeks in a 'butterfly' distribution. *Telangiectases*, minute capillary tortuosities, or *naevi*, may be seen on the face in liver disease and, rarely, as a hereditary disorder (Fig. 1.1).

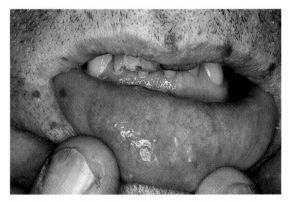

Fig. 1.1 Hereditary telangiectasia. The telangiectasia can be seen at the margin of the lips and on the lower lip.

THE SKIN

The detailed examination of the skin is described in Chapter 4. The most important abnormalities in the skin relevant to general examination are *pallor, yellowness, pigmentation, cyanosis* and *cutaneous eruptions*. In dehydration the skin is dry and inelastic so that it can be pinched up into a ridge. The skin is atrophied by age and sometimes after treatment with glucocorticoids. It is thickened, greasy and loose in acromegaly.

Pallor depends on the thickness and quality of the skin, and the amount and quality of the blood in the capillaries. Pallor occurs in persons with thick or opaque skins, who are always pale; in hypopituitarism; in states where the blood flow in the capillaries is diminished, such as shock, syncope or left heart failure; locally in a limb deprived of its blood supply; or in the fingers or toes when arterial spasm occurs on exposure to cold, as in Raynaud's disease. Generalized pallor may also occur in severe anaemia. Anaemia, however, is a feature of 'the colour of the blood rather than that of the patient' and the colour of the skin may be misleading. The colour of the mucous membranes of the mouth and conjunctivae gives a better indication, as does the colour of the creases of the palm of the hand.

Yellowness is usually due to jaundice. A pale lemon-yellow tint is characteristic of haemolytic jaundice; in obstructive jaundice, there is a dark yellow or orange tint. In obstructive jaundice there may be scratch marks from itching evoked by bile salts. In rare cases yellowness may be due to carotenaemia. Are there tobacco stains on the fingers, face or hair?

Pigmentation (see Ch. 4) is most commonly racial or actinic. The pigmentation of Addison's disease affects the buccal mucous membranes as well as exposed skin and parts subject to friction. In Von Recklinghausen's disease (neurofibromatosis type 1) patches of café au lait (milky coffee) pigment patches, ranging from freckling of the axillae to large (greater than 5 cm in length) areas on the limbs, trunk or face are a characteristic feature.

Cyanosis is a bluish colour of the skin and mucous membranes due to the presence of reduced haemoglobin in the blood. There are two physiological types: central and peripheral. *Central cyanosis* results from imperfect oxygenation of blood, as in heart failure and some lung diseases, or from admixture of desaturated venous blood with arterial oxygenated blood due to right-to-left (venous-arterial) shunts in the heart. In this case the cyanosis is general and the cyanosed extremities are warm. It characteristically affects the tongue as well as the limbs. *Peripheral cyanosis* is due to excessive reduction of oxyhaemoglobin in the capillaries when the flow of blood is slowed. This may happen on exposure to cold, when there is venous obstruction, or in heart failure. The cyanosed extremity or extremities are cold, and the tongue is unaffected. The cyanosis of heart failure is often due to both central and peripheral causes. A similar bluish or leaden colour rarely may be produced by methaemoglobinaemia or sulphaemoglobinaemia, usually due to the taking of drugs such as phenacetin. This should be considered in any patient who is cyanosed but not breathless. Carbon monoxide poisoning produces a generalized cherry-red discoloration, due to the presence of carboxyhaemoglobin.

Cutaneous eruptions are described in Chapter 4.

An excess of fluid in the subcutaneous tissue causing swelling of the tissues is known as *oedema*. Thus in acute nephritis an early symptom is oedema of the face, which is most marked when the patient rises in the morning. In *dependent oedema*, however, which is typically present in congestive heart failure, and in conditions associated with a low plasma protein level, the swelling first appears at the ankles and over the dorsum of the foot, and only gradually involves the legs, thighs and trunk. In local *venous obstruction* the oedema is confined to the parts from which the return of blood is impeded. Thus, oedema of an arm occurs when malignant glands constrict the axillary vein; and oedema of a leg occurs in thrombosis of the popliteal or femoral vein. Oedema of the whole upper part of the body may result from intrathoracic tumours. Oedema can be recognized by the pallid and glossy appearance of the skin over the swollen part, by its doughy feel, and by the fact that it pits on finger pressure. In recumbent patients oedema often appears first over the sacrum. In recognizing pitting oedema it is important to press firmly and for a sustained period, or slight oedema

may be missed. The oedema of lymphatic obstruction does *not* pit on pressure.

Localized oedema may be due to local changes in capillary permeability, as in angioneurotic oedema and giant urticaria. Oedema is also a feature of cutaneous or subcutaneous inflammation.

Subcutaneous emphysema is uncommon, but if present can be recognized by the crackling sensation produced by lightly compressing the part affected.

THE HANDS

The hands of the patient should be examined carefully. Notice the strength of grip as you shake hands; this is a rough indicator of abnormality. Note the general shape of the hands, the state of the joints, the character of the nails, the presence or absence of finger clubbing, the presence of nailbed infarcts, and of staining with nicotine.

In *osteoarthrosis* the finger joints are often implicated, and bony nodules, known as *Heberden's nodes* (Fig. 1.2), are formed at the bases of the terminal phalanges. In rheumatoid arthritis there is a spindle-shaped swelling of the interphalangeal joints and, later, ulnar deviation of the fingers. *Trophic changes* in the skin may be present in neurological disease and in disorders of the peripheral circulation (e.g. Raynaud's disease). *Characteristic movements or postures* of the hand may also be seen in athetosis, tetany and lead palsy. *Tremor* of the hands may occasionally be familial (essential tremor). In other cases it is due to nervousness, senility, Parkinsonism, thyrotoxicosis, alcoholism, multiple sclerosis, uraemia or hepatic failure. In *ulnar paralysis* the hand becomes deformed by overextension of the wrist, combined with excessive flexion of the ulnar two digits, so that a claw-like attitude is produced. Wasting of the small muscles of the hand, due for example to median or ulnar nerve lesions, cervical root (T1) disease or loss of anterior horn cells at the same level, gives the hand a flattened appearance. The characteristic posture of the hand in tetany is

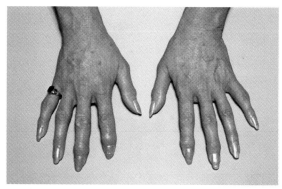

Fig. 1.2 Heberden's nodes. Reproduced with permission from M. A. Mir (1995) Atlas of Clinical Diagnosis, London, W. B. Saunders.

shown in Figs 1.3(a) and (b). In Dupuytren's contracture there is a thickening of the palmar fascia, which may lead to flexion contracture of the ring and other fingers. In acromegaly the hands are massive, the fingers spatulate with square tips and the skin thickened.

In *clubbing of the fingers* (Figs 1.4(a) and (b)), the tissues at the base of the nail are thickened, and the angle between the nail base and the adjacent skin of the finger is obliterated. The nail itself loses its longitudinal ridges and becomes convex from above downwards as well as from side to side. In extreme cases the terminal segment of the finger is bulbous, like the end of a drumstick. The toes may also be affected. Clubbing is found in association with a number of cardiopulmonary and abdominal disorders (Box 1.6). Clubbing is an important sign of

(a)

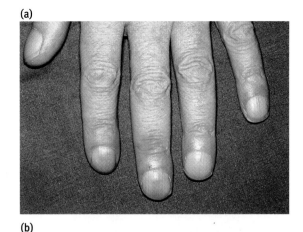

(b)

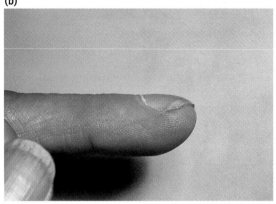

Fig. 1.4   (a) (b) Clubbing. Reproduced with permission from M. A. Mir (1995) Atlas of Clinical Diagnosis, London, W. B. Saunders.

(a)

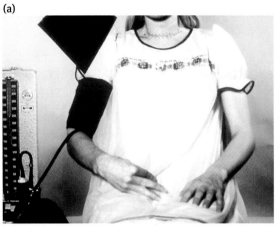

(b)

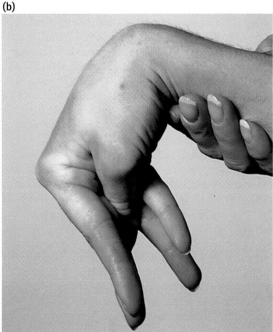

Fig. 1.3   (a) (b) Tetany. Reproduced with permission from M. A. Mir (1995) Atlas of Clinical Diagnosis, London, W. B. Saunders.

BOX 1.6   Causes of clubbing of the fingers.

Cardiopulmonary disorders
- Severe chronic cyanosis
- Congenital heart disease, e.g. Fallot's tetralogy
- Chronic fibrosing alveolitis
- emphysema
- Chronic suppuration in the lungs
  - bronchiectasis
  - empyema
- Carcinoma of the bronchus
- Pulmonary tuberculosis

Chronic abdominal disorders
- Crohn's disease
- Polyposis of the colon
- Ulcerative colitis

Subacute bacterial endocarditis

---

subacute bacterial endocarditis, when it may be associated with Osler's nodes. The latter consists of tender transient swellings about the size of a pea in the pulp of the fingers and toes. 'Splinter' haemorrhages occur beneath the nails in this condition. In hypertrophic pulmonary osteoarthropathy, besides

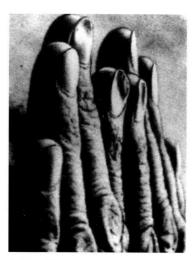

Fig. 1.5   Koilonychia.

clubbing of the fingers, there is thickening of the periosteum of radius, ulna, tibia and fibula. This gives rise to swelling above the wrist and ankle. Congenital clubbing is rare.

Koilonychia (Fig. 1.5) occurs in iron-deficiency anaemia. The nails are soft, thin, brittle and spoon-shaped. The normal convexity is lost and replaced by a concavity. *Nailbed infarcts* occur in vasculitis, especially in systemic lupus erythematosus and in polyarteritis.

THE FEET

The feet must not remain obscured under bedclothes or socks during the examination. *Pitting oedema* may be recognized only in the ankles and dorsal surfaces of the feet. The condition of the skin of the feet is especially important in diabetics and the elderly. *Peripheral vascular disease* will make the skin shiny, and hair does not grow on ischaemic legs or feet. The dorsalis pedis and posterior tibial pulses may be reduced or absent. If the toes of an ischaemic foot are compressed their dull purple colour will blanch and only slowly return. Passive elevation of an ischaemic leg will cause marked pallor of the foot as perfusion against gravity falls. Painless trophic lesions, often with deep ulceration, on the soles are seen frequently in diabetic peripheral neuropathy (the diabetic foot).

THE NECK

The neck should be inspected and palpated. Swellings in the neck are usually best felt from behind. Note the following:

THE LYMPHATIC AND SALIVARY GLANDS
In infection of the tonsils, the lymph glands at the angles of the jaws are enlarged; those below the jaw are enlarged in patients with metastases from cancer in the mouth. Glands draining an inflammatory focus are usually tender. Enlarged tuberculous glands may occur in groups or in long chains behind the sternomastoid, and scars may mark the sites of past suppuration in severe untreated cases. In human immunodeficiency virus (HIV) infection, Hodgkin's disease, other reticuloses and secondary neoplasms the glands are enlarged and discrete. In lymphatic leukaemia there may be great enlargement of the glands on both sides. In secondary syphilis the glands under the upper part of the trapezius are often palpable. If enlarged glands are found, either in the neck or elsewhere, it is important to observe whether they are firm and distinct or fused together, whether fluctuation can be elicited, and whether they are adherent to adjacent structures. The submandibular salivary glands should also be palpated when the neck is being examined from behind. If the glands are swollen and tender, the opening of their ducts into the mouth should be inspected, with the tip of the patient's tongue rolled upwards; this may reveal a salivary calculus.

THE THYROID GLAND
Inspect the neck for any general or local enlargement of the gland, and observe its movement with the larynx during swallowing. Patients find this easier if they are given a glass of water. Next, stand behind the seated patient and palpate the gland with one hand on each side of the neck. Determine if any swelling exists and, if so, whether it is uniform or nodular, hard or soft. Sometimes such an enlargement presses on the trachea and, occasionally, it may extend into the thorax behind the sternum. At other times, particularly if the disease is malignant, the recurrent laryngeal nerves may become implicated. If it is difficult to determine whether a tumour is connected with the thyroid, remember that the gland and any tumour connected with it moves up and down on swallowing. Minor degrees of enlargement of the thyroid are often better seen than felt. A bruit heard over the thyroid is a sign that the gland is hyperactive.

PULSATION IN THE NECK
Pulsations in the vessels must be noted. Any arterial pulsation is both seen and felt as a distinct thrust, whereas venous pulsation can be seen but not felt as a thrust, if it is felt at all. In aortic incompetence the carotid arteries are seen to pulsate forcibly. In aortic stenosis a systolic thrill is felt. In hypertensive patients carotid pulsation may be prominent. The jugular veins may be distended and pulsatile in congestive heart failure. In superior mediastinal obstruction due to retrosternal goitre or malignant neoplasm in the mediastinum, non-pulsatile distended veins may be seen over the neck and upper part of the body; cyanosis and oedema of the upper part of the body may accompany this sign. Distended neck veins may also be seen in large pericardial effusions.

THE BREASTS

The chance of finding a treatable cancer should make a full examination of the breasts a necessary feature of every general examination of a woman older than 35 years. With the patient reclining, arms to the sides, inspect the development and symmetry of breasts and nipples. Look for any reddening of the skin, ulceration or dimpling (*peau d'orange*). Retraction (rather than inversion) of the nipple is a sign that suggests carcinoma of the breast. Gently squeeze deeply beneath the nipple to express any milk or discharge. Determine whether it is blood, serous or milky; the patient may well have noticed this herself.

Palpate each breast with the flat part of the fingers, working over the whole breast as if it were mapped out in quardrants. Repeat this when the patient has her hands placed behind her head. If a lump is found, the characteristics to describe it are the same as those for any lump felt anywhere in the body. Determine its situation, size, shape, surface and edge; feel its consistency and mobility in relation to deep and superficial structures.

Any swelling of the male breast is likely to be seen at a glance. The swelling can be distinguished as breast tissue rather than pectoral fat by palpation when the patient's hands are behind his head. At some stage of puberty the majority of normal boys will have a palpable disc of breast tissue beneath the areola.

AXILLAE

Examine the axillae. It is difficult to feel enlarged lymph glands unless the patient's arm is raised to allow the examining fingers to be pushed high into the axilla. The arm is then lowered in the flexed position to rest across the examiner's arm and palpation is continued downwards along the chest wall.

TEMPERATURE

When taking the temperature, remember the following points:

- Before inserting the thermometer, make it an invariable rule to wash it in antiseptic or in cold water, and see that the mercury is well shaken down. Afterwards, wash it before replacing it in its case.
- The thermometer must be accurate. The centigrade (Celsius) scale is in general use in the UK, but many people are still more familiar with the Fahrenheit scale (Table 1.3).
- It must be kept in position long enough to allow the mercury to reach body temperature. It is advisable to exceed the period which the instrument professes to require. The ordinary 'half-minute' thermometer should be left in position for

TABLE 1.3   Temperature ranges in Centigrade and Fahrenheit.

	Centigrade	Fahrenheit
Normal	36.6–37.2	98–99
Subnormal	< 36.6	< 98
Febrile	> 37.2	> 99
Hyperpyrexia	> 41.6	> 107
Hypothermia	< 35	< 95

a full minute. Collapsed, comatose and elderly patients should have their rectal temperature taken with a special 'low-reading' thermometer. Accidental hypothermia is common in the elderly in winter.

- In conscious adults the temperature is taken in the mouth or in the axilla. In young children the thermometer should be placed in the fold of the groin, and the thigh flexed on the abdomen; or it may be inserted into the rectum. The temperature of the mouth and rectum is generally at least half a degree higher than that of the groin or axilla. When the temperature is taken in the mouth, the patient must breathe through the nose and keep the lips firmly closed during the observation.

In febrile disorders, there is a disturbance of heat regulation, so that the thermostatic mechanism controlling heat gain and loss is set at a level higher than normal. While the temperature is rising to this new level, heat is conserved, the skin vessels are constricted so that the body feels cold, and the patient may even shiver violently. This shivering is called a *rigor*. When the higher temperature is reached, heat loss again becomes apparent; the skin vessels dilate and the body feels warm.

FEVER

There are three classic types of fever or pyrexia: *continued*, *remittent* and *intermittent*. When fever does not fluctuate more than about 1°C (1.5°F) during 24 hours, but at no time touches the normal, it is described as *continued*. When the daily fluctuations exceed 2°C, it is called *remittent* (Fig. 1.6), and when fever is present only for several hours during the day, it is called *intermittent*. When a paroxysm of intermittent fever occurs daily, the fever is described as *quotidian*; when on alternate days, it is *tertian*; when two days intervene between consecutive attacks, it is *quartan* (Fig. 1.7). However, with the use of antibiotics and other specific drugs, these classic types of fever are less often encountered.

PULSE

Count the pulse for a full half minute when the patient is at rest and composed. Abnormalities due to cardiovascular causes, such as disturbances of the

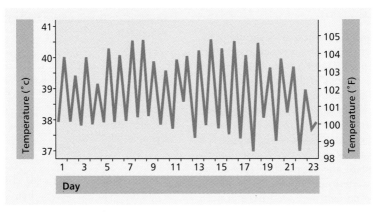

Fig. 1.6   Remittent fever. Patient died on day 23.

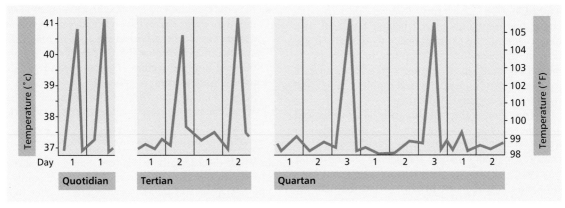

Fig. 1.7   Intermittent fever.

normal rhythm (*arrhythmia*) are described in Chapter 6. The rate in health during the stress of a medical examination varies from about 60 to 80 beats/minute. The common causes of a rapid pulse are recent exercise, excitement or anxiety, shock (e.g. bleeding), fever and thyrotoxicosis. A slow pulse is characteristic of severe hypothyroidism and of complete heart block.

RESPIRATION

Count the patient's respirations for a full half minute, starting when the patient's attention is directed elsewhere. It is convenient to do this when the patient thinks you are still counting the pulse. The normal rate in an adult is about 14–18 respirations/minute, but wide variations occur in health. The main causes of fast breathing (tachypnoea) are recent exertion, anxiety or nervousness; fever; pulmonary, pleuritic and cardiac conditions causing hypoxia; cerebral disturbance; metabolic acidosis; and hysterical over-breathing (hyperventilation). The latter may cause alkalosis and attacks of tetany.

Obstruction in different parts of the respiratory tract may give rise to recognizable varieties of noisy breathing (see Ch. 5). Obstruction in the *nasal passages* may cause sniffling or bubbling sounds. Paralysis of the soft palate causes an inspiratory snoring noise. Obstruction in the region of the *larynx* causes inspiratory stridor, as in the whoop of whooping cough. Obstruction in the *trachea* may produce growling or rattling noises when the lumen is obstructed by mucus. Obstruction in the *bronchi* may give rise to audible snoring or wheezing noises.

Obstruction of airways in the larynx or larger bronchi characteristically gives rise to *inspiratory noises*, while obstructions in the small bronchi and bronchioles produces *expiratory wheezing*. The latter is heard in bronchitis and asthma (obstructive airways disease). Alternating periods of cessation of respiration with hyperventilation (Cheyne–Stokes respiration) occur in left heart failure and in various cerebral disturbances.

The *pattern of breathing* may be characteristic of diseases quite distinct from those of the respiratory system. Examples of this are the stertorous breathing after a seizure or severe stroke, the hissing expiration of uraemia, and the 'air hunger' of diabetic ketoacidotic coma, which affects both inspiration and expiration.

ODOURS

The odours of *alcohol* and of certain drugs (e.g. paraldehyde) are easily recognizable on the breath. That of alcohol does not necessarily mean the patient's condition is due to alcoholic intoxication. The odour of *diabetic ketosis* has been described as 'sweet and sickly'; that of *uraemia* as 'ammoniacal or fishy'; and that of *hepatic failure* as 'mousy', but too much reliance on such delicate distinctions is unwise. *Halitosis* (bad breath) is common in patients whose dental hygiene has been poor, and is associated especially with *chronic gingivitis* (periodontal or gum disease).

ROUTINE PHYSICAL EXAMINATION

A schema for routine examination (Box 1.7) should be followed when it is necessary to check the various bodily systems, for example prior to surgery. Such a routine may have to be modified according to the needs of the patient—for example, the minimum necessary examination in an acutely ill patient, the examination of the nervous system in a patient with cardiac symptoms—or simply according to the circumstances—for example, in the doctor's rooms or in the patient's home.

The object of a routine examination is to check the different bodily systems to exclude abnormality. In considering symptoms related to the patient's presenting complaint a more focused and detailed examination is necessary.

General
- General appearance (does the patient look healthy, unwell or ill, well cared for or neglected?)
- Intelligence and educational level
- Mental state
- Expression and emotional state
- Build and posture
- Nutrition, obesity, oedema

BOX 1.7   Schema for routine examination.

- General appearance
- Gait
- Hair
- Eyes
- Face
- Mouth and pharynx
- Neck
- Upper limbs
- Lower limbs
- Spine and Joints
- Thorax
  - anteriorly and laterally
  - posteriorly
- Abdomen
- Examination of excreta

- Skin colour, cyanosis, anaemia, jaundice, pigmentation
- Skin eruptions, petechiae, spider naevi, vitiligo
- Body hair
- Deformities, swellings
- Temperature, pulse, respiration rate
- Features of endocrine disease, e.g. hyperlipidaemia, acromegaly, Cushing's syndrome.

Hair
- Texture and grooming.

Eyes
- Simple tests of visual acuity: compare one eye against the other
- Exophthalmos or enophthalmos
- Ptosis
- Oedema of the lids
- Conjunctivae: anaemia, jaundice or inflammation
- Pupils: size, equality, regularity, reaction to light, accommodation
- Eye movement: nystagmus, strabismus
- Ophthalmoscopic examination of the fundi and ocular chambers.

Face
- Facies
- Jaw movements
- Facial symmetry or asymmetry
- Rash
- Features of endocrine disease or hyperlipidaemia.

Mouth and pharynx
(a torch and tongue depressor should be used)

- Breath odours
- Lips: colour and eruptions
- Tongue: protrusion and appearance
- Teeth and gums (if patient has dentures, notice whether they fit and ask whether they are worn for meals or only for cosmetic reasons)
- Buccal mucous membrane: colour and pigmentation.

Pharynx
- Movement of soft palate
- State of tonsils.

Neck
- Movement, pain and range
- Veins
- Lymphatic glands
- Thyroid
- Carotid pulses and bruits.

Upper limbs
- General examination of arms and hands
- Fingernails: clubbing or koilonychia
- Pulse: rate, rhythm, volume and character

- State of arterial wall of radials and brachials
- Axillae: lymph glands
- Blood pressure
- Muscles: muscle wasting, fasciculation
- Tests for power, tone, reflexes and coordination
- Cutaneous sensation: check all modalities to exclude root or nerve lesions
- Joints: movement, pain and swelling; rheumatiod nodules and xanthelasma at elbows.

Thorax
(Table 1.4)

Anteriorly and laterally
- Type of chest, asymmetry if any
- Breasts and nipples
- Respiration: rate, depth and character
- Pulsation
- Dilated vessels
- Position of trachea by palpation
- Look for and palpate apex beat
- Palpate over precordium for thrills
- Palpate respiratory movements
- Estimate tactile vocal fremitus
- Percuss the lungs
- Auscultate the heart sounds
- Auscultate the breath sounds
- Estimate vocal resonance, cervical and axillary glands.

Posteriorly (patient sitting)
- Inspect and palpate respiratory movement
- Estimate tactile vocal fremitus
- Percuss the lung resonance
- Auscultate the breath sounds
- Estimate vocal resonance
- Note movements and deformities of the spine

TABLE 1.4 Example of CVS statement.

Pulse 76 regular, peripheral pulses normal
Neck veins not distended. No peripheral oedema
BP 130/80
Apex beat not displaced
Heart sounds I and II heard in all areas
No murmurs, lungs clear

- Palpate from behind: cervical glands, thyroid
- Look for sacral oedema.

Abdomen
- Inspection: size, distension, symmetry
- Abdominal wall: movement, scars, dilated vessels
- Visible peristalsis or pulsation
- Pubic hair
- Hernial orifices
- Palpation: tenderness, rigidity, hyperaesthesia, splashing, masses, liver, gallbladder, spleen, kidneys, bladder
- Percussion: masses, liver, spleen, bladder
- Auscultation: bowel sounds, murmurs
- Impulse on coughing at hernial orifices
- Inguinal glands
- Male genitalia: penis, scrotum, spermatic cord; female genitalia: examine if relevant
- Abdominal reflexes
- Rectal examination when indicated
- Gynaecological examination when indicated.

Lower limbs
- General examination of legs and feet
- Stance, balance and gait
- Oedema of feet and ankles
- Varicose veins
- Muscles: muscle wasting, fasciculation
- Tests for power, tone, reflexes (including plantar response) and coordination
- Joints: movement, pain and swelling
- Peripheral pulses
- Temperature of feet.

Examination of excreta
- Urine, sputum, stools, vomit: examination by naked eye, and measure or estimate amount
- Test urine for specific gravity, sugar, protein and blood.

THE NEXT STEP

The clinical assessment, or diagnosis, and the development of a plan of management for the patient following the acquisition of the database from the history and examination is addressed in the next chapter.

2
DIAGNOSIS, INVESTIGATION AND MANAGEMENT

INTRODUCTION

The purpose of the clinical database—the information obtained from the history and the physical examination—is to facilitate diagnosis and so provide a basis on which treatment can be instituted. This may require further investigation, itself suggested by the clinical data. The clinical information is not only important in relation to the diagnosis itself, but also in deciding what the objectives of effective clinical management are. *Management* is a term often used in clinical practice; it includes diagnosis, understanding of the major symptoms, planning investigation and developing means of alleviating distress and disability due to disease. It therefore includes specific treatments as a part of this process; management of the patient implies not merely drug therapy or surgery, but rather management of the whole problem confronted by the patient.

It is therefore essential that all clinical information is organized in such a way that it can readily be accessed and utilized. Data should be noted in a standardized format, using standard abbreviations that can be interpreted by other physicians if necessary. Usually, clinical data are displayed in more detail for patients admitted to hospital than for those seen only in an out-patient clinic, if only because in-patients are likely to require more complex investigations and treatments, and generally to be more sick than people seen in clinics.

ORGANIZING THE DATA

Clinical information is obtained through the history and examination. This information must be consid-ered in relation to a number of logical steps, in order that an appropriate and efficient path to management can be planned and followed. The following questions need to be considered:

- Is the patient seriously ill, or is there risk, either to life or of permanent disability?
- Is there an immediately evident diagnosis?
- If a diagnosis is not apparent, consider whether there is an organic abnormality.
- Which system is mainly affected?
- Are multiple organ systems involved?
- Is urgent assessment necessary?
- What investigations are likely to be informative?
- What is the differential diagnosis?
- What is the patient's mental state in relation to the illness?

This path of diagnosis and management can be followed in several different ways, but all depend on a logical presentation and ordering of the clinical database. For this reason the clinical data should be recorded ('written up') in a standardized format. Not only does this encourage clear thought about the patient and the problem, but it also means that other medical and non-medical staff such as physiotherapists and nurses can understand the nature of the disorder. In addition, information related to the course of the illness and its treatment can be recorded under headings derived from this initial assessment. It is a prime objective of care and treatment to anticipate events, complications and effects of therapy, so that the outcome of the disorder can be controlled as far as possible. When a serious complication develops unexpectedly, the situation becomes potentially uncontrolled. Decisions may then have to be made rapidly. It is better if a plan already exists to deal with any such a complication, from anticipation that it might occur, however unlikely this might have seemed to be. This can be termed 'risk assessment', and it is always worth thinking through at the beginning (that is, at the time of the initial diagnostic assessment).

SEVERITY OF THE ILLNESS

Ill patients deserve special attention. Accident and emergency departments are skilled at such assessments as part of their triage or initial assessment of the patient, but doctors in their consulting rooms or out-patient clinics need to be aware of the possibility that their patient may be more sick than appearances may at first suggest. The patient may not recognize the importance of certain symptoms such as tight pain in the anterior chest radiating to the left arm, a symptom that the doctor will consider as suggestive of myocardial ischaemia or incipient myocardial infarction. Haemorrhage on the other hand, a dramatic symptom, is often thought by the patient to be more important than it necessarily is. Coughing blood, even in small quantities, is likely to have a serious cause, but blood in the stools is most likely to be due to bleeding haemorrhoids, although it might also indicate an underlying carcinoma of the rectum. These possibilities will pass through the mind of the physician as the patient tells his or her story.

Acutely ill patients show signs of illness, especially major features such as high fever, shock, circulatory collapse, disturbed consciousness, severe pain, evidence of metabolic failure—for example ketosis, jaundice or uraemia—or abdominal pain and distension with vomiting. Lay persons generally recognize these signs as features of serious illness, but the patient may not present until the disorder is relatively advanced, largely because the change in function has progressed slowly over time. Some serious features, such as an acute petechial rash with drowsiness and fever, the presenting signs of meningoccal septicaemia, are often neglected until, within a few hours, the patient has become shocked, confused and stuporose.

Slowly progressive conditions, although also serious, are particularly difficult to recognize. The progressive pallor and skin haemorrhages of aplastic anaemia, often due to a myeloproliferative disorder, may be neglected until it is pointed out by an acquaintance who has not seen the person for a few weeks and therefore notes the change. Similarly, the slow onset of primary hypothyroidism or pituitary failure will often go unremarked by those in close contact with a person—even by the patient's own doctor.

People vary in their ability to cope with illness. Some people will say nothing about the onset of illness or pain until the illness has become well developed and obvious, whereas others will present with 'unbearable' symptoms very early in the natural history. The latter are much more difficult for the physician to interpret and recognize, since the symptoms may far outweigh the findings on examination, and there may even be a suspicion that the patient is anxious, concerned, depressed or simply exaggerating the symptoms. A decision must be made to investigate symptoms on the basis of their possible cause, once it has been considered that an organic disorder might explain them. Further, the investigation planned must be definitive. It is not satisfactory to plan an investigation that has a poor sensitivity and specificity in revealing an abnormality and then to rely on this unsatisfactory data.

The most satisfactory and sensitive tool in the hands of the physician is the history and examination. The experienced physician will constantly be thinking of possible physiological and anatomical explanations for the patient's symptoms as they are described, and the history especially will be used to refine the nature of these symptoms as the patient presents them.

PATTERN RECOGNITION AND LOGIC IN DIAGNOSIS

Much diagnosis is accomplished by a process of *intuitive pattern recognition* based on experience and knowledge. Certain disorders present in characteristic ways, with a sequence of symptoms, and with confirmatory signs on examination. In addition, certain key negative aspects of the history and examination can be used to exclude other conditions. This 'pattern diagnosis' can be very efficient in determining a strategy for further investigation, and for planning management, but it must be tempered by the recognition of the need for an understanding of the cause and nature of individual symptoms. The alert clinician will be on the lookout for any anomalous features that do not readily fit the diagnostic hypothesis, or which require some other explanation.

The diagnostic process is sometimes summarized in flow charts for *decision analysis*, which provide steps in the diagnostic process that invalidate a diagnosis. Such flow charts are useful as learning tools, but are rarely followed exactly by clinicians because they fail to take account of the importance of establishing the certainty of the various historical features, and the findings elicited by the clinician on examination. Only the individual clinician will know how reliable the clinical data are in any individual case; and the flow chart method of logical deductive reasoning depends absolutely on reliable data. Of course, it is the essence of clinical methods to establish a reliable database of clinical information. The clinician therefore weighs up the reliability of the evidence upon which the diagnostic assessment is to be made, and then follows a logical diagnostic path in thinking through the possible diagnosis and what investigations will be helpful that take account of the relative strength of the data as well as the deductive decision-making process indicated by the 'flow chart'. The diagnosis, in fact, can only be as good or reliable as the data on which it is based. More mistakes are made from basing a diagnosis on inaccurate clinical data than from making a logical error in following the 'flow chart' methodology.

There have been many attempts to formulate these concepts of sensitivity and specificity of clinical data in relation to diagnosis in mathematical terms, so that the accuracy of clinical decision-making and diagnosis can be refined by the use of computer analysis, but so much depends on the interpretation of the symptoms themselves, and on the validity of the signs elicited, that these methods are so far not of wide value in practice.

The student will sometimes notice an experienced clinician make an immediate diagnosis based on a few seconds' acquaintance with a patient. The consultant then uses the remainder of the consultation to explore other possibilities, to exclude other disorders and to consider various diagnostic investigations and the plan of management. Such skill comes with experience, constant practice and knowledge. Knowledge can be acquired from medical texts and from the literature, but it needs to be based on clinical experience and clinical method in order to be usable; the two skills of clinical methods and medical knowledge work together to inform medical practice.

The diagnostic process is a complex mental task in which the clinical data are weighed in the clinician's mind against the doctor's previous experience and his or her formally acquired knowledge of the medical literature. There is no substitute for knowledge, but knowledge can only be used appropriately when its significance is understood in relation to everyday clinical experience. An experienced clinician will arrive at a diagnosis on the basis of apparently minimal clues because it is clear to that clinician that certain aspects of the patient's history or physical signs have especial significance. The way in which a patient describes upper abdominal pain may be more important than the precise characteristics of the pain in suggesting a diagnosis of cardiac or oesophageal pain. On the other hand, the experienced doctor will recognize that it is possible to be misled by over-reliance on clinical intuitions, and investigation should be used as a check on diagnostic accuracy as well as in quantifying an abnormality for planning management. The role of modern computerized imaging cannot be over-estimated in this regard.

Clinicians constantly update their own personal database (i.e. their memory of patients and of the clinical features of particular disorders) in relation to the acquisition of factual knowledge derived from textbooks, medical journals, medical conferences and the Internet. There is always something new to be learned in medicine, even for the most experienced doctor. Computer-based diagnostic systems and reference databases are evolving tools in this process of informing clinicians, but they are not substitutes for learning, for wisdom and, above all, for clinical skills and easy patient relationships.

MULTIPLE CAUSATION

Although it is axiomatic that one should try to account for all of a patient's symptoms by one disease process (the principle of Occam's razor), a surprising number of patients in fact have more than one overt diagnosis, for example coronary artery disease and hiatus hernia, both of which may produce central chest pain; and still more have a disease process which either does not explain the symptoms at all or does not explain all the symptoms, for example weakness and tiredness in a patient with mild angina pectoris or mild anaemia. Moreover, an apparently simple event may have a complex medical background. For instance, an old lady gets out of bed, trips and breaks her wrist. It is possible that she was hurrying to the lavatory as she had cystitis, that she tripped because her vision was impaired by cataract, and that the wrist fracture occurred because her bones were weakened by osteoporosis.

In making a diagnosis one should try to account for a person's total disability and one should not be dismayed if this involves more than one item. Thus the diagnosis in an old lady with multiple symptoms might be:

- Loneliness
- Depression
- Mild degenerative osteoarthritis.

or in a young man with dyspepsia:

- Impending marriage
- Anxiety state
- Duodenal ulcer.

A diagnosis of this kind, which lists the patient's problems and is not confined to labelling organic disease, gives a true picture of the state of affairs. The patient's complaint forms but one part of the patient's problems. Always view the patient as a whole. Will the patient be restored to full mental and physical health when this symptom has resolved? Note that a mental adaptation to illness features in this diagnostic set, a component of the illness that arguably is that part most susceptible to be influenced by the physician and nurse.

WRITING UP THE NOTES

Carefully organized clinical notes will indicate the database with clarity, and will also reveal errors and missing data. Did you forget to take the blood pressure? Or to examine the neck for enlarged cervical lymph nodes? If you follow a rigid and stereotyped note-keeping system (Box 2.1) as you write up the clinical notes, you will notice any omission and any data that is incompatible with your initial diagnostic hypothesis will also be revealed.

Begin with *basic social data*—name, age, address, marital status, dependent family members and children, occupation—and proceed to describe the *family history*, and the *past medical history*. Note the *social history* and any relevant *past occupational history*, together with a note about *drugs* taken regularly, *alcohol* ingestion and the *smoking history*. Make a note of any doctors who have previously attended, and if there is information about previous investigations and treatments or psychiatric interventions describe these also.

Indicate the *major presenting symptom* or symptoms and their duration and then record the *current history* (history of present condition), not necessarily as given by the patient but interpreted as a conceptual and coherent narrative, starting at the beginning and running through to contemporary events. With experience it is often possible to write notes that fulfil this aim as the patient describes the problems, simply by categorizing the events and symptoms in relation to their main headings, for example, headache, dizziness and shortness of breath. Each of these would justify a separate paragraph including what the patient said and what the responses were 'on direct questioning' (ODQ). Unrelated *direct questions* designed to exclude other conditions or problems should be separately noted at the end of the narrative history. A short note about the *mental state* and intellectual level of the patient is often useful, particularly in retrospect as the illness progresses, complications develop or recovery occurs.

Sometimes the past history has relevance to the present history, for example a patient may have had a congenital heart disorder operated on in infancy and is now presenting in adult life with an aortic aneurysm. In this case it is reasonable to run together the relevant past history with the current complaint since it will be clear that the one has led to the other.

The *physical examination* should be recorded quite rigidly, since abnormal findings may be found in more than one bodily system. There are also often abnormal features on *general examination*, such as pallor, jaundice, a rash, clubbing of the fingers or lymphadenopathy. The initial statement should describe the patient briefly, without any hint of judgmental comment, in order to try to give a picture of the person. For example, 'well nourished, muscular man', or 'emaciated, frightened', or 'jaundiced, breathless, cooperative', or 'confused, agitated and restlessly wandering'. Significant general abnormalities and features of systemic illness such as abnormalities in the skin (e.g. nailbed infarcts, ecchymoses, vitiligo, etc.) should be noted.

The physical examination, whatever the order in which it is carried out, should be written up separately for each *major bodily system*. Thus there will be separate brief descriptions of the findings in the gastrointestinal system (often termed the abdomen), the cardiovascular system, the respiratory system, the nervous system, the skin and the limbs and joints. The absence of signs can be as important as their presence. Simple line drawings can often convey more information than much writing. The minimum statement about a patient's cardiovascular system, for example, might read as in Table 1.4.

The case notes should conclude with a brief *summary* of the history and the main abnormalities found on examination, followed by a tentative diagnosis, a list of *investigations* planned and arranged, and a *differential diagnosis*. The *plan of management* should be outlined, and those features to be used as an index of progress should be indicated. These might be clinical findings or might be derived from various investigations, for example the chest X-ray or the results of blood tests.

PROBLEM-ORIENTED RECORDS

The distinction between the patient's problem and the diagnosis, discussed earlier in this chapter, is sometimes stressed by the adoption of a format of case-recording in which the patient's problems are enumerated at the conclusion of the record and used to derive a notation in each follow-up note, by ascribing a number to each problem. Attention is then given to treatment and management of each problem individually. Although inclined to repetition, this problem-oriented method of medical record-keeping serves to remind the clinician to attend to all of a patient's problems individually. Certainly, it is relevant to distinguish the patient's subjective problems from the diagnosis at the outset, since the former must be relieved, if at all possible,

---

BOX 2.1   Recording the clinical findings.

- Basic personal and demographic data
- Occupational history
- Marital and sexual history
- Past history
- Social history
- Family history
- Drug history
- Alcohol, smoking and substance abuse?
- Presenting problems
- History of current problems
- Examination
- General features
- System findings
- Summary
- Plan of investigation and management
- Follow up notes (signed and dated)

even if the diagnosis is such that cure is not feasible. It is sometimes helpful to combine this approach with the traditional diagnosis-related case record in order to remind the doctor that the patient's problems are the symptoms that the medical or surgical treatment is designed to relieve.

IDENTIFICATION

All medical notes should be *signed* or *initialled*, so that the examiner can be identified. Every note must be signed. Every page of the record should have the patient's name and identifying number clearly written in the top corner, in order to avoid confusion with other patients.

PROGRESS NOTES

The progress notes should discuss the diagnosis, the patient's symptoms and signs, the results of investigations and any changes in management. Progress notes should clearly state the results of investigations, the development of the plan of management, the treatment plan and the clinical progress. The nature of information given to the patient and to the patient's family and friends must be documented, and special instructions or plans noted. If any discussion has occurred with the patient, or family, concerning resuscitation or decisions related to this, should it prove necessary, this should be carefully and frankly noted (see discussion of ethical issues, Ch. 24). If the patient has been visited or examined by doctors other than the physician signing the note, these physicians should be identified in writing and their opinions or advice should be carefully noted.

ACCESS TO CLINICAL NOTES

The case records belong to the hospital or clinic, but their content is confidential to the patient and should not be disclosed to any third party without permission from the patient. This rule can be bypassed only by court order. Patients have the right to read, see or inspect their own medical records, although they can only have copies of the records with permission of the hospital and clinician. Permission to disclose records can be withheld if it is thought that disclosure might distress the patient or be harmful, and it is sometimes allowed that certain portions—perhaps related to information concerning friends or other family members—are deleted from records disclosed to individual patients. In practice, if a patient asks to see a certain part of the record (for example a letter or report from a particular consultant), then it is almost always appropriate to let them see it immediately. Indeed, many consultants and some GPs make a habit of sending copies of their reports to patients, believing that open disclosure of their opinion and

recommendations is on the whole beneficial. Clearly, in the case of serious illness not yet certain or verified this would be inappropriate.

WRITING LETTERS AND REPORTS

It is important to communicate your findings clearly to other doctors. Any doctor receiving a referral letter from you should have a clear idea what question has arisen requiring his or her advice. A doctor receiving the result of your consultation, on the other hand, wants to know what you have found, and what plans there are for further investigation and treatment. The patient also wants to have this information.

You will probably dictate your letters and reports—this requires some skill and practice. Try to visualize the sentences as you speak them, and use the more formal grammatical constructions typical of written, rather than spoken language. Above all, *be brief*. Letters that occupy two or three sheets of paper may well not be read with great care, and probably contain uncertain advice! Set out the positive findings, the questions and the answers as you see them. Discuss any particular problems or difficulties. Be clear on your recommendations, or what you think is the nature of the underlying medical problem. State the patient's expectations and fears.

Medical reports are written as formal documents, usually for lawyers, courts, insurance companies or statutory bodies such as social security agencies. A medical report should fully identify the patient, the doctor and the source of the information used to provide the report, including a list of documents studied, and the date and place of any examination that was carried out. These data should be reviewed under appropriate headings, including conventional headings such as past medical history, current history, description of any accident, etc., and the results of the examination set out fully. The report should conclude with a discussion of the relevant findings and a clear opinion or list of conclusions. If necessary, references to textbooks or other medical literature should be given. In the case of medico-legal reports, the courts in Britain and in many other countries require a declaration of any conflict of interest, and of the doctor's overriding duty to the court. Remember that your report may be used as the basis for detailed discussion and questioning in the event that its contents are disputed.

PRESENTING A CASE

The value of a doctor's notes on a patient is greatly enhanced if they can be communicated in concise form to other doctors. Students should therefore practise making a short summary of their findings, emphasizing both important positive findings and relevant negative ones. This summary should begin with the name, age, sex and occupation of the patient, and end with a brief statement of the problem.

In addition, students should practise oral presentation of cases at every opportunity. This is an essential skill in explaining clinical problems to other physicians and surgeons. The ultimate test is the ability to communicate a difficult problem to a senior colleague on the telephone. A logical approach to the relevant aspects of the case, with only brief attention to negative data, is essential. The history and findings on examination should be communicated in temporal, coherent order, making an interesting and easily grasped story.

If you are making a formal presentation at a medical Grand Round or teaching session, try to use an overhead projector or a blackboard to present visually the most important points in the history, examination and investigation. In presenting a case, always speak as though to a single other person, rather than to a group. Try to communicate. X-rays and other medical images can often be projected using an overhead projector so that all present can easily see them.

If the patient can attend, then the important points in the history can be delineated and amplified by getting the patient to go over the history again. The salient points of the examination can also be demonstrated. Remember, this may be embarrassing or even an ordeal for the patient, so be kind, thoughtful and brief. It is generally a mistake to allow patients or their families to attend the subsequent discussion, since a number of issues not strictly relevant to the patient's actual illness will be discussed in a theoretical fashion and this may lead to unnecessary anxiety.

ASSESSMENT OF FUNCTIONAL IMPAIRMENT AFTER INJURY OR ILLNESS

In disease of any bodily system, it is useful to be able to assess the residual problem faced by the patient. In many different diseases, therefore, *rating scales* have been designed in order to try to provide some relatively objective measurement. These are weighted in relation to the most important residual problems found in the disorder under assessment. For example, in rheumatoid arthritis rating scales are particularly weighted toward stiffness, limitation of mobility of joints, ability to carry out tasks of daily living such as dressing, toileting and feeding, and joint pain; in cardiopulmonary disease the rating scales are concerned with breathlessness, exercise tolerance, sputum production and chest pain; and in multiple sclerosis most of the scales in common use rely heavily on impairment of self-caring, incontinence, visual impairment and a quantified clinical examination of the nervous system.

Clearly, these rating scales are not comparable one with another and, since they are ordinal in character, it is difficult to make statistical comparisons between two different assessments made on the same patient at two different times, although this is often done in assessing a patient's response to a treatment. Most of these rating scales were devised with specific research aims in mind, rather than for everyday clinical use, although several are now used routinely in the clinic. Despite these theoretical difficulties in handling rating scales, such scales have proven very useful in clinical practice, since they provide a relatively standardized assessment of a patient's clinical state at any given time.

In considering data from rating assessments it is well to remember that they often include assessments of clinical impairments, disabilities and handicaps, without separating these different concepts, which may overlap or even duplicate each other (Box 2.2). Functional rating scales are becoming more and more important in clinical practice, since they form one method of assessing the value of medical or other interventions in disease states. A distinction is drawn between scales that measure deficit, which are usually administered by a doctor or other health professional, and self-administered questionnaires, usually carefully structured but sometimes directed by the patients themselves, which assess 'patient-related quality of life'.

Quality of Life (QoL) is an important quantified measure that is increasingly used to determine the benefit conferred by a management strategy or treatment in a patient or group of patients with a given disease. It assesses not disability or handicap, but the person's own view of how they see their life. The quality of life is a measure determined by the patient. The doctor could regard the quality of life of a person with severe shortness of breath as poor, but to the individual a small improvement might be seen as making the difference between total helplessness and the ability to communicate with friends and family

---

BOX 2.2   Impairment, disability and handicap: definitions.

- An *impairment* is the absence or abnormality of a basic biological function, for example hand movement or vision.
- A *disability* is a lack of a normal functional ability, whether physical or psychological, and represents a lack of normal interaction between a person and the environment. Disability is easier to assess than impairment.
- A *handicap* is the disadvantage resulting from a disability. It thus often consists of dependency on others; or on some piece of equipment, and can be modified or even overcome by suitable manipulation of the environment. Measurement of handicap may not always be relevant, since it can be modified by social changes.

and therefore not only very well worthwhile but also a very considerable improvement in quality of life. Quality of life measurement is increasingly of interest in health economic studies. This kind of measurement is seen to be as valid as a quantitative measure of disability following a disease and its treatment, and perhaps more valid in everyday life.

Both disability assessment scales and quality of life scales are designed for either of two purposes: *generic* and *disease-specific* measurement. Generic scales are designed to assess disturbed function or patient-generated quality of life in general; for example some have been used to assess these concepts in the general population. Others are designed for use in certain specific diseases, such as heart failure, head and neck cancer, Parkinson's disease or multiple sclerosis. Disease-specific measurement instruments cannot be used to make comparisons across different diseases.

DISABILITY AND HANDICAP

It is useful when dealing with someone with poor physical or mental function to consider whether they suffer from an impairment, a disability or a handicap. These terms have separate meanings, defined in Box 2.1. Essentially, a *disability* is a lack of a normal functional ability, and a *handicap* is a disadvantage resulting from a disability. Handicap can therefore be modified by attention to the social and behavioral environment of the patient. Disability is a biologically determined dysfunction that may not be treatable. In other words the handicap suffered by a patient with the disability of impaired walking can be managed by the provision of a wheelchair, resulting in a measurable improvement in quality of life.

PLANNING INVESTIGATIONS

Investigations are useful in defining the nature and extent of any disease process. They may also be used for monitoring the progress of a disease during treatment. In planning investigation keep in mind the issues listed in Box 2.3.

BOX 2.3   Issues underlying the choice of investigations.

- What investigations will be informative?
- What discomforts and risks attach to each investigation?
- What information does the laboratory require?
- What specimens are required? How should they be obtained and preserved?
- What is the cost?
- Are there any risks to laboratory staff?
- How will the results be used in the patient's management?

CHOOSING THE INVESTIGATION

The result of any investigation should have a value in management that is more or less equivalent to that obtained from any other clinical data. It should complement the clinical findings from the history and examination by adding quantitative data, as in the case of blood counts in anaemia or myeloproliferative disease, or new information, as in the case of physiological data such as an ECG recording or chest X-ray. Some investigations can be used to follow the progress of a disease, for example the ESR in some autoimmune disorders such as giant cell arteritis. Automation has led to the production of 'screening tests', as for example from an autoanalyser of blood biochemistry. These automated results should be studied with care, since not all the test results will at first be thought relevant to the patient, although the discovery of unexpected abnormalities (e.g. in liver function tests) may reveal unsuspected problems such as subclinical alcoholic liver disease or hypercalcaemia due to metastatic cancer. Tests should be repeated at selected intervals, determined by clinical need in relation to treatment or the expected outcome of a disorder.

DISCOMFORTS AND RISKS

Discomfort and risk should be kept to a minimum. Discomfort can usually be alleviated by good technique, for example during invasive angiography, venepuncture or lumbar puncture. Risk may be minimized by good technique, but some risk will accompany any test, even venepuncture when, for example, a small cutaneous nerve may sometimes be damaged, causing pain. The risk should be assessed prior to the performance of the test, and fully explained to the patient in the context of the benefit expected from the information gained as a result of the test. If the information gained is not useful in clinical management, or is considered to be less than the risk, the test should not be performed.

WHAT THE LABORATORY NEEDS TO KNOW

The laboratory or imaging department needs to be fully informed as to the reasons for the test. If in any doubt, consult with laboratory staff about the value of the test—there may be other ways of approaching the problem. The laboratory ought to be informed about any possible risks (e.g. infectivity with HIV or other pathogens). Special problems such as a bleeding tendency should be made known to the phlebotomist or invasive radiologist, or to a surgeon carrying out a biopsy. Any allergies to local anaesthetic agents must be disclosed. The timing of the blood sample, its arrival in the laboratory (usually required in working hours so that it can be processed properly and not stored), and the preservative medium in which it is kept are all important. In bacteriological work these can be particularly important issues.

Every specimen must be clearly labelled with the patient's name and hospital number, the ward or clinic, and the date and time the specimen was collected. The container should also state clearly the nature of the specimen and the storage medium used for blood and bacteriological specimens. In the case of pathological specimens requiring frozen section or electron microscopy, special methods are used for storing and processing the specimen and these must be absolutely followed.

SPECIAL PROCEDURES

Venepuncture and the collection of bacteriological specimens are described in Appendix II.

MAKING THE BEST USE OF RESULTS

The interpretation of any laboratory test will depend on the relevance of the test to the presumptive diagnosis and the interpreter's knowledge of pathology, biochemistry and physiology. The task of a clinical laboratory is to put these disciplines to work in the solution of a diagnostic problem. All tests are subject to errors of performance. Fortunately these are rare, but the clinician will help the pathologist if any 'rogue' result that does not accord with other data is reported back to the laboratory. All results will depend on the precision of the method used and the variability of the quality measured amongst a healthy population.

In non-quantitative tests, as in cytology, there may be false positives and false negatives. The laboratory should be able to say with what frequency these may occur. For example, in bronchial carcinoma malignant cells are often detected in the sputum; however, in a very small proportion of examinations apparently malignant cells in the sputum will be reported when there is no bronchial carcinoma. Abnormal results are therefore often checked in the laboratory by a second observer to ensure, as far as possible, their accuracy. The clinician can give some weight to such findings by considering the patient. If the patient is a middle-aged man who smokes heavily, the report of malignant cells would be likely to be a true positive, since bronchial carcinoma is prevalent in such patients. Conversely, if the patient is a non-smoking young girl, the positive sputum report would be likely to be false, and should be reassessed.

For quantitative tests, as in biochemistry and much of haematology, the *sensitivity* and *specificity* of a test can be determined statistically in relation to their value in diagnosis. The *accuracy of the assay* must also be monitored within the laboratory and in cooperation with other laboratories. The accuracy of the assay is expressed as the variance around the mean value of multiple determinations carried out on the same specimen. The normal range of the assay is the mean value of the measurements in a population of normal subjects plus or minus two standard deviations; 95% of the results in a normal population will fall within this range but 1 in 20 of these normal subjects will show results just outside the normal range. Therefore a value just outside the range of normal does not necessarily indicate abnormality. It should also be remembered that normal ranges have to be established for the sex and age of the groups studied and also for the method as performed in each laboratory.

3
THE PSYCHIATRIC ASSESSMENT

INTRODUCTION

Psychiatric disorders are common and the range of presenting problems is wide. Every doctor must be able to carry out a psychiatric assessment. Many patients present with what are clearly psychiatric complaints. Others may present physical rather than psychiatric symptoms, although the underlying problem is emotional in origin. In some patients physical and psychiatric illness coexist.

As in physical illness, diagnosis and treatment of a mental disorder depends on a full formulation of the problem. In psychiatry, this formulation is derived virtually entirely from the history and examination. This information is obtained by interview and observation of the patient and from other witnesses such as family members and friends. Specific psychological investigations, including measures of the cognitive state and, less frequently, structured questionnaires to assess aspects of personality and mood, are also used. Laboratory tests and X-rays are used in some cases.

THE PSYCHIATRIC HISTORY

INTERVIEW TECHNIQUE

Begin by putting the patient at ease. Establish a non-threatening relationship that is warm and empathic; use words that the patient can understand. Remember that the quality and accuracy of the information gathered will determine the adequacy of the diagnostic formulation. The experience of the interview may actually be therapeutic for the patient and compliance in any treatment suggested will be enhanced by good communication. In no branch of medicine are interviewing skills so important as in psychiatry. Psychiatric patients, by the very nature of their disturbances, may be difficult to interview. Even for the most well-adjusted person the interview itself may involve searching and potentially embarrassing or even distressing issues. Be aware of these difficulties.

HISTORY-TAKING SCHEME

The psychiatric history should be carried out systematically (see Box 3.1). The full psychiatric history often requires more than one interview. The scheme must be adapted to meet the needs of the patient, and different aspects should receive different degrees of emphasis in different patients.

BOX 3.1 The psychiatric history: what topics to cover.

- Reason for referral
- Presenting complaints
- History of present illness
- Family history
- Personal history
  - childhood
  - schooling
  - occupation
  - psychosexual and marital experiences
  - forensic history
  - past medical history
  - past psychiatric history
  - drug and alcohol abuse
  - pre-morbid personality
  - social circumstances
- Witness account (with patient's permission)

HISTORY OF PRESENT ILLNESS

First, patients must be given the opportunity to explain what is worrying them. Getting patients to talk about themselves requires the doctor to be relaxed, sympathetic and, above all, a good listener. Patients must feel that their problems are respected. It is often useful to write down a patient's complaints word for word, since this is often a useful summary of the disorder. Never appear to be in haste.

Initially, let the patient do most of the talking. Clarify things later, if necessary, by asking leading questions. Try to analyse each symptom as in Box 3.2.

The date and circumstances of onset of the symptoms

Look for any precipitating factors or recent stresses. Since the illness may have been present for some time before the onset of the presenting symptoms, it may only be by asking when the patient was last well that the true date of onset of the illness can be decided.

Relieving and aggravating factors

Consistency

Any variation from day to day or during the day should be determined. This includes searching for any periodicity such as diurnal mood variation; patients with a depressive illness often feel worse in the morning.

Severity

This is often best assessed by asking the patient how the symptom interferes with normal life.

Definition

It is important to clarify what the patient means. Confusion may mean one thing to the layman and another to the doctor. Abnormal beliefs or experiences may not be clearly described but the doctor must be absolutely sure about them if the correct diagnosis is to be reached.

Effect of the complaint on the patient

The effect of the experience of each symptom on the patient's emotional state should be assessed. For instance, some patients find auditory hallucinations only mildly interfering, while others find them utterly terrifying.

Site and radiation

This is mostly relevant when the patient complains of physical symptoms but may be important when the patient is hearing voices; hearing them outside or inside the head may have a different significance.

Associated symptoms

It is important to ask in detail about any other symptoms associated with the major presenting complaint and, at this time, it is relevant to ask about sleep, appetite and weight.

Sleep disturbance may be related to physical problems, such as pain or breathlessness, or to psychological problems. Examples of the latter include initial insomnia occurring in the presence of anxiety or drug withdrawal; early morning waking and nightmares occurring with depression; excessive sleep related to drugs, substance abuse or organic illness; reversed sleep pattern (i.e. increasing during the day and decreased at night) in acute confusional states; and disturbed sleep with affective or organic illness. Sleep disturbance of recent onset is usually highly significant, whereas chronic sleep impairment, although distressing to the patient, is usually of less importance in diagnosis.

Appetite is decreased in anorexia nervosa but may be increased in anxious patients who eat for comfort. In depression, appetite may decrease or increase. It is the alteration in the pattern that is important. Associated with loss of appetite there may be a loss of weight as in depression, anorexia nervosa or self-neglect. Cycles of weight gain and weight loss sometimes occur in eating disorders. Weight gain is a feature of treatment with some psychotropic drugs.

FAMILY HISTORY

The family background is always relevant. Environmental factors are important in determining the outcome in many psychatric illnesses, and are often complex. For example, a mother's death in early life predisposes to depression in later life; failure of bonding may lead to difficulties establishing relationships in adult life, and overprotective parents may produce anxious children. The family history must be considered in detail, including information about parents and siblings and also, when relevant, about members of the extended, non-nuclear family. Remember that genetic factors are important in schizophrenia and the affective psychoses.

For each parent, if alive, ask about age and physical and psychiatric health, both present and previous. If dead, then the age of the parent at the time of death, the cause of death and the patient's age and reaction to the bereavement need to be ascertained,

---

BOX 3.2 What to consider for each complaint.

- The symptom itself
- Date and time of onset
- Aggravating and relieving factors
- Consistency (does the symptom vary in re-telling?)
- Severity
- Definitions
- Effect of the symptom on the patient
- Site and radiation of any physical symptoms
- Associated symptoms
- Any previous history of related problems

as well as the parent's health while alive. The occupations and personalities of both parents, and their relationship with each other and with the patient, including any separations from the patient in childhood are all relevant. Children whose parents have had a bad marriage are themselves vulnerable to the development of psychosexual and marital difficulties. For each sibling similar details should be obtained, including marital status.

Some idea of the family atmosphere, interfamily relationships and the position of the patient within the family will have been gained through this enquiry. It is useful to draw a family tree to facilitate understanding of the information gathered. This can vary from a simple diagram of the family members, with their ages, to a more detailed account of the emotional relationships between the various family members (Fig. 3.1). For example, in the family shown in Figure 3.1, the parents were divorced, the older two siblings were closer to their mother, and the youngest to his father, as indicated by the arrows. In some cases it may be relevant to ask about other members of the family, for example when a patient has been brought up by, or is particularly close to, a grandparent, or when a grandparent or parental sibling lives or has lived in the nuclear family home.

Finally, the family psychiatric and medical history should be discussed both in the nuclear and in the wider family. This enquiry should include psychiatric disturbance, alcoholism and suicide. An unexplained death in the family may hint at suicide. If any member of the family has had psychiatric treatment, the nature, date and place of this treatment should be ascertained.

PERSONAL HISTORY

The question to be answered is: Why have these symptoms occurred in this patient at this time?

An answer to the question requires familiarity with the patient's earlier circumstances; for example,

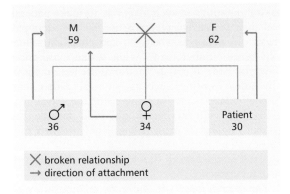

Fig. 3.1 Diagram of personal relationships. The patient was aged 30 years. The older two siblings, aged 34 and 36 years, were closer to their mother, and the patient was closer to her father. The parents were separated.

a severely anxious child with a fear of going to school and inability to separate from his or her parents may well develop symptoms of anxiety (such as agoraphobia—fear of open spaces) in later life. A systematic scheme of enquiry such as that detailed below helps to ensure that important areas are not omitted, though the weight placed on different aspects of the personal history may differ from patient to patient. A visual display of the information by means of a life chart (Fig. 3.2) may help to clarify the relationship between different areas of the patient's life and illuminate the cause of the current symptoms.

CHILDHOOD

This is the logical place to start the personal history. Begin with questions about the patient's birth. Was it planned? What was the length of gestation? Find out about the mother's health during pregnancy and whether the delivery was difficult, a happy experience or a source of contention. Note the infantile and childhood milestones. Most people are only aware of these if their parents have told them of any difficulties.

In later childhood, neurotic traits, such as recurrent fears or periods of physical or emotional disorder at times of stress, may become apparent. These and additional traits such as bed-wetting or temper tantrums must be considered in the light of relationships with peers, the atmosphere at home, relationships with family members and any bereavement or other major life event. Child abuse, whether physical, sexual or psychological, should be discussed tactfully and sympathetically when appropriate—usually when asking about childhood, the family history or the psychosexual history.

ADOLESCENCE

Assessment of adolescence includes questions that usually arise when dealing with the psychosexual history. Relevant areas of enquiry are peer and family relationships, episodes of disturbance, whether antisocial or emotional, and difficulties in growing up. Adolescence is interrelated with schooling and occupation (see below).

SCHOOLING AND HIGHER EDUCATION

Find out the dates of starting, leaving and changing schools, the level of academic achievement, relationships with peers and teachers, any difficulties in learning or behaviour, and any periods of non-attendance. The latter includes *truancy*, in which the child, usually without the parents' knowledge, indulges, often with others, in more enjoyable pastimes instead of going to school, and *school refusal*, in which the child stays at home with the knowledge of the parents because of a fear of leaving home or of going to school. *Enforced absence* is usually due to

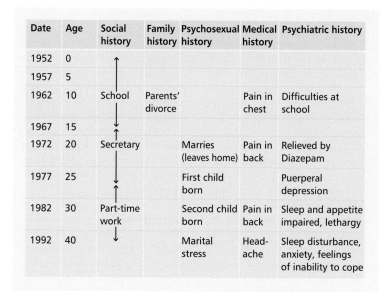

Date	Age	Social history	Family history	Psychosexual history	Medical history	Psychiatric history
1952	0					
1957	5					
1962	10	School	Parents' divorce		Pain in chest	Difficulties at school
1967	15					
1972	20	Secretary		Marries (leaves home)	Pain in back	Relieved by Diazepam
1977	25			First child born		Puerperal depression
1982	30	Part-time work		Second child born	Pain in back	Sleep and appetite impaired, lethargy
1992	40			Marital stress	Head-ache	Sleep disturbance, anxiety, feelings of inability to cope

Fig. 3.2   Life chart of a 40-year-old married mother of two from a broken home referred to the orthopaedic department with backache, for which no cause could be found. Associated symptoms included sleep disturbance, poor appetite and lethargy. Given this patient's background, in particular the divorce of her parents, one would not be surprised if she were vulnerable in psychosexual areas, and this is shown clearly in the chart to be the case by the development of emotional disturbance at the time of her marriage and the birth of her first child. One would therefore anticipate that the birth of her second child would also be a traumatic time for her. The presentation with physical symptoms—pain in the back—as a manifestation of psychiatric disorder is consistent both with her symptomatology after her parents' divorce, and at the time of her marriage, and the presence of the associated symptoms of sleep and appetite disturbance and lethargy, all common manifestations of emotional upset. The life chart clearly displays these links.

illness, although it must be remembered that illness may also be a manifestation of school refusal, and agoraphobic parents may keep children off school to help them cope with their own anxieties.

OCCUPATIONAL HISTORY

A comprehensive work history entails asking about every job the patient has had since leaving school. Enquiry should concentrate on duration of job, level of achievement and promotion, attendance and ability, enjoyment or difficulties, relationships with peers and superiors, reasons for leaving and the duration of any period of unemployment.

If the person has had numerous jobs this may become a repetitive and tedious process. Use a shortened approach by asking about the number of jobs, the length of time unemployed in total and in the last five years, the longest job, the highest level of achievement, any difficulties at work including being dismissed from a job, general relationship with colleagues and employers, and the general work record, while asking in more detail about the present job.

Where relevant, military service can be dealt with in much the same way as any other occupation.

PSYCHOSEXUAL HISTORY

This is often the most difficult area to assess, but it is essential in understanding the patient and the illness. It may be as embarrassing for the doctor as the patient, but it is important not to allow this potential difficulty to harm the doctor–patient relationship. Although in some cases it may be necessary to leave some of the questions to later interviews, sensitive and skilful interviewing usually enables adequate exploration of this area in the first interview, and this is usually the best time to deal with sexual matters.

Information gathering can be facilitated by shaping the enquiry so as to lead from easy to difficult questions, for example by taking a menstrual history before the sexual history, and by asking questions in such a way as to make patients feel their sexual behaviour is normal, for example: 'How old were you when you had your first sexual experience?' rather than: 'What sexual experiences have you had?' It may be tactful to use less emotionally laden wording, such as 'physical' rather than 'sexual' relationship. Remember that the social, religious and cultural background will fashion the patient's approach to revealing details of their psychosexual experience.

A full *sexual history* should consider all aspects of sexual experience (Box 3.3)

The *marital history* includes the relationship with the spouse from the time of meeting through the development of their relationship, engagement and marriage. Note the age and occupation of the spouse (Box 3.4).

BOX 3.3   The sexual history.

- Puberty
- Menstrual history
- Sex education
- Masturbation and fantasies
- Relationships with members of the opposite sex, especially the duration and intensity of sexual contact and enjoyment
- Engagement and marriage (see below)
- Any homosexual feelings and experiences
- Any deviant sexual experiences and fantasies, including sexual abuse in childhood or adolescence

BOX 3.4   The marital history (the same questions should be asked concerning stable non-marital relationships).

- Parental attitudes to the marriage
- Quality of marriage; disagreements, separations
- Current sexual relationship, including frequency and quality of sexual intercourse
- Extramarital affairs, if any
- Pregnancies, terminations and miscarriages
- Stillbirths and live births
- Ages and behaviour of children
- Was child rearing delayed? If so, why?
- Is there difficulty conceiving?
- Are both partners employed? Is this necessary financially? Or are there other reasons?
- Have there been previous marriages? Divorce or death of partner?
- If not married or in a stable relationship is there a reason for this?

FORENSIC HISTORY

This encompasses any and all confrontations with the law and includes juvenile delinquency as well as antisocial behaviour later in life. Details of offences committed and punishment received should be noted.

PAST MEDICAL HISTORY

Ask about: illnesses or operations in childhood or during adult life; periods of hospitalization or incapacity and any resulting disability and interference with the patient's life; the reaction of the patient and family to these episodes; and any remaining medical problems, including current symptoms and medication. It is, for example, illuminating to find out that the patient who now presents with physical symptoms has had a number of previous episodes of similar symptoms at times of stress and has recovered when the stress was resolved, or that the anxious patient awaiting surgery has always reacted badly in the past to major illnesses or operations. It is useful to ask about the frequency and nature of contact with the family doctor.

PAST PSYCHIATRIC HISTORY

Include any episodes of emotional upset, even those thought not severe enough to need medical attention. Note any minor neuroses or depressions treated by the family doctor, as well as severe psychiatric disorders needing expert psychiatric treatment. Record whether out-patient, day-patient or in-patient care was arranged, on a voluntary or compulsory basis. Ask about circumstances, precipitating factors, place of treatment, duration and response to treatment and any continuing symptoms or medication. It is often worth asking if the patient has ever taken psychotropic medication in the past, whether prescribed by the family doctor or obtained in other ways, not necessarily as any form of drug abuse but perhaps from other members of the family. Finally, it is also worth asking about contact with any voluntary organizations, such as the Samaritans, or with social services.

ALCOHOL ABUSE

Alcohol abuse (Box 3.5) may lead to physical, psychiatric and social sequelae, and it affects an increasingly large number of people. Yet it is a problem only too frequently neglected in the medical history. All patients should be asked whether they drink and, if so, roughly how much and in what circumstances, remembering that the answers frequently bear little resemblance to actual alcohol consumption.

Where there is any suspicion of alcohol-related problems, a thorough and systematic drinking history must be obtained:

- Construct an account of the patient's drinking habits through a typical day, including how they feel when they wake up in the morning, and how much sleep they have had.
- Do they remember what happened the night before?
- Were there withdrawal symptoms on getting up in the morning, such as shaking, nausea, retching, anxiety or craving for alcohol?

BOX 3.5 Features that suggest alcohol abuse.

- Excessive weekly intake
- Inability to stop drinking
- Craving for alcohol
- Primacy of drinking behaviour
- Secret drinking and drinking alone
- Morning drinking
- Withdrawal symptoms
- Drinking to avoid withdrawal
- Amnesia for events during a drinking binge
- Conviction for drunken driving, or other alcohol-related crime
- Violent behaviour
- Marital problems
- Employment problems
- Alcohol-related physical illness

- Detailed questions about the content, time, place, type and circumstances of first and all subsequent drinks and whether the patient drinks alone or in company are often revealing.
- When asking about the first drink of the day, find out about the speed at which it is drunk, (people with physical dependence often gulp rather than sip their first drink).
- Another helpful pointer to the current level of drinking is the amount of money the patient spends on drink, especially when related to income.

Enquire about:

- Any family history of drinking
- The age at which the patient started drinking, and when the patient's alcohol consumption increased
- The pattern of drinking, whether daily or in bouts, the type of alcohol consumed, and any precipitating factors (e.g. whether related to stress or mood)
- Personal difficulties caused by drinking, including its impact on the family; physical or psychiatric illness; loss of work or being drunk at work; antisocial behaviour; previous treatment or periods of abstinence or reduction in alcohol intake.

A history of serious medical or social complications, such as alcoholic hallucinosis, delirium tremens, antisocial behaviour resulting in encounters with the police or alcohol-related marital problems are especially significant.

It is also important, for treatment, to ascertain whether the patient feels he or she is drinking too much and would like to cut down or even stop drinking, and what sort of help might be necessary, or acceptable, to achieve this.

DRUG ABUSE (SUBSTANCE ABUSE)

This term implies not only drugs of addiction, whether major (e.g. morphine, heroin, cocaine, amphetamines) or minor (e.g. cannabis), but also 'recreational drugs' such as Ecstasy, prescribed drugs (commonly benzodiazepines) and non-prescribed drugs not normally considered addictive (e.g. cough linctus, analgesics). Information concerning the route of drug intake should be obtained. An assessment similar to that outlined above for alcohol abuse should be used. Particular attention should be paid to the development of any psychiatric symptoms that have developed at times of drug use. The financial consequences of the substance abuse are important indications of its importance in the patient's life.

PERSONALITY

Personality is defined as the sum of those characteristics that make a person into the individual he or she is (Box 3.6).

BOX 3.6 Points to consider when assessing personality.

- Behaviour
  - actions and reactions
- Attitude to self
- Relations with others
  - social
  - sexual
- Attitude to authority
- Level of independence
- Mood, e.g. usually happy, cheerful, sad, etc.
- Religious beliefs and moral attitudes
- Interests and hobbies
- Fantasy life

Personality may change with illness, for example disinhibition occurs with frontal lobe brain damage. The pre-morbid personality is most reliably assessed from an informant familiar with the patient before the onset of the illness. If such an objective opinion is unavailable it is worth asking the patient how others see them, for example: 'Would other people say you were a worrier?' Some features of personality, such as histrionic behaviour, will be obvious during the interview; others will already have been elicited in the history. Though many of the characteristics which make up the personality overlap—manipulative behaviour, for example, is both a manifestation of behaviour itself and a way of relating to others—they are best dealt with separately.

BEHAVIOUR

Think of behaviour in terms of *actions* and *reactions*.

Actions include level of achievement, histrionic or manipulative behaviour, deliberate self-harm or aggression towards others, disinhibition, obsessional behaviour (e.g. excessive tidiness, being overly houseproud, perfectionist, over-conscientious or obsessionally checking) and dependence on alcohol or drugs. Many of these behaviours will have been noted in the occupational, past psychiatric, forensic, and alcohol or drug abuse histories.

Reactions occur in response to stressful life events, such as illness, bereavement and other losses, or to examinations, promotion at work, failure and disappointment, and inability to cope with change. Reactions are often rather stereotyped, including being panicky or unflappable and slow to react, placid or short-tempered and easily angered. Both actions and reactions can be assessed under the following headings:

Attitude to self

- Self-interested or thoughtful about others
- Level of self-esteem and self-criticism
- Self-consciousness and sensitivity

- Self-confidence, whether high or low and constantly needing reassurance.

Relationship to others

Social
- Ease of making and keeping social relationships
- Introverted or extroverted
- Suspiciousness
- Assertiveness
- Warm and affectionate or cold and undemonstrative
- Tolerant or authoritarian and intolerant
- Relationships at work and with the family
- Psychosexual issues
- Level of psychosexual development, especially the capacity to make sexual relationships
- Direction of sexual attraction
- Other areas of difficulty.

Attitude to authority
- Well-adjusted and accepting
- Anxious and uncertain
- Generally tolerant or intolerant.

Level of independence
- Has the patient left home
- Still living with parents
- Accepting of responsibility for own actions
- Capable of making decisions.

Usual mood
- Prone to anxiety and if so, about what (e.g. illness, work, family)
- Pessimistic or optimistic
- Cyclothymic (i.e. swinging from elation to depression without reaching illness proportions)
- Calm or irritable
- Bottles up or shares feelings and emotions
- Easy-going or short-tempered and easily angered.

Religious beliefs and moral attitudes
- Which religion
- Whether practising or not
- Whether tolerant of beliefs and attitudes of others
- Ability to show regret or remorse and limit actions according to conscience.

Interests or hobbies
- What types
- Time spent on them
- Passive spectator or active participant
- Social or solitary pastimes
- Energetic or sedentary.

Fantasy life
- Sexual fantasies
- Non-sexual fantasies
- Dreams
- Nightmares.

SOCIAL CIRCUMSTANCES
Ask patients about home and how they get on with other members of the household, neighbours, and social contacts. Are there any financial problems or other stresses, including bereavement?

SUMMING UP
At the end of the history, try to sum up with the patient how you understand the problem. Ask whether you have grasped it in its entirety, left out any important areas or perhaps even totally failed to understand what the patient has been trying to put over. Besides clarifying the history, this summary also shows the patient that you have been listening and have understood.

WITNESS ACCOUNTS
Patients with severe psychiatric illnesses may be unable to give an accurate history. Those who are psychotic will have lost insight into the abnormal nature of their disturbed mental phenomena and so may not identify these experiences as anything to tell the doctor about. Alternatively, they may be suffering from a persecutory delusional state and may not want to tell anybody about what has been happening to them. Finally, patients' accounts of both the present and the past may be coloured by their current prevailing mental state, hence somebody with depression may report that their life has always been isolated and awful, even if this is not what they would have said when well. For these reasons it is often helpful to get an account of the patient's present and past mental states from a witness or informant, such as a partner, who knows them well. However, it is important to maintain medical confidentiality and to first obtain the patient's permission to speak to the informant.

THE PSYCHIATRIC EXAMINATION

This consists of physical and psychiatric examinations.

PHYSICAL EXAMINATION

A full physical examination of patients presenting with symptoms suggestive of psychiatric disorder is often both relevant and necessary. The combination of psychiatric symptoms and physical disease is common. Acutely anxious patients may have signs of thyrotoxicosis. Evidence of liver disease may suggest alcoholism. Needle marks in the arms point to drug abuse; scars of slashed wrists or other signs of self-mutilation may point to psychiatric illness. Leave the physical examination to the last; but note general features as you talk with the patient.

PSYCHIATRIC OR MENTAL STATE EXAMINATION

This should be covered systematically (Box 3.7).

APPEARANCE AND BEHAVIOUR

The patient's appearance and behaviour often reveal much about the underlying psychiatric disorder. Important points to look for include dress, personal hygiene and general grooming. Note the shabbily dressed elderly man with food stains on his clothes, perhaps indicative of an underlying dementia or schizophrenic illness.

The *facial expression* is one of the outward signs of a person's mood. Tearfulness or poverty of expression occur in depression, elation in mania, tenseness in anxiety, perplexity in schizophrenia. The *affect* may be inappropriate, such as the schizophrenic patient who laughs when relating upsetting material. It must be remembered, nonetheless, that anxious people may also laugh in similar circumstances. The emotional expression may be abnormally labile as in mania or organic brain disease.

The way the patient sits gives important clues:

- Is the patient relaxed and obviously at ease, or sitting tensely and fidgeting?
- The agitated depressive or the excited manic or schizophrenic may be so agitated that he or she gets up from the seat and paces up and down the room.
- The demented or confused patient may wander around uncomprehendingly.
- Delusions of persecution may cause the patient to feel threatened and to become angry or to terminate the interview.
- The patient with retarded depression may show little movement during the interview.
- The patient who drifts off to sleep repeatedly may be confused, with fluctuating levels of consciousness—consider over-sedation as a cause.

Observe gait and demeanour as the patient walks into the interview room:

BOX 3.7   How to examine the mental state.

Use the following headings:
- Appearance and behaviour
- Speech
- Mood
- Thought content
- Abnormal beliefs
- Abnormal experiences
- Cognitive state
- Intelligence
- Insight and rapport
- Specific tests of cerebral function
  - questionnaires
  - structured interview schedules

- Ataxia suggests organic brain disease, drug effect or alcoholism. The breath may smell of alcohol.
- There may be signs of *hysterical ataxia* that improves with suggestion or exhortation, or ataxia due to *malingering* or *simulation* in which the limp varies from moment to moment and is most marked when the patient knows he or she is being watched.

There may be other abnormal movements:

- Dystonia may be caused by major tranquilizers
- Choreiform movements are a feature of Huntington's chorea
- Tic-like mannerisms, odd postures or other bizarre disorders of movement occur in patients with schizophrenia or in organic brain disease, or may represent psychogenic disturbance. Tics are also quite frequent in normal adolescence during periods of emotional stress.

In schizophrenia, perseveration of posture may occur so that the patient's limbs can be moved into an abnormal position, maintained despite being allowed freely to revert to the previous posture (*catatonia*). When this movement is met by a waxy resistance it is termed *waxy flexibility*. The patient may repeatedly start and stop certain purposeful actions, for example shaking hands with the interviewer, or show *negativism*, in which he or she opposes the examiner's intention. In *echopraxia* the interviewer's actions are copied; these abnormal postures and movements often occur in organic brain disease as well as in non-organic catatonia. There may be slowing or *retardation of movement*, even to the extent of stupor.

Stupor is commonly caused by organic disorders but may also be a result of functional psychoses such as schizophrenia and depression. Stupor may also occur in hysteria, or in uncontrolled anxiety following extreme stress; or it may be simulated by malingerers.

Behaviour

The patient's behaviour during the interview may be disinhibited, as in the manic patient who strips or the patient with frontal brain disease who starts to urinate or masturbate during the interview. Manipulative, seductive or violent behaviour may be seen if the patient's wishes are not met. There may be verbal aggression or physical violence, the latter against either the interviewer or objects in the room. On the other hand, the patient may appear to be unduly submissive or self-critical, or may show little or no eye contact with the interviewer. He or she may appear to be suspicious of questions due to an underlying personality disorder or paranoid illness. Somtimes the patient may seem to be paying little attention to the interviewer or to be listening to someone else when there is no one else in the room; this suggests that he or she is experiencing auditory hallucinations (i.e. hearing voices). The patient may even be talking to or arguing with these voices. Undue terror without any obvious cause, or attempts to touch or shoo away non-existing objects, suggests that the patient is experiencing visual hallucinations.

Remember that bizarre behaviour or inability to relate to the interviewer may be signs of subnormality, and not of psychiatric illness.

SPEECH

It is important to assess the form of speech as well as its content. Does the patient speak at all or is he or she *mute* and, if so, is this deliberate, organic, hysterical or part of a depressive or catatonic stupor? In the mute patient it is important to assess all aspects of speech production, including the ability to produce sounds and communicate non-verbally. If the patient does speak, is this spontaneous or only in answer to questions, with monosyllabic or fuller and more elaborate replies? Is speech unduly slow as in depressive illness or so quick and continuous, with *flight of ideas*, that it is impossible to interrupt, as in hypomania and mania? Are there long pauses before the patient replies or are there arrests of speech in mid-sentence (e.g. in schizophrenia)?

Are the words normal or are there neologisms as in some types of schizophrenia or organic brain disease? Is there evidence of dysphasia or dysarthria? When the words themselves are normal, are the phrases and sentences normal and do they fit together, or does the patient seem to jump from topic to topic; if the latter occurs, is it possible to understand the link between topics, as in *flight of ideas* in mania, or is there no recognizable link, as in the formal *thought disorder* of schizophrenia? Is the link, if present, not one of content but of form as in rhyming or punning, usually features of mania? Is there evidence of *echolalia*, in which the patient repeats what the interviewer says, or *perseveration*, when the patient continues with the same theme even if this is no longer appropriate? As an example of the latter, a 60-year-old man, replying to the question 'How old are you?' answers '60, 61, 62, 63, 64, 65, 66' and so on; when asked the subsequent question, 'What year were you born?', he answers '1960' and to the next question, 'What year is it?', now also answers '1960' (perseveration on a theme of 60). Both echolalia and perseveration are found in organic brain disease and in some types of schizophrenia.

When the speech is abnormal, samples of it should be written down verbatim, or recorded on tape, as this is the only reliable way of recording the abnormality for future assessment. Two doctors may differ in what they call formal thought disorder and therefore writing in the case notes: 'There was evidence of formal thought disorder' is not helpful. A recorded sample of the patient's speech gives much less room for disagreement.

MOOD

Mood has both a subjective component, which is reflected in the way someone describes their emotional state, and an objective component, i.e. what the interviewer sees, for example, tears.

The subjective and objective components of mood are usually, but not always, congruent. An example of incongruence is the smiling face of some severely depressed patients. Subjective mood is assessed by asking the patient how he feels in himself, what his mood is, or what his spirits are like. If necessary, leading questions such as 'Are you anxious or depressed?' may be used. Abnormal mood includes, most commonly, depression and anxiety but also elation, irritability, anger and perplexity. When the mood is abnormal it should be evaluated in detail in the same way as any other presenting symptom. In affective disorders the content of any hallucinations or delusions are generally mood-congruent—depressed patients may think that they are evil while manic patients may believe that they are God.

Depression

This may be mild and influenced by daily activities, or severe. The clinical features are characteristic (Box 3.8). In severe depression, symptoms may be worse in the morning and associated with early morning waking, appetite and weight disturbance, lethargy, loss of concentration and loss of interest and enjoyment in life. There may also be ideas of worthlessness, self-deprecation, poverty, guilt, persecution, bodily ill-health, nihilism and other morbid ideas. These may sometimes be delusional in intensity (see section on abnormal experiences). The patient may be agitated or retarded, sometimes even to the point of stupor, and may be mute or, in lesser cases, show retardation of speech.

Suicide

The depressed patient may see no future, feel despairing and hopeless, and have thoughts of suicide. Suicidal ideation must always be sought for in depressed patients and very often it is also appropriate to ask about suicidality in those with other

---

BOX 3.8   Features supporting a diagnosis of depression.

- Loss of interest/enjoyment in life
- Lethargy
- Poor concentration
- Early morning waking
- Appetite and weight disturbance
- Ideas of worthlessness, guilt, persecution, nihilism
- Self-deprecation
- Retardation, leading to depressive stupor
- Retardation of speech, or muteness
- Paradoxical agitation and delusional state

psychiatric disorders such as schizophrenia, alcohol dependence, hypomania and severe anxiety disorders. Not only is it incorrect that discussing suicide with patients encourages them to commit suicide, but failure to discuss it may lead to tragedies that could have been prevented (Box 3.9). It can be asked for directly or approached through a series of questions such as: 'How do you see the future?' 'Have you felt it would be nice to escape or be able to sleep and not wake up?' 'Do you feel at times that you would rather be dead or that you are such a burden to others that they would be better off if you were dead?' 'Have you had thoughts of suicide, however fleeting?' 'Have you made any plans?' Where it is felt that the patient is suicidal but denies it, it is worth asking the question: 'What stops you killing yourself?' or: 'What do you have to live for?' Some patients admit to having suicidal thoughts but deny that they would do anything because of the impact it would have on the family or because it is against their religion or they do not have the courage. Suicide, however, is not a respecter of family feelings, religious beliefs or personal bravery. Homicidal thoughts may also be present, as in some mothers with puerperal depressive illnesses who kill their children because they are convinced they have passed on some terrible illness and death is better for them than a life of suffering.

Sometimes patients report that they have thought about suicide but say that they would not actually kill themselves because things are not quite bad enough. In this case it is appropriate to enquire as to what would need to happen in order for things to become that bad. Occasionally only very small changes would lead to clear risk of suicide.

Anxiety

Anxiety states may present with somatic symptoms related mainly to autonomic nervous system arousal or hyperventilation (Box 3.10), or to psychic symp-

---

> **BOX 3.10   Somatic symptoms of anxiety.**
>
> - Headaches and other muscular aches and pains
> - Palpitations
> - Tremor
> - Breathlessness
> - Chest pain
> - Urinary frequency
> - Faintness and lightheadedness
> - Fatigue
> - Pins and needles
> - Diarrhoea
> - Dry mouth
> - Abdominal discomfort
> - Flushes
> - Sweating

> **BOX 3.11   Psychic symptoms of anxiety.**
>
> - Feelings of anxiety
> - Irritability
> - Inability to relax
> - Inability to concentrate
> - Initial insomnia—difficulty getting off to sleep
> - Feeling of impending doom
> - Depersonalization

toms (Box 3.11), or both. The anxiety may be free-floating or situation-dependent as in phobic disorders (e.g. agoraphobia), social phobias and other specific phobias.

The patient may complain of panic attacks with sudden surges of extreme anxiety, with physical symptoms and the desire to run away, sometimes coupled with an inability to move.

Elation

Elated patients describe themselves as being on top of the world, feeling happier than they have ever done before. This is a feature of *hypomania* and *mania* when it is associated with overactivity, pressure of speech with flight of ideas, sleep impairment, irritability and grandiose ideas. Manic patients may also have moments of tearfulness or the mental state may show signs of both depression and elation, as in mixed affective states.

Other abnormal states

Irritability may occur in many psychiatric disorders, especially anxiety states and hypomania, and in situational and relationship disturbances, such as marital problems. It may also be part of the usual mood in some personalities, such as the intolerant person who does not suffer fools gladly. *Anger* may be related to a specific person or situation or may be part of an underlying psychiatric disturbance, in particular when ideas of persecution are present. Irritability and anger are common after closed head

---

> **BOX 3.9   Features suggesting increased risk of suicidal behaviour.**
>
> - Previous self-harm, especially
>   - poison
>   - stabbing
>   - hanging
>   - jumping from heights
>   - falling under vehicles
> - Continuing suicidal thoughts
> - Current depressive or schizophrenic psychosis
> - Male sex, aged > 40 years
> - Social isolation, especially in adolescence or the recently bereaved or divorced
> - Chronic painful illness
> - Alcoholism and drug abuse
> - Family history of suicide

injuries with frontal contusions. *Perplexity* is usually found in schizophrenic patients who are suspicious that something is going on but cannot quite put their finger on what it is.

THOUGHT CONTENT

Patients should be asked what their main worries are and whether they are preoccupied by any thoughts, for example morbid thoughts or obsessional ruminations. The latter are thoughts that the patient recognizes as his or her own, realizes are silly and tries to resist, but is unable to do so. They occur in obsessive compulsive neuroses and may be associated with obsessional rituals—acts which the patient feels compelled to carry out, despite recognizing their absurdity. In obsessional rituals the patient realizes that the compulsion comes from within, unlike in delusions of influence in which the impulse is felt to come from outside forces. An example of obsessional rumination is the man who knows that his wife is not unfaithful but has doubts about her which continuously run through his mind and which he is unable to suppress. Common obsessional rituals include hand-washing; the patient may wash his or her hands 40 or 50 times a day until they are raw. Obsessional checking is another common manifestation; for example, the woman who switches off her bedroom lights before leaving the house, gets to the bottom of the stairs and repeatedly has to go back up again to check the lights are off. If not followed exactly, these obsessional rituals lead to extreme anxiety.

ABNORMAL BELIEFS

These range from delusions (Box 3.12), in which the patient has false and unshakeable beliefs which are out of keeping with the social milieu from which the patient comes, to overvalued ideas, in which the patient has false beliefs which, although of major concern to him or her, are not completely unshakeable. These abnormal beliefs include misinterpretations, in which the patient concocts false explanations for various normal events which may or may not be delusional in extent. Record abnormal ideas verbatim.

BOX 3.12   Examples of abnormal beliefs.

- Delusions
  - of persecution (paranoid delusions)
  - of grandeur
  - of poverty (depressive delusions)
  - of reference
  - of love
  - of infidelity
  - of interference (alienation)
  - nihilistic delusions (e.g. that the internal organs are dead and rotten)

Though abnormal beliefs usually denote the presence of a psychiatric illness, they may also occur in certain situations in normal people, as in the case of ideas of reference, in which people can feel that what others are saying refers to them, or that other people are laughing at them behind their back. This is commonly seen in sensitive people, especially in anxiety-provoking situations, such as parties where most of the other guests are strangers.

Delusions may be *primary*, like sudden bolts from heaven, or *secondary*. In the latter their existence is understandable in terms of the rest of the patient's psychopathology, as in affective psychoses. Primary delusions may be delusional ideas—fully formed delusions that suddenly enter into the patient's mind, as in the person who for no reason suddenly believes that their food is being poisoned. This is often preceded by a delusional mood, in which the patient feels that there is something going on and that things are not quite right, but is unable to elaborate this feeling. In delusional perceptions the object is perceived normally but is interpreted in a delusional way, for example the man who sees an ashtray on the table, recognizes it as an ashtray, but believes that it has been put there to show people that he is a spy. This is not understandable in terms of the rest of the patient's psychopathology. Primary delusions should be diagnosed with caution as, by the time the patient has presented, it may be very difficult to differentiate primary from secondary.

Delusions of persecution

Also called *paranoid delusions*, these are probably the most common delusions and may occur alone or with other abnormal mental signs. They occur in organic psychoses such as confusional states, dementia, and alcohol- and drug-induced psychoses, and associated with various organic illnesses such as some endocrine disorders and systemic lupus erythematosus. They also occur in functional psychoses such as paranoid schizophrenia, paraphrenia of the elderly, depressive illness and mania, in stress-induced, psychogenic psychoses or hysterical pseudopsychoses, and in some people with paranoid personality developments.

Delusions of grandeur

These delusions occur in the now uncommon syphilitic general paralysis of the insane and in mania and schizophrenia. Patients may believe they are on a special mission or that they are Napoleon or Christ.

Delusions of poverty and other depressive delusions

Depressed patients may insist that they are destitute and have no clothes. Other common depressive delusions include self-deprecation, worthlessness and guilt: 'I have done something terrible and should be in prison and not in hospital.' Delusions of ill-health may occur and persist despite every assurance of the patient's physical health. These delusions occur both in depression and schizophrenia. Some people develop isolated abnormal ideas about their own appearance which may sometimes be delusional in intensity, for example that their nose is too long or their hair is falling out. These patients often have sensitive personalities, some may be depressed and some may become schizophrenic with time.

Nihilistic delusions

These occur mainly in severe depressive illnesses but can also occur in schizophrenia and organic brain disease. The patient with nihilistic delusions says that they are dead or that part of their body is dead. This may lead to self-harm.

Delusions of love

Erotomania is another name for this symptom, in which the patient is convinced that someone is in love with them, despite the other person having shown no signs of this. The patient may act upon this misguided belief and pester the individual so that a legal injunction may be necessary to restrain them. These delusions may occur in schizophrenia and occasionally in organic psychoses.

Delusions of infidelity

With these the patient is morbidly jealous, and convinced that their spouse is having an extramarital affair. The patient may go to extreme lengths to confirm these abnormal beliefs, often pressing the spouse to admit his or her errant ways. These arguments may lead to violence that can end in murder. These delusions occur in people with suspicious personalities, especially when associated with alcohol abuse, and in schizophrenia and affective psychoses.

Delusions of influence (passivity or alienation phenomenon)

This is one of Schneider's first-rank symptoms—those symptoms which, in the absence of organic brain disease, are highly suggestive of schizophrenia (see Box 3.13).

BOX 3.13   How to diagnose schizophrenia.

Are there any of Schneider's first-rank symptoms of schizophrenia?

- Hearing voices in the third person arguing or commenting on what the patient is doing
- Hearing one's own thoughts spoken out loud
- Thought alienation (insertion, withdrawal or broadcast)
- Delusional perceptions (a primary delusion)
- Passivity phenomena—everything in the spheres of feeling, sensations, volition and actions experienced as imposed on the patient or influenced by others

---

Delusions of influence are when patients say that their mind or body is being controlled by outside forces such as laser beams transmitted by a neighbour. When the mind rather than the body is affected, patients may complain that thoughts are being forced either into or out of their head. Another form of thought alienation is thought broadcast, in which the patient's thought leaves his or her head, travels through the air and enters into other people's heads, so that when the patient thinks something, everyone else thinks the same. Alienation, or passivity, may also affect perception, as in patients who experience somatic hallucinations which they say are being caused by other people or by external forces. These are known as 'made' experiences.

ABNORMAL EXPERIENCES

These may be divided into abnormal perceptions and abnormal experiences of the self or the environment.

Abnormal perceptions

Abnormal perceptions may occur in any of the sensory modalities—hearing, vision, smell, taste and touch (Box 3.14). Objects may be distorted while remaining recognizable or there may be a new perception, as in illusions or hallucinations. Distortions in intensity, either increased or decreased, may be due to functional or organic disorders; distortions in quality (e.g. colour) are often due to toxic substances; distortions in form, (e.g. micropsia, when the object appears smaller or further away) or macropsia, may be due to organic lesions of the visual pathway.

Illusions

Illusions occur when the object is real but perception is disturbed. They are usually related, in the psychiatric sense, to disorders of the perceptual environment of the object, thereby leading to decrease in visual clarity coupled with a state of high emotion in the perceiver. A common example is the experience of walking through a lonely alley on a dark night and perceiving a tree in the distance to be the figure of a man. Vision is impaired by the poor illumination and the lonely alley induces a feeling of fear, thus leading to the illusion. Illusions are common in psychiatric illness, particularly acute confusional states.

Hallucinations

Hallucinations occur in the absence of an appropriate object yet the patient still insists that he or she has perceived something. The commonest hallucina-

---

BOX 3.14   Examples of abnormal perceptions.

- Distortions—an abnormally perceived object
- Illusions—a disturbance of perception of a real object
- Hallucinations—an apparent perception: the object does not exist (the patient may be aware of the unreality of the perception)

tions are auditory and visual but, as with normal perceptions, they can occur in all sensory modalities. They may be due to organic disease of the nervous system or to extreme environmental disturbances as in sensory deprivation. In certain instances they may be non-pathological phenomena, as in *hypnogogic* and *hypnopompic* hallucinations experienced by a person going to sleep or waking up. Hypnogogic hallucinations also occur in narcolepsy.

In psychiatric illness, hallucinations occur in organic and functional psychoses, for example in schizophrenia and affective illnesses, severely raised levels of anxiety due to hyperventilation, grief reactions and hysterical illnesses. They are occasionally displayed by malingerers. They may occur wherever the patient is or may only be present in certain places. Thus the paranoid patient who hears the neighbours' voices plotting against him or her at home does not hear them while in hospital, yet the voices return when the patient is at home again.

Auditory hallucinations
The patient may complain of hearing noises, music, distant mumbling which he or she cannot identify, words, phrases or more elaborate speech. When patients hear voices rather than sounds they may sometimes be able to recognize them as belonging to people they know. The voices may be talking to the patient, or talking about him or her (see below). They may be persecutory, neutral or pleasing. The patient may talk back to the voices, or may appear to be listening to them intently. In some cases the voices direct the patient to certain actions which they may feel they must follow.

Second-person voices
Second-person voices with distressing content— 'You stink, you're horrible, go kill yourself'—are found in severe depressive illnesses. Third-person voices, which discuss or argue about the patient or comment on what he or she is doing, are suggestive of schizophrenia in the absence of organic brain disease (see Box 3.13), as is hearing one's own thoughts spoken out loud (echo des pensées). In grief reactions, the bereaved person may hear the footsteps or other stigmata of the dead person.

Visual hallucinations
These vary in complexity from simple flashes of light to sophisticated 'visions' of people or animals. They occur more commonly in organic psychoses, especially acute confusional states, than in functional psychoses. The opposite is true of auditory hallucinations. Visual hallucinations may be frightening, as in the case of hallucinations of spiders, insects and rats which occur especially in delirium tremens, or pleasing, as with Lilliputian hallucinations, in which the patient sees tiny people. They may coexist with auditory hallucinations as in temporal lobe epilepsy.

Olfactory hallucinations
These may occur in temporal lobe epilepsy, when an unpleasant smell may be the initial symptom of the attack, in schizophrenia (as in the patient who said that people were making cars emit noxious smells at him) and in depressive illnesses (in which the patients insist that they emit a foul odour which they can smell).

Hallucinations of taste
These are rare in psychiatric practice but may occur in temporal lobe epilepsy.

Tactile and somatic hallucinations
In cocaine psychosis patients may complain that insects are crawling over them (formication). Other patients insist that they are experiencing odd sensations in various parts of their body which are produced by other people, as in the man who complained that his neighbour's laser gun was producing a cold feeling which travelled up his legs. In the absence of organic brain disease tactile hallucinosis is a first-rank symptom of (Box 3.13). These hallucinations may have a sexual content, as in the patient who insisted that someone was having intercourse with her and she could feel it happening all the time.

Other hallucinations and illusions
Some people complain that, when alone, they feel the presence of someone else beside them. This may occur in grief reactions; as illusions when the patient is frightened; as a manifestation of hysteria; in organic brain disease and schizophrenia. Finally, *vestibular hallucinations* may occur, usually in acute organic brain disease, such as the patient with delirium tremens who has the sensation of flying through the air.

Abnormal experiences of self and environment
Déjà vu
This may occur in normal people but it is often associated with temporal lobe epilepsy, and is characterized by the patient feeling that they have been in their current situation before.

Capgras' syndrome
In this syndrome, which occurs most commonly in schizophrenia but may also occur in dementia, the patient asserts that people are not who they claim to be, but are their double.

Depersonalization
This symptom is often a manifestation of heightened anxiety levels. The patient does not feel his or her normal self and may describe this unpleasant experience as if floating above their own body looking down on it. The patient may also complain of losing the capacity to feel at an emotional level. This may be one of the most marked symptoms in depressed patients.

Derealization

This often accompanies depersonalization. Patients say that their surroundings feel unreal or gray or colourless.

COGNITIVE STATE

In elderly people, or where organic brain disease is suspected (e.g. in acute confusional states), the assessment of cognitive state is extremely important. Semiquantitative tests of cognitive function based on the general approach described here are often used, for example the *Mental Status Questionnaire* (MSQ) (Table 3.1) and the *Mini-mental State Examination* (MMSE) (Table 3.2). The MSQ consists of 10 simple questions that relate to alertness, orientation for time and space, and recent and long-term memory. Normal subjects achieve 9 or 10 correct answers; scores less than 8 imply some degree of mental confusion. Patients with severe confusion score less than 3. The MMSE (Table 3.2) differs from the MSQ in that it is more detailed and scores are, to some extent, dependent on educational level. The test has subcategories related to orientation, registration, attention, recall and language. The maximum score is 30, and scores lower than 21 are associated with cognitive impairment. Neither the MSQ nor the MMSE is capable of differentiating multifocal from diffuse organic brain disease, but both provide useful baseline assessment of a patient's cognitive performance.

Level of consciousness

An assessment of the level of alertness of the patient or, if unconscious, of the level of unconsciousness may be made. Some patients appear to have fluctuating levels of consciousness; the mental state may then fluctuate between lucidity and gross abnormality. This is a manifestation of an acute confusional state and is characteristic of states of delirium such as the delirium tremens that may be seen in alcohol-dependent patients who are acutely withdrawing

---

TABLE 3.1   Mental Status Questionnaire.

1. What is the name of this place (where are we now)?
2. What is the address of this place?
3. What is the date?
4. What month is it?
5. What year is it?
6. How old are you?
7. When is your birthday?
8. What year were you born?
9. Who is the Prime Minister?
10. Who was the previous Prime Minister?

Each question is scored: 0 for incorrect, and 1 for a correct response.
Normal subjects score 9 or 10; scores less than 8 imply a degree of mental confusion.

TABLE 3.2   Mini-mental State Examination.

Orientation
1 point for each correct answer

What is the:
  time
  date
  day
  month
  year   5 points

What is the name of this:
  ward
  hospital
  district
  town
  country   5 points

Registration
Name three objects
  1, 2, 3 points according to how many are repeated
  Re-submit list until patient word perfect in order to use this for a later test of recall
  Score only first attempt   3 points

Attention and calculation
  Have the patient subtract 7 from 100 and then from the result a total of five times
  1 point for each correct subtraction   5 points

Recall
  Ask for three objects used in the registration test, one point being awarded for each correct answer   3 points

Language
  1 point each for two objects correctly named (pencil and watch)   2 points
  1 point for correct repetition of 'No ifs, ands and buts'   1 point
  3 points if three-stage commands correctly obeyed: 'Take this piece of paper, in your right hand, fold it in half, and place it on the floor'   3 points
  1 point for correct response to a written command, such as 'close your eyes'   1 point
  Have the patient write a sentence. Award 1 point if the sentence is meaningful, has a verb and a subject   1 point
  Test the patient's ability to copy a complex diagram of two intersecting pentagons   1 point

                      Total score 30

from alcohol. For a full account of the examination of the unconscious patient see Chapter 15.

Orientation

The patient's orientation in time, place and person should be formally assessed by direct questioning and the patient's answers written down verbatim. Disorientation is an important sign of organic brain disease, whether chronic or acute, but may also occur in chronic, uninterested, institutionalized schizophrenics and in hysterical dissociative states.

Time

Ask about the day, date, month, year and time of day. If the patient does not know the month, ask about the season. All patients should know the year and either the month or season and the approximate time of day (e.g. morning, afternoon, evening or night). Long stays in hospital, where one day is much like the next, however, are not conducive to an awareness of which particular day it is or the exact date of the month.

Place

Patients should know where they are (e.g. home or hospital) and approximately where it is situated (e.g. what town or part of the town). Depending on how long they have been in the place where they are interviewed, whether at home or in a hospital ward, they should know the way to such places as the bathroom or toilet. Some patients with acute confusional states may say they are in hospital but that the hospital is part of their own home.

Person

If disorientation is suspected the patient should be asked his or her name and address.

Attention and concentration

The patient's behaviour during the interview will have shown whether they are easily distracted or have been paying attention to and concentrating on the questions you have asked. This can be tested more formally by asking the patient to subtract serial sevens from 100 or, as this may be difficult even for normal people, serial threes from 20. Tasks such as recounting the months of the year and days of the week backwards or repeating a sequence of digits (digit span) forwards are also useful. Repetition of digits backwards (e.g. the doctor says 165 to which the patient should reply 561) is dependent not only on attention and concentration but also on the ability to register the numbers 165 and remember them long enough to reverse them and is thus a test of immediate memory. Normal people should be able to manage seven digits forward and five backwards; telephone numbers in most large cities consist of seven digits. Another useful test is to ask the patient to spell 'world' backwards; the impaired patient often transposes the central letters of the word.

Memory

In chronic organic brain disease, *memory for recent events* is diminished, whereas early in the illness the patient often remains able to remember events which have happened in the past and is thus able to give a coherent account of the family and early personal history. Some patients with memory impairment—as in Korsakov's psychosis, which is usually due to thiamine deficiency following poor nutrition or associated with heavy drinking—may confabulate. An example is the alcoholic with Korsakov's psychosis seen after a 6-week stay in hospital, who when asked how long he had been an in-patient stated that he had come in that day and been at work the day before, which he then described in great detail down to what he had for his lunch that day. Confabulation is not invention, but consists of the inappropriate recall of recent or distant past experiences, illustrating a defect in the process of recall of memories.

In the case of head injuries or in epileptic attacks, an attempt should be made to assess the presence of *retrograde and anterograde amnesia*, if any, in some detail. Memory impairment may be simulated for gain by some manipulative patients, some of whom may give approximate answers. For example, if the date is Monday 11 November 2002 they may say it is Tuesday 14 October 2000 and then correct themselves to Sunday 16 December 2002. Hysterical amnesia may occur in dissociative states in which there is a sudden total loss of memory. In contrast, in organic amnesia, long-term memory and personal identity are usually spared until the later stages of the disorder. This is so even in dementing illnesses. Patients who are apathetic or depressed may appear to have memory impairment, in the latter case called *depressive pseudodementia*. This may only become apparent when the depression lifts and the memory improves.

Past memory will already have been assessed while asking about the family and personal history, but recent memory will need more specific testing. A useful approach is to ask the patient about recent television programmes, such as the events in a popular soap opera, or the fortunes of a favourite football team. Other recent events will include details about the hospital itself, and how the patient got there. Current affairs should also be asked about, such as the names of top politicians and details of any recent happenings of major importance. A less direct question is to ask the patient what has been going on in the world or in this country recently.

A more systematic approach to memory testing is to ask the patient to repeat a name and address immediately and again after about 5 minutes. Or give the patient a sentence—for example 'The one thing a nation needs in order to be rich and great is a large, secure supply of wood'—and see how many repetitions are necessary for accurate reproduction. Where relevant, visual as well as auditory memory should be tested. This can be done by giving the patient a picture depicting a series of objects and a few minutes later asking them to recall as many of the objects as they can.

The patient's answers to all specific questions about memory should be recorded verbatim.

INTELLIGENCE

An assessment of the patient's intelligence is one of the most important objectives of the interview. Not only will this help to determine suitable treatment (e.g. for psychotherapy the patient must be articulate and intelligent) but it will also affect the interpretation of the mental state examination itself. In the subnormal patient bizarre behaviour and abnormal ideas occurring as part of a normal fantasy life may be mistaken for psychiatric illness, when it really represents only an attention-seeking device. An approximate assessment of intelligence can be obtained from the educational and occupational history and from an assessment of general knowledge. Alternatively this can be tested more formally especially by using the National Adult Reading Test (NART), since reading ability correlates closely with intelligence in the absence of other disabilities (see below). If in doubt, enquire whether the patient can read and write, and see whether the patient is able to solve simple mathematical problems, especially where these are related to daily activities, such as shopping.

INSIGHT

It is important to make an assessment of the insight patients have into their own problems and this can be considered at a number of different levels. First, there is the patient who has no insight at all and does not accept that he or she is ill. Such lack of insight is one of the hallmarks of a psychotic illness where the patient is out of touch with reality. The second type of patient may accept that he or she is ill but perceives the illness on a physical rather than a psychiatric basis, as occurs with hysterical disorders and some anxiety states. Often a full explanation as to the cause of the symptoms will lead to insight, though this is not always the case. Such patients may deny there are any problems in any areas of their life despite there being obvious difficulties. Thirdly, some patients accept their need of psychiatric help but are unable fully to unravel the complexities of their problems.

RAPPORT

The rapport established in the interview between doctor and patient depends not only on the interview technique but also on the personality and mental attitude of the two participants. The doctor must not force his or her own personality and attitudes onto the patient. The way the patient relates to the doctor (see section on behaviour, p. 34) offers an insight into the patient's internal psychological state, enabling the doctor to make an evaluation of such points as dependence, relationships to others, especially those in authority (including parent figures), mood and paranoid ideation. With the patient suffering from a psychotic illness the doctor may feel that meaningful contact has never really been achieved. With the neurotic patient, or in the absence of personality problems, the doctor–patient relationship forms an important element in psychotherapy. The patient may displace onto the doctor feelings directed to other important people in his or her own life. For example, anger more appropriately directed towards a spouse or parent may instead manifest itself in the interview setting, with the doctor the recipient of this displaced emotion. Finally, patients may project their feelings onto the doctor. An angry patient may not overtly show this anger but may leave the doctor feeling angry; similarly depression and elation may be transmitted to the doctor in the interview. Thus noting how you feel during the interview may give valuable added information for the assessment of the patient's mental state.

FURTHER TESTS OF CEREBRAL FUNCTION

In patients in whom organic brain disease is suspected, a more detailed assessment of cerebral function should be carried out. In addition to the above, this includes an assessment of: speech, both verbal and written; spatial, visual, motor and numerical abilities; awareness of body image; and presence of released primitive reflexes. These comprise part of the neurological examination (see Chapter 11).

FURTHER INVESTIGATIONS

In psychiatry these consist of extended information gathering, clarification and continuing assessment of the mental state, laboratory investigations, psychological testing, social enquiry and occupational therapy assessment. In addition, EEG, CT and MRI are sometimes appropriate when exploring the possibility of a demonstrable organic cause for behavioural signs and symptoms, such as epilepsy or a space-occupying lesion. Indications for these techniques include an unusual periodicity to the behavioural changes, the presence of an altered level of consciousness and the finding of abnormalities on neurological examination.

INFORMATION GATHERING

Many patients will need more than one interview to evaluate the full psychiatric history. Other sources of information are needed to clarify and validate parts of the history. Spouse, family, friends and people at work or school may be able to help, but before they are contacted this should be discussed with the patient and verbal or, in some cases, written consent obtained. In addition to separate interviews with the patient, spouse and family, it is often necessary to bring these people together in order to carry out diagnostic and therapeutic marital and family interviews. These interviews often provide information unavailable from either party on their own as well as affording an opportunity to see how the couple or family relate to each other. In addition, when feeding back your conclusions, it allows you to give all concerned parties the same information at the same time, thus avoiding potentially divisive miscommunication. If the other informant cannot be interviewed in person it may still be possible to communicate by telephone or by letter.

It is obviously important to obtain detailed medical records from the family doctor and from any hospital concerned; the grounds for previous diagnoses can be scrutinized and the response to past treatment assessed. Conditions in the patient's home may be assessed by a social worker or occupational therapist, who may be able to see relatives who refuse to see a doctor. The patient's problems can be further assessed by suggesting that a diary of the symptoms, daily activities and emotional state would be helpful. This often indicates links which may illuminate the aetiology of the current disorder. When one is dealing with a specific behavioural disorder, for example nervous diarrhoea, overeating or aggressive behaviour, more systematic behavioural analysis may be necessary.

MENTAL STATE EVALUATION

The evaluation of the mental state is a continuous process and should be assessed at each interview. The behaviour on the ward of patients admitted to hospital should be observed and documented. This includes an account of the way they relate to other patients, to staff and visitors, and whether there are any signs of sleep or appetite disturbance or other abnormal behaviour. Questionnaires and structured interview schedules may aid quantitative assessment of the mental state and may be useful in evaluating progress.

NEUROPSYCHOLOGICAL TESTING

Psychological tests can be used to assess the patient's cognitive state, behaviour, personality and thinking process. Tests can be given to assess the level of intelligence—either briefly with the Mill Hill test or Raven's Progressive Matrices, or in more detail with the WAIS (Wechsler Adult Intelligence Scale). In behavioural disorders it is useful to carry out a thorough behavioural analysis; this must be designed to be relevant to the individual problem. These investigations require specialized skills and should be carried out by the clinical psychologist.

If there is a question of localized organic brain dysfunction, then specialized neuropsychological tests, of which there are many, that aim to explore specific cognitive processes or the functions of individual brain regions, will be employed by the clinical neuropsychologist.

THE SKIN, NAILS AND HAIR

INTRODUCTION

The skin is a large organ of the human body. Forming a major interface between man and his environment, it covers an area of approximately 2 m² and weighs about 4 kg. The structure of human skin is complex (Figs 4.1 and 4.2), consisting of a number of layers and tissue components with many important functions (Box 4.1). Reactions may occur in any of the components of human skin and their clinical manifestations reflect, among other factors, the level in the skin in which they occur.

Dermatology is a visual clinical specialty. The accurate diagnosis of most skin lesions requires an adequate history, careful examination of the patient and, occasionally, laboratory investigation.

BOX 4.1   Functions of the human skin.

- Protection: physical, chemical, infection
- Physiological: homeostasis of electrolytes, water and protein
- Thermoregulation
- Sensation: specialized nerve endings
- Lubrication and waterproofing: sebum
- Immunological: Langerhans cells, lymphocytes, macrophages
- Vitamin D synthesis
- Body odour: apocrine glands
- Psychosocial: cosmetic

HISTORY

Detailed information should be sought concerning the present skin condition. This should include the site of onset, mode of spread and duration of the disorder. Any personal history or family history of skin disease, including atopy, is important. Previous medical conditions should be noted, and a full drug history obtained, including any use of over-the-counter preparations. The social and occupational history should be noted and, in some circumstances, details of recent travel and sexual activity may be important.

EXAMINATION

The whole skin, including hair, nails and assessable mucosae, should be fully exposed, preferably in natural light. Sometimes a magnifying lens is useful.

COLOUR AND PIGMENTATION

Before inspecting any rash or lesion notice the *colour* of the skin. The normal skin colour varies, depending on lifestyle and light exposure as well as constitutional and ethnic factors.

Pallor can have many causes. It may be:

- Temporary, due to shock, haemorrhage or intense emotion
- Persistent, due to anaemia or peripheral vasoconstriction.

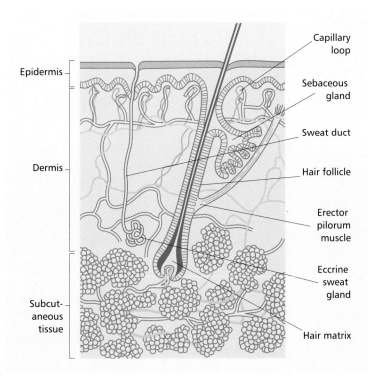

Epidermis

Dermis

Subcut-
aneous
tissue

Capillary
loop

Sebaceous
gland

Sweat duct

Hair follicle

Erector
pilorum
muscle

Eccrine
sweat
gland

Hair matrix

Fig. 4.1 The anatomy of the full
thickness of the skin in section.

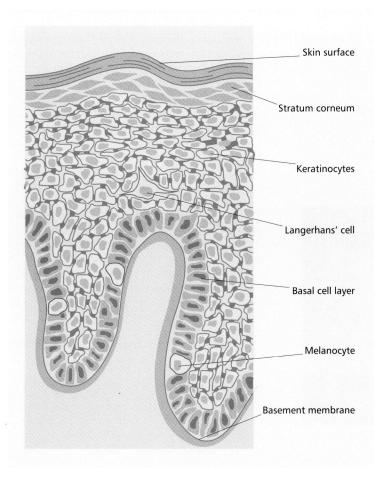

Skin surface

Stratum corneum

Keratinocytes

Langerhans' cell

Basal cell layer

Melanocyte

Basement membrane

Fig. 4.2 The anatomy of the
epidermis.

Vasoconstriction is seen in patients with severe atopy—an inherited susceptibility to asthma, eczema and hay fever. Although pallor is a feature of *anaemia*, not all pale persons are anaemic; conjunctival and mucosal colour is a better indication of anaemia than skin colour. A pale skin resulting from diminished pigment occurs with *hypopituitarism* and *hypogonadism*.

Normal skin contains varying amounts of brown *melanin* pigment. Brown pigmentation due to the presence of *haemosiderin* is always pathological. *Albinism* is an inherited generalized absence of pigment in the skin; a localized form is known as *piebaldism*. Patches of white and darkly pigmented skin are seen in *vitiligo* (Fig. 4.3). In vitiligo there is a complete absence of melanocytes. Several autoimmune endocrine disorders are associated with vitiligo.

Abnormal redness of the skin (*erythema*) is seen after overheating, extreme exertion, sunburn and in febrile, exanthematous and inflammatory skin disease. *Flushing* is a striking redness, usually of the face and neck, which may be transient or persistent. Local redness may be due to telangiectasia, especially on the face. *Cyanosis* is a blue or purple-blue tint due to the presence of excessive reduced haemoglobin, either locally, as in impaired peripheral circulation, or generally, when oxygenation of the blood is defective. The skin colour in methaemoglobinaemia is more leaden than in ordinary cyanosis; it is caused by drugs, such as dapsone, and certain poisons.

Jaundice varies from the subicteric, lemon-yellow tints seen in pernicious anaemia and acholuric jaundice, to various shades of yellow, orange or dark olive-green in obstructive jaundice. Jaundice, which stains the conjunctivae, must be distinguished from the orange-yellow of *carotenaemia*, which does not. Slight degrees of jaundice cannot be seen in artificial light.

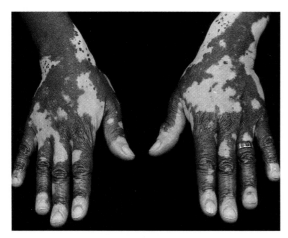

Fig. 4.3 Vitiligo: a disorder of cutaneous pigmentation that is often autoimmune in origin and associated with other autoimmune disorders.

Increased pigmentation may be racial, or due to sunburn or connected with various diseases. In *Addison's disease* there is a brown or dark-brown pigmentation affecting exposed parts and parts not normally pigmented, such as the axillae and the palmar creases; the lips and mouth may exhibit dark bluish-black areas. Note, however, that mucosal pigmentation is a normal finding in a substantial proportion of negroid people.

More or less generalized pigmentation may also be seen in the following:

- *Haemochromatosis*, in which the skin has a peculiar greyish-bronze colour with a metallic sheen, due to excessive melanin and iron pigment
- *Chronic arsenic poisoning*, in which the skin is finely dappled; affects covered more than exposed parts
- *Argyria*, in which the deposition of silver in the skin produces a diffuse slatey-grey hue
- The *cachexia* of advanced malignant disease.

In *pregnancy* there may be pigmentation of the nipples and areolae, of the linea alba, and sometimes a mask-like pigmentation of the face (*chloasma*). Chloasma may also be induced by oral contraceptives containing oestrogen. A similar condition, *melasma*, may be seen in Asian and African males.

Localized pigmentation may be seen in pellagra and in scars of various kinds, particularly those due to X-irradiation therapy. *Venous hypertension* in the legs is often associated with chronic purpura, leading to haemosiderin pigmentation. The mixture of punctate and fresh purpura and haemosiderin may produce a golden hue on the lower calves and shins. Pigmentation may also occur with chronic infestation by *body lice*. *Erythema ab igne*, a reticular pattern of pigmentation of the legs of women who habitually sit too near a fire, used to be common. When seen on the belly or back it indicates prolonged use of a hot water bottle to relieve pain, for example from malignant disease. *Livedo reticularis*, a web-like pattern of reddish-blue discoloration, mostly involving the legs, occurs in autoimmune vasculitis, especially in systemic lupus erythematosus and antiphospholipid syndrome, when it is associated with cerebral stroke. The lesions of *lichen planus* are slightly raised, flat-topped, and have a violaceous hue (Fig. 4.4). *Keloid* consists of raised and slightly pigmented, overgrown scar tissue (Fig. 4.5).

SKIN LESIONS AND ERUPTIONS

Skin eruptions and lesions should be examined with special reference to their morphology, distribution and arrangement. The terminology of skin lesions is summarized in Boxes 4.2 and 4.3. *Colour, size, consistency, configuration, margination* and *surface characteristics* should be noted.

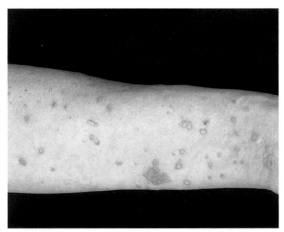

Fig. 4.4   Flat-topped papules of lichen planus.

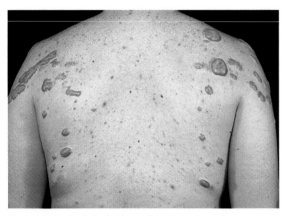

Fig. 4.5   Multiple keloid scarring of the back due to acne vulgaris. There is a genetic predisposition to the formation of keloid in scar tissue.

BOX 4.2 Primary skin lesions: a glossary of dermatological terms.	
Macule	Non-palpable area of altered colour
Papule	Palpable elevated small area of skin (< 0.5 cm)
Plaque	Palpable flat-topped discoid lesion (> 2 cm)
Nodule	Solid palpable lesion within the skin (> 0.5 cm)
Papilloma	Pedunculated lesion projecting from the skin
Vesicle	Small fluid-filled blister (< 0.5 cm)
Bulla	Large fluid-filled blister (> 0.5 cm)
Pustule	Blister containing pus
Wheal	Elevated lesion often white with red margin due to dermal oedema
Telangiectasia	Dilatation of superficial blood vessel
Petechiae	Pinhead-sized macules of blood
Purpura	Larger petechiae, which do not blanch on pressure
Ecchymosis	Large extravasation of blood in skin (bruise)

BOX 4.2 (continued)	
Haematoma	Swelling due to gross bleeding
Poikiloderma	Atrophy, reticulate hyperpigmentation and telangiectasia
Erythema	Redness of the skin
Burrow	Linear or curved elevations of the superficial skin due to infestation of female scabies mite
Comedo	Dark horny keratin and sebaceous plugs within pilo-sebaceous openings

BOX 4.3 Secondary skin lesions which evolve from primary lesions.	
Scale	Loose excess normal and abnormal horny layer
Crust	Dried exudate
Excoriation	A scratch
Lichenification	Thickening of the epidermis with exaggerated skin margin
Fissure	Slit in the skin
Erosion	Partial loss of epidermis which heals without scarring
Ulcer	At least the full thickness of the epidermis is lost. Healing occurs with scarring
Sinus	A cavity or channel that allows the escape of fluid or pus
Scar	Healing by replacement of fibrous tissue
Keloid scar	Excessive scar formation (see Fig. 4.5)
Atrophy	Thinning of the skin due to shrinkage of epidermis, dermis or subcutaneous fat
Stria	Atrophic pink or white linear lesion due to changes in connective tissue

MORPHOLOGY OF SKIN LESIONS

Inspection and palpation

Assessment of morphology requires *visual and tactile examination*. Do not be afraid to feel the lesions. You will rarely be exposed to any danger in doing so, with the exception of herpes simplex, herpes zoster, syphilis and human immunodeficiency virus (HIV) disease. If infections such as these are suspected it is wise to wear disposable plastic gloves when examining open or bleeding cutaneous lesions. Begin palpation of the skin. Pass the hand gently over it, pinching it up between the forefinger and thumb, and note the following points:

- Is it smooth or rough, thin or thick?
- Is it dry or moist?
- Is there any visible sweating, either general or local?

The *elasticity* of the skin should be investigated. If a fold of healthy skin is pinched up, it immediately flattens itself out again when released. Sometimes, however, it only does so very slowly, remaining creased for a considerable time. This is found frequently in healthy old people but may be an important sign of dehydration, for example in prolonged vomiting and diarrhoea, or in the subacute presentation of diabetes mellitus.

Subcutaneous oedema

When *oedema* (see Ch. 1) is present, firm pressure on the skin with a finger produces a shallow pit that persists for some time. In some cases no pitting is produced, especially when the oedema is of very long standing. The best place to look for slight degrees of oedema in cardiac disease is behind the malleoli at the ankles in patients who are ambulant, and over the sacrum in those who are confined to bed. The pressure of the finger should be maintained for 20–30 seconds, or slight degrees of oedema will be overlooked. Pitting is minimal or absent in oedema due to lymphatic obstruction, where the skin is usually thickened and tough.

Subcutaneous emphysema

Air trapped under the skin gives rise to a characteristic crackling sensation on palpation. It starts in, and is usually confined to, the neighbourhood of the air passages. On rare occasions it may result from the clostridial infection of soft tissues after injury or gunshot wounds (*gas gangrene*).

DISTRIBUTION OF SKIN LESIONS

Consider the distribution of an eruption by looking at the whole skin surface.

- Is it *symmetrical* or *asymmetrical*? Symmetry often implies an internal causation whereas asymmetry may imply external factors.
- Is the eruption *centrifugal* or *centripetal*? Certain common diseases such as chickenpox and pityriasis rosea are characteristically centripetal whereas erythema multiforme and erythema nodosum are centrifugal. Smallpox, now eradicated, was also centrifugal.
- A disease may exhibit a *flexor* or an *extensor* bias in its distribution: atopic eczema in childhood is characteristically flexor whereas psoriasis in adults tends to be extensor.
- Are only exposed areas affected, implicating sunlight or some other external causative factor?
- If sunlight is suspected, are areas normally in shadow involved?
- Are the genitalia involved?
- Localized distributions may point immediately to an external contact as cause, for example contact dermatitis from nickel earrings, lipstick dermatitis, etc.

Swelling of the eyelids is an important sign. Without redness and scaling, bilateral periorbital oedema may indicate acute nephritis, nephrosis or trichinosis. If there is irritation, contact dermatitis is the probable diagnosis. *Dermatomyositis* often produces swelling and heliotrope erythema of the eyelids without scaling of the skin. In *Hansen's disease* (leprosy) the skin lesions may be depigmented or reddened, with a slightly raised edge; they are also anaesthetic to pinprick testing (Fig. 4.6) and mainly located in skin that is normally cooler than body temperature.

CONFIGURATION OF SKIN LESIONS

Once the morphology of individual lesions and their distribution has been established, it is useful to describe their configuration on the skin (see Box 4.4).

THE HAIR

Hair colour and texture are racial characteristics that are genetically determined. The yellow-brown mongol race has black straight hair, negroid people have black, curly hair and white caucasians have fair, brown, red or black hair. *Secondary sexual hair* begins to appear at puberty and has characteristic

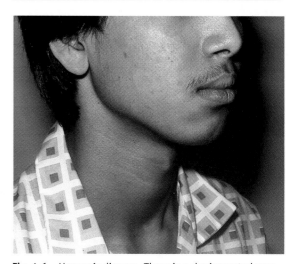

Fig. 4.6 Hansen's disease. There is a depigmented area of anaesthetic and slightly pink skin on the exposed cheek. In this lepromatous lesion acid-fast bacilli were found in scrapings.

BOX 4.4 Configuration of individual lesions.	
Nummular/discoid	Round or coin-like
Annular	Ring-like
Circinate	Circular
Arcuate	Curved
Gyrate/serpiginous	Wave-like
Linear	In a line
Grouped	Clustered
Reticulate	Net-like

male and female patterns. Common baldness in men is genetically determined but requires adequate levels of circulating androgens for its expression. It occurs in women only in old age.

GROWTH

Unlike other epithelial mitotic activity which is continuous throughout life, the growth of hair is cyclic (Fig. 4.7), the hair follicle going through alternating phases of growth (*anagen*) and rest (*telogen*). *Anagen* in the scalp lasts 3–5 years; *telogen* is much shorter at about 3 months. *Catogen* is the conversion stage from active to resting and usually lasts a few days. The length of the anagen phase determines the length to which hair in different body areas can grow. On the scalp there are about 100 000 hairs. As many as 100 hairs may be shed from the normal scalp every day as a normal consequence of growth cycling. These proportions can be estimated by looking at plucked hairs (trichogram); the 'root' of a telogen hair is non-pigmented and visible as a white, club-like swelling. Normally 85% of scalp hairs are in anagen and 15% in telogen.

ALOPECIA

Hair loss (*alopecia*) has many causes. It is convenient to subdivide alopecia into localized and diffuse types. In addition, the clinician should determine whether the alopecia results in scarring and therefore in permanent hair loss (Box 4.5).

Any inflammatory or destructive disease of the scalp skin may destroy hair follicles in its wake. Thus, burns, heavy X-ray irradiation or herpes zoster infection in the first division of the trigeminal nerve may cause a scarring alopecia. Alopecia in the presence of normal scalp skin may be patchy and localized as in traction alopecia in nervous children,

BOX 4.5 Causes of alopecia.	
Non-scarring	**Scarring**
Alopecia areata	Burns, radiodermatitis
Trichotillomania	Aplasia cutis
Traction alopecia	Lupoid erythema
Scalp ringworm (human)	Necrobiosis
Sarcoidosis	
Pseudopelade	
Kerion (see Fig. 4.26)	

ringworm infections (tinea capitis) or autoimmune alopecia areata. Secondary syphilis is a rare cause of a patchy 'moth-eaten' alopecia.

Scalp hair loss at the temples and crown, with growth of male-type body hair is characteristic of women with virilizing disorders. Metabolic causes of diffuse hair loss in women include hypothyroidism and severe iron-deficiency anaemia. Antimitotic drugs may affect the growing hair follicles, producing a diffuse loss of anagen hairs, which are pigmented throughout their length. Dramatic metabolic upsets, such as childbirth, starvation and severe toxic illnesses may precipitate follicles into the resting phase, producing an effluvium of telogen hairs 3 months later when anagen begins again. This is called *telogen alopecia*. The root of a telogen hair is non-pigmented and has a white club-like shape. In *alopecia totalis* (Fig. 4.8) there is complete loss of body hair.

THE NAILS

The nails should be examined carefully. The structure of the nail and nail bed is shown in Figs 4.9 and 4.10. The nail consists of a strong, relatively inflexible, keratinous nail plate over the dorsal surface of the end of each digit, protecting the finger tip.

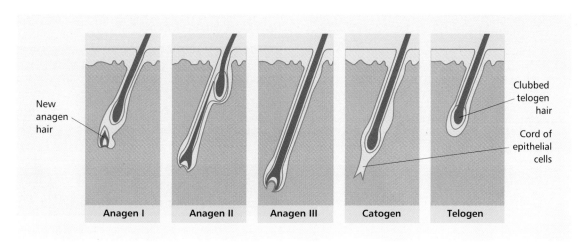

Fig. 4.7 Hair follicle growth stages.

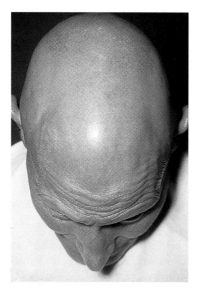

Fig. 4.8   Alopecia totalis.

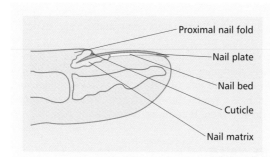

Fig. 4.9   Structure of the nail (lateral view).

- Proximal nail fold
- Nail plate
- Nail bed
- Cuticle
- Nail matrix

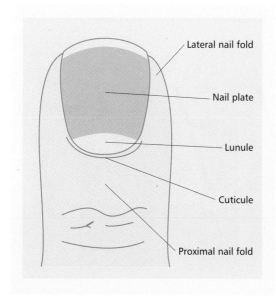

- Lateral nail fold
- Nail plate
- Lunule
- Cuticule
- Proximal nail fold

Fig. 4.10   Structure of the nail (dorsal view).

NAIL MATRIX ABNORMALITIES

Thimble pitting of the nails is characteristic of psoriasis (Fig. 4.11), but eczema and alopecia areata may also produce pitting. A severe illness may temporarily arrest nail growth; when growth starts again transverse ridges develop. These are called *Beau's lines* and can be used to date the time of onset of an illness. Inflammation of the cuticle or nail fold (*chronic paronychia*) may produce similar changes. The changes described above arise from disturbance of the nail matrix.

NAIL AND NAILBED ABNORMALITIES

Disturbance of the nail bed may produce thick nails (*pachyonychia*) or separation of the nail from the bed (*onycholysis*). This may occur in psoriasis, but may be idiopathic. Tetracyclines may induce separation when the fingers are exposed to strong sunlight (*photo-onycholysis*). The nail may be destroyed in severe lichen planus (Fig. 4.12) or epidermolysis bullosa (a genetic abnormality in which the skin blisters in response to minor trauma). Nails are missing in the inherited nail-patella syndrome. *Splinter haemorrhages* under the nails may result from trauma, psoriasis, rheumatoid arthritis or other 'collagen vascular' diseases, bacterial endocarditis and trichinosis.

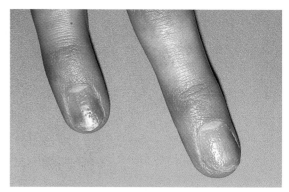

Fig. 4.11   Psoriasis of the nail beds.

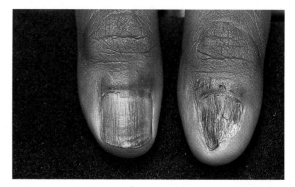

Fig. 4.12   Lichen planus, showing longitudinal ridging of the nails and overgrowth of the cuticle on the nail plate (pterigium).

THE NAILS IN SYSTEMIC DISEASE

In *iron-deficiency states*, the fingernails and toenails become soft, thin, brittle and spoon-shaped. They lose their normal transverse convex curvature, becoming flattened or concave (*koilonychia*). The 'half and half' nail, with a white proximal and red or brown distal half, is seen in some patients with *chronic renal failure*. Whitening of the nail plates may be related to *hypoalbuminaemia*, as in cirrhosis of the liver. Some drugs, notably antimalarials, antibiotics and phenothiazines, may discolour the nail. *Nail-fold telangiectasia* or *erythema* is a useful physical sign in dermatomyositis, systemic sclerosis and systemic lupus erythematosus. In dermatomyositis the cuticle becomes ragged. In systemic sclerosis loss of finger pulps may lead to curvature of the nail plates. An impaired peripheral circulation, as in Raynaud's phenomenon, can lead to thinning and longitudinal ridging of the nail plate, sometimes with partial onycholysis. In bronchiectasis the nails may take on a curved, yellow appearance (Fig. 4.13).

CLUBBING

This is probably caused by hypervascularity and the opening of anastomotic channels in the nail bed (see Ch. 1). Clubbing may, rarely, be congenital. The distal end of the digit becomes expanded, with the nail curved excessively in both longitudinal and transverse planes. Viewed from the side, the angle at the nail plate is lost and may exceed 180°. In normal nails, when both thumb nails are placed in apposition, there is a lozenge-shaped gap, whereas in clubbing there is a reduction in this gap (Schamroth's window test, see Fig. 4.14). In hypertrophic pulmonary osteoarthropathy there is clubbing of the fingers with thickening of the periosteum of the radius, ulna, tibia and fibula. (The causes of clubbing are listed in Box 1.6.)

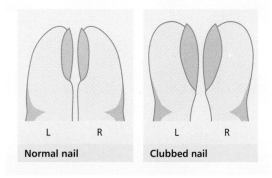

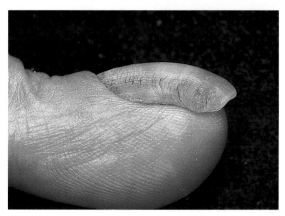

Fig. 4.13   Yellow nail syndrome in bronchiectasis.

Fig. 4.14   Schamroths' window test.

CUTANEOUS MANIFESTATIONS OF INTERNAL DISEASE

GENODERMATOSES (LESIONS OF INHERITED ORIGIN)

White macules shaped like small ash leaves which are present at birth may be the first sign of *tuberous sclerosis*. Sometimes they are difficult to see by natural light but show up under the Wood's light (ultraviolet light). They should be looked for in infants with seizures. *Pigmentation of the lips* is a feature of Peutz–Jeghers syndrome, genetically determined, in which multiple polyps of the stomach or colon appear which may later undergo malignant transformation. *Café au lait* type macules are a common sign of *neurofibromatosis*: (NF1); they may be multiple. Another valuable sign in Von Recklinghausen's neurofibromatosis is bilateral freckling of the axillary skin. The characteristic soft neurofibromata may be solitary or few, or hundreds may be scattered over the body. *Ichthyosis* (scaly fish skin) is usually present from childhood and is genetic, but if ichthyosis is acquired in adult life, a search should be made for malignancy or other underlying disease.

NON-ORGAN-SPECIFIC AUTOIMMUNE DISORDERS

Several of the so-called collagen vascular diseases show characteristic cutaneous eruptions. *Systemic lupus erythematosus*, seen in females between puberty and the menopause, may show a symmetrical 'butterfly' erythema of the nose and cheeks. In *discoid lupus* the cutaneous lesion is localized (Fig. 4.15). In *polyarteritis nodosa*, reticular livedo of the limbs, with purpura, vasculitic papules and ulceration, occurs. In *scleroderma* (systemic sclerosis), acrosclerosis of the fingertips with scarring, ulceration and calcinosis, follows a Raynaud's phenomenon of increasing severity. *Dermatomyositis* often presents with a heliotrope discoloration and oedema of the eyelids, and with fixed erythema over

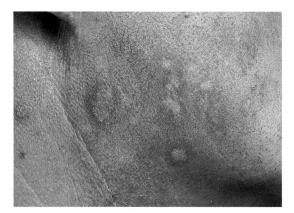

Fig. 4.15   Discoid lupus erythematosus, showing atrophic scars.

the dorsa of the knuckles and fingers and over the bony points of the shoulders, elbows and legs. There is usually weakness of the proximal limb muscles. Dermatomyositis in the middle-aged is associated in about 10% of cases with internal malignancy.

SKIN PIGMENTATION

Acanthosis nigricans is a brownish velvety thickening of the axillae, groins and sides of the neck. Sometimes there is thickening of the palms and soles, and warty excrescences may develop on the skin, eyelids and oral mucosa. In the middle-aged, acanthosis nigricans is strongly associated with internal malignancy but benign minor forms are seen in obese young women, especially Arabs, and in children with endocrinopathies characterized by insulin resistance. Patchy depigmented macules which are hypoanaesthetic and associated with enlargement of the peripheral nerves are features of certain types of *leprosy*.

Generalized, severe persistent *pruritus* in the absence of obvious skin disease may be due to sys-

BOX 4.6   Causes of pruritus in systemic disease.

- Iron deficiency anaemia
- Diabetes mellitus
- Thyrotoxicosis or hypothyroidism
- Renal failure
- Hepatic failure
- Obstructive jaundice
- Lymphoma and other malignancies
- Drugs: cocaine, morphine, etc.
- Parasites, e.g. onchocerciasis, etc.
- Psychogenic

temic disease (Box 4.6). However, in old people with dry skin it is common and of no systemic significance. *Diabetes mellitus* has a number of skin manifestations: of these pruritus vulvae, pruritus ani, balanoposthitis and angular stomatitis are due to *Candida* overgrowth. Boils, follicular pustules or ecthyma are staphylococcal. Impetigo and erysipelas, a streptococcal infection, are uncommon (Fig. 4.16). *Eruptive xanthomata* are a rare feature of uncontrolled diabetes mellitus. *Necrobiosis lipoidica diabeticorum* (Fig. 4.17) produces reddish-brown plaques, usually on the shins, with central atrophy of the skin. It has to be distinguished from *peri-tibial myxoedema* (which is hypertrophic, not atrophic), the *dermatoliposclerosis* of chronic venous disease in the legs and the *epidermal hypertrophy* of chronic lymphatic obstruction.

Neuropathic ('perforating') ulcers are found on pressure points of the heel, ball of foot, or toes and are characteristically painless. *Arteriopathic ulceration* resulting from large vessel disease is seen on the foot, and due to small vessel disease on the calves. *Spider naevi* consist of a central arteriole feeding a cluster of surrounding vessels. Many young people have up to seven naevi on the face, shoulders or

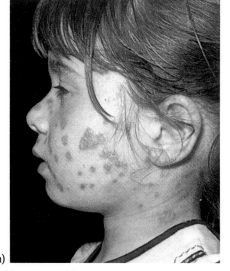

(a)

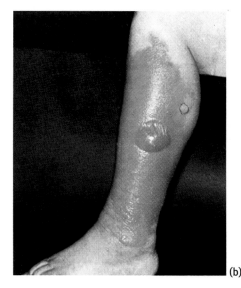

(b)

Fig. 4.16   **(a)** Impetigo. **(b)** Erysipelas.

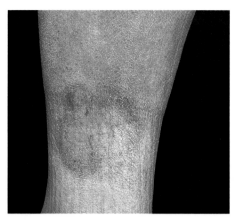

Fig. 4.17   Necrobiosis lipoidica diabeticorum.

arms. In older age-groups pregnancy, the administration of oestrogens (as in oral contraceptives) and liver disease may cause multiple lesions. Pregnancy and liver disease may also produce erythema of the thenar and hypothenar eminences ('*liver palms*'). *Leuconychia* is also seen in liver disease.

Erythema nodosum is a condition in which tender, painful, red nodules appear, typically on the shins. They fade slowly over several weeks, leaving bruising, but never ulcerate. *Sarcoidosis* and *drug sensitivity* are the commonest causes, but other systemic disorders should be considered (Box 4.7).

Xanthomata are yellow or orange papules or nodules in the skin due to dermal aggregations of lipid-loaded cells. Different patterns of hyperlipoproteinaemia may induce varying patterns of xanthomatosis. Thus, the *type IIa (hypercholesterolaemia)* pattern typically causes tuberose xanthomata on the extensor aspects of the knees and elbows and on the buttocks, sometimes associated with tendon xanthomata. Widespread eruptive xanthomata are more characteristic of *hypertriglyceridaemia*. White deposits of lipid (*arcus senilis*) in the cornea may have a similar explanation but may be a normal feature in those over 60 years. Flat lipid deposits around the eyes (*xanthelasma*) may be due to hyperlipidaemia but are also seen in the middle-aged and elderly without any general metabolic upset.

Carotenaemia produces an orange-yellow colour of the skin, especially of the palms and soles. It occurs in those who eat great quantities of carrots and other vegetables, in hypothyroidism, in diabetic patients, and also in those taking beta-carotene for the treatment of porphyria.

HAEMORRHAGE IN THE SKIN

Aggregations of extravasated red blood cells in the skin cause *purpura* (see Fig. 4.18). Purpura may be punctate, from capillary haemorrhage, or may form larger macules according to the extent of haemorrhage and the size of vessels involved. The *Hess test* for capillary fragility involves deliberately inducing punctate purpura on the forearm by inflating a cuff above the elbow at 100 mmHg for 3 minutes. Sensitivity to drugs may cause widespread 'capillaritis'.

The term *ecchymosis* implies a bruise, usually with cutaneous and subcutaneous haemorrhage causing a palpable lump. A frank fluctuant collection of blood is a *haematoma*. Unlike erythema and telangiectasia, purpura cannot be blanched by pressure. It must not be confused with *senile haemangioma* (cherry angioma or Campbell de Morgan spot), which is common in later life on the trunk and has no pathological significance. Haemorrhage into the thick epidermis of the palm or sole due to trauma (e.g. '*jogger's heel*') may induce brown or almost black macules which take weeks to disappear, inviting confusion with melanoma.

THE SKIN IN SEXUALLY TRANSMITTED DISEASES

The skin is involved in various sexually transmitted diseases. The *primary chancre* of syphilis may occur

---

BOX 4.7   Causes of erythema nodosum.

- Sarcoidosis
- Sulphonamides
- Streptococcal infection
- Tuberculosis
- Inflammatory bowel disease
- Behçet's disease
- Other infections, e.g. leprosy, systemic mycoses, toxoplasmosis, lymphogranuloma venereum

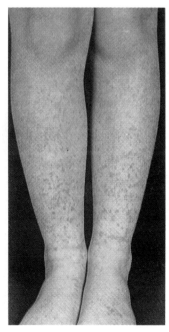

Fig. 4.18   Purpura in Henoch–Schönlein disease.

on the genitalia of either sex, at or near the anus, on the lip or, rarely, elsewhere. The rash of *secondary syphilis* is brownish-red, maculopapular and typically involves the palms and soles. It does not itch. Other manifestations of the secondary stage are condylomata lata around the anogenital area, snail-track ulceration and 'mucous patches' in the mouth. There may be low-grade fever, lymphadenopathy and splenomegaly.

Septicaemia is a rare complication of *gonorrhoea*, which particularly occurs in pregnant women, presenting with pustular skin lesions. *Recurrent type II herpes simplex* is common on the penis; it occurs less often on the buttocks where relapses may be heralded by a radiating neuralgia. *Genital viral warts* are common in both sexes. They are particularly important in females because there is evidence that certain viral subtypes are responsible for chronic cervical dysplasia with malignant potential.

AIDS and other *HIV-related syndromes* have many cutaneous manifestations including disseminated *Kaposi's sarcoma* (see Fig. 20.6), candidiasis molluscum contagiosum, seborrhoeic dermatitis, folliculitis and oral hairy leucoplakia (Fig. 4.19).

VIRAL INFECTION OF THE SKIN

Several of the commonest viral infections and illnesses of childhood are characterized by fever and a distinctive rash (*exanthem*), including measles, varicella and rubella. In measles, upper respiratory symptoms are quickly followed by a characteristic maculopapular erythematous rash. In rubella (German measles), the rash is more transient, micropapular and associated with occipital lymphadenopathy and only slight malaise. The exanthem of varicella (chickenpox) is papulovesicular and centripetal, and there may be lesions in the mouth. In herpes zoster (Fig. 4.20) and herpes simplex infections there is a non-follicular papulovesicular rash in which the vesicles are planted in an inflamed base. The rash is painful. In

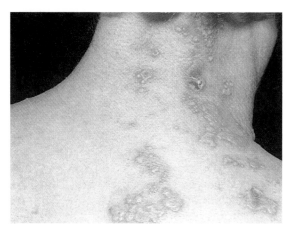

Fig. 4.20   Herpes zoster.

herpes zoster the rash follows a segmental distribution, in the skin of a dermatome. The vesicular lesion becomes encrusted (Fig. 4.21) and, later, secondary infection may occur.

Other less common viral infections associated with a rash include erythema infectiosum, due to a parvovirus, in which the exanthem on the face gives a 'slapped-cheek' appearance, and roseola infantum, a disease of toddlers, which mimics rubella.

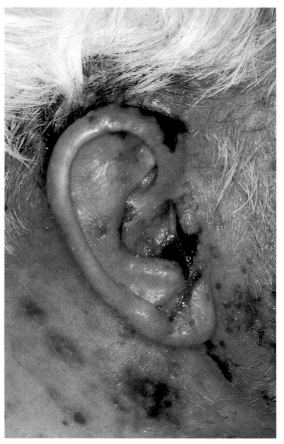

Fig. 4.21   Herpes zoster vesicles on the ear lobe involving the C2 dermatome.

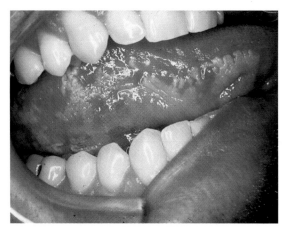

Fig. 4.19   Hairy leucoplakia.

DRUG ERUPTIONS

In the last 30 years, eruptions caused by drugs have become common. Most, but not all, such rashes are due to allergic hypersensitivity.

Drug rashes can mimic almost every pattern of skin disease. Thus *urticaria* may be caused by penicillin; a measles-like (*morbilliform*) rash may be induced by ampicillin, especially when given in infectious mononucleosis; *eczema-like* rashes are seen with methyldopa and phenylbutazone therapy: whereas gold and chloroquine rashes *mimic lichen planus*. Generalized *exfoliative dermatitis* may be induced by sulphonylureas, indomethacin and allopurinol.

Drugs which may sensitize the skin to sunlight (*phototoxic reaction*) include tetracyclines, sulphonamides and nalidixic acid. *Acne-like* rashes may follow high-dose prednisolone therapy, and are common with phenytoin therapy. Certain cytotoxic drugs and sodium valoproate cause *hair loss*. Both *erythema nodosum* and *erythema multiforme* may be induced by sulphonamides, including co-trimoxazole. Laboratory tests are of almost no value in the diagnosis of drug eruptions. Careful history-taking and knowledge of the common patterns of drug reactions usually allow accurate diagnosis.

TUMOURS IN THE SKIN

Exposure to the sun may result, after many years, in the development of skin tumours, for example *squamous or basal cell carcinoma*, or *melanoma*. These tumours are especially common in fair-skinned people. Basal cell carcinoma arises especially on the face, near the nose, or on the forehead (Fig. 4.22). The lesion may be ulcerated with a firm, rounded edge, or papular. Melanomas occur especially on skin that has been burned by the sun (e.g. torso, ears, forearms). They may be pigmented or unpigmented, and may develop rapidly in a mole that has been present for many years. *Seborrhoeic keratosis* is a raised pigmented lesion found in the sun-exposed elderly (Fig. 4.23).

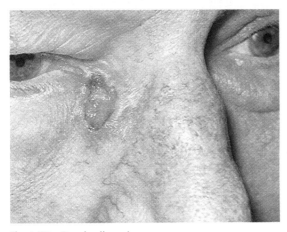

Fig. 4.22   Basal cell carcinoma.

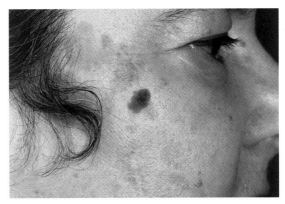

Fig. 4.23   A pigmented basal cell papilloma (seborrhoeic keratosis) on the face. This is a benign lesion.

SPECIAL TECHNIQUES IN EXAMINATION OF THE SKIN

The skin is uniquely available to the examining physician. There are a number of diagnostic procedures.

TZANCK PREPARATION

This technique is useful for rapid diagnosis of vesicular infections or blistering eruptions such as pemphigus. The intact blister is opened and the base gently scraped. The material obtained is smeared onto the microscope slide, allowed to air-dry and then stained. Viral lesions will show typical multinucleated giant cells and pemphigus will show acantholytic cells.

MICROSCOPICAL EXAMINATION

Microscopical examination is useful in the diagnosis of scabies, pediculosis and fungal infection (tinea and candidiasis).

SCABIES
Scabies is caused by the mite *Acarus (Sarcoptes) scabei*. The female *Acarus* is larger than the male and burrows in the epidermis, depositing eggs. These burrows should be looked for between the fingers, on the hands or wrists and sides of the feet. They can be recognized with the naked eye as short dark lines terminating in a shining spot of skin. The eggs lie in the dark line, the *Acarus* in the shining spot. It may be picked out by means of a flat surgical needle and placed on a slide under the microscope for more detailed examination.

PEDICULOSIS
Three forms of pediculosis or louse infestation occur: *Pediculus capitis* on the head, *Pediculus corporis* on the trunk and *Pediculus pubis* on the pubic and axillary hairs. The eggs or nits of *P. pubis* and *P. capitis* adhere to the hairs. From their position on the hairs one can judge roughly the duration of the condition, for they are fixed at first near the root of the hair, and

are carried up as the hair grows, so the higher the nits are, the longer the pediculi have been present. *P. corporis* should be looked for in the seams of the clothes, especially where the clothes come into contact with the skin, for example over the shoulders. The bites of the parasite produce haemorrhagic spots, each with a dark centre and a paler areola. Marks of scratching should be looked for on parts accessible to the patient's nails. *P. pubis* is venereally acquired and causes intense pubic itching. The nits are laid on the pubic hair and the lice themselves are easily visible.

P. corporis is seen only in the grossly deprived, in vagrants, in those living rough, and in conditions of war and social upheaval. In contrast, *P. capitis* is common in schoolchildren, however clean they and their families may be, and is endemic in many schools.

FUNGUS INFECTIONS

Fungus may grow in the skin, nails or hair and can cause disease (*ringworm* or *tinea*), for example *athlete's foot*.

Skin

The skin between the toes, the soles of the feet and the groin are the commonest sites of fungal infection. The lesions may be scaly or vesicular, tending to spread in a ring form with central healing (Fig. 4.24); macerated, dead-white, offensive-smelling epithelium is found in the intertriginous areas such as the toe clefts.

Nails

Discoloration, deformity, hypertrophy and abnormal brittleness may result from fungus infection.

Hair

Ringworm of the scalp is most common in children. It presents as round or oval areas of baldness covered with short, broken-off, lustreless hair stumps. These hair stumps may fluoresce bright green under Wood's ultraviolet light. Some fungi do not produce fluorescence with Wood's light, however, and these can be detected only by microscopy and culture (Fig. 4.25).

Microscopical examination for fungus infection

Scales from the active edge of a lesion are scraped off lightly with a scalpel, or the roofs of vesicles are snipped off with scissors. The material is placed in a drop of 10–20% aqueous potassium hydroxide solution on a microscope slide, covered with a coverslip and left for 30 minutes to clear. It is then examined under the light microscope with the 8-mm or 4-mm objective using low illumination. The mycelia are recognized as branching, refractile threads which boldly transgress the outlines of the squamous cells. Nails are examined in much the same way but it is necessary to break up the snippings and shavings into small fragments. These are either heated in potassium hydroxide or are left to clear in it overnight before being examined.

A scalp lesion is cleaned with 70% alcohol or with 1% cetrimide: infected stumps and scales are removed by scraping with a scalpel. The hairs are cleaned in potassium hydroxide in the same way as skin scales. Examination under the microscope reveals spores on the outside of the hair roots, and mycelia inside the hair substance. The species of fungus responsible may be established by culture on Sabouraud's glucose–agar.

WOOD'S LIGHT

Wood's light lamp emits long-wave ultraviolet light at a peak of 360 nm. Wood's light examination is performed in a darkened room and is useful in identifying fluorescence of fungi and corynebacterial infection (erythrasma), elevated porphyrins in urine or in the localization of pigmentary abnormalities.

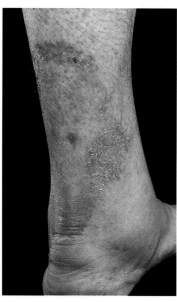

Fig. 4.24 Tinea rubrum (ringworm infection).

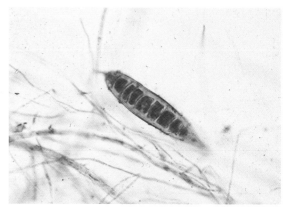

Fig. 4.25 Lactophenol blue preparation showing macronidia of *Microsporum* spp. isolated from skin scrapings from a patient with ringworm.

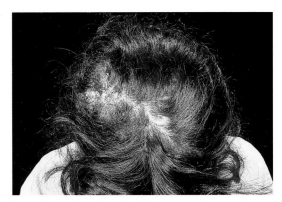

Fig. 4.26 Kerion, due to localized deep dermatophyte infection in scalp.

PATCH TESTING

This is an important and valuable tool for diagnosis of suspected allergic dermatitis due to contact (contact dermatitis).

The formulation of the allergens is critical and various standard contact allergen batteries have been developed in different countries and clinics to include the commonest culprits. Patch testing is simple but results are not always easy to interpret. Allergens are placed in shallow aluminium wells of 1 cm^2 and applied in strips to the patient's back for 48 hours for initial reading and a second reading at 96 hours. This ensures that any delayed type hypersensitivity (e.g. Coombe's type IV reaction to an allergen) can be identified.

SKIN BIOPSY

Biopsy of the skin is used to identify the nature of expanding or inflammatory lesions. The biopsy can be studied by conventional histology, often supplemented by molecular biology to identify specific proteins or genetic abnormalities. Skin biopsy is increasingly used in diagnosis and in assessing the progress of skin diseases.

5
THE RESPIRATORY SYSTEM

INTRODUCTION

Diseases of the respiratory system account for up to a third of deaths in most countries and for a major proportion of visits to the doctor and time away from work or school. As with every aspect of diagnosis in medicine, the key to success is a clear and carefully recorded history; symptoms may be trivial or extremely distressing, but either may indicate serious and life-threatening disease.

THE HISTORY

Most patients with respiratory disease will present with one or more of the following symptoms:

BREATHLESSNESS

Everyone becomes breathless on strenuous exertion. Breathlessness inappropriate to the level of physical exertion, or even occurring at rest is called *dyspnoea*. Its mechanisms are complex and not fully understood. It is not simply due to a lowered blood oxygen tension (*hypoxia*) or to a raised blood carbon dioxide tension (*hypercapnia*), although these may play a significant part. People with cardiac disease (Ch. 6) may become dyspnoeic as well as those with primarily respiratory problems.

Is the dyspnoea related only to exertion? How far can the patient walk at normal pace on the level? This may take some skill to elicit as few people note their symptoms in this form, but a brief discussion about what they can do in their daily lives usually gives a good estimate of their mobility.

Is there variability in the symptom? Are there good days and bad days and, very importantly, are there any times of day or night that are usually worse than others? Variable airways obstruction due to asthma is very often worse at night and in the early morning. By contrast, people with predominantly irreversible airways obstruction due to chronic obstructive pulmonary disease will often say that as long as they are sitting in bed they feel quite normal; it is exercise which troubles them.

COUGH

A cough may be dry or it may be productive of sputum.

- How long has the cough been present? A cough lasting a few days following a cold has less significance than one lasting several weeks in a middle-aged smoker, which may be the first sign of a malignancy.
- Is the cough worse at any time of day or night? A dry cough at night may be an early symptom of asthma, as may cough which comes in spasms lasting several minutes.
- Is the cough aggravated by anything, for example dust, pollen or cold air? The increased reactivity of the airways seen in asthma, and in some normal people for several weeks after viral respiratory infections, may present in this way. Severe coughing, whatever its cause, may be followed by vomiting.

SPUTUM

- Is sputum produced?
- What does it look like? Children and some adults swallow sputum, but it is always worth asking for a description of its colour and consistency. Yellow or green sputum is usually purulent. People with asthma may produce small amounts of very thick or jelly-like sputum, sometimes in the shape of a cast of the airways. Eosinophils may accumulate in the sputum in asthma causing a purulent appearance, even when no infection is present.
- How much is produced? When severe lung damage in infancy and childhood was common, bronchiectasis was often found in adults. The amount of sputum produced daily often exceeded a cupful. Bronchiectasis is now rare, and chronic bronchitis causes the production of smaller amounts of sputum.

HAEMOPTYSIS

Haemoptysis means the coughing of blood in the sputum. It should *never* be dismissed without very careful evaluation of the patient. The potentially serious significance of blood in the sputum is well known, and fear often leads patients to not mention it: a specific question is always necessary.

- Is there any blood in the sputum? Is it fresh or altered blood? How often has it been seen and for how long?

Blood may be coughed up alone or sputum may be bloodstained. It is sometimes difficult for the patient to describe whether or not the blood has originated from the chest or whether it comes from the gums or nose, or even from the stomach. The patient should always be asked about associated conditions such as epistaxis (nosebleeds), or the subsequent development of melaena (altered blood in the stool), which occurs in the case of upper gastrointestinal bleeding. Usually, however, it is clear that the blood originates from the chest and this is an indication for further investigation.

WHEEZING

Always ask whether the patient hears any noises coming from the chest. Even if a wheeze is not present when you examine the patient, it is useful to know that he or she has noticed it on occasions. Sometimes, wheezing will have been noticed by others (especially by a partner at night, when asthma is present) but not by the patient.

Sometimes *stridor* (see below) may be mistaken for wheezing—by both patient and doctor. This serious finding usually indicates narrowing of the larynx, trachea or main bronchi.

PAIN IN THE CHEST

Apart from musculoskeletal aches and pains consequent upon prolonged bouts of coughing, chest pain caused by lung disease usually arises from the pleura. Pleuritic pain is sharp and stabbing, and is made worse by deep breathing or coughing. It occurs when the pleura is inflamed, most commonly by infection in the underlying lung.

More constant pain, unrelated to breathing, may be caused by local invasion of the chest wall by a lung tumour.

A spontaneous pneumothorax causes pain which is worse on breathing but may have more of an aching character than the stabbing pain of pleurisy. If a pulmonary embolus causes infarction of the lung, pleurisy—and hence pleuritic pain—may occur, but an acute pulmonary embolus can also cause pain which is not stabbing in nature.

OTHER SYMPTOMS

Quite apart from the common symptoms of respiratory disease, there are some other aspects of the history which are particularly relevant to the respiratory system:

EAR, NOSE AND THROAT

Some questions related to the *ear, nose and throat* are often relevant. Recurrent sinusitis and rhinitis may be linked with asthma or, less commonly, with bronchiectasis. A change in the voice may indicate involvement of the left recurrent laryngeal nerve by a carcinoma of the lung. Sometimes patients using inhalers for asthma, and especially inhaled steroids, develop hoarseness or weakness of the voice which improves on changing the treatment. Do not ascribe hoarseness to this cause in older patients, since carcinoma of the vocal cords can also be present with hoarseness or a change in the quality of the voice. Laryngoscopy is always indicated.

THE SMOKING HISTORY

Always take a full smoking history—and do so in a sympathetic and non-condemnatory way, or you are unlikely to get an accurate picture. The time for advice about smoking cessation is after completion of your assessment, not at its outset. Simply asking 'Do you smoke?' is not enough. Novices will be astonished at how often closer probing of the answer 'no' reveals that the patient gave up yesterday, or that they state their intention of doing so from the time of your consultation. Age of starting and stopping if an ex-smoker and average consumption for both current and ex-smokers are the bare minimum information needed.

Identification of an individual as a current or ex-smoker will greatly influence the interpretation which you place on your findings upon history and examination. Almost all cases of lung cancer and chronic obstructive pulmonary disease occur in those who have smoked.

THE FAMILY HISTORY

There is a strong inherited susceptibility to asthma. Associated conditions like eczema and hay fever may also be present in relatives of those with asthma, particularly in those who develop the condition when young.

THE OCCUPATIONAL HISTORY

No other organ is as susceptible to the working environment as the lungs. Several hundred different substances have now been recognized as causing occupational asthma. Paint sprayers, workers in the electronics, rubber or plastics industries and woodworkers are relatively commonly affected. Always ask about a relationship between symptoms and work.

Damage from inhalation of asbestos may take decades to become manifest, most seriously as malignant mesothelioma. In industrialized countries, this once extremely rare tumour of the pleura has become more common, and will become even more common in the next 20 years. In middle-aged individuals who present with a pleural effusion—often the first sign of a mesothelioma—you will need to ask about possible asbestos exposure in jobs right back to the time of leaving school.

THE EXAMINATION

GENERAL ASSESSMENT

An examination of the respiratory system is incomplete without a simultaneous general assessment (Box 5.1). Watch the patient as he or she comes into the room, during your history taking, and while the patient is undressing and climbing onto the couch. If a hospital in-patient, is there breathlessness just on moving in bed? What is on the bedside table—inhalers, tissues, a sputum pot, an oxygen mask? What is the physique and state of general nourishment of the patient?

For your examination, patients should be comfortably resting on a bed or examination couch, and

---

BOX 5.1   Points to note in a general assessment.

- Physique
- Voice
- Breathlessness
- Clubbing
- Cyanosis or pallor
- Intercostal recession
- Use of accessory respiratory muscles
- Venous pulses
- Lymph nodes

---

supported by pillows so that they can lean back comfortably at an angle of 45 degrees.

Hands should be inspected for *clubbing, pallor* or *cyanosis*. Lips and tongue should be inspected for central cyanosis. A breathless patient may be using the accessory muscles of respiration (e.g. sternomastoid), and in the presence of severe chronic obstructive pulmonary disease many patients find it easier to breathe through pursed lips (Fig. 5.1).

As well as your general visual assessment, *listen* to the patient. What is the nature of the voice—is it hoarse? Is the patient capable of producing a normal, explosive cough—or is the voice weak or non-existent even when the patient is asked to cough? Is there *wheezing* audible, usually loudest in expiration, or is there *stridor*, a high-pitched *inspiratory* noise?

EXAMINATION OF THE CHEST

RELEVANT ANATOMY

Interpretation of signs in the chest often causes problems for the beginner. A revision of the relevant anatomy may help set the scene.

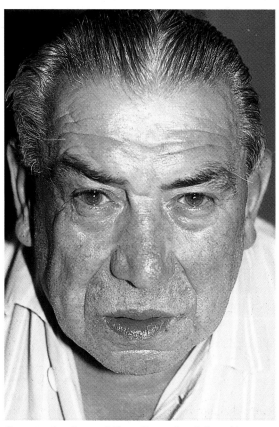

Fig. 5.1   Respiratory failure. The patient is breathless at rest and there is central cyanosis with blueness of the lips and face. The lips are pursed during expiration, a characteristic feature of chronic obstructive pulmonary disease (COAD). This facial appearance is often accompanied by heart failure with peripheral oedema (cor pulmonale).

The *bifurcation of the trachea* corresponds on the anterior chest wall with the sternal angle, the transverse bony ridge at the junction of the body of the sternum and the manubrium sterni. Posteriorly, the level is at the disc between the fourth and fifth thoracic vertebrae. The ribs are most easily counted downwards from the second costal cartilage, which articulates with the sternum at the extremity of the sternal angle.

A line from the second thoracic spine to the sixth rib in the mammary line corresponds to the upper border of the lower lobe (major interlobar fissure). On the right side a horizontal line from the sternum at the level of the fourth costal cartilage, drawn to meet the line of the major interlobar fissure, marks the boundary between the upper and middle lobes (the minor interlobar fissure). The greater part of each lung, as seen from behind, is composed of the lower lobe; only the apex belongs to the upper lobe. The middle and upper lobes on the right side and the upper lobe on the left occupy most of the area in front (Fig. 5.2) This is most easily visualized if the lobes are thought of as two wedges fitting together, not as two cubes piled one on top of the other (Fig. 5.3).

The stethoscope is so much part of the 'image' of a doctor that it is very easy for the student to forget that listening is only one part of the examination of the chest. Obtaining the maximum possible information from your examination requires you to *look*, then to *feel* and only then to *listen*.

LOOKING: INSPECTION OF THE CHEST

Appearance of the chest

First, are there any obvious scars from previous surgery? Are there any lumps visible beneath the skin, or any lesions on the skin itself?

The normal chest is bilaterally symmetrical and elliptical in cross-section. The chest may be distorted by disease of the ribs or spinal vertebrae as well as by underlying lung disease (Box 5.2).

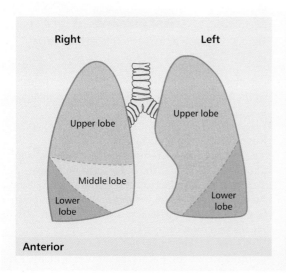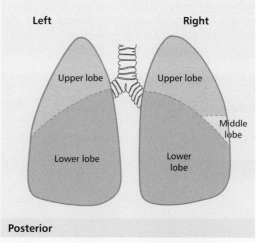

Fig. 5.2 Anterior and posterior aspects of the lungs.

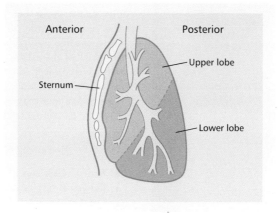

Fig. 5.3 Lateral aspect of the left lung.

Kyphosis (forward bending) or *scoliosis* (lateral bending) of the vertebral column will lead to asymmetry of the chest and if severe may significantly restrict lung movement.

A normal chest X ray is seen in Figure 5.4.

Severe airways obstruction, particularly long term, as in chronic obstructive pulmonary disease (COPD) (Figs 5.1, 5.5) may lead to an overinflated and barrel-shaped chest. The ribs are set less obliquely than normal.

Movement of the chest

Look at the *chest movements*. Are they symmetrical? If they seem to be diminished on one side, that is likely to be the side on which there is an abnormality. Intercostal recession—a drawing in of the intercostal spaces with inspiration—may indicate severe upper airways obstruction, as in laryngeal disease, or tumours of the trachea. In COPD, the lower ribs often move inwards on inspiration instead of the normal outwards movement.

Venous pulses

The *venous pulses* in the neck (see Ch. 86) should be inspected. A raised venous pressure is usually indica-

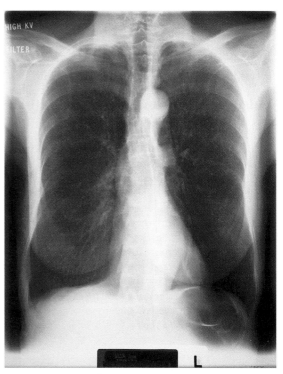

Fig. 5.5   Chest X-ray in severe chronic obstructive pulmonary disease.

tive of right heart failure but can be due to obstruction of the superior vena cava, usually due to malignancy in the upper mediastinum.

Respiratory rate and rhythm

The normal rate of respiration in a relaxed adult is about 14–16 breaths per minute (Box 5.3). *Tachypnoea* is an increased respiratory rate observed by the doctor, while *dyspnoea* is the symptom of breathlessness experienced by the patient. *Apnoea* means cessation of respiration.

Cheyne–Stokes breathing is the name given to a disturbance of respiratory rhythm in which there is cyclical deepening and quickening of respiration, followed by diminishing respiratory effort and rate, sometimes associated with a short period of complete apnoea, the cycle then being repeated. This is often observed in severely ill patients and particularly in severe cardiac failure, narcotic drug poisoning, and neurological disorders. It is occasionally seen, especially during sleep, in elderly patients without any obvious serious disease.

Some patients may have apnoeic episodes during sleep due to complete cessation of respiratory effort

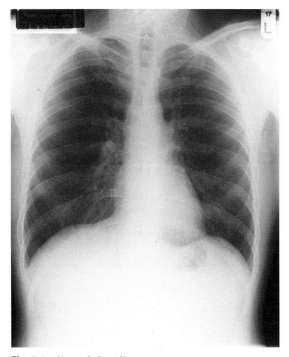

Fig. 5.4   Normal chest X-ray.

(*central apnoea*), or, much more commonly, apnoea despite continuation of respiratory effort. This is known as obstructive apnoea and is due to obstruction of the upper airways by soft tissues in the region of the pharynx.

FEELING: PALPATION OF THE CHEST

Lymph nodes
The *lymph nodes* in the supraclavicular fossae, cervical regions and axillary regions should be palpated. They are often enlarged secondary to the spread of malignant disease from the chest, and this finding will influence decisions regarding treatment.

Swellings and tenderness
It is useful to palpate any part of the chest which presents an obvious *swelling*, or where the patient complains of pain (Box 5.4). Feel gently, as pressure may increase the pain. It is often important, particularly in the case of musculoskeletal pain, to identify a site of tenderness (Box 5.5).

Trachea and heart
The *positions* of the cardiac impulse and trachea should then be determined. Feel for the trachea in the suprasternal notch and decide whether it is central or deviated to one side by its relation to the suprasternal notch and the insertion of the sternomastoids. Avoid heavy-handedness in this situation—it is uncomfortable for the patient if the examiner is rough. A slight deviation of the trachea to the right may be found in healthy people.

Displacement of the cardiac impulse without displacement of the trachea may be due to scoliosis, to a congenital funnel depression of the sternum or to enlargement of the left ventricle. In the absence of these conditions, a significant displacement of the cardiac impulse or trachea, or of both together, suggests that the position of the mediastinum has been altered by disease of the lungs or pleura. The mediastinum may be *pushed* away from the affected side by a pleural effusion or pneumothorax. Fibrosis or collapse of the lung will *pull* the mediastinum towards the affected side.

Chest expansion
As well as by simple inspection, possible asymmetrical expansion of the chest may be further explored by palpation. Face the patient and place the fingertips of both hands on either side of the lower rib cage, so that the tips of the thumbs meet in the midline in front of, but not touching, the chest. A deep breath by the patient will increase the distance between the thumbs and indicate the degree of expansion. If one thumb remains closer to the midline, this suggests diminished expansion on that side.

Tactile vocal fremitus is detected by palpation but this is not a commonly used routine examination technique. It is discussed further under auscultation, below.

FEELING: PERCUSSION OF THE CHEST
The technique of percussion was probably developed as a way of ascertaining how much fluid remained in barrels of wine or other liquids. Auenbrugger applied percussion to the chest having learned this method in his father's wine cellar. Effective percussion is a knack which requires consistent practice; do so upon yourself or on willing colleagues, as percussion can be uncomfortable for patients if performed repeatedly and inexpertly.

The middle finger (the pleximeter finger) of the left hand is placed on the part to be percussed and the back of its middle phalanx is then struck with the tip of the middle finger of the right hand (vice versa if you are left-handed). The movement should be at the *wrist* rather than at the elbow. The percussing finger is bent so that its terminal phalanx is at right angles and it strikes the pleximeter finger perpendicularly. As soon as the blow has been given, the striking finger is raised: the action is a tapping movement.

The two commonest mistakes made by the beginner are, first, failing to ensure that the finger of the left hand is flatly and firmly applied to the chest wall and, second, striking the percussion blow from the elbow rather than from the wrist.

The character of the sound produced varies both qualitatively and quantitatively (Box 5.6). When the air in a cavity of sufficient size and appropriate shape is set into vibration, a resonant sound is produced and there is also a characteristic sensation felt by the

---

BOX 5.4   Points to note on palpation of the chest.

- Swelling
- Pain and tenderness
- Tracheal position
- Cardiac impulse
- Asymmetry
- Tactile vocal fremitus

BOX 5.5   Causes of pain and tenderness in the chest.

- A recent injury of the chest wall, or inflammatory conditions
- Intercostal muscular pain—as a rule, localized painful spots can be discovered on pressure
- A painful costochondral junction
- Secondary malignant deposits in the rib
- Herpes zoster before the appearance of the rash

BOX 5.6   Points to note on percussion of the chest.

- Resonance
- Dullness
- Pain and tenderness

finger placed on the chest. Try tapping a hollow cupboard and then a solid wall—the feeling is different, as well as the sound. The sound and feel of resonance over a healthy lung has to be learned by practice, and it is against this standard that possible abnormalities of percussion must be judged.

The normal degree of resonance varies between individuals, and in different parts of the chest in the same individual, being most resonant below the clavicles anteriorly and the scapulae posteriorly where the muscles are relatively thin, and least resonant over the scapulae. On the right side, there is loss of resonance inferiorly as the liver is encountered. On the left side, the lower border overlaps the stomach so there is a transition from lung resonance to tympanitic stomach resonance.

Always systematically compare the percussion note on the two sides of the chest, moving backwards and forwards from one side to the other, not all the way down one side and then down the other. Percuss over the clavicles; traditionally, this is done without an intervening finger on the chest, but there is no reason for this, and it is more comfortable for the patient if the finger of the left hand is used in the usual way. Percuss three or four areas on the anterior chest wall, comparing left with right. Percuss the axillae, then three or four areas on the back of the chest.

Reduction of resonance (i.e. the percussion note is said to be *dull*) occurs in two important circumstances:

- When the underlying lung is more solid than usual, usually due to consolidation
- When the pleural cavity contains fluid, i.e. a pleural effusion is present.

Less commonly, a dull percussion note may be due to a thickened pleura. The percussion note is most dull when there is underlying fluid, as in a pleural effusion. Pleural effusion causes the sensation in the percussed finger to be similar to that felt when a solid wall is percussed. This is often called *stony dullness*. By comparing side with side, it is usually easy to detect a unilateral pleural effusion. Effusions may occur bilaterally in some patients, and this may be more difficult to detect clinically. Pleural effusion usually leads to decreased chest wall movement.

An *increase in resonance*, or hyperresonance, is more difficult to detect than dullness. It may be noticeable when the pleural cavity contains air, as in pneumothorax. Sometimes, however, in this situation one is tempted to think that the slightly duller side is the abnormal side. Further examination and chest X-ray will reveal the true situation.

LISTENING: AUSCULTATION OF THE CHEST
Listen to the chest with the diaphragm, not the bell, of the stethoscope (chest sounds are relatively high-pitched, and therefore the diaphragm is more sensitive than the bell). Ask the patient to take deep breaths in and out *through the mouth*. Demonstrate what you would like the patient to do, and then check visually that they are doing it while you listen to the chest.

As with percussion, you should listen in comparable positions to each side alternately, switching back and forth from one side to the other to compare (Box 5.7).

The breath sounds
Breath sounds have *intensity* and *quality*. The intensity (or loudness) of the breath sounds may be normal, reduced or increased. The quality of normal breath sounds is described as *vesicular*.

Breath sounds will be of normal intensity when the lung is inflating normally but may be reduced if there is localized airway narrowing, if the lung is extensively damaged by a process such as emphysema, or if there is intervening pleural thickening or pleural fluid. Breath sounds may be of increased intensity in very thin subjects.

Breath sounds probably originate from turbulent airflow in the larger airways. When you place your stethoscope upon the chest, you are listening to how those sounds have been changed on their journey from their site of origin to the position of your stethoscope diaphragm. Normal lung tissue makes the sound quieter, and selectively filters out some of the higher frequencies. The resulting sound that you hear is called a *vesicular* breath sound. There is usually no distinct pause between the end of inspiration and the beginning of expiration.

When the air underlying the stethoscope is airless, as in consolidation, the sounds generated in the large airways are transmitted more efficiently, so they are louder and there is less filtering of the high frequencies. The resulting breath sounds heard by the stethoscope are termed *bronchial breathing*, classically heard over an area of consolidated lung in cases of pneumonia. The sound resembles that obtained by listening over the trachea, although the noise there is much louder. The quality of the sound is rather harsh, the higher frequencies being heard more clearly. The expiratory sound has a more sibilant (hissing) character than the inspiratory one and lasts for most of the expiratory phase.

BOX 5.7   Points to note on auscultation of the chest.

- Vesicular breath sounds
- Bronchial breath sounds
- Vocal fremitus and resonance
  —bronchophony
  —whispering pectoriloquy
  —aegophony

Added sounds
  —pleural rub
  —wheezes
  —crackles

The intensity and quality of all breath sounds is so variable from patient to patient and in different situations that it is only by repeated auscultation of the chests of many patients that one becomes familiar with the normal variations and learns to recognize the abnormalities.

Added sounds

Added sounds are abnormal sounds that arise in the lung itself or in the pleura. The added sounds most commonly arising in the lung are best referred to as *wheezes* and *crackles*. Older terms such as *râles* to describe coarse crackles, *crepitations* to describe fine crackles, and *rhonchi* to describe wheezes are poorly defined, have led to confusion, and are best avoided.

Wheezes are musical sounds associated with airway narrowing. Widespread *polyphonic wheezes*, particularly heard in expiration, are the commonest and are characteristic of diffuse airflow obstruction, especially in asthma and chronic obstructive pulmonary disease. These wheezes are probably related to dynamic compression of the bronchi, which is accentuated in expiration when airway narrowing is present. A fixed *monophonic* wheeze can be generated by localized narrowing of a single bronchus, as may occur in the presence of a tumour or foreign body. It may be inspiratory or expiratory or both and may change its intensity in different positions.

Wheezing generated in smaller airways should not be mistaken for *stridor* associated with laryngeal disease or localized narrowing of the trachea or the large airways. Stridor almost always indicates a serious condition requiring urgent investigation and management. The noise is often both inspiratory and expiratory. It may be heard at the open mouth without the aid of the stethoscope. On auscultation of the chest, stridor is usually loudest over the trachea.

Crackles are short, explosive sounds often described as bubbling or clicking noises. When the large airways are full of sputum, a coarse rattling sound may be heard even without the stethoscope. However, crackles are not usually produced by moistness in the lungs. It is more likely that they are produced by sudden changes in gas pressure related to the sudden opening of previously closed small airways. Crackles at the beginning of inspiration are common in patients with chronic obstructive pulmonary disease. Localized loud and coarse crackles may indicate an area of bronchiectasis. Crackles are also heard in pulmonary oedema. In diffuse interstitial fibrosis, crackles are characteristically fine in character and late inspiratory in timing.

The *pleural rub* is characteristic of pleural inflammation and usually occurs in association with pleuritic pain. It has a creaking or rubbing character and in some instances can be felt with the palpating hand as well as being audible with the stethoscope.

Take care to exclude false added sounds. Sounds resembling pleural rubs may be produced by movement of the stethoscope on the patient's skin or of clothes against the stethoscope tubing. Sounds arising in the patient's muscles may resemble added sounds; in particular, the shivering of a cold patient makes any attempt at auscultation almost useless. The stethoscope rubbing over hairy skin may produce sounds resembling fine crackles.

Vocal resonance

You will note from the above that when listening to the breath sounds, you are detecting—with your stethoscope—vibrations which have been made in the large airways. Vocal resonance is the resonance of sounds in the chest made by the voice. When testing vocal resonance, you are detecting vibrations transmitted to the chest from the vocal cords as the patient repeats a phrase, usually the words 'ninety-nine'. The ear perceives not the distinct syllables but a resonant sound, the intensity of which depends on the loudness and depth of the patient's voice and the conductivity of the lungs. As always in examining the chest, each point examined on one side should be compared at once with the corresponding point on the other side.

Not surprisingly, conditions which increase or reduce conduction of the breath sounds to the stethoscope have similar effects upon the vocal resonance. Consolidated lung conducts sounds better than air-containing lung, so in consolidation, the vocal resonance is increased and the sounds are louder and often clearer. In such circumstances, even when the patient whispers a phrase (e.g. 'one, two, three') the sounds may be heard clearly; this is known as *whispering pectoriloquy*. Above the level of a pleural effusion, or in some cases over an area of consolidation, the voice may sound nasal or bleating; this is known as *aegophony*, but is an unusual physical finding.

Vocal fremitus

Vocal fremitus is detected with the hand on the chest wall. It should therefore perhaps be regarded as part of palpation, but it is usually carried out after auscultation (see below). As with vocal resonance, the patient is asked to repeat a phrase such as 'ninety-nine'. The examining hand feels distinct vibrations when this is done. Some examiners use the ulnar border of the hand, but there is no good reason for this: the flat of the hand, including the fingertips, is far more sensitive.

From the above, it should be clear that listening to the breath sounds, listening to the vocal resonance, and eliciting vocal fremitus are all doing essentially the same thing: they are investigating how vibrations generated in the larynx or large airways are transmitted to the examining instrument—the stethoscope in the first two cases and the fingers in the third.

It follows that in the various pathological situations, all three physical signs should behave in similar ways. Where there is consolidation, the breath sounds are better transmitted to the stethoscope, so they are louder and there is less attenuation of the higher frequencies, 'bronchial breathing' is heard. Similarly, the vocal resonance and the vocal fremitus are increased. Where there is a pleural effusion, the breath sounds are quieter or absent, and the vocal resonance and the vocal fremitus are reduced.

The intelligent student should now ask: 'Why try and elicit all three signs?' The experienced physician will answer: 'Because it is often difficult to interpret the signs that have been elicited'.

PUTTING IT TOGETHER: AN EXAMINATION OF THE CHEST

There is no single perfect way of examining the chest, and most doctors develop their own minor variations of order and procedure. The following is one scheme for examining the chest which combines efficiency with thoroughness:

- Observe the patient generally, and the surroundings
- Ask the patient's permission for the examination, and ensure lying back comfortably at 45 degrees
- Examine the hands
- Check the face for anaemia or cyanosis
- Observe the respiratory rate
- Inspect the chest movements and the anterior chest wall
- Feel the position of the trachea, and check for lymphadenopathy
- Feel the position of the apex beat
- Check the symmetry of the chest movements by palpation
- Percuss the anterior chest and axillae.

Sit the patient forward;

- Inspect the posterior chest wall
- Percuss the back of the chest
- Listen to the breath sounds
- Check the vocal resonance
- Check the tactile vocal fremitus.

If you are examining a hospital in-patient, *always* take the opportunity of turning the pillow over before lying the patient back again; a cool, fresh pillow is a great comfort to an ill person.

- Listen to the breath sounds on the front of the chest
- Check the vocal resonance
- Check the tactile vocal fremitus.

Stand back for a moment and reflect upon whether you have omitted anything:

- Thank the patient and ensure they are dressed or appropriately covered.

PUTTING IT TOGETHER: INTERPRETING THE SIGNS

Developing an appropriate differential diagnosis on the basis of the signs you have elicited requires thought and practice. Keeping the following in mind will help:

- If movements are diminished on one side, there is likely to be an abnormality on that side
- The percussion note is dull over a pleural effusion and over an area of consolidation—the duller the note, the more likely it is to be a pleural effusion
- The breath sounds, the vocal resonance and the tactile vocal fremitus are quieter or less obvious over a pleural effusion, and louder or more obvious over an area of consolidation
- Over a pneumothorax, the percussion note is more resonant than normal but the breath sounds, vocal resonance and tactile vocal fremitus are quieter or reduced. Pneumothorax is easily missed.

OTHER INVESTIGATIONS

SPUTUM EXAMINATION

AT THE BEDSIDE

Hospital in-patients should have a sputum pot and this must be inspected (Box 5.8). *Mucoid sputum* is characteristic in patients with chronic bronchitis when there is no active infection. It is clear and sticky and not necessarily produced in a large volume. Sputum may become *mucopurulent* or *purulent* when bacterial infection is present in patients with bronchitis, pneumonia, bronchiectasis or a lung abscess. In these last two conditions the quantities may be large and the sputum is often foul-smelling.

Occasionally asthmatics have a yellow tinge to the sputum, due to the presence of many eosinophils. A particularly tenacious form of mucoid sputum may also be produced by people with asthma, and sometimes they cough up casts of the bronchial tree, particularly after an attack. Patients with bronchopulmonary aspergillosis may bring up black sputum or sputum with black parts in it; this is the fungal element of the *Aspergillus* (Fig. 5.6).

When sputum is particularly foul-smelling, the presence of anaerobic organisms should be suspected. Pink or white frothy sputum may be brought up by patients in pulmonary oedema, for example in acute left heart failure. Rusty-coloured sputum is characteristic of lobar pneumonia. Blood may be coughed up alone, or bloodstained sputum produced, with bronchogenic carcinoma, pulmonary

---

BOX 5.8   Characteristics to note when assessing sputum.

- Mucoid
- Purulent
- Frothy
- Bloodstained
- Rusty

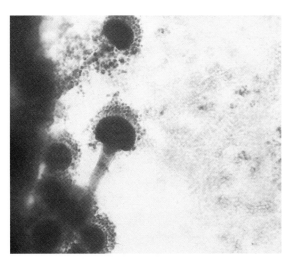

Fig. 5.6 *Aspergillus* spp. from bronchial aspirate, after culture on Saburaud's medium.

tuberculosis, pulmonary embolism, bronchiectasis or pulmonary hypertension (e.g. with mitral stenosis).

IN THE LABORATORY

Sputum may be examined under the microsope in the laboratory for the presence of pus cells and organisms and may be cultured in an attempt to identify the causative agent of an infection. It is seldom practical to wait for the results of such examinations and most clinical decisions have to be based on the clinical probability of a particular infection being present.

Pulmonary tuberculosis, a disease becoming more common in all parts of the world, requires specialized techniques of laboratory microscopy and culture to identify the responsible organisms, and if the diagnosis is suspected these tests must be specifically requested.

Sputum examination for malignant cells is a useful test in establishing a diagnosis of carcinoma of the lung.

LUNG FUNCTION TESTS

Measurements of respiratory function may provide valuable information. First, in conjunction with the clinical assessment and other investigations they may help establish a diagnosis. Secondly, they will help indicate the severity of the condition. Thirdly, serial measurements over time will show changes indicating disease progression or, alternatively, a favourable response to treatment. Finally, regular monitoring of lung function in chronic diseases such as idiopathic pulmonary fibrosis, cystic fibrosis or obstructive airways disease may warn of preclinical deterioration.

Simple respiratory function tests fall into three main groups:

- Measuring the size of the lungs
- Measuring how easily air flows into and out of the airways
- Measuring how efficient the lungs are in the process of gas exchange.

A *spirometer* will measure how much air can be exhaled after a maximal inspiration; the patient breathes in as far as he or she can, then blows out into the spirometer until no more air at all can be breathed out. This volume is called the *vital capacity* (VC). The amount of air in the lungs at full inspiration is a measure of the *total lung capacity*, and that still remaining after a full expiration is called the *residual volume*.

The actual value of total lung capacity cannot be measured with a spirometer. The simplest way of determining it is to get the patient to inspire a known volume of air containing a known concentration of helium. Measuring the new concentration of helium which exists after mixing with the air already in the lungs enables calculation of the total lung capacity. Subtraction of the vital capacity from this value gives the residual volume.

Usually, vital capacity is measured after the patient has blown as hard and fast as possible into the spirometer, when the measurement is known as the *forced vital capacity* or FVC. In normal lungs, VC and FVC are almost identical, but in chronic obstructive pulmonary disease (COPD) compression of the airways during a forced expiration leads to closure of airways earlier than usual and FVC may be less than VC.

Figure 5.7(a) shows the trace produced by a spirometer. Volume in litres is on the x-axis and time in seconds is on the y-axis. Thus, the trace moves *up* during expiration assessing FVC, and *along* the y-axis as time passes during expiration.

The volume of air breathed out in the first second of a forced expiration is known as the *forced expiratory volume in the first second*—almost always abbreviated to FEV_1. In normal lungs, the FEV_1 is over 70% of FVC. When there is obstruction to airflow, as in COPD, the time taken to fully expire is prolonged and the FEV_1/FVC ratio is reduced. An example is shown in Figure 5.7(b). A trace like this is described as showing an obstructive ventilatory defect. As noted above, the FVC may be reduced in severe airways obstruction, but in such cases the FEV_1 is reduced even more and the FEV_1/FVC ratio remains low.

Some lung conditions restrict expansion of the lungs, but do not interfere with the airways. In such individuals, both the FEV_1 and the FVC are reduced in proportion to each other, so the ratio remains normal even though the absolute values are reduced. Figure 5.7(c) shows a trace of this kind, a restrictive ventilatory defect in a patient with diffuse pulmonary fibrosis.

Look again at the normal expiratory spirogram (Fig. 5.7(a)). The slope of the trace is steepest at the onset of expiration. The trace thus shows that the

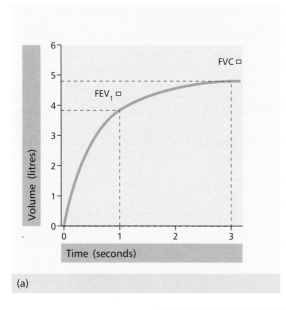

(a)

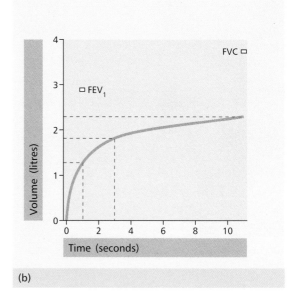

(b)

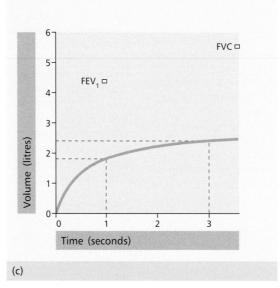

(c)

Fig. 5.7 **(a)** Normal expiratory spirometer trace. **(b)** Spirometer trace showing an obstructive defect. Note the very prolonged (10 second) expiration. **(c)** Spirometer trace showing a restrictive defect.

rate of change of volume with time is greatest in early expiration; in other words, the rate of airflow is greatest then. This measurement, the *peak expiratory flow rate* (PEFR) is readily measured with a *peak flow meter*. A simplified version of this device is shown in Figure 5.8. This Mini-Peak flow meter is light and inexpensive, and people with asthma can use it to monitor themselves and alter their medication, as suggested by their doctor, at the first signs of any fall in peak flow measurements which indicate a deterioration in their condition.

Normal gas exchange consists of the uptake of oxygen into the pulmonary capillary blood and the release of carbon dioxide into the alveoli. For this to be achieved, the ventilation of the lungs by air and

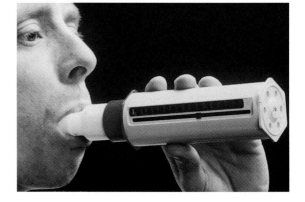

Fig. 5.8   A Mini-Wright peak flow meter.

their perfusion by blood need to be anatomically matched. An approximation of the efficiency of the process of gas exchange may be obtained by measuring the pulmonary transfer factor for carbon monoxide. This is assessed with similar apparatus to the helium-dilution technique for measuring lung volumes. Instead of using helium, which does not easily enter the blood, a known and very low concentration of carbon monoxide is used. This gas is very readily bound by the haemoglobin in the pulmonary capillaries. The patient inspires to total lung capacity (TLC), holds the breath for 10 seconds, then fully expires. The difference between the inspired carbon monoxide concentration and the expired concentration is a measure of the efficiency of gas exchange, and can be expressed per unit lung volume if TLC is simultaneously measured by the helium dilution technique.

ARTERIAL BLOOD SAMPLING

In a sample of arterial blood, the partial pressures of oxygen (Pa_{O_2}) and of carbon dioxide (Pa_{CO_2}), and the pH, can be measured. The arterial Pa_{CO_2} will reflect the effective ventilation of alveoli that are adequately perfused with blood so that efficient gas exchange can take place. Provided the rate of production of carbon dioxide by the body remains constant, the Pa_{CO_2} will be directly related to the level of alveolar ventilation. The normal range is 4.7–6.0 kPa (36–45 mm Hg). When alveolar ventilation is reduced, then the Pa_{CO_2} will rise. A number of different conditions may reduce alveolar ventilation.

Alveolar ventilation rises, and Pa_{CO_2} may fall, in response to a metabolic acidosis, in very anxious individuals, and in many lung conditions which tend to reduce the oxygenation of the blood.

The Pa_{O_2} is normally in the range 11.3–14.0 kPa (80–100 mm Hg). Any lung disease that interferes with gas exchange may reduce arterial Pa_{O_2}.

IMAGING THE LUNG AND CHEST

ANATOMY
See p. 63.

THE CHEST X-RAY
The chest X-ray is an important extension of the clinical examination (Box 5.9). This is particularly so in patients with respiratory symptoms, and a normal X-ray taken some time before the development of symptoms should therefore not be accepted as a reason for not performing an up-to-date film. In many instances it is of great value to have previous X-rays for comparison, but if these are lacking then careful follow-up with subsequent films may provide the necessary information.

The standard chest X-ray is a posteroanterior view (PA) which is taken with the film against the front of

---

> **BOX 5.9   Points to note when assessing the chest X-ray.**
>
> - Bony skeleton
> - Position of the patient
> - Position of the trachea
> - Outline of heart
> - Outline of mediastinum
> - Diaphragm
> - Lung fields

the patient's chest and the X-ray source 2 m behind the patient (Fig. 5.4). The X-ray is examined systematically on a viewing box according to the following plan:

The position of the patient
- Is the patient straight or rotated? If straight, the inner ends of the clavicles will be disposed symmetrically with reference to the vertebral column. Any rotation will tend particularly to alter the appearance of the mediastinum and the hilar shadows.

The outline of the heart and the mediastinum
- Is this normal in size, shape and position?

The position of the trachea
- This is seen as a dark column representing the air within the trachea. The cartilaginous rings are not visible.
- Is the trachea centrally placed or deviated to either side?

The diaphragm
- Can the diaphragm be seen on each side?
- Is it normal in shape and position? Normally, the anterior end of the sixth or seventh rib crosses the mid-part of the diaphragm on each side, although the diaphragm on the right may be a little higher than on the left.
- Are the cardiophrenic angles clearly seen?

The lung fields
For radiological purposes, the lung fields are divided into three zones:

- The *upper zone* extends from the apex to a line drawn through the lower borders of the anterior ends of the second costal cartilages.
- The *mid-zone* extends from this line to one drawn through the lower borders of the fourth costal cartilages.
- The *lower zone* extends from this line to the bases of the lungs.
- Each zone is systematically examined on both sides and any area which appears abnormal is carefully compared with the corresponding area on the opposite side.

- The minor interlobar fissure, which separates the right, upper and middle lobes, may sometimes be seen running horizontally in the third and fourth interspace on the right side.

The bony skeleton

- Is the chest symmetrical?
- Is scoliosis present?
- Are the ribs unduly crowded or widely spaced in any area?
- Are cervical ribs present?
- Are any ribs eroded or absent?

As well as the standard anteroposterior view, lateral views are carried out to help localize any lesion that is seen. In examining a lateral view, as in Figure 5.9, follow this plan:

- Identify the sternum anteriorly and vertebral bodies posteriorly. The cardiac shadow lies anteriorly and inferiorly.
- There should be a lucent (dark) area retrosternally which has approximately the same density as the area posterior to the heart and anterior to the vertebral bodies. Check for any difference between the two, or for any discrete lesion in either area.
- Check for any collapsed vertebrae.
- The lowest vertebrae should appear darkest, becoming whiter as they progress superiorly. Interruption of this smooth gradation suggests an abnormality overlying the vertebral bodies involved.

THE CT SCAN

The routine chest X-ray consists of shadows at all depths in the chest superimposed on one another. In computed tomography (CT) scanning, X-rays are passed through the body at different angles and the resulting information is processed by computer to generate a series of cross-sectional images. A thoracic CT scan thus comprises a series of cross-sectional 'slices' through the thorax at various levels. Figure 5.10(a) shows a CT scan, with the numerical data having been processed to generate an image showing details of the mediastinal structures. In Figure 5.10(b), the data have been processed so that the lung parenchyma is well seen, but the mediastinal structures are not. Interpreting these figures is easier if you keep carefully in mind the orientation of the patient: in effect, the patient is lying on his or her back, with the feet towards you, and you are looking up 'through' the soles of the feet to the level of the mid-thorax.

The CT scan is a vital part of the staging of carcinoma of the bronchus, and inoperability may be demonstrated by evidence on CT of mediastinal involvement. CT scanning will demonstrate the presence of dilated and distorted bronchi, as in bronchiectasis. Diffuse pulmonary fibrosis will be shown by a

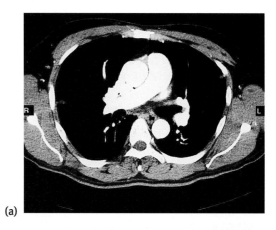

(a)

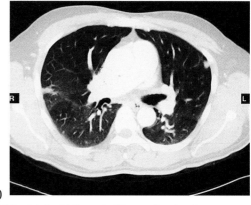

(b)

Fig. 5.10   (a) A mid-thoracic CT scan showing the mediastinal structure and soft tissues. (b) A mid-thoracic CT scan showing details of the lung parenchyma.

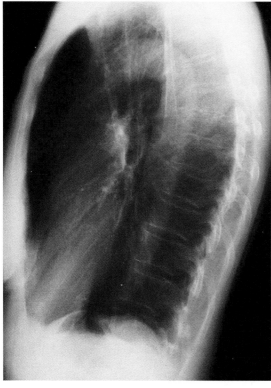

Fig. 5.9   A lateral chest X-ray.

modified high resolution/thin section scan technique. Emboli in the pulmonary arteries can be demonstrated by a rapid data acquisition spiral CT technique, and in some hospitals CT is replacing isotope lung scanning (see below) for the diagnosis of pulmonary embolism. Additionally, some machines can now generate three-dimensional representations of the thoracic structures (Fig. 5.11)

RADIOISOTOPE IMAGING

Within the lung, the most widely used radioisotope technique is combined *ventilation and perfusion scanning*, used to aid the diagnosis of pulmonary embolism.

The perfusion scan is performed by injecting intravenously a small dose of macroaggregated human albumin particles labelled with technetium-99m. A gamma-camera image is then built up of the radioactive particles impacted in the pulmonary vasculature. The distribution of perfusion in the lung can then be seen. The ventilation scan is obtained by inhalation of a radioactive gas such as krypton-81m, again using scanning to identify the distribution of the radioactivity.

Blood is usually diverted away from areas of the lung which are unventilated, so a *matched* defect on both the ventilation and perfusion scans usually indicates parenchymal lung disease. If there are areas of ventilated lung which are not perfused (i.e. an *unmatched* defect), then this is evidence in support of

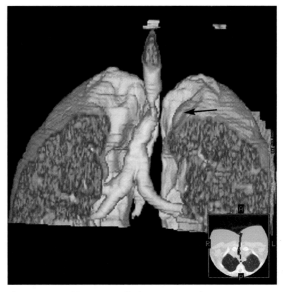

Fig. 5.11   A CT-generated 3D reconstruction demonstrating that the patient has a tracheal stenosis (arrowed). (Courtesy of Professor R. H. Reznek.)

an embolism to the unperfused area. Figure 5.12 shows a ventilation/perfusion isotope scan. The unmatched defects (areas ventilated by the inspired air but not perfused by blood) suggest a high probability of pulmonary embolism.

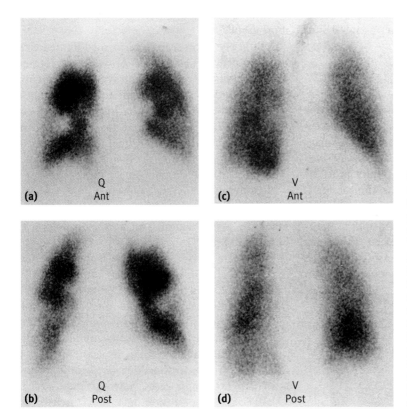

(a)   Q   Ant

(b)   Q   Post

(c)   V   Ant

(d)   V   Post

Fig. 5.12   Ventilation (V)/perfusion (Q) isotope scan of the lungs. Segmental and subsegmental loss of perfusion (a & b) can be seen with relatively normal ventilation (c & d). The clear punched-out areas in the perfusion (Q) scans indicate areas of reduced isotope concentration during the perfusion scan. Thus these are areas of reduced blood flow. The ventilation scans show normal aeration of the lungs as depicted by the isotope distribution in the pulmonary airways. These sequences of scans are suggestive of pulmonary embolism because they show impaired perfusion with normal ventilation.

MAGNETIC RESONANCE IMAGING

Magnetic resonance imaging (MRI) is useful in demonstrating mediastinal abnormalities and can help evaluate invasion of the mediastinum and chest wall by tumour. Apart from the fact that it does not use ionizing radiation, at present it has few other advantages over CT scanning in imaging the thorax. MRI is particularly degraded by movement artefact in imaging the chest, because of the relatively long acquisition time necessary for this technique.

ULTRASOUND

Ultrasound scanning reveals much less detail than CT scanning, but has the advantages that it does not involve radiation and that it gives 'real-time' images—the operator can visualize what is happening as it happens.

Ultrasound is used for examining diaphragmatic movement. A paralysed hemidiaphragm—usually a result of damage to the phrenic nerve by a mediastinal tumour—does not move downward during inspiration. If the patient is asked to make a sudden inspiratory effort, as in sniffing, the non-paralysed side of the diaphragm moves down, so intrathoracic pressure drops, and the paralysed side moves *up*.

Ultrasound is also valuable in distinguishing pleural thickening from pleural fluid—with real-time imaging the latter can be seen to move with changes in posture. When such fluid is present, ultrasound may be used to aid placement of a catheter to drain the collection, and also to accurately steer a draining catheter into an intrapulmonary abscess.

FIBRE-OPTIC BRONCHOSCOPY

Fibre-optic bronchoscopy is an essential tool in the investigation of many forms of respiratory disease (Fig. 5.13). For discrete abnormalities, such as a mass seen on chest X ray and suspected to be a carcinoma, bronchoscopy is usually indicated to investigate its nature. Under local anaesthesia, the flexible bronchoscope is passed through the nose, pharynx and larynx, down the trachea, and the bronchial tree is then inspected. Figure 5.14 shows a carcinoma of the bronchus seen down the bronchoscope. Flexible biopsy forceps are passed down a channel inside the bronchoscope, and are used to obtain tissue samples for histological examination. Similarly, aspirated bronchial secretions and brushings of any endobronchial abnormality can be sent to the laboratory for cytological examination.

At bronchoscopy, specimens are also taken for microbiological examination in order to determine the nature of any infecting organisms. In diffuse interstitial lung disease, such as sarcoidosis or pulmonary fibrosis, the technique of transbronchial biopsy can be used to obtain small specimens of lung parenchyma for histological examination and confirmation of the diagnosis.

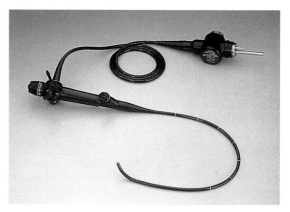

Fig. 5.13   A fibre-optic bronchoscope. (Courtesy of Key Med Ltd)

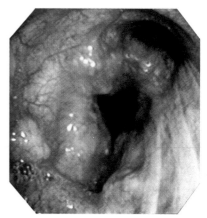

Fig. 5.14   A carcinoma of the bronchus, seen down the bronchoscope.

PLEURAL ASPIRATION AND BIOPSY

A pleural effusion can give rise to diagnostic problems and, sometimes, management problems when the amount of fluid causes respiratory embarrassment. When a pleural effusion is seen as a presenting feature in a middle-aged or older patient, the most likely cause is carcinoma. Less commonly, particularly in younger patients, it may be due to tuberculosis. In either case the diagnosis is best obtained by both aspiration of the fluid and pleural biopsy. Aspiration alone has a lower diagnostic yield.

After anaesthetizing the skin, subcutaneous tissues and pleura, pleural fluid may be aspirated by syringe and needle for microbiological examination and cytological examination. Large pleural effusions may need drainage by the placement of an indwelling catheter, left in situ until the fluid has been fully removed. As noted above, ultrasound guidance can be helpful, particularly if the fluid is *loculated* in various pockets.

Cytological examination of pleural fluid may demonstrate the presence of malignant cells. Many polymorphs may be seen if the effusion is secondary to an underlying pneumonic infection. With tuberculosis the fluid usually contains many lymphocytes, although tubercle bacilli themselves are rarely seen. In empyema, pus is present in the pleural cavity; this pus has a characteristic appearance and will be full of white cells and organisms.

The pleural fluid should also be examined for protein content. A transudate resulting from cardiac or renal failure can be distinguished from an exudate, usually resulting from pleural inflammation, by its lower protein content (less than 30 g/litre). Frankly blood-stained effusions occur with malignancy, pulmonary infarction and trauma.

Biopsies of the pleura can be obtained percutaneously and under local anaesthesia with an *Abram's pleural biopsy needle*. This technique can be used when there is pleural fluid present to obtain pleural tissue for histological examination and, whenever tuberculosis is a possibility, for microbiological culture. If ultrasound examination shows the pleura to be thickened, biopsies may be obtained with the aid of ultrasound screening by Abram's needle, Tru-cut needle and similar techniques.

THORACOSCOPY

This technique enables the pleural cavity to be directly examined and biopsies to be taken under direct vision. The procedure is commonly performed under a general anaesthetic by a surgeon who uses a rigid thoracoscope after the lung has been deflated. More recently, flexible thoracoscopes have been developed which can sometimes be used under local anaesthetic.

LUNG BIOPSY

As noted above, the technique of transbronchial biopsy can be used to obtain samples of lung parenchyma. Such specimens are often too small for diagnosis. In this circumstance, biopsies of the lung taken at thoracoscopy may be of value. Occasionally, a formal open lung biopsy obtained at thoracotomy may be necessary.

When there is a discrete, localized lesion it may be possible to obtain a biopsy percutaneously with the aid of CT scanning to direct the insertion of the biopsy needle (Fig. 5.15)

IMMUNOLOGICAL TESTS

Sometimes asthma is related to the development of type I hypersensitivity to certain allergens. Part of the assessment of such patients might include skin sensitivity tests, in which minute quantities of the suspected allergen are introduced intradermally. Delayed (type IV, cell-mediated) hypersensitivity is shown by the Mantoux and Heaf tests used to detect the presence of sensitivity to tubercular protein.

Precipitating antibodies in the circulating blood are present in patients with some fungal diseases, such as

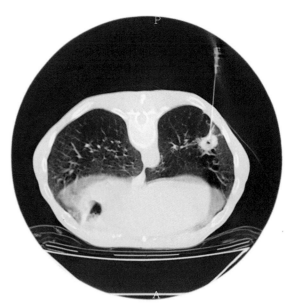

Fig. 5.15 A CT-guided percutaneous biopsy in progress. The radio-dense (white) structure is the biopsy needle.

bronchopulmonary aspergillosis or aspergilloma. In patients suspected of having an allergic alveolitis antibodies may be demonstrated to the relevant antigens. Immunoglobulin E levels are often raised in patients with asthma.

CONCLUSION

Evaluation of the respiratory system, as with all other organ systems, requires a careful assessment of the history, the findings on physical examination and the results of appropriately chosen special investigations. As the conclusion to this chapter, a series of case histories are presented below, together with the findings on clinical examination and the results of investigations.

CASE HISTORIES

Patient 1

A 25-year-old woman presented with a history of recurrent, wheezy breathlessness. This was worse at night and in the early morning. Physical examination was normal at the time she was seen, as was her chest X-ray. Measurements of peak expiratory flow, obtained with a peak flow meter, were recorded over a 2-week period (Fig. 5.16). These showed a daily (diurnal) variation in her peak flow, worse in the morning, typical of asthma. She was treated with inhaled steroids and inhaled bronchodilators, and her symptoms resolved.

Patient 2

A 70-year-old woman, a smoker throughout her adult life, presented with haemoptysis. Physical

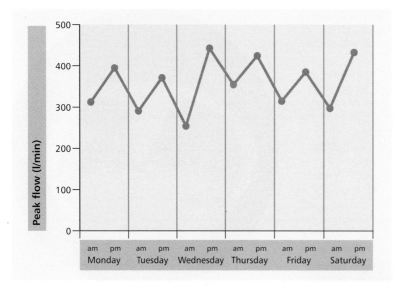

Fig. 5.16   A peak-flow chart.

examination revealed widespread expiratory wheezing suggestive of airways obstruction, which was confirmed on spirometry: her FEV_1 was 1.4 litres (40% of the predicted value for her age and height) and FVC 3.2 litres (80% predicted); FEV_1 was therefore 44% of FVC (normal > 70%).

A chest X-ray showed a mass in the right upper lobe (Fig. 5.17). At bronchoscopy, a tumour was seen (Fig. 5.18) which on histological examination was found to be a squamous cell carcinoma.

Patient 3

A 66-year-old woman, a long-term smoker, presented with a 5-year history of increasing breathlessness. Physical examination showed hyperinflation on the left, reduced movement on the right, and tracheal deviation to that side. The breath sounds were quiet but with a wheeze audible. A chest X-ray (Fig. 5.19) confirmed the hyperinflation and tracheal deviation, and showed fibrosis in the right upper lobe. The findings are compatible with chronic obstructive pulmonary disease (confirmed by an obstructive spirometry trace, similar to Fig. 5.7b) in a patient with apical scarring due to previous tuberculosis.

Patient 4

A 55-year-old woman had a long history of rheumatoid arthritis. She became gradually breathless over the course of 2 years.

Physical examination showed symmetrical limitation of respiratory movement. Fine, late inspiratory crackles were audible at both lung bases. Spirometry showed a marked restrictive ventilatory defect, similar to that seen in Figure 5.7(c), both the FEV_1 and the FVC being reduced but the ratio between them being normal. The diagnosis of diffuse interstitial fibrosis secondary to lung disease was confirmed by the typical appearances seen on high resolution CT scanning.

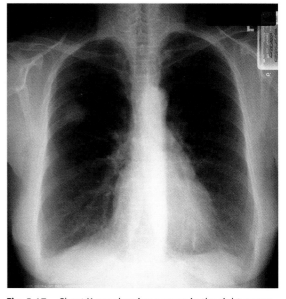

Fig. 5.17   Chest X-ray showing a mass in the right upper lobe.

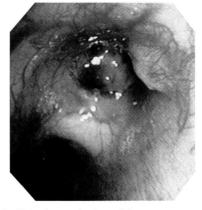

Fig. 5.18   Bronchoscopic view of the tumour seen radiologically in Figure 5.17.

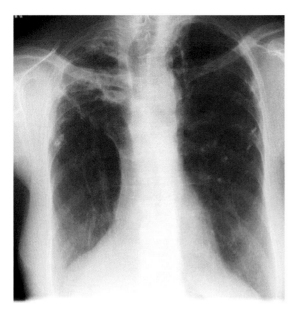

Fig. 5.19   Chest X-ray of patient 3, showing hyperinflation, tracheal deviation and fibrosis in the right upper lobe.

The patient suddenly became more short of breath, and presented to the accident and emergency department. Chest movements were diminished on the right, where the percussion note was more resonant than the left, but the breath sounds, vocal resonance and tactile vocal fremitus were all reduced. Chest X-ray (Fig. 5.20) confirmed that she had developed a pneumothorax which required intercostal tube drainage.

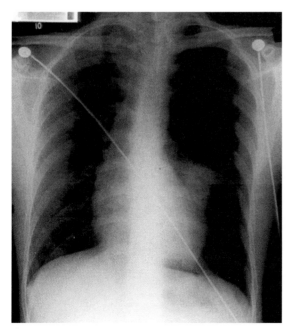

Fig. 5.20   Chest X-ray of patient 4, showing a right pneumothorax, with a lucent area (absent lung markings) and the denser collapsed lung.

Patient 5
A 22-year-old man had a 4-month history of malaise, weight loss, fevers and night sweats. Over the course of the past 4 weeks he had developed increasing breathlessness.

Physical examination showed a thin young man. Chest movements were diminished on the left, and the trachea was deviated to the right. The percussion note was very dull on the left, where the breath sounds were almost absent, and both the vocal resonance and the tactile vocal fremitus were markedly reduced.

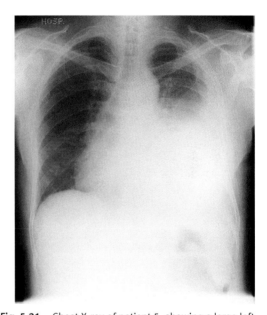

Fig. 5.21   Chest X-ray of patient 5, showing a large left pleural effusion.

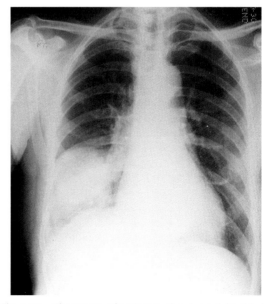

Fig. 5.22   Chest X-ray of patient 6, showing a right-sided pneumonia, with consolidation.

Chest X-ray (Fig. 5.21) confirmed the presence of a very large left pleural effusion. Pleural aspiration obtained fluid of high protein content, and an Abram's pleural biopsy showed histological changes highly suggestive of tuberculosis, a diagnosis later confirmed when microbiological cultures of the pleural fluid were available.

Patient 6

A previously fit 40-year-old man developed a fever, and within 24 hours was very ill with breathlessness and right sided chest pain, which was worse whenever he breathed in.

Physical examination showed him to have a respiratory rate of 40, and to be centrally cyanosed. The percussion note was dull at the right base posteriorly, but breath sounds were bronchial in character at this site and both vocal resonance and tactile vocal fremitus were increased. A pleural rub could be heard.

The clinical diagnosis of right basal consolidation due to pneumonia, along with pleural involvement as evidenced by the pleuritic pain and the pleural rub, was confirmed by chest X-ray (Fig. 5.22). The clinical impression of cyanosis was confirmed by blood gas analysis which, while he was breathing air, showed a PaO_2 of only 7.8 kPa. This was despite a slightly low $PaCO_2$ of 4.0 kPa which demonstrated that he was breathing harder than usual and accordingly that those alveoli which were not involved by the pneumonia were clearing carbon dioxide efficiently.

Blood cultures grew *Streptococcus pneumoniae*, and with intravenous antibiotics as well as full supportive care he made a slow but steady recovery.

6
THE CARDIOVASCULAR SYSTEM

INTRODUCTION

The 20th century saw major changes in patterns of cardiovascular disease. In the developed world, syphilitic and tuberculous involvement of the cardiovascular system became rare, and the incidence of rheumatic disease declined considerably. Myocardial and conducting tissue disease, on the other hand, were diagnosed with increasing frequency and the importance of arterial hypertension became well recognized. Coronary artery disease emerged as the major cardiovascular disorder of the era, becoming the most common cause of premature death throughout Europe, North America, and Australasia. As the new millennium begins, coronary artery disease shows signs of loosening its grip on the developed world. Elsewhere, however, its prevalence is in steep ascent, and in the third world it now threatens to overtake malnutrition and infectious disease as the major cause of death.

As patterns of cardiovascular disease changed, so did the cardiologist's diagnostic tools. A century that started with the stethoscope, the sphygmomanometer, the chest X-ray and a very rudimentary electrocardiogram saw the development of a variety of new imaging modalities, utilizing ultrasound, radioisotopes, X-rays and magnetic resonance. This noninvasive capability was complemented by introduction of the catheterization laboratory, permitting angiographic imaging, electrophysiological recording and tissue biopsy of the heart. Add to this the resources of the chemical pathology, bacteriology and molecular biology laboratories, and the array of diagnostic technology available to the modern cardiologist becomes almost overwhelming. Nevertheless, most of the common cardiac disorders encountered in clinical practice can still be diagnosed at the bedside on the basis of a careful history and physical examination. Indeed, this simple fact defines the true art of cardiology and remains as relevant now as it was before recent technological advances.

THE CARDIAC HISTORY

This should record details of presenting symptoms, of which the most common are chest pain, fatigue and dyspnoea, palpitations, and presyncope or syncope (see below). Previous illness should also be recorded, since this may provide important clues about the cardiac diagnosis—thyroid, connective tissue and neoplastic disorders, for example, can all affect the heart. Rheumatic fever in childhood is important because of its association with valvular heart disease and hypertension; and diabetes and dyslipidaemias because of their association with coronary artery disease. Smoking is a major risk factor for coronary artery disease. Alcohol abuse may predispose to cardiac arrhythmias and cardiomyopathy. The cardiac history should quantify both habits in terms of pack-years smoked and units of alcohol consumed. The family history should always be documented because coronary artery disease and hypertension often run in families, as do some of the less common cardiovascular disorders such as hypertrophic cardiomyopathy. Indeed, in the the patient with hypertrophic cardiomyopathy, a family history of sudden death is probably the single most important indicator of risk. Finally, the drug history should be recorded, as many commonly prescribed drugs are potentially cardiotoxic. Beta-blockers and some calcium channel blockers (diltiazem, verapamil), for example, can cause symptomatic bradycardias while tricyclic antidepressants and beta-agonists can cause tachyarrhythmias. Vasodilators cause variable reductions in blood pressure which can lead to syncopal attacks, particularly in patients with aortic stenosis. The myocardial toxicity of certain cytotoxic drugs (notably doxorubicin and related compounds) is an important cause of cardiomyopathy.

CHEST PAIN

Myocardial ischaemia, pericarditis and aortic dissection are common cardiovascular causes of chest pain.

Myocardial ischaemia and infarction
(Boxes 6.1–6.5)
Ischaemia of the heart results from an imbalance between myocardial oxygen supply and demand, producing pain called *angina*. Angina is usually a symptom of atherosclerotic coronary artery disease which impedes myocardial oxygen supply. Other causes of coronary artery disease (see Box 6.5) are rare. The history is diagnostic if the location of the pain, its character, its relation to exertion and its duration are typical. The patient describes retrosternal pain which may radiate into the arms, the throat or the jaw. It has a constricting character, is provoked by exertion and relieved rapidly by rest. When coronary occlusion produces myocardial infarction

the pain is similar in location and character but is usually more severe, more prolonged, and unrelieved by rest.

Pericarditis
This also causes central chest pain which is sharp in character and aggravated by deep inspiration, cough or postural changes. It is usually idiopathic or caused by Coxsackie B infection. It may also occur as a complication of myocardial infarction, but other causes are seen less commonly (Box 6.6).

Aortic dissection (Boxes 6.7)
This produces severe tearing pain in either the front or the back of the chest. The onset is abrupt, unlike the crescendo quality of ischaemic cardiac pain.

Rare cardiovascular causes of chest pain include mitral valve disease associated with massive left atrial dilatation. This causes discomfort in the back which is sometimes associated with dysphagia due to oesophageal compression. Aortic aneurysms can also cause pain in the chest due to local compression.

BOX 6.1   Angina.

Typical patient
- Middle-aged (male) or elderly (either sex) often with family history of coronary heart disease and one or more of the major reversible risk factors (smoking, hypertension, hypercholesterolaemia)

Major symptoms
- Exertional chest pain and shortness of breath. Pain often described as 'heaviness' or 'tightness' and may radiate into arms, neck or jaw

Major signs
- None, although hypertension and signs of hyperlipidaemia (xanthelasmata, xanthomas) may be present
- Peripheral vascular disease, evidenced by absent pulses or arterial bruits, is commonly associated with coronary heart disease

Diagnosis
- Typical history is most important diagnostic tool
- *ECG*: often normal; may show Q waves in patients with previous myocardial infarction
- *Stress test*: exertional ST depression
- *Isotope perfusion scan*: exertional perfusion defects
- *Coronary arteriogram*: confirms coronary artery disease

Additional investigations
- Blood sugar and lipids to rule out diabetes and dyslipidaemia

Comments
- A careful history is the single most important means of diagnosing angina

BOX 6.2   Unstable angina.

Typical patient
- Middle-aged (male) or elderly (either sex) often with family history of coronary heart disease and one or more of the major reversible risk factors (smoking, hypertension, hypercholesterolaemia)

Major symptoms
- Chest pain and shortness of breath. Pain may wax and wane but is often prolonged and indistinguishable from myocardial infarction

Major signs
- Often none apart from those attributable to sympathetic activation; tachycardia and sweating

Diagnosis
- *ECG*: Often normal. May show regional ST depression
- *Markers of injury*: CKMB usually normal but raised troponins indicate high risk of progression to myocardial infarction

Additional investigations
- *Biochemistry*: Blood sugar and lipids to rule out diabetes and dyslipidaemia

Comments
- Clinically may be indistinguishable from myocardial infarction. Differential diagnosis depends on ECG findings and cardiac enzymes

BOX 6.3   Acute myocardial infarction.

Typical patient
- Middle-aged (male) or elderly (either sex) often with family history of coronary heart disease and one or more of the major reversible risk factors (smoking, hypertension, hypercholesterolaemia)
- In many patients there is no preceding history of angina

Major symptoms
- Chest pain and shortness of breath. Pain usually prolonged and often described as 'heaviness' or 'tightness' with radiation into arms, neck or jaw. Alternative descriptions include 'congestion' or 'burning' which may be confused with indigestion

Major signs
- *Ischaemic myocardial damage*, fourth heart sound, dyskinetic precordial impulse
- *Autonomic disturbance*, Tachycardia (anterior MI), bradycardia (inferior MI), sweating, vomiting, syncope

Diagnosis
- *ECG*: regional ST elevation
- *Markers of injury*: raised CKMB and troponins

BOX 6.3   (continued)

Additional investigations
- *Biochemistry*: Blood sugar and lipids to rule out diabetes and dyslipidaemia
- *Risk stratification*: Echocardiogram (LV function) and stress testing (reversible ischaemia)

Comments
- History and ECG remain most useful diagnostic tools

BOX 6.4   Causes of angina.

Impaired myocardial oxygen supply
- Coronary artery disease
  - atherosclerosis
  - arteritis in connective tissue disorders
  - diabetes mellitus
- Coronary artery spasm
- Congenital coronary artery disease
  - arteriovenous fistula
  - anomalous origin from pulmonary artery
- Severe anaemia

Increased myocardial oxygen demand
- Left ventricular hypertrophy
  - hypertension
  - aortic valve disease
  - hypertrophic cardiomyopathy
- Tachyarrhythmias

BOX 6.5   Causes of coronary artery disease.

- Atherosclerosis
- Arteritis
  - systemic lupus erythematosus
  - polyarteritis nodosa
  - rheumatoid arthritis
  - ankylosing spondylitis
  - syphilis
  - Takayasu disease
- Embolism
  - infective endocarditis
  - left atrial/ventricular thrombus
  - left atrial/ventricular tumour
  - prosthetic valve thrombus
  - complication of cardiac catheterization
- Coronary mural thickening
  - amyloidosis
  - radiation therapy
  - Hurler's disease
  - pseudoxanthoma elasticum
- Other causes of coronary luminal narrowing
  - aortic dissection
  - coronary spasm
- Congenital coronary artery disease
  - anomalous origin from pulmonary artery
  - arteriovenous fistula

BOX 6.6   Causes of acute pericarditis.

- Idiopathic
- Infective
  - viral (Coxsackie B, influenza, *Herpes simplex*)
  - bacterial (*Staphylococcus aureus, Mycobacterium tuberculosis*)
- Connective tissue disease
  - systemic lupus erythematosus
  - rheumatoid arthritis
  - polyarteritis nodosa
- Uraemia
- Malignancy (e.g. breast, lung, lymphoma, leukaemia)
- Radiation therapy
- Acute myocardial infarction
- Post myocardial infarction/cardiotomy (Dressler's syndrome)

BOX 6.7   Aortic dissection.

Typical patient
- Middle-aged or elderly patient with history of hypertension or arteriosclerotic disease
- Occasionally younger patient with aortic root disease (e.g. Marfan's syndrome)

Major symptoms
- Chest pain

Major signs
- Often none
- Sometimes, regional arterial insufficiency (e.g. coronary or vertebral artery occlusion causing myocardial infarction or stroke); aortic regurgitation; cardiac tamponade; sudden death

Diagnosis
- *CXR*: Widened mediastinum, occasionally with left pleural effusion
- *Transoesophageal echocardiogram*: confirms dissection
- *CT scan*: confirms dissection
- *MRI scan*: confirms dissection

Additional investigations
- None

Comments
- Having established the diagnosis, emergency surgery is usually necessary, particularly if the dissection involves the ascending thoracic aorta

DYSPNOEA

Dyspnoea is an abnormal awareness of breathing occurring either at rest or at an unexpectedly low level of exertion. It is a major symptom of many cardiac disorders, particularly left heart failure (Table 6.1), but its mechanisms are complex. In acute pulmonary oedema and orthopnoea, dyspnoea is due mainly to

the elevated left atrial pressure that characterizes left heart failure (Box 6.8). This produces a corresponding elevation of the pulmonary capillary pressure and increases transudation into the lungs, which become oedematous and stiff. The extra effort required to ventilate the stiff lungs causes dyspnoea. In exertional dyspnoea, however, other mechanisms apart from changes in left atrial pressure are also important.

TABLE 6.1   Causes of heart failure.

Ventricular pathophysiology	Clinical examples
Restricted filling	Mitral stenosis Hypertrophic cardiomyopathy
Pressure loading	Hypertension Aortic stenosis Coarctation of the aorta
Volume loading	Mitral regurgitation Aortic regurgitation
Contractile impairment	Coronary artery disease Dilated cardiomyopathy Myocarditis
Arrhythmia	Severe bradycardia Severe tachycardia

BOX 6.8   Acute LVF.

Typical patient
- Patient with acute myocardial infarction or known left ventricular disease

Major symptoms
- Severe dyspnoea and variable circulatory collapse

Major signs
- Low output state (hypotension, oliguria, cold periphery); tachycardia; S3; sweating; crackles at lung bases

Diagnosis
- *CXR*: bilateral air space consolidation with typical perihilar distribution
- *Echocardiogram*: usually confirms left ventricular disease

Additional investigations
- *ECG*: may show evidence of acute or previous myocardial infarction
- *Blood gas analysis*: shows variable hypoxaemia

Comments
- Although most cases are caused by acute myocardial infarction or advanced left ventricular disease, it is vital to exclude valvular disease or myxoma which are potentially correctable by surgery

Exertional dyspnoea

This is the most troublesome symptom in heart failure (Box 6.9). Exercise causes a sharp increase in left atrial pressure and this contributes to the pathogenesis of dyspnoea by causing pulmonary congestion (see above). However, the severity of dyspnoea does not correlate closely with exertional left atrial pressure and other factors must therefore be important. These include respiratory muscle fatigue and the effects of exertional acidosis on peripheral chemoreceptors. As left heart failure worsens, exercise tolerance deteriorates. In advanced disease the patient is dyspnoeic at rest.

Orthopnoea

Lying flat causes a steep rise in left atrial pressure in patients with heart failure, resulting in pulmonary congestion and severe dyspnoea. To obtain uninterrupted sleep extra pillows are required, and in advanced disease the patient may choose to sleep sitting in a chair.

BOX 6.9   Congestive heart failure.

Typical patient
- Middle-aged (male) or elderly (either sex) patient with history of myocardial infarction or long-standing hypertension
- In cases where there is no clear cause, always inquire about alcohol consumption

Major symptoms
- Exertional fatigue and shortness of breath, with orthopnoea in advanced cases

Major signs
- *Fluid retention*: basal crackles, raised JVP, peripheral oedema
- *Reduced cardiac output*: cool skin, peripheral cyanosis
- *Other findings*: third heart sound

Diagnosis
- *ECG*: usually abnormal; often shows Q waves (previous myocardial infarction) or left ventricular hypertrophy (hypertension)
- *CXR*: cardiac enlargement, congested lung fields
- *Echocardiogram*: LV dilatation with regional (coronary heart disease) or global (cardiomyopathy) contractile impairment

Additional investigations
- Renal function as prelude to diuretic and ACE-inhibitor therapy
- Blood count to rule out anaemia

Comments
- The echocardiogram is the single most important diagnostic test in the patient with heart failure

---

Paroxysmal nocturnal dyspnoea

Frank pulmonary oedema on lying flat wakens the patient from sleep with distressing dyspnoea and fear of imminent death. The symptoms are corrected by standing upright, which allows gravitational pooling of blood to lower the left atrial pressure.

FATIGUE

Exertional fatigue is an important symptom of heart failure and is particularly troublesome towards the end of the day. It is caused partly by deconditioning and muscular atrophy but also by inadequate oxygen delivery to exercising muscle, reflecting impaired cardiac output.

PALPITATION

Awareness of the heart beat is common during exertion or heightened emotion. Under other circumstances it may be indicative of an abnormal cardiac rhythm. A description of the rate and rhythm of the palpitation is essential. Extrasystoles are common but rarely signify important heart disease. They are usually experienced as 'missed' or 'dropped' beats; the forceful beats that follow may also be noticed. Rapid irregular palpitation is typical of atrial fibrillation. Rapid regular palpitation of abrupt onset occurs in atrial, junctional and ventricular tachyarrhythmias.

DIZZINESS AND SYNCOPE

Cardiovascular disorders produce dizziness and syncope by transient hypotension resulting in abrupt cerebral hypoperfusion. Recovery is usually rapid, unlike with other common causes of syncope (e.g., stroke, epilepsy, overdose).

Postural hypotension

Syncope on standing upright reflects inadequate baroreceptor-mediated vasoconstriction. It is common in the elderly. Abrupt reductions in blood pressure and cerebral perfusion cause the patient to fall to the ground, whereupon the condition corrects itself.

Vasovagal syncope

This is caused by autonomic overactivity, usually provoked by emotional or painful stimuli, less commonly by coughing or micturition. Only rarely are syncopal attacks so frequent as to be significantly disabling ('malignant' vasovagal syndrome). Vasodilatation and inappropriate slowing of the pulse combine to reduce blood pressure and cerebral perfusion. Recovery is rapid if the patient lies down.

Carotid sinus syncope

Exaggerated vagal discharge following external stimulation of the carotid sinus (e.g. shaving, or a tight shirt collar) causes reflex vasodilatation and slowing of the pulse. These may combine to reduce blood pressure and cerebral perfusion in some elderly patients, causing loss of consciousness.

Valvar obstruction

Fixed valvar obstruction in aortic stenosis may prevent a normal rise in cardiac output during exertion, such that the physiological vasodilatation that occurs in exercising muscle produces abrupt reduction in blood pressure and cerebral perfusion, resulting in syncope. Vasodilator therapy may cause syncope by a similar mechanism. Intermittent obstruction of the mitral valve by left atrial tumours (usually myxoma) may also cause syncopal episodes (Fig. 6.1).

Stokes–Adams attacks

These are caused by self-limiting episodes of asystole (Fig. 6.2) or rapid tachyarrhythmias (including ventricular fibrillation). The loss of cardiac output causes syncope and striking pallor. Following restoration of normal rhythm recovery is rapid and is associated with flushing of the skin as flow through the dilated cutaneous bed is re-established.

THE CARDIAC EXAMINATION

A methodical approach is recommended, starting with inspection of the patient and then proceeding to examination of the radial pulse, measurement of heart rate and blood pressure, examination of the neck (carotid pulse, jugular venous pulse), palpation of the anterior chest wall, auscultation of the heart, percussion and auscultation of the lung bases, and, finally, examination of the peripheral pulses and auscultation for carotid and femoral arterial bruits.

INSPECTION OF THE PATIENT

Chest wall deformities such as pectus excavatum should be noted, since these may compress the heart and displace the apex, giving a spurious impression of cardiac enlargement. Large ventricular or aortic aneurysms may cause visible pulsations. Superior vena caval obstruction is associated with prominent venous collaterals on the chest wall. Prominent venous collaterals around the shoulder occur in axillary or subclavian vein obstruction.

Anaemia

This may exacerbate angina and heart failure. Pallor of the mucous membranes is a useful but sometimes misleading physical sign and diagnosis requires laboratory measurement of the haemoglobin concentration.

Cyanosis

This is a blue discoloration of the skin and mucous membranes caused by increased concentration of reduced haemoglobin in the superficial blood vessels.

Peripheral cyanosis may result when cutaneous vasoconstriction slows the blood flow and increases oxygen extraction in the skin and the lips. It is

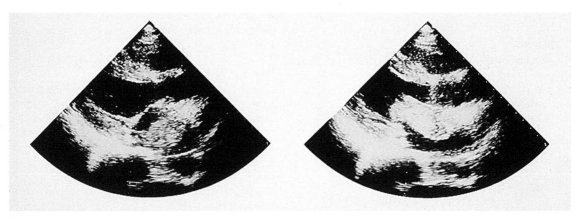

Fig. 6.1   Left atrial myxoma: 2D echocardiogram (long axis view). During diastole, the tumour (arrowed) prolapses through the mitral valve and obstructs left ventricular filling.

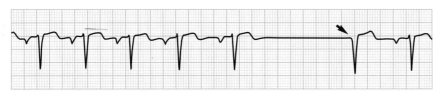

Fig. 6.2   Prolonged sinus arrest. After the fifth sinus beat there is a pause of about 1.8 s terminated by a nodal escape beat (arrowed) before sinus rhythm resumes.

physiological during cold exposure. It also occurs in heart failure when reduced cardiac output produces reflex cutaneous vasoconstriction. In mitral stenosis, cyanosis over the malar area produces the characteristic mitral facies.

Central cyanosis may result from the reduced arterial oxygen saturation caused by cardiac or pulmonary disease. It affects not only the skin and the lips but also the mucous membranes of the mouth. Cardiac causes include pulmonary oedema (which prevent adequate oxygenation of the blood) and congenital heart disease. Congenital defects associated with central cyanosis include those in which desaturated venous blood bypasses the lungs by ('reversed') shunting through septal defects or a patent ductus arteriosus (e.g. Eisenmenger's syndrome, Fallot's tetralogy).

Clubbing of the fingers and toes

In congenital cyanotic heart disease clubbing is not present at birth but develops during infancy and may become very marked. Infective endocarditis is the only other cardiac cause of clubbing.

Other cutaneous and ocular signs of infective endocarditis

These are caused by immune complex deposition in the capillary circulation. A vasculitic rash is common, as are splinter haemorrhages in the nail bed although these are a very non-specific finding. Other 'classic' manifestations of endocarditis, including Osler's nodes (tender erythematous nodules in the pulps of the fingers), Janeway lesions (painless erythematous lesions on the palms) and Roth's spots (erythematous lesions in the optic fundi) are now rarely seen.

Coldness of the extremities

In patients hospitalized with severe heart failure this is an important sign of reduced cardiac output. It is caused by reflex vasoconstriction of the cutaneous bed. Measurement of skin temperature provides a useful indirect means of monitoring cardiac output in the intensive care unit.

Pyrexia

Infective endocarditis is invariably associated with pyrexia which may be low grade or 'swinging' in nature if paravalvar abscess develops. Pyrexia also occurs for the first three days after myocardial infarction.

Oedema

Subcutaneous oedema which pits on digital pressure is a cardinal feature of congestive heart failure. Pressure should be applied over a bony prominence (tibia, lateral malleoli, sacrum) to provide effective compression. Oedema is caused by salt and water retention by the kidney. Two mechanisms are responsible:

- *Reduced sodium delivery to the nephron.* This is caused by reduced glomerular filtration caused by constriction of the preglomerular arterioles in response to sympathetic activation and angiotensin II production.
- *Increased sodium reabsorption from the nephron.* This is the more important mechanism. It occurs particularly in the proximal tubule early in heart failure but, as failure worsens, renin angiotensin activation stimulates aldosterone release which increases sodium reabsorption in the distal nephron.

Salt and water retention expands plasma volume and increases the capillary hydrostatic pressure. Hydrostatic forces driving fluid out of the capillary exceed osmotic forces reabsorbing it, so that oedema fluid accumulates in the interstitial space. The effect of gravity on capillary hydrostatic pressure ensures that oedema is most prominent around the ankles in the ambulant patient and over the sacrum in the bedridden patient. In advanced heart failure oedema may involve the legs, genitalia and trunk. Transudation into the peritoneal cavity (ascites) and the pleural and pericardial spaces may also occur.

ARTERIAL PULSE

The arterial pulses should be palpated for evaluation of rate, rhythm, character and symmetry.

Rate and rhythm

By convention, both are assessed by palpation of the right radial pulse. Rate, expressed in beats per minute, is measured by counting over a timed period of 15 seconds. Normal sinus rhythm is regular, but in young patients may show phasic variation in rate during respiration (*sinus arrhythmia*). An irregular rhythm usually indicates atrial fibrillation but may also be caused by frequent ectopic beats, or self-limiting paroxysmal arrhythmias. In patients with atrial fibrillation the rate should be measured by auscultation at the cardiac apex because beats that follow very short diastolic intervals may create a 'pulse-deficit' by not generating sufficient pressure to be palpable at the radial artery.

Character

This is defined by the volume and waveform of the pulse and should be evaluated at the right carotid artery (i.e. the pulse closest to the heart and least subject to damping and distortion in the arterial tree). Pulse volume provides a crude indication of stroke volume, being small in heart failure and large in aortic regurgitation. The waveform of the pulse is of greater diagnostic importance (Fig. 6.3). Aortic stenosis produces a slowly rising carotid pulse; in aortic regurgitation, on the other hand, the large stroke volume vigorously ejected produces a rapidly

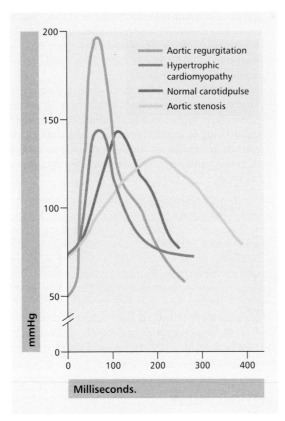

Fig. 6.3 The waveform of the pulse is characterized by the rate of rise of the carotid upstroke. Note in aortic regurgitation the upstroke is rapid and followed by abrupt diastolic 'collapse'. In hypertrophic cardiomyopathy the upstroke is also rapid and the pulse has a jerky character. In aortic stenosis the upstroke is slow with a plateau.

rising carotid pulse which collapses in early diastole owing to back flow through the aortic valve. In mixed aortic valve disease a *biphasic pulse* with two systolic peaks is occasionally found. *Alternating pulse*—alternating high and low systolic peaks—occurs in severe left ventricular failure but the mechanisms is unknown. *Paradoxical pulse*—an inspiratory decline in systolic pressure greater than 10 mmHg—occurs in cardiac tamponade and, less frequently, in constrictive pericarditis and obstructive pulmonary disease (Fig. 6.4). It represents an exaggeration of the normal inspiratory decline in systolic pressure and is not, therefore, truly paradoxical.

Symmetry
Symmetry of the radial, brachial, carotid, femoral, popliteal and pedal pulses should be confirmed. A reduced or absent pulse indicates an obstruction more proximally in the arterial tree, caused usually by atherosclerosis or thromboembolism, less commonly by aortic dissection. Coarctation of the aorta causes symmetrical reduction and delay of the femoral pulses compared with the radial pulses.

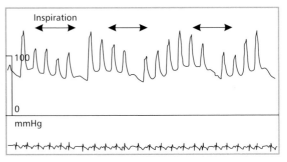

Fig. 6.4 Paradoxical pulse (radial artery pressure signal). The patient had severe tamponade. Note the exaggerated (> 10 mmHg) decline in arterial pressure during inspiration.

MEASUREMENT OF BLOOD PRESSURE

Blood pressure is measured indirectly by sphygmomanometry. Supine and erect measurements should be obtained to provide an assessment of baroreceptor function. A cuff (of width at least 40% the arm circumference) is attached to a mercury or aneroid manometer and inflated around the extended arm. Auscultation over the brachial artery reveals five phases of *Korotkoff sounds* as the cuff is deflated:

- *Phase 1*: the first appearance of the sounds marking systolic pressure
- *Phase 2 and 3*: increasingly loud sounds
- *Phase 4*: abrupt muffling of the sounds
- *Phase 5*: disappearance of the sounds.

Phase 5 provides a better measure of diastolic blood pressure than phase 4, not only because it corresponds more closely with directly measured diastolic pressure, but also because its identification is less subjective. Nevertheless, in those conditions where Korotkoff sounds remain audible despite complete deflation of the cuff (aortic regurgitation, arteriovenous fistula, pregnancy) phase 4 must be used for the diastolic measurement.

JUGULAR VENOUS PULSE

Fluctuations in right atrial pressure during the cardiac cycle generate a pulse which is transmitted backwards into the jugular veins. It is best examined while the patient reclines at 45 degrees. If the right atrial pressure is very low, however, visualization of the jugular venous pulse may require a smaller reclining angle. Alternatively, manual pressure over the upper abdomen may be used to produce a transient increase in venous return to the heart which elevates the jugular venous pulse (hepatojugular reflux).

Jugular venous pressure
The normal upper limit is 4 cm vertically above the sternal angle. This is about 9 cm above the right atrium and corresponds to a pressure of 6 mmHg. Elevation of the jugular venous pressure indicates

elevation of the right atrial pressure unless the superior vena cava is obstructed, producing engorgement of the neck veins (Box 6.10). During inspiration the pressure within the chest falls and there is a fall in the jugular venous pressure. In constrictive pericarditis, and less commonly in tamponade, inspiration produces a paradoxical rise (*Kussmaul's sign*) in the jugular venous pressure (JVP) because the increased venous return cannot be accommodated within the constricted right side of the heart (Fig. 6.5).

Waveform of jugular venous pulse

The jugular venous pulse has a flickering character caused by '*a*' and '*v*' waves separated by '*x*' and '*y*' descents. The '*a*' wave produced by atrial systole precedes tricuspid valve closure. It is followed by the '*x*' descent (marking descent of the tricuspid valve ring) which is interrupted by the diminutive '*c*' wave as the tricuspid valve closes. Atrial pressure then rises again, producing the '*v*' wave as the atrium fills passively during ventricular systole. The decline in atrial pressure as the tricuspid valve opens to allow ventricular filling

---

BOX 6.10   Causes of elevated jugular venous pressure.

- Congestive heart failure
- Cor pulmonale
- Pulmonary embolism
- Right ventricular infarction
- Tricuspid valve disease
- Tamponade
- Constrictive pericarditis
- Hypertrophic/restrictive cardiomyopathy
- Superior vena cava obstruction
- Iatrogenic fluid overload, particularly in surgical and renal patients

---

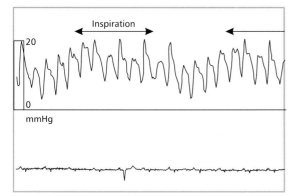

Fig. 6.5   Kussmaul's sign. Jugular venous pressure recording in a patient with tamponade. The venous pressure is raised and there is a particularly prominent systolic 'x' descent, giving the waveform of the JVP an unusually dynamic appearance. Note the inspiratory rise in atrial pressure (Kussmaul's sign) reflecting the inability of the tamponaded right heart to accommodate the inspiratory increase in venous return.

produces the '*y*' descent. Important abnormalities of the pattern of deflections are shown in Figure 6.6.

PALPATION OF THE CHEST WALL

The location of the apical impulse inferior or lateral to the fifth intercostal space or the mid-clavicular line, respectively, usually indicates cardiac enlargement. Palpable third and fourth heart sounds give the apical impulse a double thrust. In the past, considerable importance has been attached to the character of the apical impulse ('thrusting' in aortic valve disease, 'tapping' in mitral stenosis) but this is of very limited practical value in the modern era.

Left ventricular aneurysms can sometimes be palpated medial to the cardiac apex. Right ventricular enlargement produces a systolic thrust in the left parasternal area. The turbulent flow responsible for heart murmurs may produce palpable vibrations ('*thrills*') on the chest wall, particularly in aortic stenosis, ventricular septal defect and patent ductus arteriosus.

AUSCULTATION OF THE HEART

The diaphragm and bell of the stethoscope permit appreciation of high- and low-pitched auscultatory events respectively. The apex, lower left sternal edge, upper left sternal edge and upper right sternal edge should be auscultated in turn. These locations correspond to the mitral, tricuspid, pulmonary and aortic areas respectively, and loosely identify sites at which sounds and murmurs arising from the four valves are best heard.

First sound (S1)

This corresponds to mitral and tricuspid valve closure at the onset of systole. It is accentuated in mitral stenosis because prolonged diastolic filling through the narrowed valve ensures that the thickened leaflets are widely separated at the onset of systole. Thus valve closure generates unusually vigorous vibrations. In advanced mitral stenosis the valve is rigid and immobile and S1 becomes soft again.

Second sound (S2)

This corresponds to aortic and pulmonary valve closure following ventricular ejection. S2 is single during expiration. Inspiration, however, causes physiological splitting into aortic followed by pulmonary components because increased venous return to the right side of the heart delays pulmonary valve closure. Important abnormalities of S2 are illustrated in Figure 6.7.

Third and fourth sounds (S3, S4)

These low frequency sounds occur early and late in diastole respectively. When present they give a characteristic 'gallop' to the cardiac rhythm. Both sounds

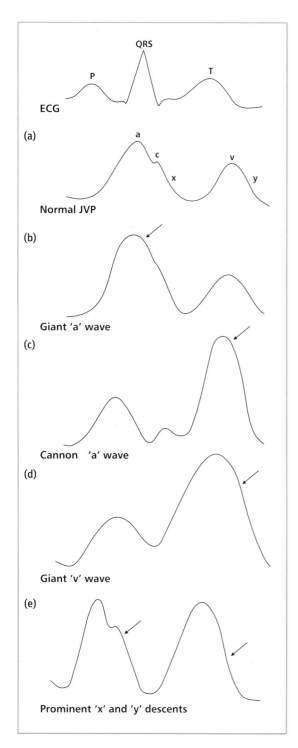

Fig. 6.6 Waveform of the jugular venous pulse. The ECG is portrayed at the top of the illustration. Note how electrical events precede mechanical events in the cardiac cycle. Thus the P wave (atrial depolarization) and QRS complex (ventricular depolarization) precede the 'a' and 'v' waves, respectively, of the JVP.
(a) Normal JVP. The 'a' wave produced by atrial systole is the most prominent deflection. It is followed by the 'x' descent interrupted by the small 'c' wave marking tricuspid valve closure. Atrial pressure then rises again ('v' wave) as the atrium fills passively during ventricular systole. The decline in atrial pressure as the tricuspid valve opens produces the 'y' descent.
(b) Giant 'a' wave. Forceful atrial contraction against a stenosed tricuspid valve or a noncompliant hypertrophied right ventricle produces an unusually prominent 'a' wave.
(c) Cannon 'a' wave. This is caused by atrial systole against a closed tricuspid valve. It occurs when atrial and ventricular rhythms are dissociated (complete heart block, ventricular tachycardia) and marks coincident atrial and ventricular systole.
(d) Giant 'v' wave. This is an important sign of tricuspid regurgitation. The regurgitant jet produces pulsatile systolic waves in the JVP.
(e) Prominent 'x' and 'y' descents. These occur in constrictive pericarditis and give the JVP an unusually dynamic appearance. In tamponade only the 'x' descent is usually exaggerated.

are best heard with the bell of the stethoscope at the cardiac apex. They are caused by abrupt tensing of the ventricular walls following rapid diastolic filling. Rapid filling occurs early in diastole (S3) following atrioventricular valve opening and again late in diastole (S4) due to atrial contraction. S3 is physiological in children and young adults but usually disappears after the age of 40. It also occurs in high-output states caused by anaemia, fever, pregnancy and thyrotoxi-

cosis. After the age of 40, S3 is nearly always pathological, usually indicating left ventricular failure or, less commonly, mitral regurgitation or constrictive pericarditis. S4 is sometimes physiological in the elderly. More commonly, however, it is pathological and occurs when vigorous atrial contraction late in diastole is required to augment filling of a hypertrophied, non-compliant ventricle (e.g. hypertension, aortic stenosis, hypertrophic cardiomyopathy).

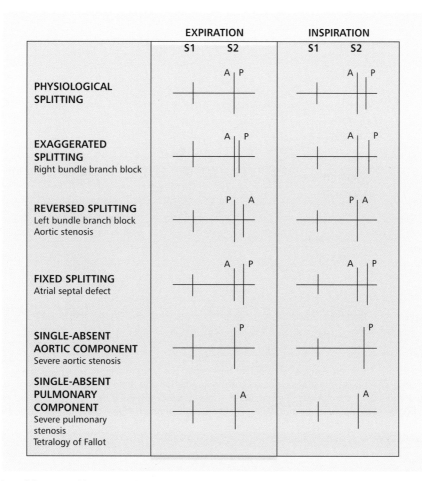

	EXPIRATION	INSPIRATION

Fig. 6.7 Splitting of the second heart sound. The first sound representing mitral and tricuspid closure is usually single but the aortic and pulmonary components of the second sound normally split during inspiration as increased venous return delays right ventricular emptying. Abnormal splitting of the second heart sound is an important sign of heart disease.

Systolic clicks and opening snaps

Valve opening, unlike valve closure, is normally silent. In aortic stenosis, however, valve opening produces a click in early systole which precedes the ejection murmur. The click is only audible if the valve cusps are pliant and non-calcified and is particularly prominent in the congenitally bicuspid valve. A click later in systole suggests mitral valve prolapse, particularly when followed by a murmur. In mitral stenosis, elevated left atrial pressure causes forceful opening of the thickened valve leaflets. This generates a snap early in diastole which precedes the mid-diastolic murmur.

Heart murmurs (Fig. 6.8)

These are caused by turbulent flow within the heart and great vessels. Occasionally the turbulence is caused by increased flow through a normal valve—usually aortic or pulmonary—producing an 'innocent' murmur. However, murmurs may also indicate valve disease or abnormal communications between the left and right sides of the heart (e.g. septal defects). Heart murmurs are defined by four characteristics: *loudness, quality, location* and *timing*.

The *loudness* of a murmur reflects the degree of turbulence. This relates to the volume and velocity of flow and not the severity of the cardiac lesion. Loudness is graded on a scale of 1 (barely audible) to 6 (audible even without application of the stethoscope to the chest wall). The *quality* of a murmur relates to its frequency and is best described as low-, medium- or high-pitched. The *location* of a murmur on the chest wall depends on its site of origin and has led to the description of four valve areas (see above). Some murmurs radiate, depending on the velocity and direction of blood flow. The sound of the high-velocity systolic flow in aortic stenosis and mitral regurgitation, for example, is directed towards the neck and the axilla respectively; that of the high-velocity diastolic flow in aortic regurgitation is directed towards the left sternal edge. Murmurs are *timed* according to the phase of systole or diastole during which they are audible (e.g. mid-systolic, pansystolic, early diastolic). It is inadequate to describe the timing of a murmur as systolic or diastolic without more specific reference to the length of the murmur and the phase of systole or diastole during

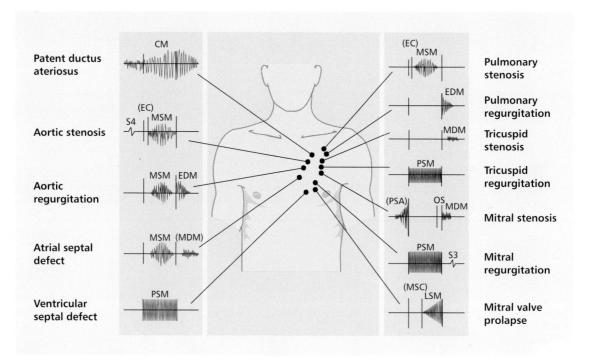

Fig. 6.8   Heart murmurs. These are caused by turbulent flow within the heart and great vessels, and may indicate valve disease. Heart murmurs (defined by loudness, quality, location, radiation and timing) may be depicted graphically as shown in this illustration. CM = continuous murmur. MSM = mid systolic murmur. PSM = pansystolic murmur. LSM = late systolic murmur. EDM = early diastolic murmur. MDM = mid diastolic murmur. PSA = presystolic accentuation of murmur. EC = ejection click. MSC = mid systolic click. OS = opening snap. S3 = third heart sound. S4 = fourth heart sound. Parentheses indicate those auscultatory findings which are not constant.

which it is heard: *systolic* murmurs are either mid-systolic, pansystolic or late systolic; *diastolic* murmurs are either early diastolic, mid-diastolic or presystolic in timing. Continuous murmurs are audible in both phases of the cardiac cycle.

A *mid-systolic* ('*ejection*') murmur is caused by turbulence in the left or right ventricular outflow tracts during ejection. It starts following opening of the aortic or pulmonary valve, reaches a crescendo in mid-systole, and disappears before the second heart sound. The murmur is loudest in the aortic area (with radiation to the neck) when it arises from the left ventricular outflow tract, and in the pulmonary area when it arises from the right ventricular outflow tract. It is best heard with the diaphragm of the stethoscope while the patient sits forward. Important causes of *aortic ejection murmurs* are aortic stenosis and hypertrophic cardiomyopathy. Aortic regurgitation also produces an ejection murmur due to increased stroke volume and velocity of ejection. *Pulmonary ejection murmurs* may be caused by pulmonary stenosis or infundibular stenosis (Fallot's tetralogy). In atrial septal defect the pulmonary ejection murmur results from right ventricular volume loading and does not indicate organic valvular disease. '*Innocent*' *murmurs* unrelated to heart disease are always mid-systolic in timing and are caused by turbulent flow in the left (sometimes right)

ventricular outflow tract. In most cases there is no clear cause but they may reflect a hyperkinetic circulation in conditions such as anaemia, pregnancy, thyrotoxicosis or fever. They are rarely louder than grade 3, often vary with posture, may disappear on exertion, and are not associated with other signs of organic heart disease.

Pansystolic murmurs are audible throughout systole from the first to the second heart sounds. They are caused by regurgitation through incompetent atrioventricular valves and by ventricular septal defects. The pansystolic murmur of *mitral regurgitation* is loudest at the cardiac apex and radiates into the left axilla. It is best heard with the diaphragm of the stethoscope with the patient lying on the left side. The murmurs of *tricuspid regurgitation* and *ventricular septal defect* are loudest at the lower left sternal edge. Inspiration accentuates the murmur of tricuspid regurgitation because the increased venous return to the right side of the heart increases the regurgitant volume. *Mitral valve prolapse* may also produce a pansystolic murmur but, more commonly, prolapse occurs in mid-systole producing a click followed by a late-systolic murmur.

Early diastolic murmurs are high pitched and start immediately after the second heart sound, fading away in mid-diastole. They are caused by regurgitation through incompetent aortic and pulmonary valves and are best heard using the diaphragm of the stethoscope while the patient leans forward. The early diastolic murmur of *aortic regurgitation* radiates from the aortic area to the left sternal edge where it is usually easier to hear. *Pulmonary regurgitation* is loudest at the pulmonary area.

Mid-diastolic murmurs are caused by turbulent flow through the atrioventricular valves. They start following valve opening, relatively late after the second sound, and continue for a variable period during mid-diastole. *Mitral stenosis* is the principal cause of a mid-diastolic murmur which is best heard at the cardiac apex using the bell of the stethoscope while the patient lies on the left side. Increased flow across a non-stenotic mitral valve occurs in *ventricular septal defect* and *mitral regurgitation* and may produce a mid-diastolic murmur. In severe *aortic regurgitation*, preclosure of the anterior leaflet of the mitral valve by the regurgitant jet may produce mitral turbulence associated with a mid-diastolic murmur (Austin Flint murmur). A mid-diastolic murmur at the lower left sternal edge, accentuated by inspiration, is caused by *tricuspid stenosis* and also by conditions which increase tricuspid flow (e.g. atrial septal defect, tricuspid regurgitation).

In *mitral or tricuspid stenosis*, atrial systole produces a presystolic murmur immediately before the first heart sound. The murmur is perceived as an accentuation of the mid-diastolic murmur associated with these conditions. Because presystolic murmurs are generated by atrial systole they do not occur in patients with atrial fibrillation.

Continuous murmurs are heard during systole and diastole, and are uninterrupted by valve closure. The commonest cardiac cause is *patent ductus arteriosus* in which flow from the high-pressure aorta to the low-pressure pulmonary artery continues throughout the cardiac cycle, producing a murmur over the base of the heart which, though continuously audible, is loudest at end systole and diminishes during diastole. Ruptured sinus of Valsalva aneurysm also produces a continuous murmur.

Friction rubs and venous hums
A friction rub occurs in pericarditis. It is a high-pitched scratching noise audible during any part of the cardiac cycle and over any part of the left precordium. A continuous venous hum at the base of the heart reflects hyperkinetic jugular venous flow. It is particularly common in infants and usually disappears on lying flat.

THE ELECTROCARDIOGRAM

The electrocardiogram (ECG) records the electrical activity of the heart at the skin surface. A good-quality 12-lead ECG is essential for the evaluation of almost all cardiac patients.

ELECTROPHYSIOLOGY

Generation of electrical activity
The wave of depolarization that spreads through the heart during each cardiac cycle has vector properties defined by its direction and magnitude. The net direction of the wave changes continuously during each cardiac cycle and the ECG deflections change accordingly, being positive as the wave approaches the recording electrode and negative as it moves away. Electrodes orientated along the axis of the wave record larger deflections than those orientated at right-angles. Nevertheless, the size of the deflections is determined principally by the magnitude of the wave, which is a function of muscle mass. Thus the ECG deflection produced by depolarization of the atria (P wave) is smaller than that produced by the depolarization of the more muscular ventricles (QRS complex). Ventricular repolarization produces the T wave.

Inscription of the QRS complex
The ventricular depolarization vector can be resolved into two components:

- Septal depolarization—spreads from left to right across the septum
- Ventricular free wall depolarization—spreads from endocardium to epicardium.

Left ventricular depolarization dominates the second vector component, the resultant direction of which is from right to left. Thus electrodes orientated to the left ventricle record a small negative deflection (Q wave) as the septal depolarization vector moves away, followed by a large positive deflection (R wave) as the ventricular depolarization vector approaches. The sequence of deflections for electrodes orientated towards the right ventricle is in the opposite direction (Fig. 6.9).

Any positive deflection is termed an R wave. A negative deflection before the R wave is termed a Q

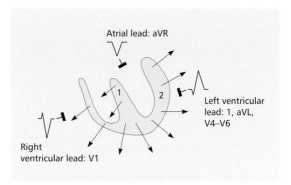

Fig. 6.9 Inscription of the QRS complex. The septal depolarization vector (1) produces the initial deflection of the QRS complex. The ventricular free-wall depolarization vector (2) produces the second deflection which is usually more pronounced. Lead aVR is orientated towards the cavity of the left ventricle and records an entirely negative deflection.

wave (this must be the first deflection of the complex), while a negative deflection following the R wave is termed an S wave.

Electrical axis

Because the mean direction of the ventricular depolarization vector (the electrical axis) shows a wide range of normality, there is corresponding variation in QRS patterns consistent with a normal ECG. Thus correct interpretation of the ECG must take account of the electrical axis. The frontal plane axis is determined by identifying the limb lead in which the net QRS deflection (positive and negative) is least pro-

nounced. This lead must be at right-angles to the frontal plane electrical axis, which is defined using an arbitrary hexaxial reference system (Fig. 6.10).

NORMAL 12-LEAD ECG

This is illustrated in Figure 6.11. Leads I–III are the standard bipolar leads, which each measure the potential difference between two limbs:

● *Lead I*: left arm to right arm
● *Lead II*: left leg to right arm
● *Lead III*: left leg to left arm.

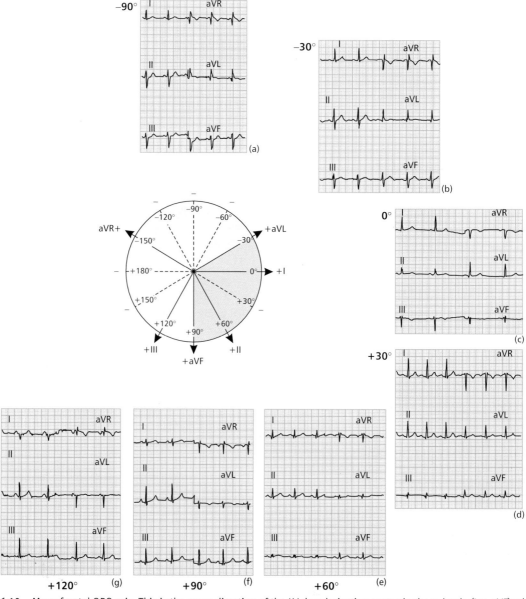

Fig. 6.10   Mean frontal QRS axis. This is the mean direction of the LV depolarization vector in those leads (I to aVF) which lie in the frontal plane of the heart. It lies at right angles to the lead in which the net QRS deflexion is least pronounced. It is quantified using a hexaxial reference system. The QRS axis shows a wide range of normality from −30° to 90°. Thus, despite the different ECG patterns in this illustration, only recordings **(a)** and **(g)** are abnormal, due to left and right axis deviation respectively.

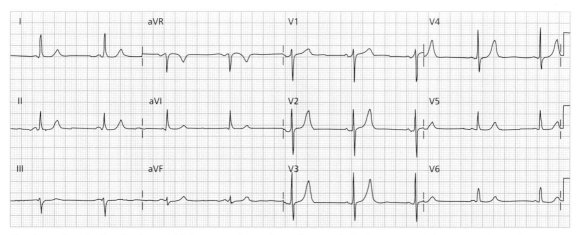

Fig. 6.11   Standard 12-lead ECG. This is a normal recording. The QRS deflections are equiphasic in lead aVF. This is at right-angles to lead I (see Fig. 6.10) which is dominantly positive. The frontal plane QRS axis is, therefore, 0°. The square wave calibration signal is 1mV.

The remaining leads are unipolar connected to a limb (aVR to aVF) or to the chest wall (V_1–V_6). Because the orientation of each lead to the wave of depolarization is different, the direction and magnitude of ECG deflections is also different in each lead. Nevertheless, the sequence of deflections (P wave, QRS complex, T wave) is identical. In some patients a small U wave can be seen following the T wave. Its orientation (positive or negative) is the same as the T wave but its cause is unknown.

ANALYSIS OF THE ECG

Heart rate
The ECG is usually recorded at a paper speed of 25 mm/s. Thus each large square (5 mm) represents 0.20 seconds. The heart rate (beats/minute) is conveniently calculated by counting the number of large squares between consecutive R waves and dividing this into 300.

Rhythm
In normal sinus rhythm, P waves precede each QRS complex and the rhythm is regular. Absence of P waves and an irregular rhythm indicate atrial fibrillation.

Electrical axis
Evaluation of the frontal place QRS axis is described above.

P wave morphology
The duration should not exceed 0.10 seconds. Broad-notched 'mitral' P waves indicate left atrial dilatation caused usually by mitral valve disease or left ventricular failure. Tall-peaked 'pulmonary' P waves indicate right atrial enlargement caused usually by pulmonary hypertension and right ventricular failure.

PR interval
The normal duration is 0.12 to 0.20 seconds measured from the onset of the P wave to the first deflection of the QRS complex. Prolongation indicates delayed atrioventricular conduction (first degree heart block). Shortening indicates rapid conduction through an accessory pathway bypassing the atroventricular node (Wolff–Parkinson–White syndrome).

QRS morphology
The QRS duration should not exceed 0.12 seconds. Prolongation indicates slow ventricular depolarization due to bundle branch block (Fig. 6.12), pre-excitation

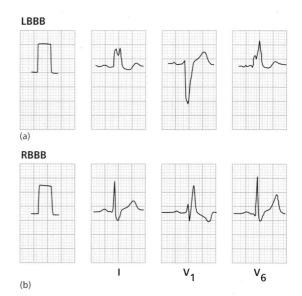

Fig. 6.12   Bundle branch block. **(a)** Left bundle branch block (LBBB); the entire sequence of ventricular depolarization is abnormal, resulting in a broad QRS complex with large slurred or notched R waves in I and V_6. **(b)** Right bundle branch block (RBBB); right ventricular depolarization is delayed, resulting in a broad QRS complex with an 'rSR' pattern in V_1 and prominent S waves in I and V_6.

(Wolff–Parkinson–White syndrome), ventricular tachycardia or hypokalaemia.

Exaggerated QRS deflections indicate ventricular hypertrophy (Fig. 6.13). Voltage criteria for left ventricular hypertrophy are fulfilled when the sum of the S and R wave deflections in leads V_1 and V_6 respectively exceeds 35 mm (3.5 mv). Right ventricular hypertrophy causes tall R waves in right ventricular leads (V_1 and V_2). Diminished QRS deflections occur in myxoedema and also when pericardial effusion or obesity electrically insulate the heart. The presence of pathological Q waves (duration greater than 0.04 seconds) should be noted because this usually indicates previous myocardial infarction.

ST segment morphology

Minor ST elevation reflecting early repolarization may occur as a normal variant (Fig. 6.14) particularly in patients of African or West Indian origin. Pathological elevation (> 2.0 mm above the isoelectric line) occurs in acute myocardial infarction, variant angina and pericarditis. Horizontal ST depression

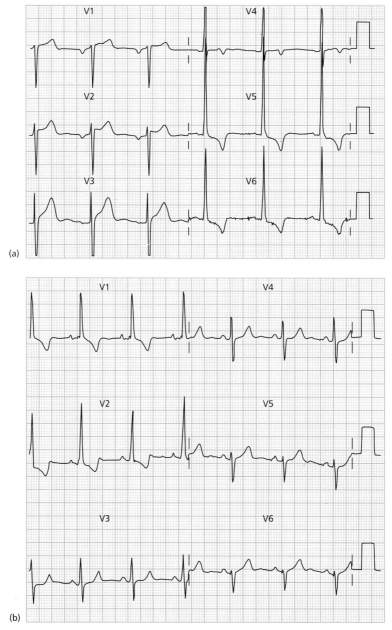

(a)

(b)

Fig. 6.13   Ventricular hypertrophy. **(a)** Left ventricular hypertrophy. The QRS voltage deflections are exaggerated such that the sum of S and R waves in V_1 and V_6, respectively, exceeds 35 mm. T wave inversion in V_5 and V_6 indicates left ventricular 'strain'. **(b)** Right ventricular hypertrophy. Prominent R waves in V_1 and V_2 associated with T wave inversion are shown.

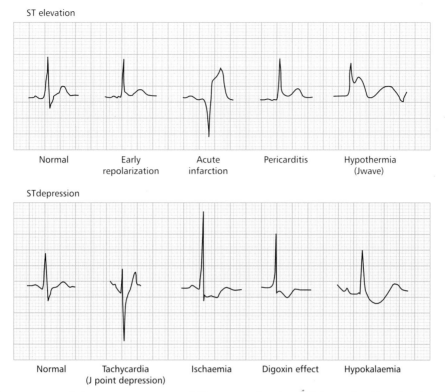

ST elevation

| Normal | Early repolarization | Acute infarction | Pericarditis | Hypothermia (Jwave) |

ST depression

| Normal | Tachycardia (J point depression) | Ischaemia | Digoxin effect | Hypokalaemia |

Fig. 6.14 ST segment morphology: common causes of ST segment elevation and depression. Note that depression of the J point (junction between the QRS complex and ST segment) is physiological during exertion and does not signify myocardial ischaemia. Planar depression of the ST segment, on the other hand, is strongly suggestive of myocardial ischaemia.

indicates myocardial ischaemia. Other important causes of ST depression are digitalis therapy and hypokalaemia.

T wave morphology
The orientation of the T wave should be directionally similar to the QRS complex. Thus T wave inversion is normal in leads with dominantly negative QRS complexes (aVR, V_1, and sometimes lead III). Pathological T wave inversion occurs as a nonspecific response to various stimuli (e.g. viral infection, hypothermia). More important causes of T wave inversion are ventricular hypertrophy, myocardial ischaemia and myocardial infarction. Exaggerated peaking of the T wave is the earliest ECG change in acute myocardial infarction. It also occurs in hyperkalaemia.

CLINICAL APPLICATIONS OF ECG

DIAGNOSIS OF CORONARY HEART DISEASE
Territories supplied by the three major coronary arteries, although variable, are highly circumscribed, the left anterior descending artery supplying the anterior wall, the circumflex artery the lateral wall, and the right coronary artery the inferior wall of the left ventricle. The regional distribution of coronary flow has important implications for electrocardiography (and diagnostic imaging), patients with cor-

onary heart disease showing *regional* electrocardiographic (or wall motion) abnormalities while patients with diffuse myocardial disease (e.g., cardiomyopathy) show more widespread changes.

Stable angina
The ECG is often normal in patients with stable angina unless there is a history of myocardial infarction, when pathological Q waves or T wave inversion may be present.

Exercise stress testing
This is one of the most widely used tests for evaluating the patient with chest pain. The patient is usually exercised on a treadmill, the speed and slope of which can be adjusted to increase the workload gradually. The exercise ECG provides important *diagnostic* information. Thus, in patients with coronary artery disease, exercise-induced increases in myocardial oxygen demand may outstrip oxygen delivery through the atheromatous arteries, resulting in regional ischaemia. This causes planar or downsloping ST segment depression with reversal during recovery (Fig. 6.15). The diagnostic accuracy of stress testing is not 100% and Bayes' theorem predicts that false positive and false negative results will be common when the probability of coronary disease is very low (as in young women) or very high (as in elderly patients with typical symptoms) respectively.

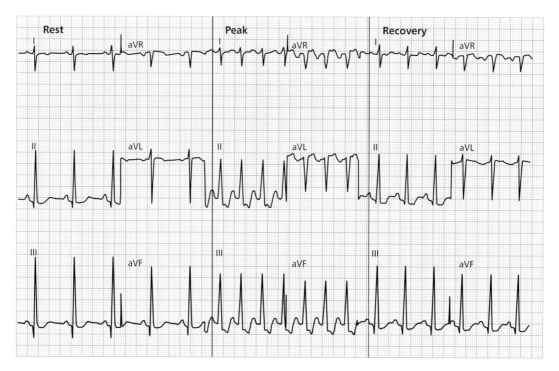

Fig. 6.15 Exercise ECG: ischaemic changes in inferior standard leads (II, III and aVF). At rest the ST segments are isoelectric. Exercise causes tachycardia and provokes 3 mm of down-sloping ST depression in leads II, III and aVF. The changes reverse during recovery. The findings suggest exertional ischaemia affecting the inferior wall of the heart. The probability of coronary artery disease is high.

The exercise ECG also provides important *prognostic* information: a high risk of myocardial infarction or sudden death is indicated by ST depression very early during exercise, by an exertional fall in blood pressure or by exercise-induced ventricular arrhythmias. In these cases, urgent coronary arteriography is required.

Acute coronary syndromes

Unstable angina and acute myocardial infarction both present with unprovoked ischaemic cardiac pain, and reliable differential diagnosis cannot be made using clinical criteria. However, the 12-lead ECG usually resolves this important question, since in unstable angina it is either normal or shows regional ST depression which is typically planar in configuration (Fig. 6.16). Regional T wave changes may also occur, although these are less specific. In acute myocardial infarction the ECG is nearly always diagnostic. Peaking of the T wave followed by ST segment elevation occur during the first hour of pain (Fig. 6.17). The changes are regional, and reciprocal ST depression may be seen in the opposite ECG leads. Usually a pathological Q wave occurs during the following 24 hours and thereafter persists indefinitely. The ST segment returns to the isoelectric line within 2–3 days and T wave inversion may occur. Occasionally T wave inversion is the only ECG change; it is usually attributed to limited subendocardial infarction if other criteria for infarction

are fulfilled. The ECG is a valuable indicator of infarct location. Changes in leads II, III and aVF indicate inferior infarction (Fig. 6.18), while changes in leads V_1–V_6 indicate anteroseptal (V_1–V_3) or anterolateral (V_1–V_6) infarction (Fig. 6.19). When the infarct is located posteriorly, ECG changes may be difficult to detect, but dominant R waves in leads V_1 and V_2 often develop (Fig. 6.18).

DETECTION OF CARDIAC ARRHYTHMIAS

Electrocardiographic documentation of the arrhythmia should be obtained prior to instituting treatment. In patients with sustained arrhythmias a 12-lead recording at rest is usually diagnostic, but a long continuous recording of the lead showing the clearest P wave (if present) should also be obtained. In patients with paroxysmal arrhythmias special techniques may be required for electrocardiographic documentation.

In-hospital ECG monitoring

Patients who have had out-of-hospital cardiac arrest or severe, arrhythmia-induced heart failure should undergo ECG monitoring in hospital under the continuous surveillance of trained staff.

Ambulatory (Holter) ECG monitoring

Patients with intermittent palpitation or dizzy attacks should have a continuous 24-hour ECG recording while engaging in normal activities.

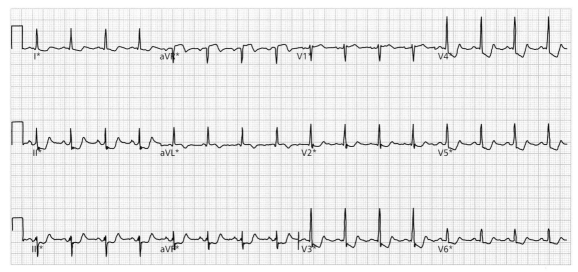

Fig. 6.16   Unstable angina: 12-lead ECG showing planar/down-sloping ST depression in the inferolateral territory.

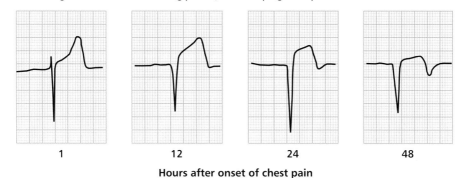

1   12   24   48

Hours after onset of chest pain

Fig. 6.17   AMI: evolution of ECG changes. Elevation of the ST segment occurs during the first hour of chest pain. The Q wave develops during the subsequent 24 hours and usually persists indefinitely. Within a day of the attack the ST segment usually returns to the isoelectric line and T wave inversion may occur.

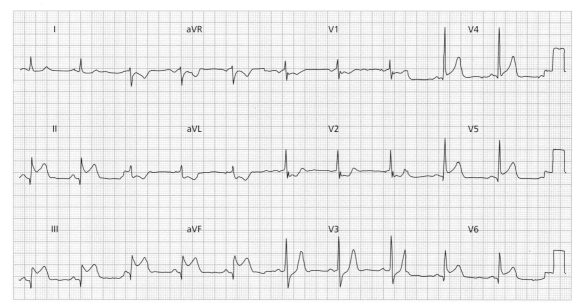

Fig. 6.18   Acute inferoposterior infarction. ECG 2 hours after the onset of chest pain. Typical ST elevation in leads II, III and aVF with reciprocal ST depression in aVL is diagnostic of inferior myocardial infarction. Prominent R waves in leads V_1 and V_2 associated with ST depression indicate posterior extension of the infarct. This pattern may reflect occlusion of the right coronary artery or a dominant circumflex coronary artery.

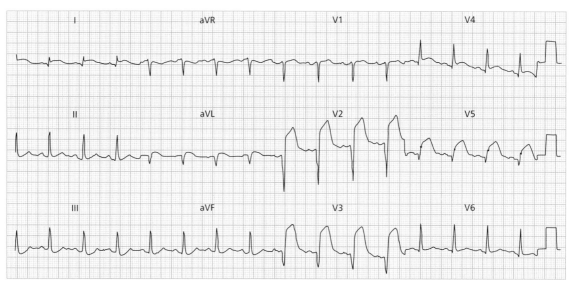

Fig. 6.19   Acute anterior infarction. ECG 1 hour after the onset of chest pain. Typical ST elevation in leads V_1–V_5 is diagnostic of anterior myocardial infarction. Additional ST elevation in standard leads I and aVL indicates lateral extension of the infarct This pattern usually reflects proximal occlusion of the left anterior descending coronary artery.

Portable cassette recorders are available for this purpose. Analysis of the tape often identifies the cardiac arrhythmias, particularly if symptoms were experienced during the recording (Fig. 6.20).

Patient-activated ECG recording
For patients with very infrequent symptoms, the detection rate with 24-hour ambulatory monitoring is low and patient-activated recorders are therefore more useful. When symptoms occur the patient applies the recorder to the chest wall. The recorder may then transmit the ECG by telephone to the hospital for scrutiny by the physician.

Exercise testing
The ECG recorded during exercise may be helpful when there is a history of exertional palpitation. Arrhythmias provoked by ischaemia or increased sympathetic activity are more likely to be detected during exercise.

Tilt testing
When malignant vasovagal syndrome is suspected, ECG and blood pressure recordings during tilt from supine to erect posture can be helpful. Abnormal bradycardia and hypotension sufficient to produce presyncope or syncope is strongly suggestive of the diagnosis.

Programmed cardiac stimulation
This technique requires cardiac catheterization with electrodes catheter-mounted. Premature stimuli are introduced into the atria or ventricles with a view to stimulating re-entry arrhythmias. In the normal heart sustained arrhythmias are rarely provoked by premature stimuli. Thus arrhythmia provocation during programmed stimulation is usually diagnostic, particularly when the arrhythmia reproduces symptoms. To test the efficacy of treatment the test can be repeated after administration of antiarrhythmic drugs.

DIAGNOSIS OF ATRIAL ARRHYTHMIAS (Fig. 6.21)
The ECG in atrial arrhythmias shows a narrow and morphologically normal QRS complex when ventricular depolarization occurs by normal His–Purkinje pathways. Rate-related or pre-existing bundle branch block, however, results in broad ventricular complexes that are difficult to distinguish from ventricular tachycardia.

Atrial ectopic beats
These rarely indicate heart disease. They often occur spontaneously but may be provoked by toxic stimuli such as caffeine, alcohol and cigarette smoking. They are caused by the premature discharge of an atrial ectopic focus; is an early and often bizarre P wave is essential for the diagnosis. The premature impulse enters and depolarizes the sinus node such that a partially compensatory pause occurs before the next sinus beat during resetting of the sinus node.

Atrial fibrillation
This is often idiopathic. It is common in hypertensive heart disease, mitral valve disease, thyrotoxicosis and left ventricular failure. It also occurs after major surgery and in response to various toxic stimuli, particularly alcohol. Atrial activity is chaotic and mechanically ineffective. P waves are therefore absent and are replaced by irregular fibrillatory waves (rate 400–600 per minute). The long refractory period of the atrioventricular node ensures that only some of the atrial impulses are conducted to produce an

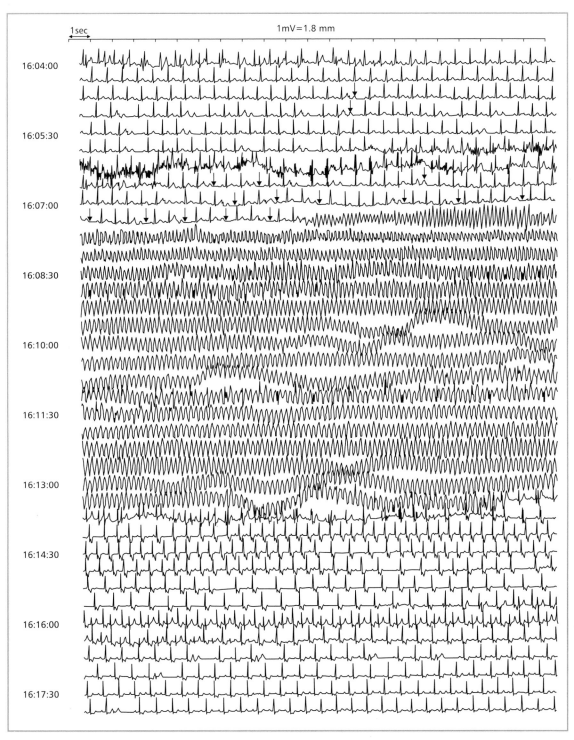

Fig. 6.20 Ventricular tachycardia: Holter recording. When tachycardias are paroxysmal in nature, continuous ECG monitoring is often necessary to document the arrhythmia. Here a Holter recording illustrates a long burst of rapid VT lasting a total of 6 min. Preceding the VT there is second degree heart block (arrows).

irregular ventricular rate of 130–200 beats per minute. If the atrioventricular node is diseased the ventricular rate is slower, but in the presence of a rapidly conducting accessory pathway in Wolff–Parkinson–White syndrome dangerous ventricular rates above 300 beats per minute may occur.

Atrial flutter

This is less common than atrial fibrillation but occurs under exactly similar circumstances. Re-entry mechanisms produce an atrial rate close to 300 beats per minute. The normal atrioventricular node conducts with 2:1 block giving a ventricular rate of 150 beats

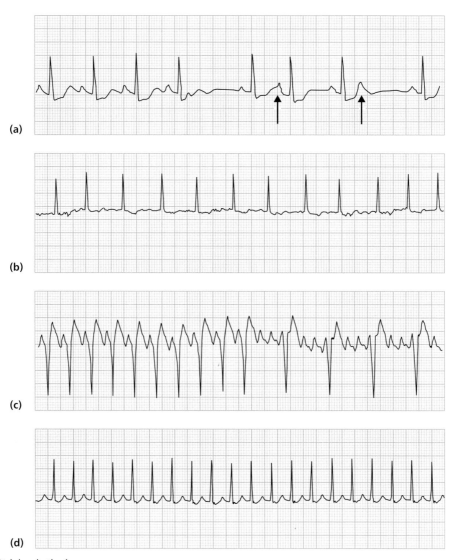

Fig. 6.21 Atrial arrhythmias:
(a) Ectopic beats. After the 4th sinus beat there is a very early P wave which, finding the AV node refractory, is not conducted to the ventricle. This produces a pause before the next sinus beat which itself is followed by a somewhat later atrial ectopic (arrowed) which is conducted normally. This is followed by a sinus beat following which the T wave is distorted by another early atrial ectopic (arrowed) which is also blocked.
(b) Atrial fibrillation. Note the irregular fibrillatory waves (best seen in V_1) and the irregular ventricular response. The ventricular rate is fairly slow because the patient was treated with a beta-blocker.
(c) A flutter. AV conduction is first with 2:1 block, giving a ventricular rate of about 150/min and then gives way to 4:1 block. Saw-tooth flutter waves at a rate of 300/min are clearly visible.
(d) AV junctional re-entrant tachycardia (AVJRT). Often called supraventricular tachycardia (SVT) this arrhythmia causes a regular tachycardia, rate 180/min.

per minute. Higher degrees of block may reflect intrinsic disease of the atrioventricular node or the effects of nodal blocking drugs. The ECG characteristically shows saw-tooth flutter waves which are most clearly seen when block is increased by carotid sinus pressure.

DIAGNOSIS OF JUNCTIONAL ARRHYTHMIAS

These are often called supraventricular tachycardias (SVTs) and are usually paroxysmal without obvious cardiac or extrinsic causes. They are re-entry arrhythmias caused either by an abnormal pathway between the atrium and the atrioventricular node (atrionodal pathway) or by an accessory atrioventricular pathway (bundle of Kent) as seen in Wolff–Parkinson–White syndrome. Like atrial arrhythmias, ventricular depolarization usually occurs by normal His–Purkinje pathways, producing a narrow QRS complex which confirms the supraventricular origin of the arrhythmia. Rate-related or pre-existing bundle branch block, on the other hand, produces broad ventricular complexes difficult to distinguish from ventricular tachycardia.

Atrioventricular junctional re-entry tachycardia (AVJRT)

The abnormal atrionodal pathway provides the basis for a small re-entry circuit. In sinus rhythm, the electrocardiogram is usually normal although occasionally the PR interval is short (Lown–Ganong–Levine syndrome). During tachycardia the rate is 150–250 beats per minute (Fig. 6.21). The arrhythmia is usually self-limiting but will sometimes respond to carotid sinus pressure. If this fails, intravenous verapamil or adenosine are usually effective by blocking the re-entry circuit within the atrioventricular node. Anti-tachycardia pacing or DC cardioversion may also be used. Many patients are now being treated by catheter ablation to destroy the abnormal atrionodal pathway and avoid the need for long-term drug therapy (see below).

Wolff–Parkinson–White syndrome (WPW)

This congenital disorder, affecting 0.12% of the population, is caused by an accessory pathway (bundle of Kent) between the atria and ventricles. During sinus rhythm, atrial impulses conduct more rapidly through the accessory pathway than the atrioventricular node such that the initial phase of ventricular depolarization occurs early (pre-excitation) and spreads slowly through the ventricles by abnormal pathways. This produces a short PR interval and slurring of the initial QRS deflection (delta wave). The remainder of ventricular depolarization, however, is rapid because the the delayed arrival of the impulse conducted through the atrioventricular node rapidly completes ventricular depolarization by normal His–Purkinje pathways (Fig. 6.22). Cardiac arrhythmias affect about 60% of patients with Wolff–Parkinson–White syndrome and are usually re-entrant (rate 150–250 beats per minute) triggered by an atrial premature beat (Fig. 6.23). In most patients the re-entry arrhythmia is 'orthodromic', with anterograde conduction through the atrioventricular node and retrograde conduction through the accessory pathway. This results in a narrow complex tachycardia (without pre-excitation) that is indistinguishable from AVJRT. Occasionally, the re-entry circuit is in the opposite direction ('antidromic'), producing a very broad, pre-excited tachycardia.

Patients with Wolff–Parkinson–White syndrome are more prone than the general population to atrial fibrillation. If the accessory pathway is able to conduct the fibrillatory impulses rapidly to the ventricles, it may result in ventricular fibrillation and sudden death. Digoxin (and to a lesser extent verapamil) should be avoided because it shortens the refractory period of the accessory pathway and can heighten the risk. Patients with dangerous accessory pathways of this type require ablation of the pathway either surgically or, preferably, by catheter techniques. Ablation therapy is also being used increasingly in patients with frequent re-entry arrhythmias which, though not dangerous, are often very troublesome.

DIAGNOSIS OF VENTRICULAR ARRHYTHMIAS
Ventricular premature beats

These may occur in normal individuals either spontaneously or in response to toxic stimuli such as caffeine or sympathomimetic drugs. They are caused by the premature discharge of a ventricular ectopic

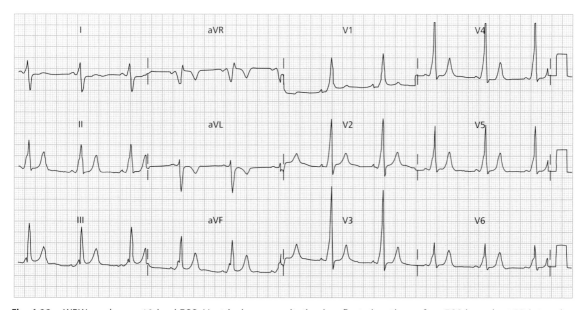

Fig. 6.22 WPW syndrome: 12-lead ECG. Ventricular pre-excitation is reflected on the surface ECG by a short PR interval and a slurred upstroke to the QRS complex (delta wave). The remainder of the QRS complex is normal because delayed arrival of the impulse conducted through the AV node rapidly completes ventricular depolarization through normal His–Purkinje pathways.

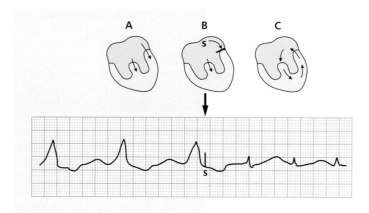

Fig. 6.23 Wolff–Parkinson–White syndrome—re-entry tachycardia recorded at fast paper speed. Just after the third pre-excited (broad) complex a premature atrial pacing stimulus (S) initiates an impulse that is blocked in the bundle of Kent but is conducted normally through the AV node producing ventricular depolarization without pre-excitation. Thus the QRS complex is narrow and lacks a delta wave. The impulse is conducted retrogradely through the bundle of Kent, re-enters the proximal conducting system, and completes the re-entry circuit, initiating a self-sustaining orthodromic re-entry tachycardia (last three complexes).

focus which produces an early and broad QRS complex (Fig. 6.24). The premature impulse may be conducted backwards into the atria, producing a retrograde P wave, but penetration of the sinus node is rare. Thus, resetting of the sinus node does not usually occur and there is a fully compensatory pause before the next sinus beat.

Ventricular tachycardia

This is always pathological. It is defined as three or more consecutive ventricular beats at a rate above 120 per minute. Ventricular depolarization inevitably occurs slowly by abnormal pathways, producing a broad QRS complex. This distinguishes it from most atrial and junctional tachycardias which have a narrow QRS complex, although differential diagnosis may be more difficult for atrial or junctional tachycardias with a broad QRS complex caused by rate-related or pre-existing bundle branch block (Fig. 6.25). Nevertheless, ventricular tachycardia can usually be identified by careful scrutiny of the 12-lead ECG (Fig. 6.26). *Support* for the diagnosis is provided by a very broad QRS complex (>140 ms), extreme left or right axis deviation, concordance of the QRS deflections in V_1–V_6 (either all positive or all negative), and configurational features of the QRS complex, including an 'rSR' complex in V_1 and a QS complex in V_6. *Confirmation* of the

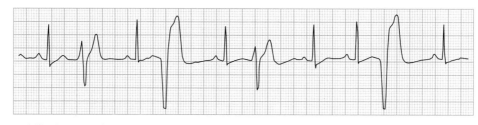

Fig. 6.24 Multifocal, ventricular ectopic beats. Frequent broad complex ectopic beats are seen early after the sinus beats. Note, however, that the ectopic beats have two different morphologies, indicating that they arise from different foci. Note also that the coupling interval (interval between QRS complex and ectopic beat) is identical for beats arising from any particular focus.

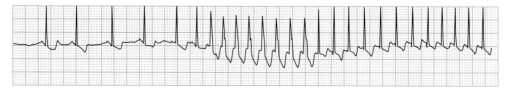

Fig. 6.25 Paroxysmal AV nodal re-entrant tachycardia. This Holter recording shows sinus rhythm giving way to a broad complex tachycardia. However, this is clearly the result of temporary bundle branch block because it converts spontaneously to a narrow complex tachycardia confirming that the arrhythmia is junctional not ventricular in origin.

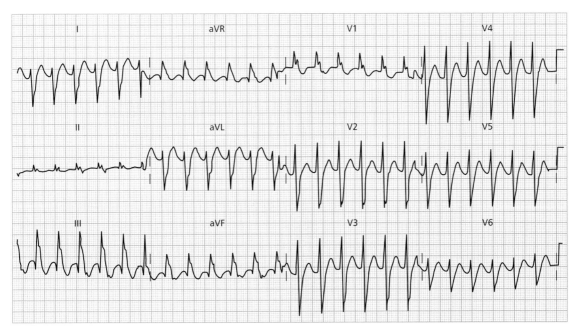

Fig. 6.26 Ventricular tachycardia: 12-lead ECG. The recording shows a broad complex tachycardia. The following features suggest or confirm the ventricular origin of the tachycardia: very broad QRS complex (> 140ms); extreme right axis deviation; atrioventricular dissociation—note the dissociated P waves seen clearly in leads II and V_1; the 'rSR' complex in V_1.

diagnosis is provided by any evidence of AV dissociation: either P waves, at a slower rate than the QRS complexes, 'marching through' the tachycardia (Fig. 6.27(a)), or ventricular capture and/or fusion beats, in which the dissociated atrial rhythm penetrates the ventricle by conduction through the AV node and interrupts the tachycardia, producing sometimes a normal ventricular complex (capture, Fig. 6.27(a)) or, more commonly, a broad hybrid complex (fusion) that is part sinus and part ventricular in

origin (Fig. 6.27(b)). *Torsades de pointes*, a broad complex tachycardia with changing wavefronts, also provides unequivocal evidence of ventricular tachycardia and is particularly characteristic of the arrhythmia that complicates long QT syndrome, often resulting in sudden death. The syndrome may be inherited as an autosomal dominant (Romano–Ward syndrome) or as an autosomal recessive (Lange–Nielsen syndrome) trait, when it is associated with congenital deafness.

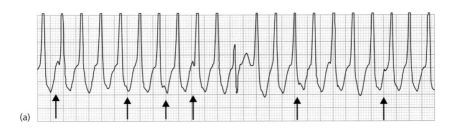

(a)

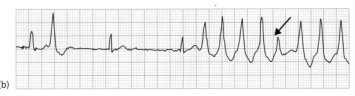

(b)

Fig. 6.27(a) Ventricular tachycardia: AV dissociation. P waves (arrowed) can be seen 'marching through' the tachycardia, confirming its ventricular origin. The tachycardia is interrupted by a narrow capture beat.

Fig. 6.27(b) Ventricular tachycardia: fusion. In this example VT is initiated by a very early ventricular ectopic beat (morphologically similar to the previous isolated ectopic beat) and is interrupted by a fusion beat (arrowed) confirming the ventricular origin of the tachycardia.

Ventricular fibrillation

This occurs most commonly in severe myocardial ischaemia, either with or without frank infarction. It is a completely disorganized arrhythmia characterized by irregular fibrillatory waves with no discernible QRS complexes. There is no effective cardiac output and death is inevitable unless resuscitation with direct current cardioversion is instituted rapidly.

DIAGNOSIS OF SINOATRIAL DISEASE
(Fig 6.28 and Box 6.11)

Sinus node discharge is not itself visible on the surface ECG, but the atrial depolarization it triggers produces the P wave. The spontaneous discharge of the normal sinus node is influenced by a variety of neurohumoral factors, particularly vagal and sympathetic activity which respectively slow and quicken the heart rate. In *sinoatrial disease*, sinus node discharge may be abnormally slow, blocked (with failure to activate atrial depolarization), or absent altogether (Box 6.12). Under these circumstances the sinus rate may be very slow, the atrium may fibrillate or pacemaker function may be assumed by foci lower in the atrium, the atrioventricular node or the His–Purkinje conducting tissue in the ventricles. The intrinsic rate of these 'escape' pacemaker foci is slower than the normal sinus rate.

Sinus bradycardia (less than 50 beats per minutes)

This is physiological during sleep and in trained athletes but in other circumstances often reflects sinoatrial disease, particularly when the heart rate fails to increase normally with exercise.

Sinoatrial block

If the sinus impulse is blocked and fails to trigger atrial depolarization, a pause occurs in the ECG. No P wave is seen during the pause owing to the absence of atrial depolarization. The electrically 'silent' sinus discharge, however, continues uninterrupted. Thus the pause is always a precise multiple of preceding P–P intervals. Sinoatrial block that cannot be abolished by atropine-induced vagal inhibition usually indicates sinoatrial disease, particularly with pauses longer than 2 seconds.

Sinus arrest

Failure of sinus node discharge produces a pause on the ECG that bears no relation to the preceding P–P interval. Pauses longer than 2 seconds are usually pathological. Prolonged pauses are often terminated by an escape beat from a 'junctional' focus in the bundle of His.

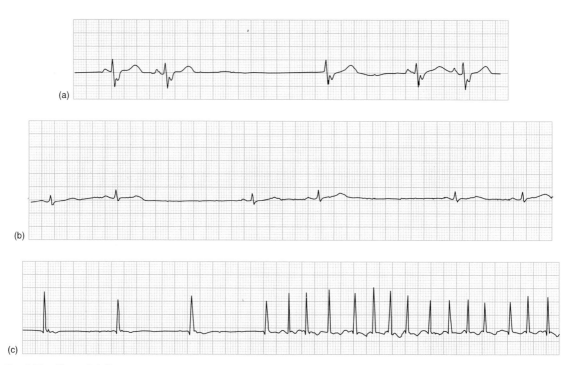

Fig. 6.28 Sinoatrial disease.
(a) Sinus arrest with late junctional escape. After the second sinus beat there is a long pause interrupted by a single junctional escape beat before sinus rhythm is re-established.
(b) Sinoatrial block. Pauses after the second and fourth complexes are the result of sinoatrial block which has prevented sinus impulses from depolarizing the atrium. No P waves are seen but, because the sinus discharge continues uninterrupted, the pauses are each a precise multiple of the preceding PP interval. Sinoatrial block is probably rare.
(c) Bradycardia–tachycardia syndrome. A slow junctional rhythm gives way to rapid atrial fibrillation.

BOX 6.11   Sinoatrial disease.

Typical patient
- Elderly, often with no previous cardiac history

Major symptoms
- Intermittent syncopal or presyncopal attacks
- Patients may also complain of exertional fatgue (chronotropic incompetence) or palpitations (tachycardia—bradycardia syndrome)

Major signs
- Often none
- Sometimes sinus bradycardia or slow atrial fibrillation

Diagnosis
- *ECG*: Often normal. May show sinus bradycardia or slow atrial fibrillation
- *Ambulatory ECG*: 24 hour Holter recording may show pauses diagnostic of sinoatrial disease

Additional investigations
- None

Comments
- Documentation of the sinus pauses (or very slow AF) during an attack of symptoms provides the most robust diagnostic information

BOX 6.12   Causes of sinoatrial disease.

Acute
- Myocardial infarction
- Coronary artery disease
- Drugs (e.g. beta-blockers, digitalis)
- Hypothermia
- Atrial surgery

Chronic
- Idiopathic fibrotic disease
- Congenital heart disease
- Ischaemic heart disease
- Amyloid

Bradycardidia–tachycardia syndrome

In this syndrome atrial bradycardias are interspersed by paroxysmal tachyarrhythmias, usually atrial fibrillation. Nevertheless, it is the bradycardia that usually causes symptoms, particularly dizzy attacks and blackouts.

DIAGNOSIS OF ATRIOVENTRICULAR BLOCK

In *atrioventricular block* (Fig. 6.29), conduction is delayed or completely interrupted, either in the atrioventricular node or in the bundle branches (Box 6.13). When conduction is merely delayed (e.g. first-degree atrioventricular block, bundle branch block), the heart rate is unaffected. When conduction is completely interrupted, however, the heart rate may slow sufficiently to produce symptoms. In second-

BOX 6.13   Causes of atrioventricular heart block.

Acute
- Myocardial infarction
- Drugs (e.g. beta-blockers, verapamil, digitalis, adenosine)
- Surgical or catheter ablation of the His bundle

Chronic
- Idiopathic fibrosis of both bundle branches
- Ischaemic heart disease
- Congenital heart disease
- Calcific aortic valve disease
- Chagas' disease
- Infiltrative disease (amyloid haemochromatosis)
- Granulomatous disease (sarcoid, tuberculosis)

degree atrioventricular block, failure of conduction is, by definition, intermittent, and if sufficient sinus impulses are conducted to maintain an adequate ventricular rate symptoms may be avoided. In third-degree atrioventricular block there is complete failure of conduction and continuing ventricular activity depends on the emergence of an escape rhythm. If the block is within the atrioventricular node the escape rhythm usually arises from a focus just below the node in the bundle of His (junctional escape), and is often fast enough to prevent symptoms. If both bundle branches are blocked, however, the escape rhythm must arise from a focus lower in the ventricles. Ventricular escape rhythms of this type are nearly always associated with symptoms because they are not only very slow but also unreliable, and may stop altogether, producing prolonged asystole.

First-degree atrioventricular block

Delayed atrioventricular conduction causes prolongation of the PR interval (> 0.20 seconds). Ventricular depolarization occurs rapidly by normal His–Purkinje pathways and the QRS complex is usually narrow.

Second-degree atrioventricular block: Mobitz type I (Wenckebach).

This occurs commonly in inferior myocardial infarction. Successive sinus beats find the atrioventricular node increasingly refractory until failure of conduction occurs. The delay permits recovery of nodal function and the process may then repeat itself. The ECG shows progressive prolongation of the PR interval, culminating in a dropped beat. Block is within the atrioventricular node itself and ventricular depolarization occurs rapidly by normal pathways. Thus the QRS complex is usually narrow.

Second-degree atrioventricular block: Mobitz type II

This always indicates advanced conducting tissue disease affecting the bundle branches. The ECG

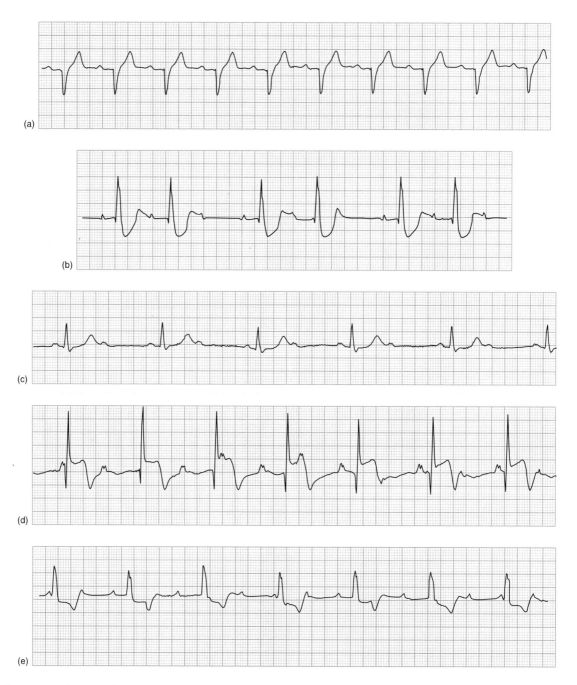

Fig. 6.29   Atrioventricular conducting tissue disease.

(a) 1° AV block. Delayed AV conduction causes a prolonged PR interval (greater than 0.20 s).

(b) 2° AV block—Wenckebach type. This is also called Mobitz type I block and occurs within the AV node. Three Wenckebach cycles are shown. Successive sinus beats find the AV node increasingly refractory until failure of conduction occurs. This delay permits recovery of nodal function and the process repeats itself.

(c) 2° AV block at bundle branch level (Mobitz type II). This is standard lead I. Note the PR interval of conducted beats is normal but the QRS complex shows right bundle branch block. Intermittent block in the left bundle results in failure of conduction of alternate P waves.

(d) 3° (complete) AV block at level of AV node. In this patient with acute inferior myocardial infarction, there is complete failure of AV conduction as reflected by the dissociated atrial and ventricular rhythms. Note the regular P waves and the regular slower QRS complexes occurring independently of one another. Because block is at the level of the AV node a junctional escape rhythm has taken over with a narrow QRS complex.

(e) 3° (complete) AV block at bundle branch level. The atrial and ventricular rhythms are dissociated because none of the atrial impulses are conducted. The ECG shows regular P waves and regular but slower QRS complexes. Because the escape rhythm is ventricular in origin the QRS complexes are broad and the rate is slow.

typically shows a normal PR interval with bundle branch block in conducted beats, intermittent block in the other bundle branch resulting in complete failure of atrioventricular conduction and dropped beats.

Third-degree (complete) atrioventricular block

The atrial and ventricular rhythms are 'dissociated' because none of the atrial impulses are conducted. Thus the ECG shows regular P waves (unless the atrium is fibrillating) and regular but slower QRS complexes occurring independently of each other. When block is within the atrioventricular node (e.g. inferior myocardial infarction, congenital atrioventricular block), a junctional escape rhythm with a reliable rate (40–60 beats per minute) takes over (see Fig. 6.29). Ventricular depolarization occurs rapidly by normal pathways, producing a narrow QRS complex. However, when block is within the bundle branches (e.g. idiopathic fibrosis) there is always extensive conducting tissue disease. The ventricular escape rhythm is slow and unreliable, with a broad QRS complex (Fig. 6.29).

Right bundle branch block

This may be a congenital defect but is more commonly the result of organic conducting tissue disease. Right ventricular depolarization is delayed, resulting in a broad QRS complex with an 'rSR' pattern in lead V_1 and prominent S waves in leads I and V_6.

Left bundle branch block

This always indicates organic conducting tissue disease. The entire sequence of ventricular depolarization is abnormal, resulting in a broad QRS complex with large slurred or notched R waves in leads I and V_6.

THE CHEST X-RAY

Good-quality posteroanterior (PA) and lateral chest X-rays are always helpful in the assessment of the cardiac patient (Fig. 6.30).

CARDIAC SILHOUETTE

Though the PA chest X-ray exhibits a wide range of normality, the transverse diameter of the heart should not exceed 50% of that of the lung fields. Cardiac enlargement is caused either by dilatation of the cardiac chambers or by pericardial effusion (Fig. 6.31). Myocardial hypertrophy only affects heart size if very severe.

Ventricular dilatation

The PA chest X-ray does not reliably distinguish left from right ventricular dilatation. For this, the lateral chest X-ray is more helpful. Dilatation of the post-

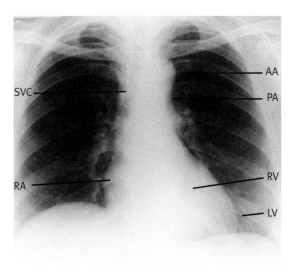

Fig. 6.30   Normal chest X-ray: posteroanterior projection. Note the heart is not enlarged (cardiothoracic ratio less than 50%) and the lung fields are clear.
SVC = superior vena cava. RA = right atrium. AA = aortic arch. LV = left ventricle. PA = pulmonary artery. RV = right ventricle.

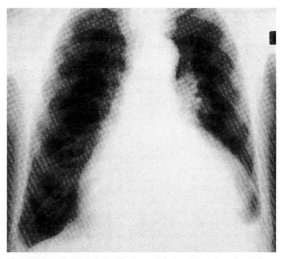

Fig. 6.31   Pericardial effusion with tamponade: chest X-ray. There is a left hilar mass caused by carcinoma. Pericardial infiltration has produced effusion and tamponade evidenced by the severe cardiac enlargement. Malignant disease is now the most common cause of tamponade in most developed countries.

eriorly located left ventricle encroaches on the retrocardiac space, while dilatation of the anteriorly located right ventricle encroaches on the retrosternal space.

Atrial dilatation

Right atrial dilatation is usually due to right ventricular failure but occurs as an isolated finding in tricuspid stenosis and Ebstein's anomaly. It produces cardiac enlargement without specific radiographic signs.

Left atrial dilatation occurs in left ventricular failure and mitral valve diseae (Fig. 6.32). Radiographic signs are:

- Flattening and later bulging of the left heart border below the main pulmonary artery
- Elevation of the left main bronchus, with widening of the carina
- Appearance of the medial border of the left atrium behind the right side of the heart (double-density sign).

Vascular dilatation

Aortic dilatation caused by aneurysm or dissection may produce widening of the entire upper mediastinum. Localized dilatation of the proximal aorta occurs in aortic valve disease and produces a prominence in the right upper mediastinum (Fig. 6.33). Dilatation of the main pulmonary artery occurs in pulmonary hypertension and pulmonary stenosis and produces a prominence in the right upper mediastinum. Dilatation of the main pulmonary artery occurs in pulmonary hypertension and pulmonary stenosis and produces a prominence below the aortic knuckle (Fig. 6.34).

Intracardiac calcification

Because the radiodensity of cardiac tissue is similar to that of blood, intracardiac structures can rarely be identified unless they are calcified. Valvar, pericardial or myocardial calcification may occur, and usually indicates important disease of these structures. Calcification is best appreciated on the deeply penetrated lateral chest X-ray.

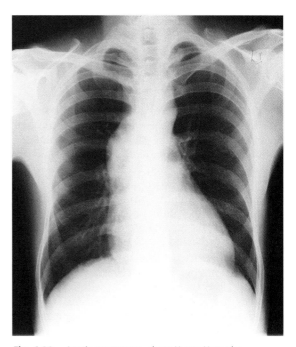

Fig. 6.33 Aortic aneurysm: chest X-ray. Note the dilatation of the ascending aorta in this patient with Marfan's syndrome.

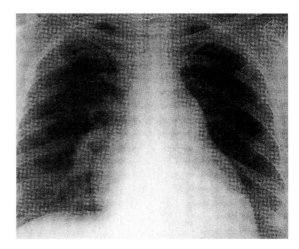

Fig. 6.34 Pulmonary hypertension caused by chronic pulmonary embolic disease. The chest X-ray shows cardiac enlargement (caused by right ventricular dilatation) with dilatation of the main pulmonary artery. The lung fields are relatively oligaemic reflecting reduced pulmonary flow.

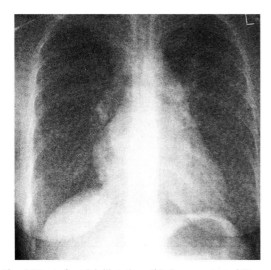

Fig. 6.32 Left atrial dilatation. This is a penetrated PA chest X-ray in a patient with mitral stenosis. The dilated, posteriorly located left atrium is clearly visible. Note flattening of the left heart border, the widening of the carina and the double-density sign at the right heart border.

LUNG FIELDS

Common lung field abnormalities in cardiovascular disease are caused either by altered pulmonary flow or by increased left atrial pressure.

Altered pulmonary flow

Increments in pulmonary flow sufficient to cause radiographic abnormalities are caused by left-to-right intracardiac shunts (e.g. atrial septal defect, Fig. 6.35), ventricular septal defect, patent ductus arteriosus). Prominence of the vascular markings gives the lung fields a plethoric appearance. Reductions in pulmonary flow, on the other hand, cause reduced vascular markings. This may be regional (e.g. pulmonary embolism) or global (e.g. severe pulmonary hypertension, see Fig. 6.34).

Increased left atrial pressure

This occurs in mitral stenosis and left ventricular failure and produces corresponding rises in pulmonary venous and pulmonary capillary pressures. Prominence of the upper lobe veins is an early radiographic finding. As the left atrial and pulmonary capillary pressures rise above 18 mmHg, transudation into the lung produces interstitial pulmonary oedema, characterized by prominence of the interlobular septa, particularly at the lung bases (Kerley B lines). Further elevation of pressure leads to alveolar pulmonary oedema characterized by perihilar 'bat's wing' shadowing (Fig. 6.36).

Other lung field abnormalities

Pulmonary infarction

Localized and typically wedge-shaped areas of consolidation are occasionally seen in pulmonary embolic disease, although more often the bronchial circulation protects against ischaemic damage.

Pneumonic consolidation and abscess

In patients with right sided endocarditis infected pulmonary emboli commonly cause septic foci within the lung fields.

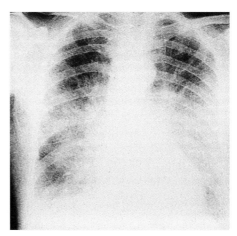

Fig. 6.36   Chest X-ray in acute left ventricular failure: the patient had severe pulmonary oedema caused by acute myocardial infarction. The heart is not yet enlarged but there is prominent alveolar pulmonary oedema in a perihilar ('bat's-wing') distribution. Note the bilateral pleural effusions.

Interstitial lung disease

In longstanding pulmonary hypertension complicating rheumatic mitral valve disease, haemosiderosis (stippled shadowing throughout the lung fields) was once a common X-ray finding. It is now rarely seen.

BONY ABNORMALITIES

Bony abnormalities are unusual in cardiovascular disease, apart from coarctation of the aorta and thoracic outlet syndromes. In coarctation, dilated bronchial collateral vessels erode the inferior aspect of the ribs to produce notches although they are rarely present before adolescence. Cervical ribs may compress the neurovascular bundle in the thoracic outlet, and special thoracic outlet views are necessary for radiographic diagnosis.

ECHOCARDIOGRAPHY

Echocardiography is one of the most versatile non-invasive imaging techniques in clinical cardiology. Because it does not utilize ionizing radiation, it is free of known risk and can be used safely throughout pregnancy. Transthoracic imaging with the transducer applied to the chest wall is usually satisfactory, but better quality information is obtained by the transoesophageal approach in which the transducer is mounted on a probe and positioned in the oesophagus, directly behind the heart. This provides better quality images because there are no intervening ribs or lung tissue and the probe is closely applied to the posterior aspect of the heart. It is particularly useful for imaging the left atrium, aorta and prosthetic heart valves.

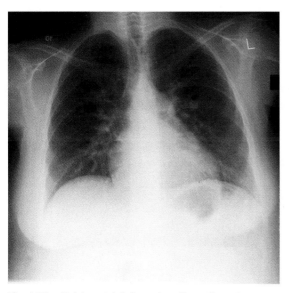

Fig. 6.35   Atrial septal defect: chest X-ray. Note the prominent proximal pulmonary arteries and the pulmonary plethora reflecting increased pulmonary flow.

PRINCIPLES

Physics

A transducer containing a piezoelectric element converts electrical energy into an ultrasound beam which can be directed towards the heart. The beam is reflected when it strikes an interface between tissues of different density. The reflected ultrasound, or *echo*, is converted back to electrical energy by the piezoelectric element, which permits construction of an image using two basic units of information:

- The *intensity* of the echoes which defines the density difference at tissue interfaces within the heart
- The *time* taken for echoes to arrive back at the transducer which defines distance of the cardiac structures from the transducer.

Density differences within the heart are greatest between the blood-filled chambers and the myocardial and valvular tissues, all of which are clearly visible on the echocardiogram. Because the depth of the myocardial and valvular tissues with respect to the transducer changes constantly throughout the cardiac cycle, the time taken for echo reflection changes accordingly. Thus, real-time imaging throughout the cardiac cycle provides a dynamic record of cardiac function.

M-mode echocardiogram (Fig. 6.37(a))

This provides a unidimensional 'ice-pick' view through the heart. Continuous recording on photographic paper provides an additional time dimension, thereby permitting appreciation of the dynamic component of the cardiac image. By convention, cardiac structures closest to the transducer are displayed at the top of the record and more distant structures are displayed below. Thus, on the transthoracic M-mode echocardiogram, anteriorly located ('right-sided') structures lie above the posteriorly located ('left-sided') structures, but on the transoesophageal echocardiogram the display is reversed.

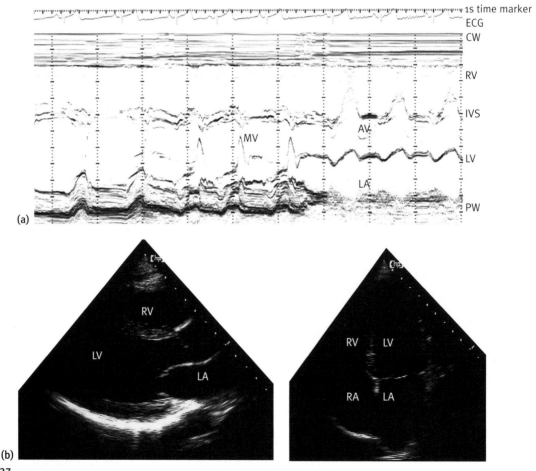

Fig. 6.37

(a) M-mode echocardiography. The figure shows a sweep as the transducer is angulated from the left ventricle to the aortic root.

(b) Transthoracic 2D echocardiography. Parasternal long axis and apical 4 chamber views are shown.

The dots are a 1 cm scale. CW = chest wall. RV = right ventricle. IVS = interventricular septum. LV = left ventricle. PW = posterior LV wall. MV = mitral valve. AV = aortic valve. LA = left atrium.

Two-dimensional echocardiogram (Fig. 6.37(b))
This provides more detailed information about morphology than the M-mode recording. By projecting a fan of echoes in an arc of up to 80°, a two-dimensional 'slice' through the heart can be obtained, the precise view depending on the location and angulation of the transducer.

CLINICAL APPLICATIONS

Congenital heart disease
Echocardiography, particularly the two-dimensional technique, has revolutionized the diagnosis of congenital heart disease, in the majority of cases obviating the need for invasive investigation by cardiac catheterization (Fig. 6.38). The relationships of the cardiac chambers and their connections with the great vessels are readily determined. Valvular abnormalities and septal defects can also be recognized. Recent technology has permitted in utero fetal imaging for the antenatal diagnosis of cardiac defects.

Myocardial disease
Echocardiography permits accurate assessment of cardiac dilatation, hypertrophy and contractile function. Congestive cardiomyopathy produces ventricular dilatation with *global* contractile impairment (Fig. 6.39). This must be distinguished from the *regional* contractile impairment which follows myocardial infarction in patients with coronary artery disease (Fig. 6.40). Hypertrophic cardiomyopathy is characterized by thickening (hypertrophy) of the left ventricular myocardium, usually with disproportionate involvement of the interventricular septum (asymmetric septal hypertrophy). In aortic and hypertensive heart disease, on the other hand, left ventricular hypertrophy is usually symmetrical (Fig. 6.41).

Valvular disease (Boxes 6.14–6.17)
Echocardiography is of particular value for identifying both structural and dynamic valvular abnormalities and any associated chamber dilatation or hypertrophy. The severity of valvular involvement in congenital, rheumatic, degenerative and infective disease may thus be defined; the technique is diagnostic of bicuspid aortic valve and mitral valve prolapse, and readily identifies valve thickening and calcification in rheumatic and calcific disease (Figs 6.41, 6.42). Vegetations in infective endocarditis can usually be visualized if they are large enough (> 3 mm, Fig. 6.43). The transoesophageal approach is usually necessary for endocarditis involving prosthetic heart valves.

Pericardial disease
Although the echocardiogram is of little value in constrictive pericarditis, it is the most sensitive technique

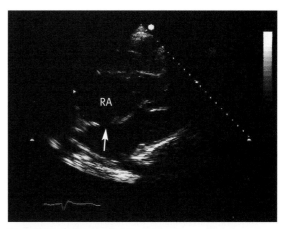

Fig. 6.38 Atrial septal defect: 2D echocardiogram (subcostal view). In this view, good views of the interatrial septum can usually be obtained without resorting to transoesophageal echocardiography. Note the ASD (arrowed) and the dilatation of the right atrium (RA).

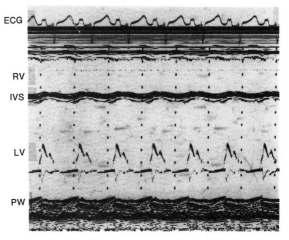

Fig. 6.39 Dilated cardiomyopathy: echocardiogram. This M-mode study shows severe dilatation of the left ventricular cavity with severe global contractile impairment. The patient later underwent successful heart transplantation.

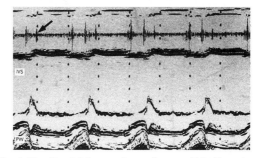

Fig. 6.40 Heart failure: echocardiogram. This M-mode study shows considerable dilatation of the left ventricle. Note that the interventricular septum (IVS) is almost akinetic, but the posterior wall (PW) is contracting normally. Regional contractile impairment of this type indicates coronary heart disease. The phonocardiogram recorded simultaneously shows normal first and second heart sounds and also a third heart sound (arrowed).

BOX 6.14   Aortic stenosis.

Typical patient
- Middle-aged (congenitally bicuspid valve) or elderly (degenerative calcific disease) man or woman

Major symptoms
- Exertional shortness of breath is usual presenting symptom
- Angina may also occur and, in advanced cases, syncopal attacks or sudden death

Major signs
- *Carotid pulse*: slow upstroke with plateau
- *Auscultation*: fourth heart sound at cardiac apex; ejection systolic murmur at base of heart radiating to neck. The murmur may be preceded by an ejection click if the valve is mobile and not heavily calcified

Diagnosis
- *ECG*: left ventricular hypertrophy
- *CXR*: dilatation of ascending aorta
- *Echocardiogram*: calcified immobile aortic valve with left ventricular hypertrophy. Doppler studies permit quantification of the severity of stenosis

Additional investigations
- Cardiac catheterization is necessary to evelute coronary arteries in patients being considered for aortic valve replacement surgery

Comments
- Aortic stenosis is now the commonest acquired valve lesion in developed countries

BOX 6.15   Aortic regurgitation.

Typical patient
- Young men (Marfan's syndrome, etc.) or older patients (long-standing hypertension) with dilating disease of the aortic root

Major symptoms
- Exertional shortness of breath is usual presenting symptom
- Angina may also occur.

Major signs
- *Carotid pulse*: sharp upstroke with early diastolic collapse
- *Blood pressure*: systolic hypertension with wide pulse pressure
- *Auscultation*: early diastolic murmur at left sternal edge. Third heart sound at cardiac apex in severe cases. Mid-diastolic murmur (Austin Flint) may be heard at apex due to preclosure of mitral valve by regurgitant jet

BOX 6.15   (continued)

Diagnosis
- *ECG*: left ventricular hypertrophy
- *CXR*: cardiac enlargement with dilatation of ascending aorta
- *Echocardiogram*: often normal valve with dilated aortic root. Doppler studies confirm regurgitant jet

Additional investigations
- Cardiac catheterization is necessary to evelute coronary arteries in older patients (> 50) being considered for aortic valve replacement surgery

Comments
- The timing of valve replacement surgery is difficult but should anticipate irreversible left ventricular contractile failure

BOX 6.16   Mitral stenosis.

Typical patient
- Young to middle-aged woman with history of rheumatic fever in childhood

Major symptoms
- Exertional shortness of breath with orthopnoea in advanced cases
- Palpitations commonly signal the development of atrial fibrillation which puts patient at serious risk of peripheral embolism and stroke

Major signs
- *Pulse*: atrial fibrillation in many cases
- *Auscultation*: Loud S1 with early diastolic opening snap followed by low-pitched mid-diastolic murmur best heard at cardiac apex. If the patient is in sinus rhythm, there is presystolic accentuation of the murmur

Diagnosis
- *ECG*: atrial fibrillation usually
- *CXR*: Signs of left atrial enlargement (flat left heart border, widening of carenal angle, and double density sign at right heart border. Pulmonary congestion
- *Echocardiogram*: rheumatic mitral valve and left atrial dilatation. Doppler studies confirm diastolic jet

Additional investigations
- Cardiac catheterization is necessary to evelute coronary arteries in patients aged > 50 being considered for mitral valve replacement surgery

Comments
- In patients with atrial fibrillation, anticoagulation with warfarin is mandatory to protect against stroke

BOX 6.17   Mitral regurgitation.

Typical patient
- Mitral valve prolapse (floppy mitral valve) causes regurgitation of variable severity and more commonly affects women at almost any age
- Patients with subvalvar disease (papillary muscle dysfunction or chordal rupture) are usually elderly men or women

Major symptoms
- Exertional shortness of breath with orthopnoea in advanced cases
- Palpitations commonly signal the development of atrial fibrillation which puts patient at serious risk of peripheral embolism and stroke

Major signs
- *Pulse*: often sinus rhythm but may be atrial fibrillation
- *Auscultation*: pansystolic murmur at cardiac apex, radiating to axilla. Often associated with third heart sound

Diagnosis
- *ECG*: atrial fibrillation, but may be normal
- *CXR*: cardiac enlargement with variable signs of left atrial enlargement, though these are usually less marked than in mitral stenosis. Pulmonary congestion in severe cases
- *Echocardiogram*: prolapsing (floppy) mitral valve may be seen; in subvalvar disease, the valve often appears normal. Left ventricular and left atrial dilatation. Doppler studies confirm regurgitant jet

Additional investigations
- Cardiac catheterization is necessary to evalute coronary arteries in patients aged > 50 being considered for mitral valve replacement surgery

Comments
- In patients with atrial fibrillation, anticoagulation with warfarin is mandatory to protect against stroke

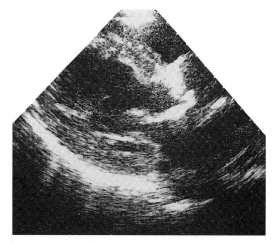

Fig. 6.41   Aortic stenosis and left ventricular hypertrophy: 2D echocardiogram (long axis view). The aortic valve is grossly thickened and highly echogenic. Concentric LV hypertrophy is present.

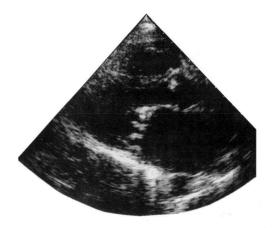

Fig. 6.42   Mitral stenosis: 2D echocardiogram (parasternal long axis view). The mitral valve leaflets are densely thickened (arrowed) and the left atrium is severely dilated.

available for the diagnosis of pericardial effusion (Fig. 6.44). The effusion appears as an echo-free space distributed around the ventricles but usually avoiding the potential space behind the left atrium.

Other clinical applications

Intracardiac tumours, particularly myxomas and thrombi, are readily visualized by echocardiography (see Fig. 6.1); and the oesophageal instrument has found important application for identifying thrombus in the left atrial appendage (Fig. 6.45). The oesophageal technique is also helpful for diagnosing aortic disease such as aneurysm and dissection since it provides better views of the thoracic aorta than are possible with conventional 2D echocardiography (Fig. 6.46). The application of stress echocardiography for diagnosis of coronary

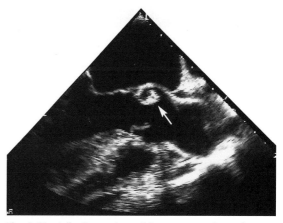

Fig. 6.43   Infective endocarditis: transoesophageal echocardiogram. A vegetation (arrowed) is adherent to the aortic valve leaflet.

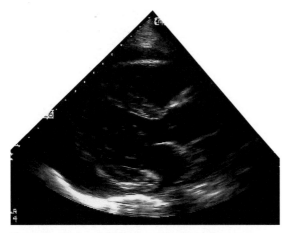

Fig. 6.44 Pericardial effusion: 2D echocardiogram (parasternal long axis view). Note the echo-free space around the heart, but not behind the left atrium.

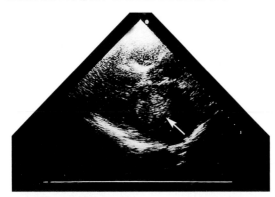

Fig. 6.45 Mitral stenosis: 2D echocardiogram (long axis view). The left atrium (LA) is severely dilated and a large thrombus (arrowed) is visible, emphasizing the importance of anticoagulation in patients with mitral valve disease and atrial fibrillation.

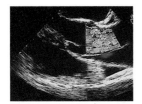 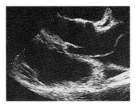

Fig. 6.46 Aortic dissection—transoesophageal echocardiogram. Right panel: this longitudinal axis transoesophageal echocardiogram reveals the dilated aortic root and an S-shaped flap traversing the lumen. Left panel: same patient with colour Doppler superimposed to show flow in the true lumen.

artery disease is currently investigational. Pharmacological stress with dobutamine is usually used, patients with coronary artery disease showing regional wall motion abnormality in response to the inotropic stimulus. A potentially interesting development of the technique is its potential for identifying 'hibernating' (and therefore potentially salvageable) myocardium in patients with previous coronary occlusions.

DOPPLER ECHOCARDIOGRAPHY

Doppler echocardiography permits evaluation of the direction and velocity of blood flow within the heart and great vessels. It is widely used for measuring the severity of valvular stenosis and identifying valvular regurgitation and intracardiac shunts through septal defects.

PRINCIPLES

Physics

According to the Doppler principle, when an ultrasound beam is directed towards the bloodstream the frequency of the ultrasound reflected from the blood cells is altered. The frequency shift or Doppler effect is related to the direction and velocity of flow. If continuous wave Doppler is used, blood flow at any point along the path of the ultrasound beam is detected, such that a 'clean' Doppler signal from the area of interest may be difficult to obtain. Pulsed Doppler, however, has a range-gating facility which permits frequency sampling from any specific point within the heart, pre-selected on the echocardiogram. This lends greater precision to the technique. Nevertheless, pulsed Doppler is less able than continuous wave Doppler to quantify very high velocity jets, such as those that occur in aortic stenosis.

Colour-flow mapping

This has been a major technological advance. Instead of the unidirectional ultrasound beam used in continuous wave and pulsed Doppler imaging, the beam is rotated through an arc. Frequency sampling throughout the arc permits construction of a colour-coded map, red indicating flow towards, and blue away from, the transducer. Colour flow data can be superimposed on the standard 2D-echocardiogram to identify precisely the patterns of flow within the four chambers of the heart. This simplifies the interpretation of Doppler imaging and provides more useful qualitative data, although it is less useful for quantitative assessment of valve gradients which requires the precision of conventional Doppler technique.

CLINICAL APPLICATIONS

In paediatric cardiology, the combination of 2D-echocardiography and colour-flow Doppler mapping has made possible the 'non-invasive' diagnosis of the large majority of congenital defects, often without the need for cardiac catheterization. These techniques have also revolutionized the diagnosis of valvular disease in all age groups. In valvular regurgitation, the retrograde flow that occurs after valve closure is readily detected by Doppler echocardiography, although only an approximate estimate of its severity is possible (Fig. 6.47). In valvular stenosis, peak velocity (as opposed to volume) of flow across the valve is directly related to the degree of stenosis. Thus measurement of Doppler flow velocity (ideally by continuous wave) permits quantification of stenosis by the application of the Bernoulli equation:

$$\text{pressure gradient} = 4 \times \text{velocity}^2.$$

CARDIOVASCULAR RADIONUCLIDE IMAGING

PRINCIPLES

All radionuclide techniques require the internal administration of a radioisotope; the distribution of radioactivity in the area of interest is then imaged with a gamma camera. Ideally, the isotope should be distributed homogeneously in that part of the cardiovascular system under investigation: thus, isotopes that remain in the intravascular space during imaging are used for radionuclide angiography. In myocardial perfusion scintigraphy, however, isotopes taken up by the myocardium are required. Because of their potential toxicity, isotopes with a short half-life are usually used.

CLINICAL APPLICATIONS

Radionuclide ventriculography

This method is used for assessment of ventricular function. Red cells labelled with technetium-99m are allowed to equilibrate in the blood pool and the heart is then imaged under the gamma camera (Fig. 6.48). The waxing and waning of radioactivity within the ventricular chambers during diastole and systole, respectively, permits construction of a dynamic ventriculogram. Left ventricular contractile function can be evaluated quantitatively, by calculation of ejection fraction, or qualitatively, by observa-

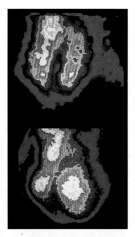

Fig. 6.48   Radionuclide ventriculography: colour coded study showing systolic and diastolic frames in a patient with dilated cardiomyopathy. The left ventricular cavity is severely dilated with contractile failure.

tion of wall movement. Global left ventricular impairment is characteristic of cardiomyopathy, while regional defects are seen following myocardial infarction. Stress radionuclide angiography using exercise or peripheral cold stimulation (cold pressor test) is used for detection of myocardial ischaemia: provocation of reversible regional-wall-motion abnormalities is strongly suggestive of coronary artery disease.

Myocardial perfusion scintigraphy

This method is used for diagnosis of coronary artery disease (Fig. 6.49). The investigation requires a standardized exercise stress test with continuous ECG monitoring in order to provoke myocardial ischaemia in susceptible subjects. Thallium-201 is used most commonly, but the more recently introduced Tc99m-labelled MIBI provides better image quality. Isotope is injected intravenously at peak exercise and the heart is imaged under a gamma camera. Isotope is distributed homogeneously in normally perfused myocardium, ischaemic or infarcted areas appearing as scintigraphic defects. If thallium-201 is used, repeat imaging after 2–4 hours rest permits reassessment of scintigraphic defects—those that disappear (reversible defects) indicate areas of exercise-induced ischaemia, those that persist (fixed defects) indicate infarcted myocardium. If Tc99m-labelled MIBI is used, resting images for assessment of reversibility require a separate injection of isotope 24 hours after (or before) the exercise images.

Hot-spot scintigraphy

This method permits diagnosis of acute myocardial infarction but in practice is rarely used. Technetium-99m pyrophosphate is taken up by recently infarcted myocardium, producing a localized 'hot spot' of radioactivity on the scintigram. Diagnostic sensitivity is greatest during the first week following infarction.

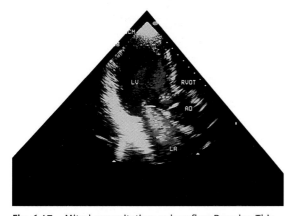

Fig. 6.47   Mitral regurgitation: colour-flow Doppler. This is an apical long axis view of the heart showing a large jet of mitral regurgitation (blue) occupying most of the left atrial cavity (LA).

STRESS   REDISTRIBUTION

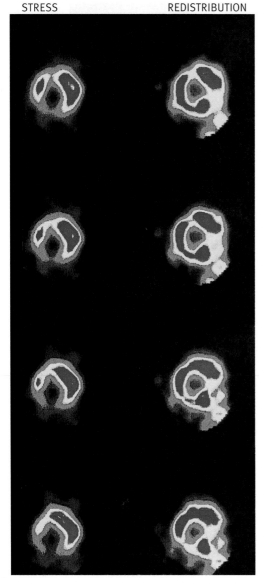

Fig. 6.49 Thallium-201 perfusion scan. These are tomographic slices across the short axis of the left ventricle. An inferior wall defect is seen during stress, but it largely disappears during rest as isotope 'redistributes' into the ischaemic area. A smaller fixed defect is seen in the anterior wall indicating infarction in that territory.

Pulmonary scintigraphy

This method is used for the diagnosis of pulmonary embolism (Fig. 6.50). Technetium-99m labelled microspheres injected intravenously become trapped within the pulmonary capillaries. The normal pulmonary perfusion scintigram shows homogeneous distribution of radioactivity throughout both lung fields. Pulmonary embolism causes regional impairment of pulmonary flow, which results in a perfusion defect on the scintigram; however, the appearance is non-specific and occurs in many other pulmonary dis-

orders, particularly chronic obstructive pulmonary disease. Specificity is enhanced by simultaneous ventilation scintigraphy. Inhaled xenon-133 is distributed homogeneously throughout the normal lung and, in pulmonary embolism (unlike other pulmonary disorders), distribution remains homogeneous. Thus a scintigraphic perfusion defect not 'matched' by a ventilation defect is highly specific for pulmonary embolism.

COMPUTED TOMOGRAPHY

PRINCIPLES

Computed tomography (CT) measures the attenuation of X-rays after they traverse body tissues. Attenuation is greatest for tissues such as bone which are relatively radio-opaque, and least for tissues such as lung or fat which are relatively radio-translucent. From X-ray attenuation measurements, taken as a sensor rotates around the chest, cross-sectional images are constructed. Image resolution is excellent and contrast injection into a peripheral vein provides adequate opacification of the blood pool for identification of intracardiac structures. In the past, the clinical application of CT in cardiology was limited by image acquisition times of up to 5 seconds, during which the constant motion of the heart degraded the image. The current generation of ultrafast CT scanners (with image acquisition times of less than 1 second) provide high resolution cardiac images in both static and video mode; measurements of blood flow can also be obtained by application of indicator dilution principles.

CLINICAL APPLICATIONS

CT (with contrast enhancement) is widely used for the non-invasive diagnosis of aortic dissection, when two contrast columns separated by an intimal flap can be clearly seen (Fig. 6.51). It is also used for accurate assessment of pericardial thickness in constrictive disease (Fig. 6.52) and in the diagnosis of cardiac tumours. Additional applications of ultrafast CT include the evaluation of graft patency following coronary bypass surgery, analysis of ventricular wall motion and blood flow quantification in congenital heart disease permitting dynamic assessment of shunts and other defects.

MAGNETIC RESONANCE IMAGING

PRINCIPLES

Magnetic resonance imaging (MRI) utilizes the fact that certain nuclei with an intrinsic spin generate magnetic fields and behave like tiny bar magnets. Placed in a magnetic field, these nuclei align and

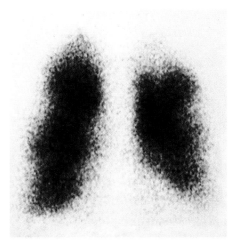

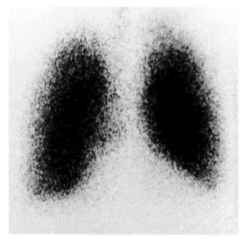

Fig. 6.50 Ventilation (right) and perfusion (left) lung scans in pulmonary embolism. Contrast the homogeneous distribution of isotope in the ventilation scan with the regional defects in the perfusion scan.

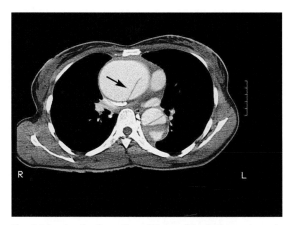

Fig. 6.51 Aortic dissection: CT scan (Marfan's syndrome). The ascending aorta is severely dilated and the intimal flap (arrowed) is clearly visible. This flap extends around the arch (not seen here) into the descending aorta where again it is clearly visible.

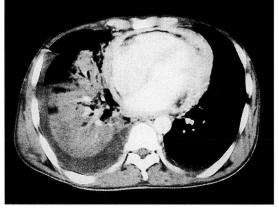

Fig. 6.52 Noncalcific pericardial constriction: CT scan. There is consolidation in the right lung and severe pericardial thickening. The patient had pulmonary tuberculosis with pericardial involvement and presented with fever and signs of constriction. Anti-tuberculous therapy caused regression of all symptoms and signs although the patient is at major risk of developing constriction later as the pericardium becomes fibrotic and calcified.

adopt a resonant frequency that is unique to that nucleus and the strength of the magnetic field. If the nuclei are exposed to pulsed radiowaves of that frequency, they resonate and release energy which allows their location to be determined.

For imaging purposes, the patient lies in a strong magnetic field which is artificially graded. The hydrogen protons of fat and water are imaged and, on exposure to pulsed radiowaves, they resonate at different frequencies in different parts of the imaging zone. Analysis of the emitted frequencies permits construction of tomographic and three-dimensional images of the heart. If data acquisition is gated to a specific part of the cardiac cycle, motion artefact is eliminated and excellent image resolution can be obtained.

CLINICAL APPLICATIONS

Already, MRI is being used for the diagnosis of aortic dissection (Fig. 6.53) and for imaging cardiac tumours. Potential applications may include coronary artery imaging without the need for contrast material, identification of histological and metabolic disorders of the myocardium, and assessment of myocardial perfusion using para-magnetic contrast agents. The realization of this exciting potential will ensure an important role for MRI in clinical cardiology.

CARDIAC CATHETERIZATION

Catheters introduced into an artery or vein may be directed into the left or right sides of the heart,

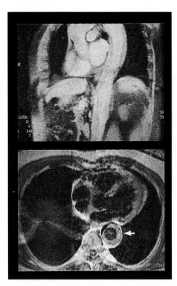

Fig. 6.53 Aortic dissection: MRI scan. The upper panel (coronal section) reveals an extensive aortic dissection extending from aortic root through arch and into descending aorta. The lower panel reveals a transverse view through the heart and descending aorta. Note the thrombus in the false lumen surrounding the true lumen in the descending aorta (arrowed).

respectively. Vascular access is usually percutaneous, using the femoral vessels, or by surgical cut-down, using the antecubital vessels. Originally developed for diagnostic purposes, catheter techniques are now being used increasingly for the interventional management of cardiovascular disease.

CARDIAC ANGIOGRAPHY

Coronary arteriography uses relatively small volumes of contrast (5–8 ml), injected manually, but other angiographic procedures require much larger amounts (up to 50 ml), introduced by power injection. Digital subtraction techniques permit reductions in contrast volume but have, at present, only a limited role in cardiovascular angiographic diagnosis (see below). Until recently, images have been recorded on high-speed cine film or video, to provide a dynamic record of ventricular wall movement, blood flow and intravascular anatomy. The current generation of angiographic laboratories, however, utilize digital technology and provide better quality images which can be stored electronically.

Aortic root angiography

Contrast injection into the aortic root demonstrates the vascular anatomy in suspected aneurysm or dissection, and also permits evaluation of aortic valve function (Fig. 6.54). The normal aortic valve prevents diastolic backflow of contrast, but in aortic regurgitation variable opacification of the left ventricle occurs, depending on the severity of the valve lesion.

Left ventricular angiography

Contrast injection into the left ventricle defines ventricular anatomy, and wall motion, and also permits evaluation of mitral valve function (Fig. 6.55). Dilatation of the ventricle and contractile dysfunction occurs in left ventricular failure. Exaggerated contractile function with systolic obliteration of the cavity occurs in hypertrophic cardiomyopathy. Filling defects within the ventricular lumen may indicate thrombus or neoplasm. The normal mitral valve prevents systolic backflow of contrast into the left atrium, but in mitral regurgitation variable atrial opacification occurs depending on the severity of the valve lesion.

Coronary arteriography

This is the only reliable technique for diagnostic imaging of the coronary arteries. Indications are summarized in Box 6.18. The technique requires selective injection of contrast into the left and right coronary arteries (Fig. 6.56) and multiple views in different projections are necessary for a complete

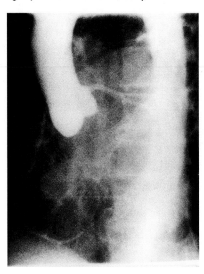

Fig. 6.54 Aortic root angiogram: normal study. Contrast injection provides an X-ray image of the ascending aorta. The coronary arteries arising from the sinuses of Valsalva are clearly seen.

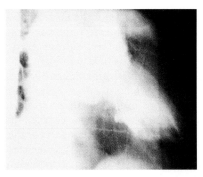

Fig. 6.55 Left ventricular angiogram showing mitral regurgitation. Contrast injection into the left ventricle has resulted in prompt opacification of the left atrium owing to back flow across the diseased mitral valve.

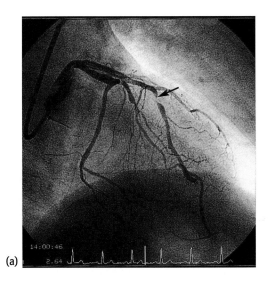

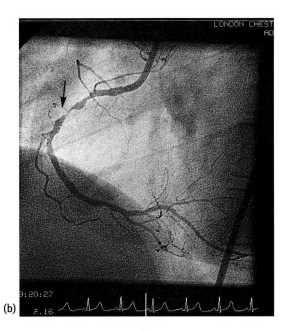

Fig. 6.56 Coronary arteriograms.
(a) Left anterior descending disease (arrowed). This tight stenosis threatens the coronary supply to the anterior wall of the left ventricle.
(b) Right coronary artery disease (arrowed). Serial stenoses in this dominant right coronary artery threaten the supply to the inferior wall of the heart.

BOX 6.18   Indications for coronary arteriography.

- Severe angina unresponsive to medical treatment
- Unstable angina
- Angina or a positive exercise test following myocardial infarction
- Cardiac arrhythmias when there is clinical suspicion of underlying coronary artery disease
- Preoperatively in patients requiring valve surgery when advanced age (>50) or angina suggest a high probability of coronary artery disease

---

study. Intraluminal filling defects or occlusions indicate coronary artery disease which is nearly always caused by atherosclerosis.

Pulmonary arteriography

Injection of contrast medium into the main pulmonary artery opacifies the arterial branches throughout both lung fields. The normal flow distribution is homogeneous. Vascular occlusions with regional perfusion defects usually indicate pulmonary thromboembolism (particularly when intraluminal filling defects are present) but may also occur in advanced emphysema.

INTRACARDIAC PRESSURE MEASUREMENT

Cardiac catheterization for measurement of blood flow and pressure within the heart and great vessels is widely used both for diagnostic purposes and to guide treatment. The fluid-filled catheter is attached to a pressure transducer which converts the pressure waves into electrical signals. For measurement of right-sided pressures, the catheter is directed by the venous route into the right atrium and then advanced through the right ventricle into the pulmonary artery. For measurement of left-sided pressures, the catheter is directed by the arterial route into the ascending aorta and advanced retrogradely through the aortic valve into the left ventricle. Because access to the left atrium is technically difficult, left atrial pressure is usually measured indirectly using the pulmonary artery wedge pressure.

The pulmonary artery wedge pressure is obtained during the right heart catheterization by advancing the catheter distally into the pulmonary arterial tree until the tip wedges in a small branch. Alternatively, a catheter with a pre-terminal balloon (Swan–Ganz catheter) may be used. Inflation of the balloon in the pulmonary artery causes the catheter tip to be carried with blood flow into a more distal branch which becomes occluded by the balloon. Regardless of which method is used, the wedge pressure recorded at the catheter tip is a more or less accurate measure of the left atrial pressure transmitted retrogradely through the pulmonary veins and capillaries.

Haemodynamic evaluation of valvular stenosis

In the normal heart there is no pressure gradient across an open valve. Such a gradient usually indicates valvular stenosis (Fig. 6.57) and, as stenosis worsens, the pressure gradient increases. This therefore provides a useful index of the severity of stenosis.

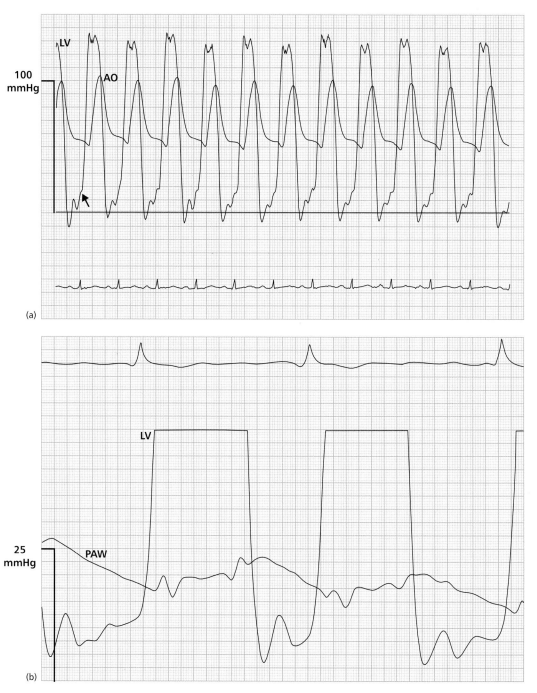

Fig. 6.57 Valvar stenosis: pressure signals.
(a) Aortic stenosis: simultaneous left ventricular (LV) and aortic (Ao) pressure signals. In the normal heart the pressure signals should be superimposed throughout systole. Here there is a peak systolic gradient of about 50 mmHg across the aortic valve. Note the prominent 'a' wave (arrowed) reflecting the major contribution that atrial systole makes to filling of the hypertrophied, noncompliant ventricle. Note also the pulsus alternans indicating left ventricular failure.
(b) Mitral stenosis: simultaneous recordings of the pulmonary artery wedge (PAW) and left ventricular (LV) pressure signals (LV). In the normal heart the pressure signals should be superimposed throughout diastole. Here there is a pressure gradient > 10 mmHg indicating severe mitral stenosis. Note that the patient is in AF and the pressure gradient varies inversely with the RR interval, tending to increase as the RR interval shortens.

However, it must be recognized that the pressure gradient is itself influenced by the flow through the valve. For example, if output is very low the gradient may be small despite the presence of severe stenosis. This applies particularly to the aortic valve because flow velocity is normally high.

Haemodynamic evaluation of intracardiac shunts

Left-to-right intracardiac shunts through atrial or ventricular septal defects introduce 'arterialized' blood into the right side of the heart. This results in an abrupt increase or step-up in the oxygen saturation of venous blood at the level of the shunt, which can be detected by right heart catheterization. Thus, by drawing serial blood samples for oxygen saturation from the pulmonary artery, right ventricle, right atrium and vena cavae, the shunt may be localized to the site at which the step-up in oxygen saturation occurs. The magnitude of the step-up is related to the size of the shunt but precise quantification of the shunt requires measurement of pulmonary and systemic blood flow. The extent to which the pulmonary–systemic flow ratio exceeds 1 is a measure of the size of the shunt.

Haemodynamic evaluation of constriction and tamponade (Boxes 6.19, 6.20)

In constrictive pericarditis and tamponade, diastolic relaxation of the ventricles is impeded, preventing adequate filling. Compensatory increments in atrial pressures occur to help maintain ventricular filling, and because these disorders usually affect both ventricles equally, the filling pressures also equilibrate. Thus simultaneous left- and right-sided recordings in constrictive pericarditis and tamponade show characteristic elevation and equalization of the filling pressures (atrial or ventricular end-diastolic) with loss of the normal differential (Fig. 6.58). Exactly similar

---

BOX 6.19   Constriction.

Typical patient
- Middle-aged or elderly patient with long history of progressive debilitation

Major symptoms
- Dyspnoea and weight loss with abdominal discomfort

Major signs
- Fluid retention with raised JVP (prominent 'x' and 'y' descents), hepatomegaly and peripheral oedema; diastolic filling sound ('pericardial knock'); paradoxical rise in JVP with inspiration (Kussmaul's sign)

Diagnosis
- This is a clinical diagnosis, confirmed by demonstration of increased pericardial thickness (± calcification) on CT or MRI scan

Additional investigations
- *CXR*: often normal but occasionally shows pericardial calcification on lateral film

Comments
- Tuberculosis no longer commonest cause in developed countries, where most cases are idiopathic

---

BOX 6.20   Tamponade.

Typical patient
- Either middle-aged or elderly patient with malignant disease (usually breast or lung), or patient of any age with tuberculosis

Major symptoms
- Dyspnoea and variable circulatory collapse

Major signs
- Low output state (hypotension, oliguria, cold periphery); tachycardia; paradoxical pulse; raised JVP with rapid 'x' descent; paradoxical rise in JVP on inspiration (Kussmaul's sign)

Diagnosis
- This is a clinical diagnosis, confirmed by echocardiographic demonstration of pericardial infusion

Additional investigations
- *ECG*: low voltage QRS complexes with alternating electrical axis
- *Tests for aetiological diagnosis*: these might include serological tests for rheumatoid and SLE, and tests for malignant or tuberculous disease

Comments
- Any cause of pericardial effusion may produce tamponade, malignant disease being the commonest cause in developed countries Pericardiocentesis relieves the tamponade. Pericardial fluid should always be sent for cytological and bacteriological analysis

---

physiology characterizes restrictive cardiomyopathy, in which infiltrative disease (usually amyloid in the UK) impedes relaxation of the ventricles.

Measurement of cardiac output

Cardiac output measurement is being used increasingly in intensive care units for characterizing cardiovascular status and monitoring responses to treatment. It is usually calculated by application of the Fick principle. A Swan–Ganz catheter with a right atrial portal and a terminal thermistor is positioned in the pulmonary artery. A known volume of cold saline (usually 10 ml) is injected into the right atrium and the temperature reduction in the pulmonary artery is recorded at the thermistor. The contour of the cooling curve is dependent upon cardiac output, which is calculated by measurement of the area under the curve using a bed-side computer.

A relatively simple non-invasive measure of cardiac output can be obtained by Doppler echocardiography using the 'area-length' method. Thus, the length of the column of blood ejected by the left ventricle during a single beat is obtained by multiplying the Doppler aortic flow velocity (cm/s) by the ejection time (s). The length of the column of blood is

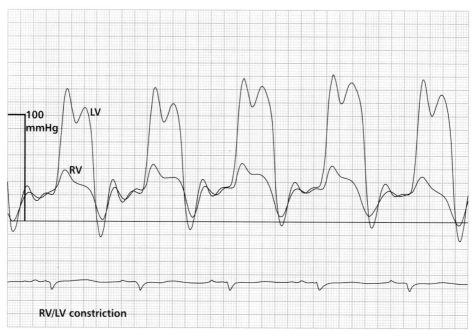

Fig. 6.58   Pericardial constriction: left (LV) and right (RV) ventricular pressure signals. Like tamponade and restrictive cardiomyopathy, constriction usually affects both ventricles equally and the diastolic pressures must rise and equilibrate to maintain ventricular filling. Thus in diastole the pressure signals are superimposed with a typical 'dip and plateau' configuration ('square root' sign).

then multiplied by the echocardiographic cross-sectional area of the aorta to yield stroke volume (ml/beat). Cardiac output is the product of stroke volume and heart rate.

INTRAVASCULAR ULTRASOUND

An ultrasound transducer mounted at the tip of a coronary catheter can now be used to provide cross-sectional images of the artery. The technique permits visualization of coronary plaques and provides information about plaque composition and structure that cannot be obtained from angiographic images (Fig. 6.59). Indeed, it is already apparent from ultrasound studies that coronary arteries which appear angiographically normal may in reality be extensively diseased. Intravascular ultrasound has already found a clinical role in coronary angioplasty and stenting when 'before and after' images can be used to document satisfactory patency of the vessel and correct deployment of the stent. Potential future developments include identification of lipid-laden, vulnerable coronary plaques which are prone to rupture, putting the patient at risk of acute coronary events.

PATHOLOGY LABORATORY SUPPORT

HAEMATOLOGY LABORATORY

Anaemia is an important diagnosis in the cardiac patient and is confirmed by measurement of the cir-

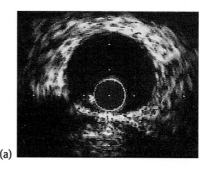

(a)

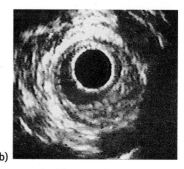

(b)

Fig. 6.59   Intravascular Ultrasound.
(a) Normal cross-sectional ultrasound scan in a distal segment of the right coronary artery. The ultrasound's transducer is clearly visible at the intersection of the horizontal and vertical centimetre scales.
(b) Coronary artery disease: a large semilunar coronary plaque extending from the 1 o'clock to the 7 o'clock position is shown severely reducing the coronary arterial lumen.

culating haemoglobin concentration. It exacerbates angina by adversely affecting the myocardial oxygen supply–demand relationship and also exacerbates heart failure by increasing the cardiac work necessary to meet oxygen demands of metabolizing tissues. Rarely, anaemia is a consequence of, rather than a contributor towards, heart disease. Thus, in infective endocarditis a normochromic normocytic anaemia is almost invariable, reflecting the adverse effects of chronic illness on erythropoiesis. Chronic haemolysis occasionally occurs in patients with mechanical prosthetic heart valves and is caused by traumatic erythrocyte damage. Anaemia is usually low grade but if severe may require removal of the prosthesis and substitution with a xenograft.

BIOCHEMISTRY LABORATORY

Cardiac enzymes and other markers of myocardial injury

Following myocardial infarction, enzymes released into the circulation by the necrosing myocytes provide biochemical evidence of injury. Creatine kinase (CK) has been the most widely used enzyme. Serum levels peak within 24 hours, but because the enzyme is also found in skeletal muscle false positive results may occur following intramuscular injections or external cardiac massage. The isoenzyme MB, however, is specific for myocardial CK and provides more accurate diagnostic information. Other enzymes such as glutamic oxaloacetic transaminase and lactic dehydrogenase peak later but are very nonspecific and are no longer used.

Newer serum markers of myocardial injury are now replacing enzymatic markers. These include the highly specific troponins T and I, and also somewhat less specific markers such as myoglobin, the principle value of which is that very early release during the process of infarction may permit early diagnosis even when the ECG is nondiagnostic.

Renal function

Renal function should always be measured in the cardiac patient. Renal dysfunction is a major cause (and consequence) of hypertension, while in heart failure progressive deterioration of renal function is almost inevitable as perfusion of the kidneys becomes threatened. Renal function may also deteriorate in response to treatment with diuretics and ACE-inhibitors and careful monitoring is essential as these drugs are introduced. Cardiac drugs that are excreted through the kidneys (e.g. digoxin) should be used cautiously if renal function is impaired. In the patient with established renal failure, accelerated coronary artery disease and heart failure commonly occur, reflecting the combined effects of dyslipidaemia, hypertension, arterial endothelial dysfunction, anaemia and volume loading on the cardiovascular system. Indeed, cardiovascular disease is the major cause of death in patients with renal failure.

Electrolytes

Serum potassium interacts importantly with the cardiac conduction system, patients with hypokalaemia being at risk of lethal cardiac arrhythmias, while hyperkalaemia may also cause bradyarrhythmias and heart block. Patients presenting with acute coronary syndromes commonly have hypokalaemia reflecting the effects of sympathoadrenal activation on membrane-bound sodium-potassium ATPase and this may require correction because of its association with lethal arrhythmias. In patients on thiazide or loop diuretics, potassium supplements (or potassium sparing diuretics) are usually necessary to protect against hypokalemia unless ACE-inhibitors are also given. Serum potassium should always be measured in patients with hypertension, not only to provide a baseline before introduction of diuretic therapy but also as a simple screening test for primary aldosteronism.

Glucose and lipids

Blood glucose and lipid profiles should be analysed in all patients with suspected vascular disease. For screening purposes, random blood samples are satisfactory but if the findings are abnormal fasting samples should be obtained for glucose, triglycerides, total cholesterol and high- and low-density lipoprotein cholesterol. In patients with acute myocardial infarction, treatment decisions must be based on the admission lipid profile as blood samples obtained up to 3 months after the acute event show spurious reductions of total and low-density lipoprotein cholesterol. Treatment of diabetes protects against microvascular complications and in hyperglycaemic patients with acute myocardial infarction, insulin and glucose infusion improves survival. Treatment of hypercholesterolaemia is effective in primary and secondary prevention of coronary artery disease.

BACTERIOLOGY LABORATORY

Blood culture (Box 6.21)

In suspected infective endocarditis, treatment must not be delayed beyond the time necessary to obtain three to four blood samples for culture (Table 6.2). Aerobic, anaerobic and fungal cultures should be performed. Occasionally, bone marrow cultures are helpful for detection of *Candida* and *Brucella* endocarditis. *Coxiella* and *Chlamydia* can never be cultured from the blood and must be diagnosed by serological tests. Failure to detect bacteraemia may be due to pretreatment with antibiotics, inadequate sampling (up to six blood samples should be taken over 24 hours) and infection with unusual microorganisms.

BOX 6.21 Infective endocarditis.

Typical patient
- Elderly man or woman with mitral or aortic valve disease (often not previously recognized)
- Younger patients with congenital heart defects (usually VSD or PDA)
- Also at risk are patients with prosthetic heart valves or a history of intravenous drug abuse

Major symptoms
- Non-specific feverish ('flu-like') illness.

Major signs
- Fever and heart murmur (usually aortic or mitral regurgitation)
- Splinter haemorrhages and vasculitic rash may occur
- Clubbing, Osler's nodes and Roth spots are rare

Diagnosis
- *Blood culture*: usually provides bacteriological diagnosis
- *Echocardiogram*: usually reveals valvular regurgitation ± vegetation

Additional investigations
- *Haematology*: leucocytosis; normochromic, normocytic anaemia
- *Inflammatory markers*: raised ESR and CRP
- *Urinalysis*: haematuria

Comments
- Formerly a disease of young adults, now seen more commonly in the elderly
- Diagnosis should always be considered in patients with fever and a heart murmur

Serology

If recent streptococcal throat infection can be confirmed by demonstration of elevated serum antistreptolysin O titre, Jones's criteria may be used for diagnosis of rheumatic fever (Box 6.22). The presence of two major criteria, or one major and two minor criteria, indicates a high probability of rheumatic fever. In suspected viral pericarditis or myocarditis, the aetiological diagnosis depends upon the demonstration of elevated viral antibody titres in acute serum samples, which decline during convalescence. Virus may sometimes be cultured from throat swabs and stools.

BOX 6.22 Jones's criteria for the diagnosis of rheumatic fever.

Major criteria
- Carditis
- Polyarthritis
- Erythema marginatum
- Chorea
- Subcutaneous nodules

Minor criteria
- Fever
- Arthralgia
- Previous rheumatic fever
- Elevated ESR
- Prolonged PR intervals

TABLE 6.2 Organisms implicated in endocarditis.

Organism	Typical source of infection	First choice antibiotics (pending sensitivity studies)
Streptococcus viridans	Upper respiratory tract	Benzylpenicillin: gentamicin
Streptococcus faecalis	Bowel and urogenital tract	Ampicillin: gentamicin
Anaerobic streptococcus	Bowel	Ampicillin: gentamicin
Staphylococcus epidermidis	Skin	Flucloxacillin: gentamicin
Fungi: *Candida, histoplasmosis,*	Skin and mucous membranes	Amphotericin B*: 5-fluorocytosine*
Coxiella burnetii	Complication of Q fever	Chloramphenicol*: tetracycline*
Chlamydia psittaci	Contact with infected birds	Tetracycline* and erythromycin
Acute disease		
Staphylococcus aureus	Skin	Flucloxacillin: gentamicin
Streptococcus pneumoniae	Complication of pneumonia	Benzylpenicillin: gentamicin
Neisseria gonorrhoeae	Venereal	Benzylpenicillin: gentamicin

* These drugs are not bactericidal, and valve replacement is nearly always necessary to eradicate infection.

7
THE GASTROINTESTINAL TRACT AND ABDOMEN

INTRODUCTION

The human gastrointestinal tract is a complex system of serially connected organs approximately 8 m in length, extending from the mouth to the anus, which, together with its connected secretory glands, controls the passage, processing, absorption and elimination of ingested material. Symptoms of gut disorders are often vague, and signs of abnormality few unless the disease is advanced. Careful analysis of the clues provided both from the gut itself and from the effect of gut disease on the body as a whole are required if diagnosis is to be achieved.

SYMPTOMS OF GASTROINTESTINAL DISEASE

In normal health there is some awareness of the functional state of the gut, and this can be related to body needs. For example, thirst and hunger are common symptoms and the latter may be associated with epigastric discomfort or pain. The state of hydration can be subjectively assessed by awareness of the sensation of dryness of the mouth. Swallowing is normally perceived, and there is temperature sensation in the upper and mid-oesophagus, as well as in the mouth. The normal gastric motility can, to some extent, be perceived, and it is common for people to experience vigorous peristaltic contractions in the gut. The movement of gas and fluid in the gut, called borborygmi, can also be perceived. The experience of a sensation of fullness in the colon and rectum prior to defaecation, or during constipation and the call to stool are, similarly, aspects of the normal sensation of gut activity.

During illness, or sometimes following the ingestion of spicy foods, epigastric discomfort or fullness and intestinal hurry may occur. These symptoms also reflect normal activity in the gut.

The common symptoms of gastrointestinal disease are listed in Box 7.1.

SYMPTOMS OF OESOPHAGEAL DISEASE

Disease of the oesophagus can cause the following symptoms:

Dysphagia
Dysphagia; the sensation of something sticking in the throat or chest during swallowing, may be due to oesophageal stricture from benign or malignant causes. Dysphagia is a potentially serious symptom that should always be investigated. Dysphagia due to a mechanical cause, such as the presence of an oesophageal tumour or peptic stricture, usually presents with initial difficulty in swallowing solids which progresses to difficulty with liquids. Neurogenic dysphagia may present with greater difficulty in swallowing liquids than solids sometimes associated with aspiration or coughing.

Heartburn
This is due to acid reflux from the stomach into the lower part of the oesophagus. It causes pain in the epigastrium, chest and neck and may be difficult to distinguish from angina pectoris. It occurs particularly at night when the patient lies flat in bed, or after bending or stooping when abdominal pressure is increased. Alcohol often induces heartburn.

Reflux
Reflux is a symptom which occurs when acid or bile regurgitates into the mouth, causing a bitter taste and a disagreeable sensation.

Painful swallowing
Painful swallowing or odynophagia, without difficulty in swallowing, is usually due to local infection. It is common in patients with AIDS in whom candida or herpes simplex often occur in the oesophagus.

SYMPTOMS OF STOMACH DISEASE

In disease of the stomach the following symptoms may occur:

Dyspepsia
Dyspepsia, or indigestion, includes epigastric pain, heartburn, distension, nausea or 'an acid feeling' occurring after eating or drinking. Patients may also use this term to describe an inability to digest food. The symptom is subjective, frequent, and usually benign in origin, although sometimes associated with peptic ulceration.

Flatulence
Flatulence describes excessive wind. It is associated with belching, abdominal distension and the passage of flatus per rectum. It is only infrequently associated with organic disease of the gastrointestinal tract, but usually represents a functional disturbance in which excessive air is swallowed. Certain foods produce relatively large amounts of gas—for example legumes—resulting in increased flatulence.

Hiccups
Hiccups are due to repeated sudden diaphragmatic contraction, often triggered by upper gastrointestinal irritation, but occasionally due to brainstem disease.

Vomiting
Vomiting is a neurogenic response triggered by chemoreceptors in the brainstem or reflexly through irritation of the stomach. Vomiting consists of a phase of nausea, followed by hypersalivation, pallor, sweating and hyperventilation. Retching, an involuntary effort to vomit, then occurs followed by expulsion of gastric contents through the mouth and sometimes through the nose. Most nausea and vomiting of gastrointestinal origin is associated with local pain in the abdomen. Painless vomiting should suggest neurological disease.

OTHER SYMPTOMS

Other symptoms associated with gastrointestinal problems include the following:

BOX 7.1   Common symptoms of gastrointestinal disease.

- Dysphagia
- Heartburn
- Indigestion
- Flatulence
- Hiccups
- Vomiting
- Constipation
- Diarrhoea
- Abnormal stools
- Abdominal pain
- Abdominal distension
- Weight loss
- Bleeding
- Haematemesis
- Rectal bleeding
- Melaena

Constipation

Constipation is a subjective complaint. Patients feel constipated when they sense that they have not adequately emptied the bowel by defaecation. The term is sometimes used to describe the passage of hard stools, irrespective of stool frequency. In clinical practice, the passage of formed stool less frequently than twice a week is usually taken to indicate an abnormality of bowel frequency.

Diarrhoea

Diarrhoea is common as a result of dietary indiscretion or from viral or bacterial infection. Diarrhoea may consist of watery stools of large volume, bloody diarrhoea, or frequent loose motions. Chronic diarrhoea should raise the possibility of inflammatory bowel disease or malabsorption with steatorrhoea. Steatorrhoea is the passage of pale, bulky stools containing excessive fats that commonly float in water and are difficult to flush away.

Abdominal pain

Abdominal pain may occur in the upper abdomen, in the hypochondrium, in the lower abdomen or in the rectum. The important features of abdominal pain are its site, intensity, character of duration and frequency, together with aggravating and relieving factors and associated features (see p. 151).

Abdominal distension

Abdominal distension has many causes. It may relate to flatulence, or more commonly to functional bowel disease in which the viscera are enlarged because their contractivity is diminished from disease of the bowel musculature, or its innervation. Distension is also a feature of steatorrhoea and malabsorption. It may result from ascites, or from enlargement of the viscera, for example in liver disease.

Weight loss

Weight loss is a feature of malabsorption, but may also result from loss of appetite (*anorexia*) or from starvation. It is a common feature of systemic diseases such as cancer, but is a late feature of cancer usually implying metastases.

Haematemesis

Haematemesis results from bleeding in the upper gastrointestinal tract, causing the vomiting of blood or blood products.

Rectal bleeding

Rectal bleeding results from bleeding in the rectum or anal canal, most commonly from piles but sometimes from anal or rectal carcinoma.

Melaena

Melaena, the passage of dark, partially digested blood, implies bleeding from a site more proximal than the gastrointestinal tract, usually in the upper colon or small intestine.

Jaundice

Jaundice (see below) implies disease of the liver or the biliary tract. It may also occur from excessive haemolysis. It causes yellowness of the skin and conjunctiva, and may be associated with other cutaneous and systemic features of liver disease, often with dark urine (see below).

GENERAL SIGNS

Certain systemic features of gastrointestinal disease may be evident on general examination. Particular note must be taken of the hands for *clubbing*, a clue to malabsorption or chronic liver impairment, and for palmar erythema and leuconychia which indicate liver disease. Other general signs which point to a diagnosis of liver disease include *jaundice*, spider naevi, gynaecomastia, loss of secondary sexual hair, testicular atrophy and parotid swelling. *Pruritis* and *scratch marks* should suggest chronic cholestasis. A facial appearance resembling Cushing's syndrome may also be found with chronic alcohol abuse.

Inflammatory bowel disease occasionally presents with extra-intestinal manifestations, for example arthritis, especially in the large joints; uveitis and skin rashes, including erythema nodosum and pyoderma gangrenosum. The nutritional state of the patient must be carefully assessed, since if food intake is normal the nutritional state is an index of the functional integrity of the gastrointestinal tract.

ASSESSMENT OF THE NUTRITIONAL STATE

Assessment of the nutritional state of a patient is an important part of the clinical examination. While gross *malnutrition* is usually easy to recognize, lesser degrees of body tissue depletion may be difficult to detect, particularly if oedema is also present, as in hypoalbuminaemia associated with severe protein loss, severe malabsorption, or kwashiorkor. Malnutrition may be due to starvation, to maldigestion of food or to malabsorption of the products of the process of digestion.

There are several ways to assess the nutritional state. The most important are the clinical history, including dietary history, and the physical examination, including anthropometric measurements. Other more subtle indices of malnutrition include muscle function tests and evaluation of creatinine excretion and serum levels of albumin. Anaemia, hypoalbuminaemia, ferritin and iron-binding capacity and the prothrombin time are also useful indices of malnutrition.

HISTORY

If starvation is excluded, patients likely to be at risk of malnutrition are those with reduced intake due to poor appetite or inability to eat. Malnutrition may also develop in patients with gastrointestinal failure and when metabolic needs exceed energy intake, as in hyperthyroidism.

Depressed appetite may accompany any severe illness, particularly malignancy and chronic renal or cardiac failure, in which nausea is often an accompanying problem. Other common causes include mental depression, viral illness, such as flu, which often causes transient loss of appetite, and chronic drug or alcohol abuse. Drug addicts may spend all their available income on drugs and neglect food. Alcoholics obtain calories from their drink but often develop protein and vitamin malnutrition syndromes. Malnutrition due to inability to eat (*dysphagia*) may occur in patients with neurological disturbances such as strokes, and in patients with oropharyngeal or oesophageal disease. A history of diarrhoea or steatorrhoea with progressive weight loss despite a good appetite should lead to consideration of alimentary disorders such as coeliac disease, bacterial overgrowth syndromes, or inflammatory bowel disease.

Increased metabolic needs arise in severely ill patients, particularly those with fever, burns or cancers, or following major trauma, including surgery. Hyperthyroidism must also be remembered as a cause of weight loss despite good appetite.

DIETARY HISTORY

A simple evaluation of diet is valuable in the assessment of any patient and is mandatory in all patients who appear malnourished. General questions about frequency of meals, types of food eaten, and methods of food preparation give a clue to dietary habits but are occasionally misleading if patients are elderly or impoverished. Recent changes in appetite or dietary patterns should be noted.

It is important to enquire whether the patient avoids certain foodstuffs for any reason. Do they follow, for instance, a strict diet, or have they been advised to avoid any foods in order to relieve gastrointestinal symptoms? Patients with gluten sensitivity, for example, will have been advised to avoid wheat products, while patients with intestinal lactase deficiency will avoid milk. A strict vegetarian or vegan diet may lead to vitamin B_{12} deficiency. Excessive dietary fibre intake leads to flatulence, bulky stools, increased bowel frequency and uncomfortable bowel distension. Low dietary fibre intake may be associated with constipation or difficult defaecation. In anorexia–bulimia, a disorder usually affecting young women, there are cyclic changes in appetite, food intake and dietary fads develop in

association with a pathological aversion to body habitus and self.

PHYSICAL EXAMINATION

In the general assessment of nutritional status careful attention must be given to the presence and distribution of body fat, the muscle bulk and the presence of oedema. Loss of muscle mass is common in *malnutrition*. Wasting of the temporalis muscles produces the characteristic gaunt appearance of the starved. Additional clues to poor nutrition are a dry, cracked skin, loss of scalp and body hair, and poor wound healing. In malnutrition the limb muscles are thin, the distal reflexes may be difficult to elicit, and the subcutaneous fat is atrophic. In *obesity* there is an increase in the proportion of fat in the body, largely in the subcutaneous compartment. In *protein-calorie malnutrition* there is a deficiency of protein with relatively good carbohydrate intake; the blood albumin level is reduced, and there may be oedema so that the body weight may be an unreliable indicator of malnutrition.

The nutritional state can be assessed semiquantitatively by measuring skinfold thickness with skin calipers, as an estimate of fat stores. A more accurate estimate of nutritional status is obtained by comparing weight with height: the Quetelet (body mass) index.

SKINFOLD THICKNESS

The skinfold thickness can be measured at standard sites, such as the biceps, triceps, infrascapular and supra-iliac regions, using a Harpenden calliper or similar device. The calliper is designed so that the jaws of the device remain parallel and constant pressure is exerted between them at different skinfold thicknesses. The triceps skinfold, midway between acromion and olecranon, is the most commonly used site. The skinfold thickness is measured in the vertical plane with the arm hanging relaxed by the side of the body. Normal values are shown in Table 7.1.

Skinfold measurements vary between the same observer by 0.3–0.6 standard deviations. If the arm circumference is measured at the same site, and it is assumed that the arm and muscle circumference are circular and circumferential respectively, a cross-sectional area for muscle and fat can be derived.

TABLE 7.1   Skinfold thickness: normal skinfold thickness measured by Schofield's callipers (mm). The 80% and 60% ranges are associated with nutritional depletion.

	Standard	80%	60%
Adult males	12.5	10.0	7.5
Adult females	16.5	13.0	10.0
Nutritional state	Normal nutrition	Moderate depletion	Severe depletion

QUETELET (BODY MASS) INDEX

The relationship between body weight and height provides a simple estimate, in adult subjects, as to whether weight is appropriate for height. The normal range of the index, calculated by the following formula, is 10–25 in men, and 18–24 in women:

$$\text{Quetelet body mass index} = \frac{\text{Weight (kg)}}{\text{height (m)}^2}.$$

The Quetelet index correlates well with three other, more technical methods of measuring body fat: total body water, body densitometry and whole body potassium measurements.

Nutritional intervention will be needed in practice if the Quetelet index is less than 18 or if weight loss during an illness is greater than 10%. Patients with a Quetelet index greater than 30 are so obese that weight loss is advisable. In malnourished children retardation of growth in height tends to lag behind that of weight and 'catch-up' growth occurs when malnutrition is corrected. The relation between weight and height in children should always, therefore, be compared with age, using the centile charts of normal ranges (Ch. 18). In *marasmus* there is severe growth retardation and wasting with a normal serum albumin, no oedema and a relatively alert child. In *kwashiorkor* growth retardation is not so severe, skin and hair changes are present, the albumin is low, there is oedema, and the child is miserable.

There are health penalties for malnutrition and for obesity (Box 7.2).

COMPOSITION OF THE BODY

The body can be considered to be composed of stores of different nutrients, which can be utilized during fasting or starvation, and increased during times of plenty (Table 7.2).

The composition of the body has been studied directly in cadavers. It can also be assessed in life, using methods that are restricted to clinical research rather than clinical practice. The lean body mass (LBM) can be calculated from measurement of the total body water (TBW), determined by a labelled water dilution method, according to the formula:

$$\text{Lean body mass} = \frac{\text{Total body water (litres)}}{0.73}.$$

BOX 7.2　Health penalties of disturbed nutrition.

Malnutrition
- Reduced ability to perform physical and mental work
- Reduced exercise tolerance
- Impaired respiratory function
- Impaired immunity
- Poor wound and fracture healing
- Increased surgical risk
- Amenorrhoea
- Osteoporosis
- Specific deficiency syndromes

Obesity
- Increased mortality indices
- Reduced quality of life
- Reduced physical fitness and mobility
- Hypertension and ischaemic heart disease
- Diabetes mellitus
- Osteoarthritis
- Hiatus hernia
- Gall stones
- Increased operative risk
- Increased risk of cancer, e.g. cancer of breast

TABLE 7.2　Body composition in health (calculated for a 70-kg man).

	kg	kcal/g	kcal stored
Water	42	0	0
Fat	10	9	90 000
Protein	10	4	40 000
Glycogen:			
muscle	0.15	4	600
liver	0.075	4	300
Circulating glucose, fatty acids, triglycerides, etc			113

Lean body mass can also be calculated by body densitometry and by gamma neutron activation analysis of total body nitrogen, calcium and other elements.

The body's composition changes with increasing age as shown in (Table 7.3).

TABLE 7.3　Body composition at different ages.

	Newborn	10 years M	10 years F	Adult M	Adult F
Weight (kg)	3.4	31	31	72	58
LBM (kg)	2.9 (85%)	27 (87%)	26 (81%)	61 (85%)	42 (72%)
Fat (kg)	0.5 (15%)	4 (13%)	6 (19%)	11 (15%)	16 (28%)

THE MOUTH AND THROAT

The examination of the mouth and throat is conducted with the patient sitting up either in bed, with the head resting comfortably back on pillows, or in a chair. A bright torch, a tongue depressor (spatula) and a pair of latex gloves are essential. The lips, teeth, gums, tongue, palate, fauces and oropharynx are then visualized systematically, and finally palpation of the sides of the tongue, floor of mouth and tonsillar regions is carried out.

INSPECTION

THE LIPS

Look closely at the philtrum (the shallow depression running from nose to upper lip) for the tell-tale scar of a repaired cleft lip. When present, particularly if associated with 'nasal speech', inspect the palate carefully for signs of a cleft. Next, look at the corners of the mouth for cracks or fissures (*angular stomatitis*). The cracks are reddish-brown, moist, superficial, linear ulcers radiating from the angles of the mouth. In children their origin is infective (*perleche*); they are common in the elderly when ill-fitting or deficient dentures result in overclosure of the mouth. Cheilosis is also seen in severe iron-deficiency anaemia; it also occurs in vitamin B_2 (riboflavin) deficiency.

Observe any desquamation or inflammation of the lips (*cheilitis*). This is common and self-limiting in cold weather. Grouped vesicles on the lips on a red base with crusted lesions are seen in herpes simplex labialis commonly associated with coryza. This infection is usually of short duration and the lack of induration and ulceration serves to distinguish it from other more serious conditions. Recurrent actinic cheilitis with small blisters and exfoliation, however, is a premalignant condition found in people constantly exposed to the sun and wind, such as sports people, farmers and fishermen.

Look for any ulcer on the lips. *Carcinoma* (epithelioma) usually occurs on the lower lip away from the midline; the ulcer is indolent, flat and shallow, although in time the edge may become heaped up and induration may be felt. Epithelioma must be differentiated from keratoacanthoma, pyogenic granuloma and the chancre of primary syphilis. A *keratoacanthoma* (molluscum sebaceum) is a lesion due to overgrowth of the stratum granulosum of the skin. It usually presents as a firm, rounded nodule sometimes with ulceration; it is more common on the upper lip and heals spontaneously without treatment. *Pyogenic granuloma* is a soft red raspberry-like nodule on the upper lip which often follows minor trauma. The upper lip is the commonest site of an extragenital chancre, which appears as a small, round lesion that is firm and indurated. A 'snail-track ulcer' in secondary syphilis has a serpiginous outline and greyish-white non-purulent exudate. In both epithelioma and chancre, enlarged painless cervical nodes may often be felt. *Rhagades*, white scars at the angles of the mouth that extend into the mouth, due to cheilosis associated with congenital syphilis, are now only of historical interest. A crack in the middle of the lower lip in cold weather is a common, painful problem, but is of no sinister significance.

Very occasionally multiple small brown or black spots are seen on the skin around the mouth (*circumoral pigmentation*) which may also extend onto the lips and buccal mucosa. This pigmentation constitutes one of the triad of cardinal features of the Peutz–Jeghers syndrome and signifies underlying small bowel polyposis, a condition inherited as a Mendelian dominant. On the buccal mucosa the pigmentation may look very like that seen in Addison's disease. Look carefully at the lips and tongue for telangiectasia (see Fig. 1.1). Their presence may signal the existence of others elsewhere in the intestine, which occasionally bleed.

Now gently grasp the lower lip with the index finger and thumb of both hands and evert it fully, to display the mucous surface of the lip. Two lesions are commonly seen in this site: aphthous ulcers and retention cysts. *Aphthous ulcers* are small, superficial, painful ulcers with a white or yellow base and a narrow halo of hyperaemia (Fig. 7.1). Such ulcers are also seen on the tongue, buccal mucosa and palate. *Retention cysts* of the mucous glands of the lips and buccal mucosa appear as round, translucent swellings, elevated from the surface with a characteristic white or bluish appearance. They are also found on the mucous surface of the lower lip.

THE TEETH

Ask the patient to grimace so as to show the teeth. If the patient wears dentures, ask him or her to remove them and open the mouth widely. Using a tongue depressor to retract first the lips and then the cheeks, note the number of teeth present and look for decay (*caries*). The tooth most commonly missing is an impacted unerupted third mandibular molar (wisdom tooth). Inspect both the buccal and lingual

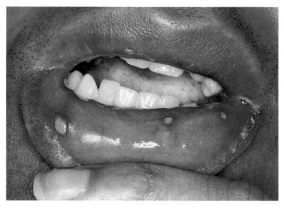

Fig. 7.1 Apthous ulcers.

aspects of the teeth. It is said that lack of teeth may cause indigestion but many edentulous people suffer no indigestion whether they wear dentures or not. Look for any changes in the following:

Colour

Tartar deposition occurs mainly on the lingual aspect of the lower incisor and canine teeth and consists of precipitated calcium salts of saliva which is stained brown in smokers. The chewing of betel nuts may also discolour the plaque of teeth a reddish-brown. Children up to the age of 8 treated with tetracycline (and children of expectant mothers so treated after the 14th week of pregnancy) are at risk of acquiring permanent staining of both the deciduous and the permanent teeth. This takes the form of disfiguring horizontal bands, which may be yellow or grey and must not be mistaken for bands of hyperplasia on the enamel due to exanthematous fevers or any serious illness occurring during the development of the crowns. In endemic fluorosis, chalk-white patches appear on the teeth or the teeth present a dull, unglazed appearance, sometimes with pitting and brown staining (*Maldon teeth*).

Shape

Ill-formed hypoplastic teeth have a broad, concave biting edge, while some notching of the incisors is seen in those who persistently bite cotton or hold hairclips between their teeth. This must not be mistaken for *Hutchinson's teeth*—a manifestation of congenital syphilis, but a very rare finding nowadays. In this condition the two central upper permanent incisors are rounded in section and notched at their biting edge. They may also be broader near the gum than at the crown, so as to be peg-shaped. The first permanent molars may be dome-shaped. The two central upper incisors are sometimes lost in leprosy. Patients who habitually induce vomiting (e.g. in anorexia nervosa) may show evidence of gastric acid-induced erosion of the inner surface of the incisors.

Ridging

Transverse ridging is sometimes seen in the permanent teeth of those who had vitamin C and D deficiency in infancy.

Enlargement of the lower jaw in acromegaly leads to alteration of the bite, so that the lower teeth may close outside the upper ones.

THE GUMS

Examine the gums at the same time as the teeth. Pink, healthy gums adhere closely to the necks of the teeth and have a sharp border. With increasing age *gingival recession* occurs, so making the teeth appear longer and exposing the cementum below the enamel. This makes it easier for infection to gain a hold.

In *chronic marginal gingivitis*, the gums are retracted, frequently bleed easily and lose their characteristic stippling. Sometimes pus can be squeezed from them (*pyorrhoea alveolaris*).

Acute herpetic gingivostomatitis due to the simplex virus occurs most commonly in infants and children. Many small vesicles appear on the gums, cheeks, palate, tongue and lips. The vesicles rupture to produce shallow ulcers with a yellowish floor and bright red margins. *Vincent's gingivostomatitis*, an infection due to fusiform spirochaetes, characteristically destroys the interdental papillae. A thick, felted, greenish-grey slough is formed and halitosis is present. In patients exposed to lead compounds, a *stippled blue line* can often be observed running along the edge of the gum, especially opposite those teeth showing gingivitis. Similar lines may be produced by bismuth or mercury but these are uncommon signs. The gums in scurvy are swollen, irregular in outline, red, spongy and bleed easily. Hypertrophy of the gums may occur in pregnancy and in patients treated for long periods with phenytoin. Haemorrhages may be observed in the buccal mucous membrane in thrombocytopenic purpura and acute leukaemia.

Pus can form in a carious tooth to form an alveolar or dental abscess with throbbing pain, exacerbated by tapping the affected tooth. Localized swelling of the gum and swelling of the face (if pus has escaped through the lateral alveolar margin) are signs associated with this condition. Ill-fitting dentures can produce a granuloma or an ulcer on the gum at the point of pressure where the denture does not fit properly. Such a lesion has to be differentiated from a carcinomatous ulcer arising in the gum; the latter presents the same macroscopic features as malignant ulcers elsewhere in the mouth.

Epulis is a general term used to describe any swelling arising in the gum of the maxilla or mandible.

THE TONGUE

Ask the patient to protrude the tongue. Inability to do so fully (*ankyloglossia*) is seen, very rarely, in infants due to tongue-tie (a congenitally short frenulum linguae) or in advanced malignancy of the tongue involving the floor of the mouth. When carcinoma involves the side of the tongue (the commonest site) and the floor of the mouth, slight deviation towards the affected side may occur. Slight deviation is not uncommon and may be due to asymmetry of the jaws. In hemiplegia, deviation towards the paralysed side may be found. In lesions of the hypoglossal nerve or its nucleus there may be fasciculation of the affected side; later this side may be wasted and deeply grooved (*lingual hemiatrophy*). The tongue is large in acromegaly, cretinism, myxoedema, lymphangioma and amyloidosis.

Tremor of the tongue may be due to nervousness, thyrotoxicosis, delirium tremens or parkinsonism.

Next examine the dorsum of the tongue.

Colour

Is the tongue pale, red or discoloured? Pallor is seen in severe anaemia. Discoloration is most often due to the ingestion of coloured foods, for example red wine or coloured sweets.

Moistness

The state of the tongue gives some indication of the state of hydration of the body, provided the patient is not a mouth breather. A dry, brown tongue may be found in the later stages of any severe illness, but is found particularly in advanced uraemia and in acute intestinal obstruction.

Fur

Furring of the tongue is of little value as an indication of disease. It is often found in heavy smokers. A brown fur, the 'black hairy tongue', is due to a fungus infection and is of no special significance, though frequently a source of great alarm to its possessor. The tongue of scarlet fever at first shows bright red papillae standing out of a thick white fur. Later the white coat disappears leaving enlarged papillae on a bright red surface—the 'strawberry tongue'. Hairy leucoplakia is a common feature in patients with HIV infection. In chronic superficial glossitis, areas of *leucoplakia* (whitish opaque areas of thickened epithelium) are separated by intervening smooth and scarred areas; there are no normal papillae to be seen and the fissures run mainly in a longitudinal direction.

The papillae

Generalized atrophy of the papillae produces a smooth or bald tongue which is characteristic of vitamin B$_{12}$ deficiency but may also sometimes be found in iron-deficiency anaemia, coeliac disease and other gastrointestinal disorders and deficiency states, especially pellagra. In severe cases smoothness may be associated with wrinkling of the mucous membrane, which has then to be distinguished from fissuring of the tongue seen in chronic superficial glossitis due to syphilis, and congenital fissuring of the tongue or 'scrotal tongue', which is common and of no pathological significance. In *congenital fissuring* the papillae are normal but the surface is interrupted by numerous irregular but more or less symmetrical folds which tend to run mainly horizontally. In *median rhomboid glossitis* a lozenge-shaped area of loss of papillae and fissuring is seen in the midline anterior to the foramen caecum. It feels nodular and may be mistaken for a carcinoma. It must also be distinguished from a lingual thyroid but this is situated posterior to the foramen caecum. *Geographical tongue* is another harmless anomaly characterized by localized irregular red areas of desquamated epithelium and filiform papillae surrounded by a whitish-yellow border; the papillae change in distribution and give the appearance of a map. The 'false geographical tongue' with a similar appearance occurs chiefly in children with fever.

The sides and undersurface

Ask the patient to open the mouth wide and protrude the tongue fully to one side. Then retract the cheek with a spatula. This displays the side and lateral undersurface well. Some patients find this impossible to do, so wrap a gauze swab around the tip of the tongue and with index finger and thumb gently pull the tongue out and to one side. Benign ulcers in this site are common and may be inflammatory or traumatic in origin, very often due to ill-fitting dentures or broken carious teeth; such ulcers tend to be painful, superficial and lack induration. However, in an elderly patient any ulcer at this site must be regarded as malignant until proved otherwise by biopsy; it is the most frequent site of carcinoma in the mouth and presents as a hard, indurated ulcer with everted raised edges.

Now ask the patient to retract the tongue fully and slightly elevate the tip with the mouth wide open. This displays the undersurface of the anterior tongue and floor of the mouth. Note the frenulum linguae and the orifice of the submandibular duct opening on either side of the base of the frenulum. The ampulla of each duct lies just proximal to the orifice and is a common site for calculi formed in the submandibular salivary gland to lodge. The calculus is seen as a white or yellow bleb distending an oedematous hyperaemic ampulla.

A small ulcer on the frenulum is sometimes seen in persistent coughing and particularly in whooping cough. Sublingual varicosities are common in the elderly. Two types of cyst may be found in the floor of the mouth:

- *Ranula*, which forms a bluish-white translucent swelling of variable size and is due to blockage of the duct of a mucous gland
- *Sublingual dermoid cyst*, a round opaque swelling lying beneath the mucosa either above or below the mylohyoid, which is due to sequestration of epidermal tissue beneath the skin along the embryological lines of fusion of the mouth.

THE BUCCAL MUCOSA

Inspect the buccal mucosa. Retract the cheek with a spatula. Note the opening of the parotid duct, which is seen as a tiny swelling opposite the upper second molar tooth. In the catarrhal stage of measles, before the appearance of the rash, small bluish-white spots, surrounded by a red areola, may be seen opposite the molar teeth. These are known as *Koplik's spots*. In the same position irregular areas of dots of slate-grey or blue pigmentation are seen in Addison's disease.

Aphthous ulcers, mucus retention cysts and *papillomata* present the same appearance on the buccal mucosa as elsewhere in the mouth. Mouth ulcerations (see Box 7.3)—either aphthous or larger, more chronic lesions—are well-recognized manifestations of inflammatory bowel disease, particularly Crohn's

---

BOX 7.3   Causes of mouth ulcers.

- Inflammatory bowel disease
- Behçet's disease
- Leucoplakia
- Lichen planus
- Thrush (candidiasis)
- Idiopathic aphthous ulcers
- Koplik's spots (measles)
- Malignant erosion

---

disease. Mouth ulcers in association with genital ulcers indicate Behçet's syndrome. White opalescent patches (rather like white paint) of *leucoplakia* may also be seen on the inner aspect of the cheek; these should be differentiated from lichen planus, an oral manifestation of a skin disease, but in this case look elsewhere, especially on the arms and legs, for similar lesions. *Thrush* (monilial stomatitis), a fungal infection due to *Candida albicans*, presents as a different sort of white patch. It is seen as small white points raised somewhat above the surrounding surface, which is usually redder than normal. As the infection gains hold so the lesions coalesce and may form extensive sheets throughout the mouth. Patches of thrush are apt to be mistaken for small milk curds, but curds can be easily detached, while thrush patches can be removed only with difficulty and then tend to leave behind a raw surface. Thrush is common in debilitated children, beneath unclean dentures and in patients on cytotoxic or immunosuppressive drugs. It is also seen frequently on surgical wards, especially in ill patients with sepsis in the postoperative period and in those treated with broad-spectrum antibiotics, which destroy the normal bacterial flora of the mouth and thus allow the fungi to flourish. Oropharyngeal candidiasis is also a feature of cellular immunodeficiency states including AIDS.

THE PALATE, FAUCES, TONSILS AND PHARYNX
Ask the patient to put the head right back and keep the mouth wide open. Inspect the hard and soft palates and note the position of the uvula. Get the patient to say 'ah', which raises the soft palate and increases visibility of the fauces, tonsils and oropharynx. (For abnormalities of movement of the soft palate during phonation see p. 251.)

If a good view of these structures has not been obtained, introduce a spatula to depress the base of the tongue and, if necessary, another spatula to retract the anterior pillar of the fauces to view the tonsils properly.

Again look for any ulcers, erythema or vesicles. *Vesicles* confined to one side of the hard palate which progress to painful oval ulcers are characteristic of herpes zoster of the maxillary division of the trigeminal nerve (fifth cranial); this disorder usually occurs in older patients and is accompanied by a character-

istic skin rash in the corresponding dermatome on the face. Herpes zoster infection of the glossopharyngeal nerve (ninth cranial) produces similar lesions in the pharynx.

Malignant ulcers do occur on the hard palate but much less frequently than elsewhere in the mouth, and present the same appearances. Ectopic salivary gland tissue may be present in the mouth; the hard palate is the commonest site. Tumours of this tissue present as a smooth, hard swelling projecting from the surface of the hard palate, sometimes with central ulceration.

If a hole is seen in the hard palate it is usually due to one of the following:

- Imperfect closure or breakdown after repair of a cleft palate
- Radionecrosis of bone following radiotherapy for treatment of local carcinoma
- Tertiary syphilis with formation of a gumma.

Petechiae on the palate are common in glandular fever but they are also features of any form of thrombocytopenia, rubella and streptococcal tonsillitis. Oral lesions may be the presenting feature of *glandular fever*: enlarged tonsils are covered with a white exudate which tends to become confluent; there is oedema of the fauces and soft palate, and erythema of the oropharynx. This contrasts with the yellow punctate follicular exudate seen in *streptococcal tonsillitis*. Whenever a membranous exudate is seen, *diphtheria* should spring to mind and, as in all cases of mouth infection, a swab should be taken for bacteriological examination. The membrane in diphtheria varies in colour from white to green and often starts on the tonsil before spreading to the fauces and pharynx.

Finally, look at the pharynx. The presence on its surface of a number of small round or oval swellings, somewhat like sago grains, is so common as to be almost normal in appearance. In pharyngitis these are much increased.

Notice any vesicles or ulcers. In *chickenpox* (herpes varicella) oral lesions may be apparent before the characteristic rash appears. There is erythema of the pharyngeal and buccal mucosae, followed by vesicles which progress to oval or round ulcers with a white slough. In *herpangina* (Coxsackie virus infection) which is also common in the young, similar lesions may be seen in the oropharynx, soft palate and uvula.

In the *common cold* (coryza), mucopus may be noticed on the posterior wall of the pharynx running down from the nasopharynx. Less common nowadays is a peritonsillar abscess (*quinsy*) and retropharyngeal abscess. The latter forms a smooth, tense, tender swelling which bulges forwards from the posterior wall of the oropharynx.

THE BREATH
Carious teeth, infection or ulceration of the gum, stomatitis, and retention and decomposition of secretion in

the follicles of enlarged tonsils are the commonest sources of offensive breath. Characteristic odours may be recognized:

- In ketosis the breath smells of acetone
- In uraemia there is a fishy or ammoniacal odour
- In hepatic failure the odour is described as 'mousy'
- In suppurative conditions of the lung the breath may have a putrid smell
- In bronchiectasis the odour has been compared to that of apple blossom with a hint of stale faeces
- Paraldehyde and alcohol also impart their characteristic smells to the breath.

Obsessional focusing on 'bad breath as a symptom' may indicate depression.

PALPATION

Palpation forms an important, frequently neglected part of the examination of the mouth, particularly in patients who complain of oral symptoms or in whom unexplained cervical lymphadenopathy is found. Although not a routine part of physical examination, palpation in the mouth is imperative in anyone with a solitary or suspected ulcer in the oral cavity and bimanual palpation provides further information about such things as swellings in the floor of the mouth or cheek.

Impress on the patient that you will be as gentle as possible. Put on a disposable glove, and ask the patient to remove any dentures and to open the mouth widely. With the tongue elevated and to one side, place the index finger of the right hand beneath the tongue on one side of the frenulum and run the finger back along the floor of the mouth. Even a small calculus can easily be felt in any part of the submandibular duct. Then come forwards, running the finger along the lingual side of the tongue to the midline and return on the buccal side of the gum towards the lower molar teeth. Now run the finger up the mucosa covering the ascending ramus of the mandible, and examine both palatal and buccal aspects of the gum of the upper jaw.

If an ulcer is present, try and decide whether any induration is present or not. To perform bimanual examination, with the index finger already inside the mouth, place the fingertips of the left hand flat beneath the mandible, or over the cheek, outside the mouth, and exert gentle pressure between your right index finger and the fingers of the left hand.

Now palpate the tongue and feel the dorsum and the lateral and undersurfaces with the index finger; it sometimes helps for the patient to protrude the tongue to one or other side to do this and, if necessary, the tongue can be held in a gauze swab between finger and thumb of the other hand.

Palpation of the posterior third of the tongue, fauces and tonsils is the least pleasant part for the patient as it usually causes gagging, and it is thus left until last. As before, the index finger is used and run over these structures as rapidly as possible. Feel for irregularity, ulceration and particularly induration, in order to detect a small or hidden carcinoma. Any abnormality felt in these sites in a patient with symptoms demands illuminated head lamp and laryngeal examination (Ch. 13).

THE ABDOMEN   (see Figs 7.2 and 7.3)

It is helpful when recording in notes or communicating information to colleagues to think of the abdomen as divided into regions (Fig. 7.4). The two *lateral vertical* planes pass from the femoral artery below to cross the costal margin close to the tip of the ninth costal cartilage. The two *horizontal* planes, the subcostal and interiliac, pass across the abdomen to connect the lowest points on the costal margin, and the tubercles of the iliac crests respectively.

Remember that the area of each region will depend on the width of the subcostal angle and the proximity of costal margin to iliac crest, in addition to other features of bodily habitus which naturally vary greatly from one patient to the next.

INSPECTION

The patient should be lying supine with arms loosely by his or her sides, on a firm couch or mattress, the head and neck supported by enough pillows, normally one or two, sufficient for comfort (Fig. 7.5). A sagging mattress makes examination, particularly palpation, difficult. Make sure there is a good light, that the room is warm and that your hands are warm. A shivering patient cannot relax and vital signs, especially on palpation, may be missed.

Stand on the patient's right side and expose the abdomen by turning down all the bedclothes except the upper sheet. The clothing should then be drawn up to just above the xiphisternum and the sheet folded down across the upper thighs to expose the groins and genitalia. This point is important; many are the patients who present with intestinal obstruction due to a strangulated femoral or inguinal hernia where the diagnosis has been missed initially due to lack of proper exposure of the groins in an effort to save embarrassment. However, once full inspection has taken place the sheet may be pulled up to the level of the symphysis pubis to allay anxiety.

Inspection is an important and neglected part of abdominal examination. It is well worthwhile spending 30 seconds observing the abdomen from different positions to note the following features:

SHAPE

Is the abdomen of normal contour and fullness, or distended? Is it scaphoid (sunken)?

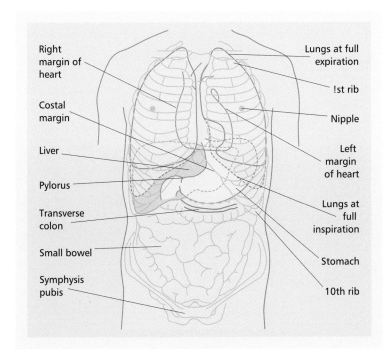

Fig. 7.2   Anterior view of external relations of the abdominal and thoracic organs.

Right margin of heart
Costal margin
Liver
Pylorus
Transverse colon
Small bowel
Symphysis pubis

Lungs at full expiration
!st rib
Nipple
Left margin of heart
Lungs at full inspiration
Stomach
10th rib

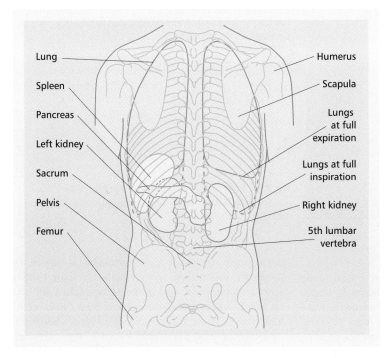

Fig. 7.3   Posterior view of the external relations of the abdominal and thoracic organs. The liver is not shown.

Lung
Spleen
Pancreas
Left kidney
Sacrum
Pelvis
Femur

Humerus
Scapula
Lungs at full expiration
Lungs at full inspiration
Right kidney
5th lumbar vertebra

- *Generalized fullness* or *distension* may be due to fat, fluid, flatus, faeces or fetus.
- *Localized distension* may be symmetrical and centred around the umbilicus, as in the case of small bowel obstruction, or asymmetrical as in gross enlargement of the spleen, liver or ovary.
- Make a mental note of the site of any such swelling or distension; think of the anatomical structures in that region and note if there is any movement of the swelling, either with or independent of respiration.
- Remember that chronic urinary retention may cause palpable enlargement in the lower abdomen.

A *scaphoid* abdomen is seen in advanced stages of starvation and malignant disease, particularly carcinoma of the oesophagus and stomach.

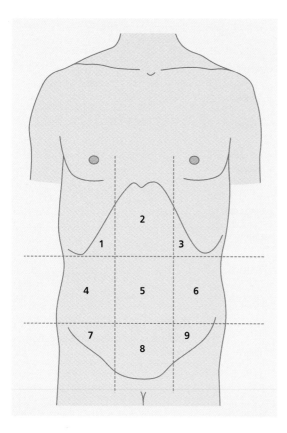

Fig. 7.4   Regions of the abdomen. 1 and 3: right and left hypochondrium; 2: epigastrium; 4 and 6: right and left lumbar; 5: umbilical; 7 and 9: right and left iliac; 8: hypogastrium or suprapubic.

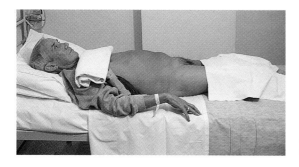

Fig. 7.5   Position of the patient and exposure for abdominal examination. Note that the genitalia must be exposed.

THE UMBILICUS

Normally the umbilicus is slightly retracted and inverted. As it is at the centre of the abdomen, one's eyes inevitably come to rest on it at the same time as noting the general shape of the abdomen. If it is everted then an umbilical hernia may be present and this can be confirmed by feeling an expansile impulse on palpation of the swelling when the patient coughs. The hernial sac may contain omentum, bowel or fluid. A common finding in the umbilicus of elderly obese women is a concentration of inspissated desquamated epithelium and other debris (*omphalolith*).

MOVEMENTS OF THE ABDOMINAL WALL

Normally there is a gentle rise in the abdominal wall during inspiration and a fall during expiration; the movement should be free and equal on both sides. In *generalized peritonitis* this movement is absent or markedly diminished, which helps to limit further spread of infection within the peritoneal cavity and the pain of peritoneal irritation (the 'still, silent abdomen'). To aid the recognition of intra-abdominal movements shine a light across the patient's abdomen. Even small movements of the intestine may then be detected by alterations in the pattern of shadows cast over the abdomen.

Visible pulsation of the abdominal aorta may be noticed in the epigastrium and is a frequent finding in nervous, thin patients. It must be distinguished from an aneurysm of the abdominal aorta, where pulsation is more obvious and a widened aorta is felt on palpation.

Visible peristalsis of the stomach or small intestine may be observed in three situations:

- *Obstruction at the pylorus.* Visible peristalsis may occur where there is obstruction at the pylorus produced either by fibrosis following chronic duodenal ulceration or, less commonly, by carcinoma of the stomach in the pyloric antrum. Peristalsis will be seen as a slow wave either passing across the upper abdomen from left to right hypochondria or, if gross gastric dilatation is present, passing down to the suprapubic region and ascending to terminate in the right epigastrium. In pyloric obstruction, a diffuse swelling may be seen in the left upper abdomen but, where obstruction is long-standing with severe gastric distension, this swelling may occupy the left mid and lower quadrants. Such a stomach may contain up to 2 litres of fluid and, on shaking the abdomen, a splashing noise is usually heard ('*succussion splash*'). This splash is frequently heard in healthy patients for up to 3 hours after a meal, so enquire when the patient last ate or drank.
- *Congenital pyloric stenosis of infancy.* Not only may visible peristalsis be apparent but also the grossly hypertrophied circular muscle of the antrum and pylorus may be felt as a 'tumour' to the right of the midline in the epigastrium. Both these signs may be elicited more easily after the infant has been given a feed. Standing behind the child's mother with the child held on her lap may allow the child's abdominal musculature to relax sufficiently to feel the walnut sized swelling.
- *Obstruction in the distal small bowel.* Peristalsis may be seen where there is intestinal obstruction in the distal small bowel or coexisting large and small bowel hold-up produced by distal colonic obstruction, with an incompetent ileocaecal valve allowing reflux of gas and liquid faeces into the ileum. Not only is the abdomen distended and tympanitic (hyperresonant) but the distended coils of small bowel may be visible in a thin patient and tend to stand out in the centre of the abdomen in a 'ladder pattern'.
- *As a normal finding* in very thin, elderly patients with lax abdominal muscles or large, wide-necked incisional herniae seen through an abdominal scar.

SKIN AND SURFACE OF THE ABDOMEN

In marked abdominal distension the skin is smooth and shiny. *Striae atrophica or gravidarum* are white or pink wrinkled linear marks on the abdominal skin. They are produced by gross stretching of the skin with rupture of the elastic fibres and indicate a recent change in size of the abdomen, such as is found in pregnancy, ascites, wasting diseases and severe dieting. Wide purple striae are characteristic of Cushing's syndrome and excessive steroid treatment.

Note any *scars* present, their site, whether they are old (white) or recent (red or pink), linear or stretched (and therefore likely to be weak and contain an incisional hernia). Common examples are given in Fig. 7.6.

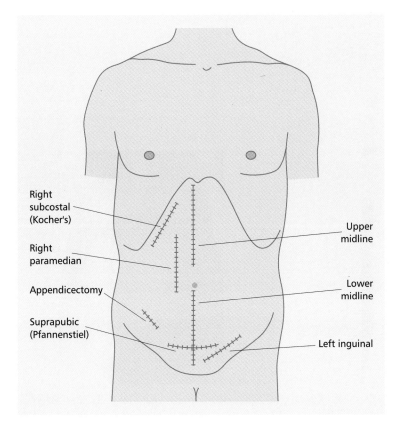

Right subcostal (Kocher's)

Right paramedian

Appendicectomy

Suprapubic (Pfannenstiel)

Upper midline

Lower midline

Left inguinal

Fig. 7.6 Some commonly used abdominal incisions. The midline and oblique incisions avoid damage to the innervation of the abdominal musculature and the later development of incisional hernia.

Look for *prominent superficial veins*, which may be apparent in three situations (Fig. 7.7): thin veins over the costal margin; occlusion of the inferior vena cava; and venous anastomoses in portal hypertension. However, small, thin veins over the subcostal margins are common and usually of no significance. *Inferior vena caval obstruction* not only causes oedema of the limbs, buttocks and groins, but in time distended veins on the abdominal wall and chest wall appear (Fig. 7.7(b)). These represent dilated anastomotic channels between the superficial epigastric and circumflex iliac veins below, and the lateral thoracic veins above, conveying the diverted blood from long saphenous vein to axillary vein; the direction of flow is therefore upwards. If the veins are prominent enough, try to detect the direction in which the blood is flowing (Fig. 7.8). Distended veins around the umbilicus (caput medusae) are uncommon but, if present, signify *portal hypertension* (Fig. 7.7(c)), other signs of which include splenomegaly and

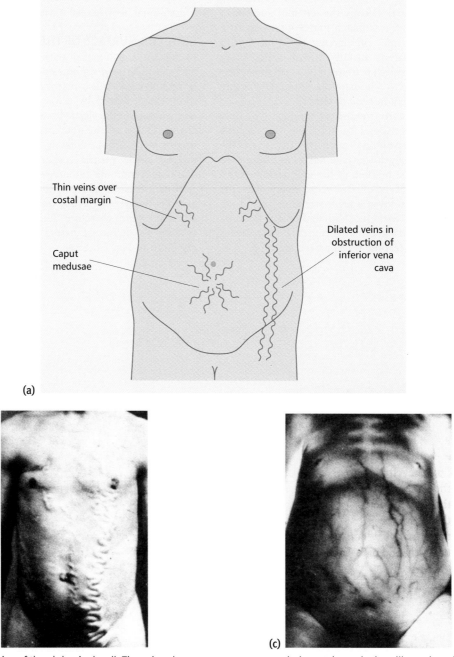

Thin veins over costal margin

Caput medusae

Dilated veins in obstruction of inferior vena cava

(a)

(b)

(c)

Fig. 7.7   **(a)** Veins of the abdominal wall. The veins shown represent venous drainage channels that dilate when there is obstruction in the inferior vena cava **(b)** or in the liver **(c)**.

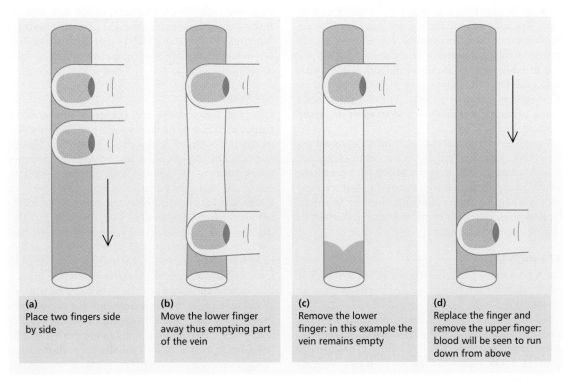

(a) Place two fingers side by side

(b) Move the lower finger away thus emptying part of the vein

(c) Remove the lower finger: in this example the vein remains empty

(d) Replace the finger and remove the upper finger: blood will be seen to run down from above

Fig. 7.8 A way of detecting the direction of blood flow in a vein. The venous valve prevents retrograde reflux **(c)** and the vein fills in its direction of flow **(d)**, after emptying **(a, b)**.

ascites. Distended veins represent the opening up of anastomoses between portal and systemic veins and are seen in other sites, such as oesophageal varices and piles.

Pigmentation of the abdominal wall may be seen in the midline below the umbilicus, where it forms the linea nigra and is a sign of pregnancy. Erythema ab igne is a brown mottled pigmentation produced by constant application of heat, usually a hot water bottle or heat pad, on the skin of the abdominal wall. It is a sign that the patient is experiencing severe pain and is most commonly associated with chronic pancreatitis.

Finally, inspect both groins, and the penis and scrotum of a male, for any swelling and to ensure that both testes are in their normal position. Then bring the sheet up just to cover the symphysis pubis.

PALPATION

Palpation forms the most important part of the abdominal examination. Tell the patient to relax as best they can and to breathe quietly, and assure them that you will be as gentle as possible. Enquire about the site of any pain and come to this region last. These points, together with unhurried palpation with a warm hand, will give the patient confidence and allow the maximum amount of information to be obtained. It is helpful to have a logical sequence to

follow and, if this is done as a matter of routine, then no important point will be omitted. The following scheme is suggested:

- Start in the left iliac region, palpating lightly, and work anticlockwise to end in the suprapubic region; repeat this using deeper palpation and with both hands if necessary
- Next feel for the left kidney
- Feel for the spleen
- Feel for the right kidney
- Feel for the liver
- Feel for the urinary bladder
- Feel for the aorta and para-aortic glands and common femoral vessels
- If a swelling is palpable, spend time eliciting its features
- Palpate both groins
- Examine the external genitalia.

Start by placing the right hand flat on the abdomen in the left iliac fossa with the wrist and forearm in the same horizontal plane where possible, even if this means bending down or kneeling by the patient's side (Fig. 7.9).

The art is to 'mould' the relaxed right hand to the abdominal wall, not to hold it rigid. The best movement is gentle but with firm pressure, with the fingers held almost straight with slight flexion at the metacarpophalangeal joints.

Avoid sudden poking with the fingertips (Fig. 7.10). Try and visualize the normal anatomical structures beneath the examining hand, and gently palpate each quadrant of the abdomen, noting any area of tenderness or localized rigidity. If necessary, repeat the palpation more slowly and deeply; in an obese or very muscular patient, putting the left hand on top of the right will allow you to exert increased pressure (Fig. 7.11).

A small proportion of patients find it impossible to relax their abdominal muscles when being examined. In such cases it may help to ask them to breathe deeply, to bend their knees up or to distract their attention in other ways. No matter how experienced the examiner, little will be gained from palpation of a poorly relaxed abdomen.

LEFT KIDNEY

The right hand is placed anteriorly in the left lumbar region while the left hand is placed posteriorly in the left loin (Fig. 7.12).

Ask the patient to take a deep breath in, press the left hand forwards, and the right hand backwards, upwards and inwards. The left kidney is not usually palpable unless either low in position or enlarged.

Its lower pole, when palpable, is felt as a rounded firm swelling between both right and left hands (i.e. bimanually palpable) and it can be pushed from one hand to the other in an action which is called 'ballotting'.

SPLEEN

Like the left kidney, the spleen is not normally palpable. It has to be enlarged to two or three times its usual size before it becomes palpable, and then is felt beneath the left subcostal margin. Enlargement takes place in a superior and posterior direction before it becomes palpable subcostally. Once the spleen has become palpable, the direction of further enlargement is downwards and towards the right iliac fossa (Fig. 7.13). Place the flat of the left hand over the lowermost rib cage posterolaterally, and the right hand beneath the costal margin well out to the left. Ask the patient to breathe in deeply, press in deeply with the fingers of the right hand beneath the costal margin, at the same time exerting considerable pressure medially and downwards with the left hand (Fig. 7.14). Repeat this manoeuvre with the right hand being moved more medially beneath the costal margin on each occasion (Fig. 7.15). If enlargement

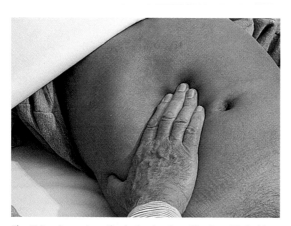

Fig. 7.9 Correct method of palpation. The hand is held flat and relaxed and 'moulded' to the abdominal wall.

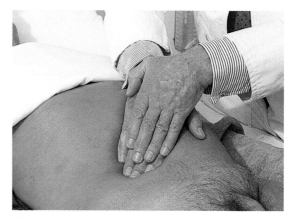

Fig. 7.11 Method of deep palpation in an obese, muscular or poorly relaxed patient.

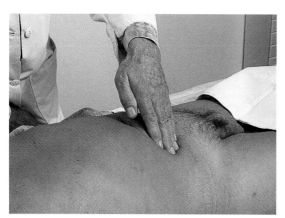

Fig. 7.10 Incorrect method of palpation. The hand is held rigid and mostly not in contact with the abdominal wall.

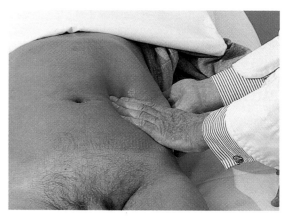

Fig. 7.12 Palpation of the left kidney.

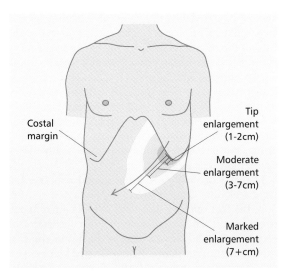

Fig. 7.13 The direction of enlargement of the spleen. The spleen has a characteristic notched shape and the organ moves downwards during full inspiration.

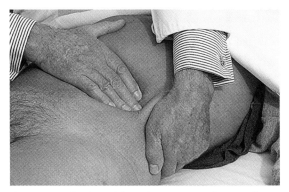

Fig. 7.14 Palpation of the spleen. Start well out to the left.

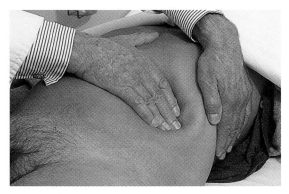

Fig. 7.15 Palpation of the spleen more medially than in Figure 7.14.

of the spleen is suspected from the history and it is still not palpable, turn the patient half on to the right side, ask them to relax back on to your left hand, which is now supporting the lower ribs, and repeat the examination as above. It may help to ask the patient to place the left hand on your right shoulder while palpating for the spleen.

In minor degrees of enlargement, the spleen will be felt as a firm swelling with smooth, rounded borders. Where considerable splenomegaly is present, its typical characteristics include a firm swelling appearing beneath the left subcostal margin in the left upper quadrant of the abdomen, which is dull to percussion, moves downwards on inspiration, is not bimanually palpable, whose upper border cannot be felt (i.e. one cannot 'get above it'), and in which a notch can often, though not invariably, be felt in the lower medial border. The last three features distinguish the enlarged spleen from an enlarged kidney; in addition there is usually a band of colonic resonance anterior to an enlarged kidney.

RIGHT KIDNEY

Feel for the right kidney in much the same way as for the left. Place the right hand horizontally in the right lumbar region anteriorly with the left hand placed posteriorly in the right loin. Push forwards with the left hand, ask the patient to take a deep breath in and press the right hand inwards and upwards (Fig. 7.16).

The lower pole of the right kidney, unlike the left, is commonly palpable in thin patients and is felt as a smooth, rounded swelling which descends on inspiration and is bimanually palpable and may be 'ballotted'.

LIVER

Sit on the couch beside the patient. Place both hands side-by-side flat on the abdomen in the right subcostal region lateral to the rectus with the fingers pointing towards the ribs. If resistance is encountered, move the hands further down until this resistance disappears. Ask the patient to breathe in deeply and, at the height of inspiration, press the fingers firmly inwards and upwards (Fig. 7.17).

If the liver is palpable it will be felt as a sharp, regular border which rides beneath the fingers. Repeat this manoeuvre working from lateral to medial regions to trace the liver edge as it passes upwards to cross from right hypochondrium to epigastrium. Another commonly employed though less accurate method of feeling for an enlarged liver is to place the right hand below and parallel to the right subcostal margin. The liver edge will then be felt against the radial border of the index finger (Fig. 7.18). The liver is often palpable in normal patients without being enlarged. If a liver edge is indefinitely felt, try to percuss in the right hypochondrium, keeping your hand still as the patient breathes deeply. Movement of the lower border together with dullness with respiration is further supporting evidence of hepatic enlargement. Hepatomegaly is conventionally described as being so many centimetres palpable below the right costal margin.

Try and make out the character of its surface (i.e. whether it is soft, smooth and tender as in heart failure, very firm and regular as in obstructive jaundice

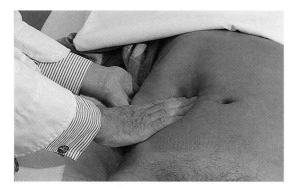

Fig. 7.16   Palpation of the right kidney.

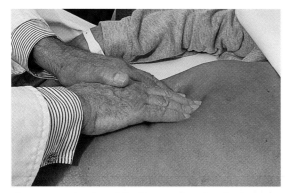

Fig. 7.17   Palpation of the liver: preferred method.

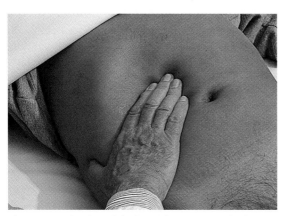

Fig. 7.18   Palpation of the liver: alternative method.

and cirrhosis, or hard, irregular, painless and sometimes nodular as in advanced secondary carcinoma). In tricuspid regurgitation the liver may be felt to pulsate. Occasionally a congenital variant of the right lobe projects down lateral to the gallbladder as a tongue-shaped process, called Riedel's lobe. Though uncommon, it is important to be aware of this because it may be mistaken either for the gallbladder itself or for the right kidney.

GALLBLADDER

The gallbladder is palpated in the same way as the liver. The normal gallbladder cannot be felt. When it is distended, however, it forms an important sign and

may be palpated as a firm, smooth, rough or globular swelling with distinct borders, just lateral to the edge of the rectus abdominis near the tip of the ninth costal cartilage. It moves with respiration. Its upper border merges with the lower border of the right lobe of the liver, or disappears beneath the costal margin and therefore can never be felt (Fig. 7.19). When the liver is enlarged or the gallbladder grossly distended, the latter may be felt not in the hypochondrium, but in the right lumbar or even as low down as the right iliac region.

The ease of definition of the rounded borders of the gallbladder, its comparative mobility on respiration, the fact that it is not normally bimanually palpable and that it seems to lie just beneath the abdominal wall helps to identify such a swelling as gallbladder rather than a palpable right kidney. This distribution may prove difficult, however, especially when the gallbladder lies in the mid or lower parts of the abdomen.

The gallbladder can usually be palpated in the following clinical situations. In *all* these situations the swelling is painless:

● In *carcinoma of the head of the pancreas* and other causes of malignant obstruction of the common bile duct, the ducts become dilated, as does the gallbladder. The patient is also deeply jaundiced.

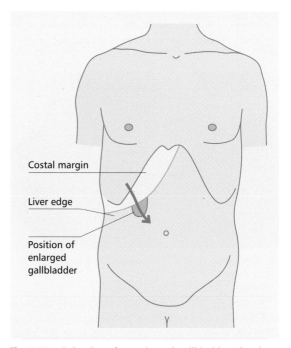

Fig. 7.19   Palpation of an enlarged gallbladder, showing how it merges with the inferior border of the liver so that only the fundus of the gallbladder and part of its body can be palpated.

- In *mucocele of the gallbladder*, a gallstone becomes impacted in the neck of a collapsed, empty, uninfected gallbladder and mucus continues to be secreted into its lumen. Finally, the uninfected wall is so distended that it becomes palpable. In this case the bile ducts are normal and the patient is not jaundiced.
- In *carcinoma of the gallbladder*, the gallbladder may be felt as a stony, hard, irregular swelling, unlike the firm, regular swelling of the two above-mentioned conditions.

Murphy's sign

In acute inflammation of the gallbladder (*acute cholecystitis*) severe pain is present. Often an exquisitely tender but indefinite mass can be palpated; this represents the underlying acutely inflamed gallbladder walled off by greater omentum. Ask the patient to breathe in deeply, and palpate for the gallbladder in the normal way; at the height of inspiration the breath is arrested with a gasp as the mass is felt. This represents Murphy's sign. The sign is *not* found in chronic cholecystitis or uncomplicated cases of gallstones.

THE URINARY BLADDER

Normally the urinary bladder is not palpable. When it is full and the patient cannot empty it (retention of urine), a smooth firm regular oval-shaped swelling will be palpated in the suprapubic region and its dome (upper border) may reach as far as the umbilicus. The lateral and upper borders can be readily made out, but it is not possible to feel its lower border (i.e. the swelling is 'arising out of the pelvis'). The fact that this swelling is symmetrically placed in the suprapubic region beneath the umbilicus, that it is dull to percussion, and that pressure on it gives the patient a desire to micturate, together with the signs above, confirm such a swelling as the bladder (Fig. 7.20).

In women, however, the palpable bladder has to be differentiated from a gravid uterus (firmer, mobile side to side and vaginal signs different), a fibroid uterus (may be bosselated, firmer and vaginal signs different) and an ovarian cyst (usually eccentrically placed to left or right side).

THE AORTA AND COMMON FEMORAL VESSELS

In most adults the aorta is not readily felt but with practice it can usually be detected by deep palpation a little above and to the left of the umbilicus. In thin patients, particularly women with a marked lumbar lordosis, the aorta is more easily palpable. Palpation of the aorta is one of the few occasions when the fingertips are used as a means of palpation. Press the extended fingers of both hands, held side by side, deeply into the abdominal wall in the position shown in Fig. 7.21; make out the left wall of the aorta and note its pulsation. Remove both hands and repeat the manoeuvre a few centimetres to the right. In this way the pulsation and width of the aorta can be estimated.

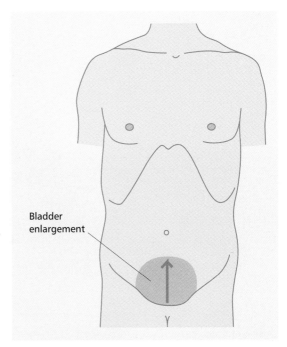

Fig. 7.20 Physical signs in retention of urine; a smooth, firm and regular swelling arising out of the pelvis which one cannot 'get below' and which is dull to percussion.

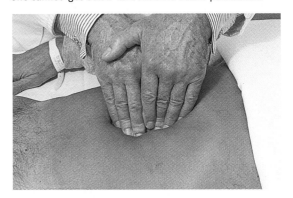

Fig. 7.21 Palpation of the abdominal aorta.

It is difficult to detect small aortic aneurysms; where a large one is present, its width may be assessed by placing a finger on either side of it and its expansile character noted by the fact that when pulsation occurs, the width between each finger increases (Fig. 7.22).

The common femoral vessels are found just below the inguinal ligament at the midpoint between the anterior superior iliac spine and symphysis pubis. Place the pulps of the right index, middle and ring fingers over this site in the right groin and palpate the wall of the vessel. Note the strength and character of its pulsation and then compare it with the opposite femoral pulse (Fig. 7.23).

Lymph nodes lying along the aorta (para-aortic nodes) are palpable only when considerably enlarged. They are felt as rounded, firm, often confluent, fixed masses in the umbilical region and epigastrium along the left border of the aorta.

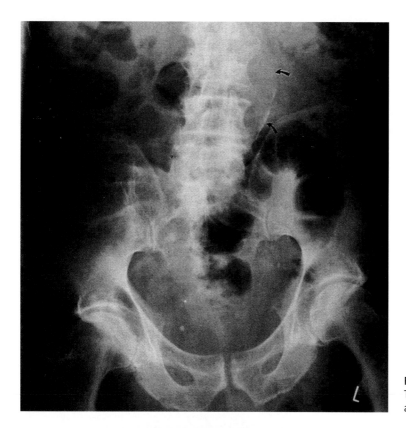

Fig. 7.22   Plain X-ray of the abdomen. The arrows mark the calcified wall of an aneurysm of the abdominal aorta.

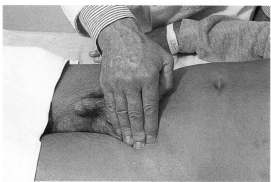

Fig. 7.23   Palpation of the right femoral artery.

CAUSES OF DIAGNOSTIC DIFFICULTY ON PALPATION

In many patients, especially those with a thin or lax abdominal wall, faeces in the colon may simulate an abdominal mass. The pelvic colon is frequently palpable, particularly when loaded with hard faeces. It is felt as a firm, tubular structure some 12 cm in length, situated low down in the left iliac fossa, parallel to the inguinal ligament. The caecum is often palpable in the right iliac fossa as a soft, rounded swelling with indistinct borders. The transverse colon is sometimes palpable in the epigastrium. It feels somewhat like the pelvic colon but rather larger and softer, with distinct upper and lower borders and a convex anterior surface. A faecal 'mass' will usually have disappeared or moved on repeat exam-

ination and may retain an indentation with pressure (not the case with a colonic malignancy).

In the epigastrium, the muscular bellies of rectus abdominis lying between its tendinous intersections can mimic an underlying mass and give rise to confusion. This can usually be resolved by asking the patient to tense the abdominal wall, when the 'mass' may be felt to contract.

WHAT TO DO WHEN AN ABDOMINAL MASS IS PALPABLE

When a swelling in the abdomen is palpable make sure first that it is not a *normal* structure, as described above. Next consider whether it could be due to enlargement of the liver, spleen, right or left kidney, gallbladder, urinary bladder, aorta or para-aortic nodes.

Now palpate the swelling again. The aim of examination is to decide the organ of origin and the pathological nature of the mass. In doing this it is helpful to bear in the mind the following points:

Site

First make sure that the swelling does indeed lie in the abdominal cavity and not in the anterior abdominal wall. Ask the patient to lift the head and shoulders off the pillow and press firmly against the forehead. Now feel the swelling again. If it disappears or becomes much less obvious, then it lies within the peritoneal cavity, whereas if it remains the same size it must be within the layers of the abdominal wall.

Note the region occupied by the swelling. Think of the organs that normally lie in or near this region and consider whether the swelling could arise from one of these organs. For instance, a swelling in the right upper quadrant most probably arises from the liver, right kidney, hepatic flexure of colon or gallbladder.

Now, if the swelling is in the upper abdomen, try and determine if it is possible to 'get above it', that is, to feel the upper border of the swelling as it disappears above the costal margin, and similarly, if it is in the lower abdomen, whether one can 'get below it'. If one cannot 'get above' an upper abdominal swelling, a hepatic, splenic, renal or gastric origin should be suspected. If one cannot 'get below' a lower abdominal mass the swelling probably arises in the bladder, uterus, ovary or occasionally upper rectum.

Size and shape

As a general rule, gross enlargement of the liver, spleen, uterus, bladder or ovary presents no undue difficulty in diagnosis. On the other hand swellings arising from the stomach, small or large bowel, retroperitoneal structures such as the pancreas, or the peritoneum (see section on mobility, below), may be difficult to diagnose. The larger a swelling arising from one of these structures, the more it tends to distort the outline of the organ of origin. For example, the characteristic outline of the kidney is retained early on, but when there is a large renal mass this outline is lost and recognition becomes difficult.

Surface, edge and consistency

The pathological nature of a mass is suggested by a number of features. A swelling that is hard, irregular in outline and nodular is likely to be a *neoplasm*, while a regular, round, smooth, tense swelling is likely to be *cystic*, but remember degeneration and softening with cyst formation occurs not infrequently in malignant tumours. A solid, ill-defined and tender mass suggests an inflammatory lesion as in Crohn's disease of the ileocaecal region.

Mobility and attachments

Considerable information can be gained from eliciting the mobility or fixity of an abdominal mass. Swellings arising in the liver, spleen, kidneys, gallbladder and distal stomach all show downward movement during inspiration, due to contraction of the diaphragm. One cannot, however, move such structures with the examining hand. In contrast, swellings originating in structures that have a mesenteric or other broad base of attachment are not influenced by respiratory movements but *can* be made to move freely by palpation, for example tumours of the small bowel and transverse colon, cysts in the mesentery, and large secondary deposits in the greater omentum.

When, on the other hand, the swelling is completely fixed it usually signifies one of three things:

- A mass of retroperitoneal origin (e.g. pancreas)
- Part of an advanced tumour with extensive spread to the anterior or posterior abdominal walls or abdominal organs
- A swelling resulting from severe chronic inflammation involving other organs (e.g. diverticulitis of the sigmoid colon or a colovesical attachment or fistula).

In the lower abdomen, the side-to-side mobility of a fibroid or pregnant uterus rapidly establishes such a swelling as uterine in origin and as not arising from bladder or ovary.

IS IT BIMANUALLY PALPABLE OR PULSATILE?

Bimanually palpable swellings in the lumbar region are usually renal in origin. Just occasionally, however, a posteriorly situated gallbladder or a mass in the posteroinferior part of the right lobe of the liver may give the impression of being bimanually palpable.

Finally, try to decide whether a swelling exhibits *pulsation*. It is often difficult to be certain whether a swelling in the upper abdomen that is pulsatile is merely transmitting pulsation from the underlying aorta or whether it is truly expansile in nature. The best way to determine this is to place two fingers on the swelling and observe what happens to them in systole. If the fingers remain parallel, then the pulsation is transmitted. If, however, the fingers tend to separate, then true expansile pulsation is present and the swelling is arterial, and may be an aneurysm (see p. 143).

PERCUSSION

Details of how to percuss correctly are given in Chapter 5. In the abdomen only light percussion is necessary—a resonant (tympanitic) note is heard throughout except over the liver, where the note is dull. Percussion is particularly useful for confirming the presence of an enlarged liver or spleen suspected on palpation. The absence of dullness over the suspected mass makes the diagnosis of hepatomegaly or splenomegaly unlikely.

DEFINING THE BOUNDARIES OF ABDOMINAL ORGANS AND MASSES

Liver

The upper and lower borders of the right lobe of the liver can be mapped out accurately by percussion. Start anteriorly, at the fourth intercostal space, where the note will be resonant over the lungs, and work vertically downwards. In the normal liver the upper border is found at about the fifth intercostal space, where the note will become dull; this dullness extends down to the lower border at or just below the right subcostal margin. The normal dullness over the upper part of the liver is reduced in severe emphysema, in the presence of a large right pneumothorax and when there is gas or air in the peritoneal cavity. The latter, occurring in a patient with severe abdominal pain, indicates perforation of a viscus (unless the patient has recently undergone laparotomy). This sign, however, is not one that should be relied on as there has to be a large volume of air or gas present to reduce the normal liver dullness, and this is not usually the case.

Percussion just below the right costal margin is useful in hepatomegaly. Ask the patient to breathe deeply while you percuss lightly, keeping the finger parallel to the rib margin. As the liver descends during inspiration a change in percussion note from resonance to dullness signals the edge of the liver. The upper margin of the liver can also be assessed, so giving a direct measure of hepatic size, normally 12–15 cm in height, i.e. extending to the fifth rib, or just below the right nipple in men.

Spleen
Percussion over an enlarged spleen provides rapid confirmation of the findings detected on palpation (page 140 and Fig. 7.14). Dullness extends from the left lower ribs into the left hypochondrium and left lumbar region. The lower border of an enlarged spleen is readily mapped out; splenic dullness gives way to the resonance of surrounding bowel.

Bladder
The findings in a patient with retention of urine are usually unmistakable on palpation (page 143 and Fig. 7.20). The dullness on percussion provides reassurance that the swelling is cystic or solid and not gaseous; its superior and lateral borders can be readily defined from adjacent bowel, which is resonant.

Other masses
The boundaries of any localized swelling in the abdominal cavity, or in the walls of the abdomen, can sometimes be defined more accurately by percussion than palpation. The dullness of a solid or cystic mass contrasts with the tympanitic note of surrounding loops of bowel.

DETECTION OF ASCITES AND ITS DIFFERENTIATION FROM OVARIAN CYST AND INTESTINAL OBSTRUCTION
Three common causes of diffuse enlargement of the abdomen are:

- The presence of free fluid in the peritoneum (*ascites*)
- A massive ovarian cyst
- Obstruction of the large bowel, distal small bowel, or both.

Percussion rapidly distinguishes between these three, as can be seen in Fig. 7.24. Other helpful symptoms or signs which are usually present are as follows.

Gross ascites
- Dull in flanks
- Umbilicus transverse and/or hernia present
- Shifting dullness positive
- Fluid thrill positive.

Large ovarian cyst
- Resonant in flank
- Umbilicus vertical and drawn up
- Large swelling felt arising out of pelvis which one cannot 'get below'.

Intestinal obstruction
- Resonant throughout
- Colicky pain
- Vomiting
- Constipation
- Increased and/or 'noisy' bowel sounds.

It is unwise and difficult to diagnose *ascites* unless there is sufficient free fluid present to give generalized enlargement of the abdomen. Two signs—shifting dullness and a fluid thrill—which present either singly or together, make the diagnosis of ascites certain. Useful as these two signs are, they can be elicited in only about half the cases of ascites. Absence of shifting dullness or of fluid thrill or both does *not* exclude a diagnosis of ascites.

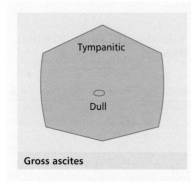
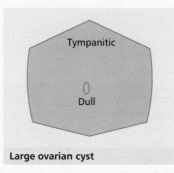
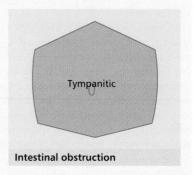

Fig. 7.24 Diffuse enlargement of the abdomen.

To demonstrate *shifting dullness*, lie the patient supine and percuss laterally from the midline, keeping your fingers in the longitudinal axis, until dullness is detected; in normal individuals dullness is detected only over the lateral abdominal musculature. Then, keeping your hand on the abdomen, ask the patient to roll away from you, on to the left side. Percuss again in this new position; if the previously dull note has now become resonant then ascitic fluid is probably present. To confirm its presence, repeat the manoeuvre on the left side of the abdomen.

To elicit a *fluid thrill* the patient is again laid supine. Place one hand flat over the lumbar region of one side, and get an assistant to put the side of the hand firmly in the midline of the abdomen. Then flick or tap the opposite lumbar region (Fig. 7.25). A fluid thrill or wave is felt as a definite and unmistakable impulse by the detecting hand held flat in the lumbar region. (The purpose of the assistant's hand is to dampen any impulse that may be transmitted through the fat of the abdominal wall.) As a rule a fluid thrill is felt only when there is a large amount of ascites present which is under tension.

AUSCULTATION

Auscultation is a useful way of listening for bowel sounds and deciding whether they are normal, increased or absent, and of detecting bruits in the aorta and main abdominal vessels.

The stethoscope should be placed on one site on the abdominal wall (just to the right of the umbilicus is best) and kept there until sounds are heard. It should not be moved from site to site. Normal bowel sounds are heard as intermittent low- or medium-pitched gurgles interspersed with an occasional high-pitched noise or tinkle.

In *simple acute mechanical obstruction of the small bowel* the bowel sounds are excessive and exaggerated. Frequent loud low-pitched gurgles (*borborygmi*) are heard, often rising to a crescendo of high-pitched tinkles and occurring in a rhythmic pattern with peristaltic activity. The presence of such

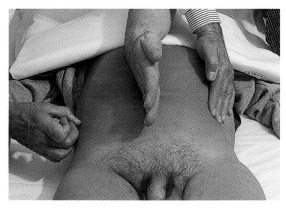

Fig. 7.25   Eliciting a fluid thrill.

sounds occurring at the same time as the patient experiences bouts of colicky abdominal pain is pathognomonic of small bowel obstruction. In between the bouts of peristaltic activity and colicky pain, the bowel is quiet and no sounds are heard on auscultation.

In an obstructed loop of bowel, when strangulation and, later, gangrene supervene, however, peristalsis ceases, and the bowel sounds rapidly become less frequent and stop altogether. In *generalized peritonitis* bowel activity rapidly disappears and a state of *paralytic ileus* ensues, with gradually increasing abdominal distension. The abdomen is 'silent' but one must listen for several minutes before being certain that such a state exists. Frequently towards the end of this period a short run of faint, very high-pitched tinkling sounds is heard. This represents fluid spilling over from one distended gas- and fluid-filled loop to another and is characteristic of ileus.

A *succussion splash* may be elicited by palpation (p. 137) and also on auscultation. It may be heard in pyloric stenosis, in advanced intestinal obstruction with grossly distended loops of bowel and in paralytic ileus. Lie the patient supine and, using the palm of the right hand, place the stethoscope over the epigastrium. Then roll the patient from side to side to agitate any fluid and gas in the stomach. If the stomach is distended with fluid a splashing sound, like the noise made by a hot water bottle partially filled with water and air, will be heard.

Vascular bruits may also be heard in the abdomen. Place the stethoscope lightly on the abdominal wall over the aorta, above and to the left of the umbilicus, and listen for a bruit. Do likewise over each iliac artery in the corresponding iliac fossa, and over the common femoral arteries in each groin. If a bruit is heard it is a significant finding which indicates turbulent flow in the underlying vessel, either due to stenosis or to aneurysm. Very occasionally bruits may be heard in the epigastrium when there is stenosis of the coeliac axis or superior mesenteric artery, or on either side of the midline in the mid-abdomen in patients with hypertension due to stenosis of the renal artery (see Ch. 9). A bruit may also be heard over a hepatoma because of increased blood flow within the tumour.

THE GROINS

Once the groins have been inspected, ask the patient to turn the head to one side and cough. Look at both inguinal canals for any expansile impulse. If none is apparent, place the left hand in the left groin so that the fingers lie over and in line with the inguinal canal; place the right hand similarly in the right groin (Fig. 7.26). Now ask the patient to give a loud cough and feel for any expansile impulse with each hand.

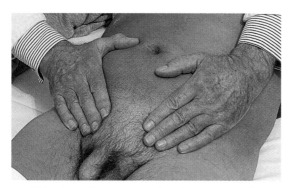

Fig. 7.26   Palpating the groins to detect an expansile impulse on coughing.

When a patient coughs, the muscles of the abdominal wall contract violently and this imparts a definite, though not expansile, impulse to the palpating hands which is a source of confusion to the inexperienced. Trying to differentiate this normal contraction from a small, fully reducible inguinal hernia is difficult, and the matter can usually be resolved only when the patient is standing up.

The femoral vessels have already been felt (Fig. 7.23) and auscultated. Now palpate along the femoral artery for enlarged inguinal nodes, feeling with the fingers of the right hand, and carry this palpation medially beneath the inguinal ligament towards the perineum. Then repeat this on the left side. A patient who complains of a lump in the groin should be examined lying down *and standing up*.

THE MALE GENITALIA

The examination of the genitalia is important in men presenting with abnormalities in the groin, and in many acute or subacute abdominal syndromes. Thus disease of the genitalia may lead to abdominal symptoms, such as pain or swelling.

Disposable gloves should be worn if there is any suspicion of venereal infection. A detailed description is given in Chapter 20.

WHAT TO DO IF A PATIENT COMPLAINS OF A LUMP IN THE GROIN

A lump in the groin or scrotum is a common clinical problem in all age-groups. Most lumps in the groin are due either to herniae or to enlarged inguinal nodes; inguinal herniae are considerably more common than femoral, with an incidence ratio of 4:1. In the scrotum, hydrocele of the tunica vaginalis or a cyst of the epididymis are common causes of painless swelling; acute epididymo-orchitis is the most frequent cause of a painful swelling.

Examination of the groins and scrotum is part of a general examination and must not be conducted in isolation. Generalized diseases such as lymphoma may present as a lump in the groin. Usually the diagnosis of a lump in the groin or scrotum can be made simply and accurately. Remember that the patient should be examined not only lying down, but also standing up.

Ask the patient to stand in front of you, get him to point to the side and site of the swelling and note whether it extends into the scrotum. Get him to turn his head to one side and give a loud cough; look for an expansile impulse and try to decide whether it is above or below the crease of the inguinal ligament. If an expansile impulse is present on inspection, it is likely to be a hernia, so move to whichever side of the patient the lump in the groin is on. Stand beside and slightly behind the patient. If the right groin is being examined, place the left hand over the right buttock to support the patient, the fingers of the right hand being placed obliquely over the inguinal canal. Now ask the patient to cough again. If an expansile impulse is felt then the lump must be a hernia.

Next decide whether the hernia is *inguinal* or *femoral*. The best way to do this is to determine the relationship of the sac to the pubic tubercle. To locate this structure push gently upwards from beneath the neck of the scrotum with the index finger (Fig. 7.27) but do not invaginate the neck of the scrotum as this is painful. The tubercle will be felt as a small bony prominence 2 cm from the midline on the pubic crest. In thin patients the tubercle is easily felt but this is not so in the obese. If difficulty is found, follow up the tendon of adductor longus, which arises just below the tubercle.

If the hernial sac passes *medial to and above* the index finger placed on the pubic tubercle, then the hernia must be inguinal in site; if it is *lateral to and below*, then the hernia must be femoral in site.

If it has been decided that the hernia is inguinal then one needs to know these further points:

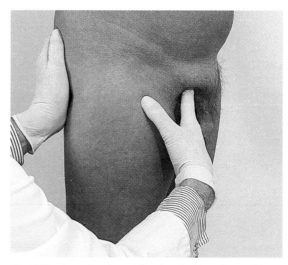

Fig. 7.27   Locating the pubic tubercle. Note the position of the examiner, at the side of the patient, with one hand supporting the buttock.

- *What are the contents of the sac*? Bowel tends to gurgle, is soft and compressible, while *omentum* feels firmer and is of a doughy consistency.
- *Is the hernia fully reducible or not*? It is best to lie the patient down to decide this. Ask the patient whether the hernia is reducible and if so get him to reduce it himself to confirm this. (It is more painful if the examiner reduces it.)
- *Is the hernia direct or indirect*? Again, it is best to lie the patient down to decide this. Inspection of the direction of the impulse is often diagnostic, especially in thin patients. A direct hernia tends to bulge straight out through the posterior wall of the inguinal canal, whilst in an indirect hernia the impulse can often be seen to travel obliquely down the inguinal canal. Another helpful point is to place one finger just above the mid-inguinal point over the deep inguinal ring (Fig. 7.28). If a hernia is fully controlled by this finger then it must be an indirect inguinal hernia.

Apart from a femoral hernia, the differential diagnosis of an inguinal hernia includes a large hydrocele of the tunica vaginalis, a large cyst of the epididymis (one should be able to 'get above' and feel the upper border of both of these in the scrotum), an undescended or ectopic testis (there will be an empty scrotum on the affected side), a lipoma of the cord, and a hydrocele of the cord.

In considering the *differential diagnosis of a femoral hernia*, one must think not only of an inguinal hernia but of a lipoma in the femoral triangle, an aneurysm of the femoral artery (expansile pulsation will be present), a saphen-ovarix (the swelling disappears on lying down, has a bluish tinge to it, there are often varicose veins present and there may be a venous hum), a psoas abscess (the mass is fluctuant, and may be compressible beneath the inguinal ligament to appear above it in the iliac fossa), and an enlarged inguinal lymph node. Whenever the latter is found, the feet, legs, thighs, scrotum, perineum and the pudendal and perianal areas must be carefully scrutinized for a source of infection or primary tumour.

The examination is completed by following the same scheme in the opposite groin.

WHAT TO DO WHEN THE PATIENT COMPLAINS OF A SWELLING IN THE SCROTUM

It is easier and better to examine the patient first lying down and afterwards standing up. *Inspection, palpation* and *transillumination* are the three keys to rapid, accurate diagnosis. After inspection of the scrotum and groins, try and answer the following questions:

Can I 'get above' the swelling?

Palpate the neck of the scrotum between fingers and thumb. If fingers and thumb cannot be approximated so that only the spermatic cord is palpable, then the swelling in question is not confined to the scrotum but is descending from the groin and is therefore an inguinoscrotal hernia, i.e. one cannot 'get above' it. (Very rarely an infantile hydrocele occurs which leads to the same signs though the testis is impalpable.) If fingers and thumb can be approximated so that one can 'get above' the swelling, that swelling can only be arising from the cord, the epididymis or the testis.

Is the swelling cystic or solid?

Is the testis palpable separately from the swelling? Palpate the swelling in the same way as the testis and scrotal contents (Chapter 20), which will give a good indication whether the swelling is cystic or solid.

What does it look like when transilluminated?

Tense the scrotal skin gently over the swelling and place a bright torch *behind* the swelling. If it transmits light then it must be a cystic swelling and is either a *cyst of the epididymis* (a spermatocele) or a *hydrocele of the tunica vaginalis*. The former lies above and a little behind the testis and the testis is palpable separately from the swelling. In the latter the testis is not palpable separately from the swelling (i.e. it is enclosed within the tunica vaginalis and therefore surrounded by fluid).

If the cyst is not translucent then its consistency is solid. Palpate the epididymis and testis again. Enlargement of the epididymis is found in inflammation (*epididymitis*): if it is tender it is acute; if it is painless it is chronic (and usually tuberculous). Enlargement of the testis is found in *orchitis* (usually acute), when it is therefore tender or, rarely, as a result of *malignancy*.

Is it visible only when the patient is standing?

A swelling that is not apparent lying down but appears on standing and which feels soft and rather like palpating a bag of worms is a *varicocele* (i.e. varicosity of the veins of the pampiniform and/or cremasteric plexi).

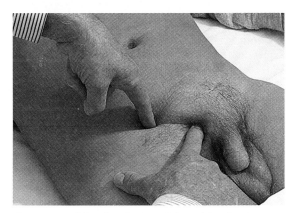

Fig. 7.28   Left hand: palpation of the pubic tubercle; index finger occluding the deep inguinal ring. Right hand: index finger on the pubic tubercle.

THE FEMALE GENITALIA

These are described in Chapter 14 and 20. As in men, examination of the genitalia may be an important part of the examination of the gastrointestinal system in acute abdominal disorders.

THE ANUS AND RECTUM

Few other regions of the body reveal such a wealth of physical signs and diagnoses on inspection and digital examination as the perianal area, anus, anal canal and rectum.

The left lateral position is best for routine examination of the rectum (Fig. 7.29). Make sure that the buttocks project over the side of the couch with the knees drawn well up, and that a good light is available. Put a disposable glove on the right hand and stand slightly behind the patient's buttocks, facing the patient's feet. Tell the patient what you are about to do and that you will be as gentle as possible.

INSPECTION

Separate the buttocks carefully and inspect the perianal area and anus. Note the presence of any abnormality of the perianal skin, such as inflammation, which may vary in appearance from mild erythema to a raw, red, moist, weeping dermatitis, or in chronic cases thickened white skin with exaggeration of the anal skin folds. The latter form *anal skin tags*, which may follow not only *severe pruritus* but also occur when prolapsing piles have been present over a period of time. Tags should not be confused with *anal warts* (condylomata acuminata), which are sessile or pedunculated papillomata with a red base and a white surface. Anal warts may be so numerous as to surround the anal verge, and even extend into the anal canal. Note any 'hole' or dimple near the anus with a tell-tale bead of pus or granulation tissue surrounding it, which represents the external opening of a *fistula-in-ano*. It is usually easy to dis-

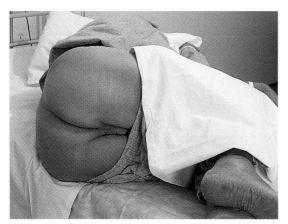

Fig. 7.29   Left lateral position for rectal examination.

tinguish a fistula-in-ano from a *pilonidal sinus*, where the opening lies in the midline of the natal cleft but well posterior to the anus.

The following acutely painful anorectal conditions can usually be diagnosed readily on inspection. An *anal fissure* usually lies directly posterior in the midline. The outward pathognomonic sign of a chronic fissure is a tag of skin at the base (sentinel pile). The fissure can easily be demonstrated by gently drawing apart the anus to reveal the tear in the lining of the anal canal.

A *perianal haematoma* (thrombosed external pile) occurs as a result of rupture of a vein of the external haemorrhoidal plexus. It is seen as a small (1 cm), tense, bluish swelling on one aspect of the anal margin and is exquisitely tender to the touch. In *prolapsed strangulated piles*, there is gross swelling of the anal and perianal skin, which looks like oedematous lips, with a deep red or purple strangulated pile appearing in between, and sometimes partly concealed by, the oedema of the swollen anus. In a *perianal abscess*, an acutely tender, red fluctuant swelling is visible which deforms the outline of the anus. It is usually easy to distinguish this from an *ischiorectal abscess* where the anal verge is not deformed, the signs of acute inflammation are often lacking and the point of maximum tenderness is located midway between the anus and ischial tuberosity.

Note the presence of any ulceration. Finally, if rectal *prolapse* is suspected, ask the patient to bear down and note whether any pink rectal mucosa or bowel appears through the anus, or whether the perineum itself bulges downwards. Downward bulging of the perineum during straining at bending down, or in response to a sudden cough, indicates weakness of the pelvic floor support musculature, usually due to denervation of these muscles. This sign is often found in women after childbirth, in women with faecal or urinary incontinence and in patients with severe chronic constipation.

DIGITAL EXAMINATION (PALPATION)

Put a generous amount of lubricant on the gloved index finger of the right hand, place the *pulp* of the finger (not the tip) flat on the anus (Figs 7.30 and 7.31) and press firmly and slowly in a slightly backwards direction. After initial resistance the anal sphincter relaxes and the finger can be passed into the anal canal. If severe pain is elicited attempting this manoeuvre then further examination should be abandoned as it is likely the patient has a fissure and unnecessary pain will be caused.

Rotate the finger through 360 degrees in the canal and feel for any thickening or irregularity of the wall of the canal. Assess the tone of the anal musculature; it should normally grip the finger firmly. If there is any doubt ask the patient to contract the anus on the examining finger or to cough. The latter induces a

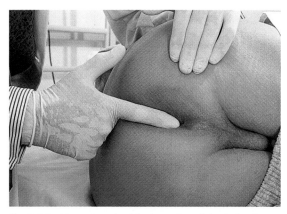

Fig. 7.30 Correct method for insertion of the index finger in rectal examination. The pulp of the finger is placed flat against the anus.

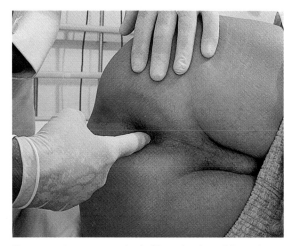

Fig. 7.31 Incorrect method of introduction of finger into the anal canal.

brisk contraction of the external anal sphincter which in the normal patient will be readily appreciated. In the old and infirm with anal incontinence or prolapse almost no appreciable contraction will be felt. With experience it is usually possible to feel a shallow groove just inside the anal canal which marks the dividing line between the external and internal sphincter. The anorectal ring may be felt as a stout band of muscle surrounding the junction between the anal canal and rectum.

Now pass the finger into the anorectum. The examiner's left hand should be placed on the patient's right hip and later it can be placed in the suprapubic position to exert downward pressure on the sigmoid colon. Try to visualize the anatomy of the rectum, particularly in relation to its anterior wall. The rectal wall should be assessed with sweeping movements of the finger through 360 degrees, 2, 5 and 8 cm inwards or until the finger cannot be pushed any higher into the rectum. Repeat these movements as the finger is being withdrawn. In this way it is possible to detect malignant ulcers, proliferative and stenosing carcinomas, polyps and villous

adenomas. The hollow of the sacrum and coccyx can be felt posteriorly. Laterally, on either side, it is usually possible to reach the side walls of the pelvis. In men one should feel anteriorly for the *rectovesical* pouch, *seminal vesicles* and the *prostate*. Normally the rectovesical pouch and seminal vesicles are not palpable. In a patient with a pelvic abscess, however, pus gravitates to this pouch, which is then palpable as a boggy, tender swelling lying above the prostate. If the pouch contains malignant deposits, hard irregular nodules may be felt. In infection of the seminal vesicles, these structures become palpable as firm, almost tubular swellings deviating slightly from the midline just above the level of the prostate.

In men, assessment of the *prostate gland* is important. It forms a rubbery, firm swelling about the size of a large chestnut. Run the finger over each lateral lobe, which should be smooth and regular. Between the two lobes lies the median sulcus, which is palpable as a faint depression running vertically between each lateral lobe. Though it is possible to say on rectal examination that a prostate is enlarged, accurate assessment of its true size is not possible. In carcinoma of the prostate, the gland loses its rubbery consistency and becomes hard, whilst the lateral lobes tend to be irregular and nodular and there is distortion or loss of the median sulcus.

In women, the cervix is felt as a firm, rounded mass projecting back into the anterior wall of the rectum. This is often a disconcerting finding for the inexperienced. The body of a retroverted uterus, fibroid mass, ovarian cyst, malignant nodule or a pelvic abscess may all be palpated in the pouch of Douglas (recto-uterine pouch), which lies above the cervix. This aspect of rectal examination forms an essential part of pelvic assessment in female patients.

On withdrawing the finger after rectal examination look at it for evidence of mucus, pus and blood. If in doubt wipe the finger on a white swab. Finally make sure to wipe the patient clean before telling him or her that the examination is completed.

THE ACUTE ABDOMEN

Diagnosis and management of acute abdominal disorders depends on information derived both from the history and from the examination.

HISTORY

The patient usually presents with *acute abdominal pain*. In considering this symptom, its site, severity, radiation, character, time and circumstances of onset, and any relieving features are all important.

SITE

Ask the patient to point to the site of maximal pain with one finger. If pain is experienced mostly in the *upper abdomen* think of perforation of a gastric or duodenal ulcer, cholecystitis or pancreatitis. If pain is located in the *mid-abdomen*, disease of the small bowel is likely. Pain in the *right iliac fossa* is commonly due to appendicitis and pain in the *left iliac fossa* to diverticulitis. In women *low abdominal pain* of acute onset is often due to salpingitis, but rupture of an ectopic pregnancy should also be considered; the menstrual history is thus important. The coexistence of *severe back and abdominal pain* may indicate a ruptured abdominal aneurysm or a dissecting aneurysm. When the parietal peritoneum is irritated, pain is felt at the site of the affected organ, but when the visceral peritoneum is predominantly involved pain is often referred in a somatic distribution. For example, in acute appendicitis pain is felt near the umbilicus at first but later, with parietal peritoneal involvement, moves towards the site of the appendix, usually in the right iliac fossa.

SEVERITY

Try to assess the severity of the pain. Ask whether it keeps the patient awake. In women who have had children, compare the severity with labour pains. Sometimes comparison to the pain of a fractured bone is useful.

RADIATION

If pain radiates from the right subcostal region to the shoulder or to the interscapular region, inflammation of the gallbladder (cholecystitis) is a likely diagnosis. If pain begins in the loin but then is felt in the lumbar region a renal stone or renal infection should be considered. Pain beginning in the loin and radiating to the groin is likely to be due to a ureteric calculus and umbilical pain radiating to the right iliac fossa is usually due to appendicitis. Central upper abdominal pain, later radiating through to the back, is common in pancreatitis.

CHARACTER AND CONSTANCY

Constant severe pain felt over many hours is likely to be due to infection. For example, diverticulitis or pyelonephritis can present in this manner. *Colicky pain*, on the other hand (i.e. pain lasting a few seconds or minutes and then passing off, leaving the patient free of pain for a further few minutes), is typical of small bowel obstruction. If such pain is suddenly relieved after a period of several hours of severe pain, perforation of a viscus should be considered. Large bowel obstruction produces a more constant pain than small bowel obstruction, but colic is usually prominent.

MODE OF ONSET

In obstruction from mechanical disorders such as that due to biliary or ureteric stone, or obstruction of the bowel from adhesions or volvulus, the onset of colicky pain is usually sudden. It is often related to activity or movement in the previous few hours. In infective and inflammatory disorders the pain usually has a slower onset, sometimes over several days, and there is no relation to activity. Recent ingestion of a rich, heavy meal sometimes precedes pancreatitis. Alcohol excess or the ingestion of aspirin or steroid therapy are sometimes precipitating features in patients presenting with perforated peptic ulcer or with haematemesis.

RELIEVING FEATURES

Abdominal pain relieved by rest suggests an infective or inflammatory disorder. If the patient cannot keep still and rolls around in agony then ureteric or biliary colic are likely diagnoses.

VOMITING

A history of vomiting is not in itself very helpful because vomiting occurs as a response to pain of any type. However, effortless projectile vomiting often denotes pyloric stenosis or high small bowel obstruction. In peritonitis the vomitus is usually small in amount but vomiting is persistent. There may be a faeculent smell to the vomitus when there is low small bowel obstruction. Persistent vomiting with associated diarrhoea strongly suggests gastroenteritis (see section on examination of vomit, p. 154).

MICTURITION

Increased frequency of micturition occurs both in urinary tract infections and in other pelvic inflammatory disorders as well as in patients with renal infections or ureteric stones. In the latter, haematuria commonly occurs.

APPETITE AND WEIGHT

In patients with a chronic underlying disorder, such as abdominal cancer, there may be a history of anorexia and weight loss, although weight loss also occurs in a variety of other disorders. Sudden loss of appetite clearly indicates a disorder of sudden onset.

OTHER FEATURES

It is important to note whether there have been previous episodes of abdominal pain and whether or not they have been severe. A tendency to improvement or worsening of the patient's symptoms after the onset is also important in deciding on management. The patient may have noticed swellings at the site of a hernial orifice, indicating the likelihood of an obstructed hernia, or there may be a history of blunt or penetrating abdominal trauma. Sometimes the patient may be aware of increasing abdominal distension, a phenomenon indicating intestinal obstruction or paralytic ileus probably associated with an inflammatory or infective underlying bowel disorder. Food poisoning may be suggested by a history of ingestion of unusual foods such as shellfish or a meal in unfamiliar surroundings. The menstrual history should never be forgotten, particularly in relation to the possibility of an ectopic pregnancy. Enquiry should always be made as to a purulent vaginal discharge, indicating salpingitis, or of discharge of mucus, pus or blood from the rectum, suggesting ulcerative colitis.

EXAMINATION

There are certain features that are important in all patients presenting with an acute abdominal crisis. The physical signs found on inspection and on auscultation (p. 146 and 151) have already been discussed.

GUARDING

Guarding is an involuntary reflex contraction of the muscles of the abdominal wall overlying an inflamed viscus and peritoneum, producing localized rigidity. It indicates localized peritonitis. What is felt on examination is spasm of the muscle, which prevents palpation of the underlying viscus. Guarding is seen classically in uncomplicated acute appendicitis. It is very important to distinguish this sign from voluntary contraction of muscle.

RIGIDITY

Generalized or 'board-like' rigidity is an indication of diffuse peritonitis. It can be looked upon as an extension of guarding, with involuntary reflex rigid-ity of the muscles of the anterior abdominal wall. It is quite unmistakable on palpation, as the whole abdominal wall feels hard and 'board-like', precluding palpation of any underlying viscus. The least downward pressure with a palpating hand in a patient with generalized rigidity produces severe pain. It may be differentiated from voluntary spasm by getting the patient to breathe: in voluntary spasm the abdominal wall will be felt to relax during expiration.

REBOUND TENDERNESS

Rebound tenderness is elicited by palpating slowly and deeply over a viscus and then suddenly releasing the palpating hand. If rebound tenderness is positive, then the patient experiences pain. This sign is explained by the fact that gradual stretching of the abdominal wall by deep palpation followed by sudden release of this pressure stimulates the parietal peritoneum which, if inflamed, produces pain. Rebound tenderness is not always a reliable sign and should be interpreted with caution, particularly in those patients with a low pain threshold.

RADIOLOGY

A plain X-ray of the abdomen is an important immediate investigation in the diagnosis of the acute abdomen, especially in suspected perforation or obstruction (Fig. 7.32).

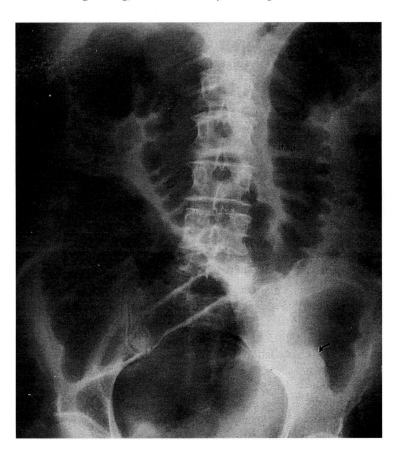

Fig. 7.32 Plain X-ray of the abdomen. Obstruction of the large bowel due to carcinoma of the sigmoid colon (curved arrow). The two small arrows indicate the transverse haustrae of the colon. The colon is dilated with gas, indicating obstruction.

EXAMINATION OF VOMIT

The character of the vomit varies with the nature of the food ingested and the absence or presence of bile, blood or intestinal obstruction. In pyloric stenosis the vomit is apt to be copious and sour-smelling, to contain recognizable food eaten many hours before and to exhibit froth on the surface after standing. The presence of much mucus gives vomit a viscid consistency. The appearance of the vomit in haematemesis varies in relation to the site and severity of the bleeding. If bleeding is copious the vomit may present the appearance of pure blood, or it may be dark red and contain clots. Such bleeding may come from a gastric ulcer or from the oesophageal varices of portal hypertension. More commonly the blood is altered to a blackish or dark brown colour by being in contact with gastric juice. The dark brown colour is due to the conversion of haemoglobin into haematin. The altered blood gives to the vomit an appearance often compared to that of 'coffee grounds'. The taking of preparations of iron or red wine may produce a similar appearance in the vomit. Vomit which contains dark green bile may resemble vomit which contains blood; however, on diluting with water the green colour of the bile becomes more apparent while blood remains dark. Remember that blood in vomit may have come from the nose or lungs and been swallowed; bright red blood that is 'vomited' nearly always originates from the naso- or oropharynx and not from the stomach. Faeculent vomit, characteristic of advanced intestinal obstruction, is brown in colour, rather like vomited tea. Its main hallmark, however, is its typically faecal odour. Vomit containing formed faeces is rare but indicates a communication between the stomach and transverse colon, i.e. gastrocolic fistula.

EXAMINATION OF FAECES

Examination of the faeces is an investigation of great importance all too easily omitted. No patient with bowel disturbance has been properly examined until the stools have been inspected. The white or grey surface of a bedpan makes an ideal background for the detection of blood, pus and mucus.

NAKED EYE INSPECTION

THE AMOUNT

Note whether the stools are copious or scanty, and whether they are hard, formed, semi-formed, or liquid.

COLOUR

Black stools may be produced by altered blood or the ingestion of iron or bismuth. In haemorrhage occurring high up in the intestine the altered blood makes the stools dark, tarry-looking and very offensive, and all chemical tests for blood are strongly positive. *Pallor* of the stools may be due to lack of entrance of bile into the intestine, as in obstructive jaundice; to dilution and rapid passage of the stool through the intestine as in diarrhoea; or to an abnormally high fat content as in malabsorption.

ODOUR

The stools in jaundice are often very offensive. Cholera stools, on the other hand, contain very little organic matter, and are almost free from odour. The stools of acute bacillary dysentery are almost odourless, while those of amoebic dysentery have a characteristic odour, something like that of semen. Melaena stools have a characteristic smell.

ABNORMAL STOOLS

Watery stools are found in all cases of profuse diarrhoea and after the administration of purgatives. In cholera the stools—known as *rice-water* stools—are colourless, almost devoid of odour, alkaline in reaction and contain a number of small flocculi consisting of shreds of epithelium and particles of mucus. Purulent or pus-containing stools are found in severe dysentery or ulcerative colitis, or in cases where an abscess has found its way into the intestines. Slimy stools are due to the presence of an excess of mucus, and point to a disorder of the large bowel. The mucus may envelop the faecal masses or may be intimately mixed with them.

Bloody stools vary in appearance according to the site of the haemorrhage. If the bleeding takes place high up, the stools look like tar. In an intussusception they may look like redcurrant jelly. If the haemorrhage is from the large intestine, the blood is less intimately mixed with faecal matter, and may even be of a bright colour. In haemorrhage from the rectum or anus it may merely streak the faecal masses. A massive duodenal bleed, however, may be red in colour when gastrointestinal transit time is brief.

The stools of bacillary dysentery consist at first of faecal material mixed with blood and pus, later of blood and pus without faecal material. Those of amoebic dysentery characteristically consist of fluid faecal material, mucus and small amounts of blood. The stools of steatorrhoea are very large, pale and putty-like or porridge-like and sometimes frothy. They are apt to stick to the sides of the lavatory pan and are difficult to flush away. If formed, they usually float.

CHEMICAL EXAMINATION

TESTS FOR FAECAL OCCULT BLOOD

Several methods are available. For reasons of ease of use and safety the guaiac test (Haemoccult®) is the most widely used. A filter paper impregnated with guaiac turns blue in the presence of haemoglobin when hydrogen peroxide is added. The test depends on the oxidation of guaiac in the presence of haemoglobin. Other substances with peroxidase activity, including dietary substances such as bananas, pineapple, broccoli and radishes can produce a false positive reaction, and ascorbic acid may cause false negative results. Therefore, dietary preparation is necessary for accurate screening testing; for example, when screening a population in the early detection of colonic cancer. In ordinary clinical use the test is sensitive to faecal blood losses of about 20 mls per day.

This test can be used on patients on a normal diet, but it may not detect small amounts of gastrointestinal bleeding.

The test is of value in indicating the presence of gastrointestinal bleeding, but may be negative in the presence of lesions which bleed intermittently or slightly, particularly those situated in the upper gastrointestinal tract. Spectroscopic methods and isotopic methods using radioactive chromium-labelled red cells that can localize the source of bleeding in the gut are also available.

TESTS FOR FAECAL FAT

Fat is present in food as neutral fat or triglyceride. It is split to greater or lesser degrees by lipases, mainly of the pancreas, into glycerol and fatty acids. Some of the fatty acids, if unabsorbed, combine with bases to form soaps. Fat may, therefore, be found in the faeces as neutral fat, fatty acids and soaps.

The estimation of the proportion of split and unsplit fats present has been found unreliable as a method of distinguishing pancreatic from non-pancreatic steatorrhoea because of the effects of bacterial activity on neutral fats.

For the estimation of the fat in the stools, the patient may be placed on a diet containing 50 g of fat per day. The fat present in the stools collected over at least 3 days is then estimated and should not exceed 6 g/day (11–18 mmol/day). It has been found that equally reliable results are obtained if the patient eats a normal diet, provided a 3–5 day collection is made. The radioactive-labelled triolein (^{14}C) ingestion/absorption test enables accurate assessment of fat transport across the gut mucosa without quantitative faecal fat measurement.

ASPIRATION OF PERITONEAL FLUID

Aspiration of peritoneal fluid (*paracentesis abdominis*) is undertaken for diagnostic and therapeutic purposes. It is essential first to make sure that the bladder is empty; if there is any doubt a catheter should be passed before paracentesis is attempted.

The patient should be lying flat or propped up at a slight angle. An abdominal binder or many-tailed bandage should be placed in position around the patient's back before paracentesis is begun. The aspiration is usually performed in the right iliac fossa, a little outside the midpoint of a line drawn from the umbilicus to the anterior superior iliac spine.

With suitable sterile precautions, the skin at the point chosen should be infiltrated with local anaesthetic and the anaesthetic then injected down to the parietal peritoneum. If the puncture is made simply for diagnostic purposes, a 10-ml syringe and a suitable needle can be used. If it is intended to drain the peritoneum, a trocar and flanged cannula (which can be fixed to the skin with adhesive tape) should be employed. A tiny incision should be made in the anaesthetized area of the skin and then the trocar and cannula inserted. Resistance is felt as the trocar perforates the parietal peritoneum. The trocar is then withdrawn from the cannula and the fluid drained into a bottle via a tube connecting the cannula to the bottle. The binder is then secured over the abdomen, which helps to promote drainage. The rate of flow, which should not be too fast, can be controlled by means of a clip on the tubing. When aspiration is complete, the cannula should be withdrawn. The puncture wound is sealed with a plastic dressing and a dry dressing applied. Therapeutic drainage should, however, be avoided if possible as diuretics are preferable.

The fluid withdrawn is sent for bacteriological and cytological examination (Fig. 7.33) and chemical analysis. Transudates, such as occur in heart failure, cirrhosis and the nephrotic syndrome, normally have a specific gravity less than 1.018 and a protein content under 25 g/litre (i.e. less than two-thirds the concentration of albumin in the plasma). Exudates occurring in tuberculous peritonitis or in the presence of secondary deposits usually have a specific gravity above 1.018 and more than 1.0 g/litre of protein. The distinction, however, is somewhat unreliable. Tubercle bacilli and an exudate of lym-

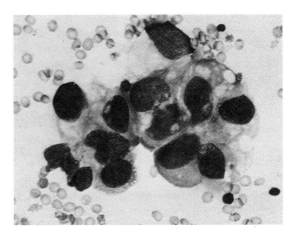

Fig. 7.33 Ascites cytology. A group of tumour cells showing random orientation and large abnormal nucleoli indicating malignancy. Ascitic fluid from patient with ovarian carcinoma. May–Grünwald–Giemsa stain. × 160.

phocytes are characteristic features of the peritoneal fluid in tuberculous peritonitis. Blood-stained fluid strongly suggests metastases. Malignant cells may also be demonstrated in the latter condition, and in malignant ascites the fluid recurs rapidly after paracentesis. In ascites due to cirrhosis the finding of 500 or more neutrophils per mm³ fluid and an unexpectedly high protein content suggests the onset of a secondary bacterial peritonitis.

SPECIAL TECHNIQUES IN THE EXAMINATION OF THE GI TRACT

There are a number of common and important methods of examining the oesophagus, stomach and duodenum, the small and large intestine, the liver, gallbladder and pancreas.

FLEXIBLE ENDOSCOPIC EXAMINATION OF THE OESOPHAGUS, STOMACH AND DUODENUM

In the last 25 years the development of the fibre-optic endoscope, and more recently of video-endoscopy, has revolutionized the inspection of the upper gastrointestinal tract (Fig. 7.34). With these instruments it is possible to inspect directly as far as the duodenal loop with or without light sedation and local pharyngeal anaesthesia. Because of the ability to photograph and biopsy any suspicious lesions, this technique is the investigation of choice for demonstrating structural abnormalities in the upper gut.

Suspected cases of oesophagitis, peptic stricture or ulcer (Fig. 7.35), neoplasia and oesophageal varices are readily confirmed by endoscopy, while therapeutic endoscopy is supplanting surgery in many cases of

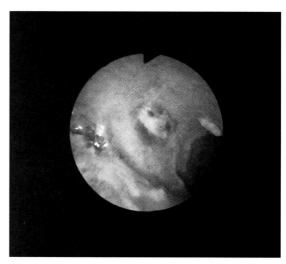

Fig. 7.35   An acute gastric erosion seen by endoscopy.

bleeding oesophageal varices, bleeding peptic ulcer and oesophageal stricture. In inoperable cancer of the oesophagus, palliative prostheses (stents) can be inserted endoscopically.

OESOPHAGEAL FUNCTION STUDIES

The oesophageal phase of swallowing can be assessed by barium swallow. Slowing or arrest of transit of the food bolus in the oesophagus can be demonstrated during fluoroscopy (p. 158). In special clinical applications manometric studies of pressure changes during swallowing are used to localize functional abnormalities in the coordination of oesophageal peristalsis, for example achalasia and oesophageal spasm. In patients with epigastric discomfort or fullness (*heartburn*) related to eating or to lying supine, reflux of acid from the stomach into the lower oesophagus should be suspected. This is common in people with hiatus hernia or other causes of incompetence of the lower oesophageal sphincter. Acid reflux can be detected by monitoring the pH in the lower oesophagus during a 24-hour period. A sudden fall of pH in this region is usually accompanied by typical heartburn pain. The pH measuring probe, attached to an oesophageal line, is placed in the lower oesophagus, 5 cm above the oesophagogastric junction, for 24 hours and the pH recorded continuously. The patient indicates when pain is experienced by pressing an electronic marker on the monitor tape recorder. This investigation has found a major clinical application in the differential diagnosis of acid reflux pain from cardiac pain.

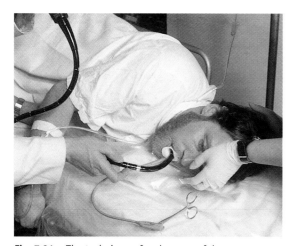

Fig. 7.34   The technique of endoscopy of the upper gastrointestinal tract. The endoscope tube is swallowed, with its attached illumination and photographic accessories. Light sedation is used by some gastroenterologists, but this is often unnecessary.

GASTRIC SECRETORY STUDIES AND SERUM GASTRIN LEVELS

Measurement of acid secretion by the stomach was formerly much used for the assessment of patients with peptic ulcer disease, and for the diagnosis of hyperacidity caused by the rare gastrin-secreting tumours (Zollinger–Ellison syndrome). However, measurement of acid secretion is not useful in the assessment of patients with peptic ulceration as, in most patients with duodenal ulceration, acid secretion is within the normal range and in many patients with Zollinger–Ellison syndrome acid secretion capacity overlaps with that of patients with idiopathic peptic ulcer disease.

In normal subjects the *basal acid output* is no more than a few millilitres per hour, containing up to 10 mmol/litre of hydrogen ion. The *maximal acid output*, measured during 1 hour after the administration of pentagastrin (6.0 µg/kg body weight), a synthetic analogue of the naturally occurring human hormone, gastrin, may reach 27 mmol/litre/h in males, and 25 mmol/litre/h in females. Patients with gastric ulcer or carcinoma have low maximal acid output.

In most patients with Zollinger–Ellison syndrome the ratio of basal to maximum acid secretion is increased to more than 0.6. In these patients the level of gastrin in the serum is increased above 100 ng/litre, and this is currently the best available screening test for this disorder. Serum gastrin levels are also increased in renal failure, pernicious anaemia, after vagotomy and during cimetidine therapy.

TESTS FOR *HELICOBACTER PYLORI*

In recent years the role of infection by *Helicobacter pylori* in the pathogenesis of gastric and duodenal ulceration has become increasingly well-documented, although the association of this infection with peptic ulceration is not fully understood. *H. pylori* is a small, 3×0.5 µm Gram-negative spiral bacillus that appears wavy under the microscope. The organism is found in the antrum in about 60% of patients with gastritis or gastric ulceration, and in almost all patients with duodenal ulceration. *H. pylori* can be detected by microscopy or culture of gastric mucosal biopsies obtained during endoscopic examination of the stomach and duodenum, but the most convenient test depends on the ability of the organism to break down urea to ammonia.

H. pylori is rich in urease. In a simple clinical test the gastric biopsy is placed in contact with a pellet or solution containing urea and a coloured pH indicator. The colour of the substrate changes when the pH is greater than 6, indicating the conversion of urea to ammonia by urease in *H. pylori*. A variant of this method utilizes ^{14}C- or ^{13}C-labelled urea, given to the patient by mouth. The patient's breath is monitored for radiolabelled carbon dioxide, indicating breakdown of the ingested urea by urease containing organisms in the upper gastrointestinal tract. Serological and saliva-based tests for *H. pylori* are also becoming available.

RADIOLOGY OF THE UPPER GASTROINTESTINAL TRACT

PLAIN RADIOGRAPHS

Plain radiographs of the chest and abdomen with the patient supine and in the erect position are of great value in cases of suspected peritonitis due to perforation of a gastric or duodenal ulcer, when gas may be seen under the diaphragm, usually on the right side (Fig. 7.36).

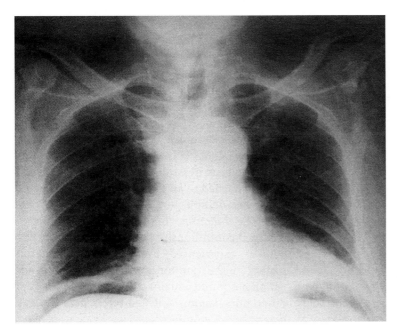

Fig. 7.36 Plain X-ray of the chest showing gas under the right and left diaphragms after perforation of the duodenal ulcer. The patient was admitted in shock with abdominal pain and rigidity.

BARIUM SWALLOW

The direct observation of the passage of a radiopaque barium solution through the pharynx and oesophagus into the stomach remains an important investigation of dysphagia. In addition to structural abnormalities such as neoplasia or stricture, disorders of motor function can be detected which might otherwise escape diagnosis. Lack of progress of barium through the lower oesophageal sphincter on swallowing in a patient with dysphagia indicates the presence of *achalasia*, a disorder of neuromuscular coordination of the oesophageal body and failure of the lower sphincter to relax. The oesophagus may be grossly dilated and unable to contract.

The barium-filled crater of a chronic gastric ulcer may be seen in the stomach as a projection from the wall (profile view) or as a rounded deposit (*en face* view) with, in either case, mucosal folds radiating towards the crater. A duodenal ulcer is usually seen *en face* with a stellate appearance of the mucosal folds. Often no definite crater is seen, but the cap is deformed as a result of scarring, characteristically producing a trefoil deformity, sometimes with pseudo-diverticula. In pyloric stenosis there is an increased amount of resting juice present and a grossly enlarged stomach which empties extremely slowly. Polypoid gastric carcinomas cause filling defects in the barium-filled stomach. Malignant ulcers may be difficult to differentiate from simple ulcers, and the radiologist therefore pays particular attention to the mucosal folds and mobility of the wall in the region of the ulcer. Infiltrating tumours produce a rigid conical shape to the stomach with absence of peristalsis and no ulceration. Carcinomas involving the cardia and pylorus cause obstruction and, if small, may be difficult to differentiate from simple lesions.

SMALL INTESTINE

BARIUM FOLLOW-THROUGH X-RAYS

The small intestine may be studied by taking films of the abdomen at intervals after a barium meal. Abnormalities in the transit time to the colon and in small bowel pattern (e.g. dilatation, narrowing, increase in transverse barring or flocculation) may be demonstrated in malabsorption. Areas of narrowing with proximal dilatation, fistulae and mucosal abnormalities may be produced by Crohn's disease. Small bowel diverticula or neoplasms may also be demonstrated.

SMALL BOWEL ENEMA

This is an alternative to the barium meal and follow-through examination and involves intubating the duodenum and passing small quantities of a non-flocculating barium suspension down the tube. This method is particularly valuable for detecting isolated focal lesions.

RADIOISOTOPE STUDIES

In inflammatory bowel disease the location of the disease, and a measure of its activity, can be obtained by radioisotope studies using indium-labelled white blood cells.

SMALL INTESTINAL ENDOSCOPY AND BIOPSY

Samples of small intestinal mucosa are valuable for histological diagnosis of suspected sprue syndromes. Direct biopsy of the lower duodenum at conventional upper gastrointestinal endoscopy is usually sufficient for diagnosis of coeliac disease but jejunal tissue can also be obtained using push type flexible enteroscopes. Biopsies can also be obtained by endoscopic laparoscopy. After the biopsy has been taken the specimen should be examined immediately by the pathologist under a low-power microscope to assess the general appearance of the intestinal villi.

The small intestinal biopsy is of particular importance in diagnosis of the malabsorption syndrome, where a flat mucosa is seen in place of the usual multiple villi. Serum antibodies to gliadin, reticulin and endomysial antigen are also useful in establishing a diagnosis of coeliac disease.

COLON, RECTUM AND ANUS

PROCTOSCOPY

The anal canal and lower rectum can be readily visualized with a rigid proctoscope. Place the patient in the position described for rectal examination and gently pass the lubricated instrument to its full depth. Remove the obturator and inspect the mucosa as the instrument is slowly withdrawn. Piles are seen as reddish/blue swellings which bulge into the lumen of the instrument. The internal opening of an anal fistula, an anal or low rectal polyp and a chronic anal fissure are other abnormalities that may be seen.

SIGMOIDOSCOPY

It is often necessary to examine the rectum and colon more fully than is possible by proctoscopy and, in such cases, the sigmoidoscope is employed. Sigmoidoscopy requires skill and experience. In accomplished hands the instrument can be passed for 30 cm. The procedure causes relatively little discomfort and anaesthesia is unnecessary.

Proctitis, polyps and carcinomas may be seen and biopsies taken. Sigmoidoscopy is particularly useful in the differential diagnosis of diarrhoea of colonic origin. Granularity, loss of vascular pattern and ulceration with bleeding may indicate the presence of ulcerative colitis, apthous ulceration may suggest Crohn's disease, multiple rounded white macules may be diagnostic of pseudo-membranous colitis due to *Clostridium difficile* toxin usually induced by antibiotics.

In suspected amoebic dysentery, the mucous membrane should be inspected and portions of mucus and scrapings from the ulcerated mucosa may be removed and examined microscopically for amoebic cysts. Urine tests for purgative abuse are useful in the investigation of persistent unexplained diarrhoea. Urine 5HIAA (5-hydroxyindole acetic acid) excretion is increased in carcinoid tumours: diarrhoea is a feature of this syndrome.

BARIUM ENEMA

A plain X-ray of the abdomen should always be taken in patients with suspected perforation or obstruction before considering a contrast study (Fig. 7.32). Barium suspension is introduced via a tube into the rectum as an enema and manipulated around the rest of the colon to fill it. Screening is performed by a radiologist and films taken. The barium is then evacuated and further films taken. By this means, obstruction to the colon, tumours, diverticular disease, fistulae and other abnormalities can be recognized.

Following evacuation, air is introduced into the colon. This improves visualization of the mucosa and is especially valuable for detecting small lesions such as polyps and early tumours (Figs 7.37 and 7.38).

FLEXIBLE ENDOSCOPIC COLONOSCOPY

As in the upper gut, the use of flexible fibre-optic and video instruments has revolutionized the investigation of the colon. Both sigmoidoscopes and colonoscopes are available. The former instrument may be employed in an out-patient setting after a simple enema preparation; the latter requires more extensive colon preparation and sedation but is also an out-patient procedure. These techniques are invaluable for obtaining tissue for diagnosis of inflammatory and neoplastic disease and for removal of neoplastic polyps (Figs 7.39 and 7.40). Dilatation of strictures, stenting, laser or other thermal treatments of obstructing tumours can also be managed by endoscopy.

THE LIVER

BIOCHEMICAL TESTS OF LIVER FUNCTION

These are used in the differential diagnosis of jaundice, to detect liver cell damage in other disorders and to monitor the results of surgery of the biliary system and pancreas. These include urinary urobilin, plasma bilirubin, alkaline phosphatase, serum

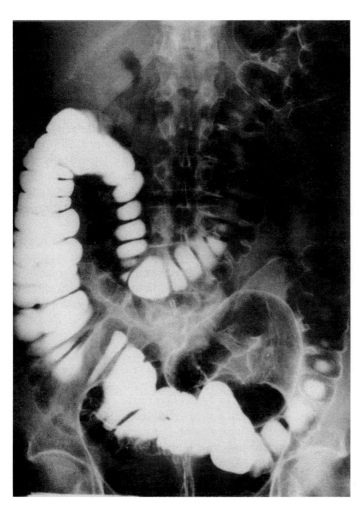

Fig. 7.37 Barium enema with air contrast. The right colon is outlined by barium sulphate, and the rectum, left colon and part of the transverse colon are outlined by air with a thin mucosal layer of barium sulphate. Note the normal haustral pattern in the colon and the smooth appearance of the rectum. The anal canal can also be seen.

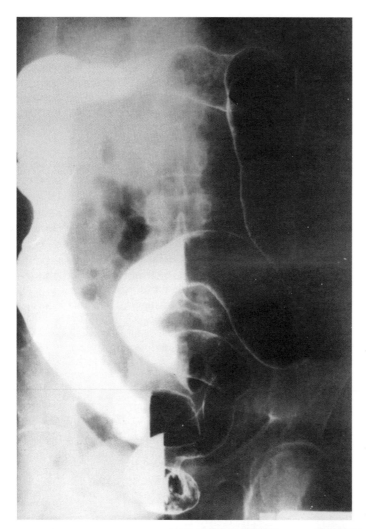

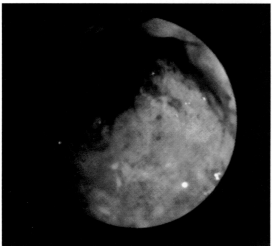

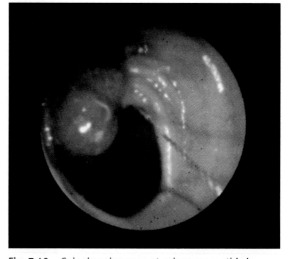

Fig. 7.38   Barium enema with air contrast. In this patient with ulcerative colitis, the normal mucosal pattern, and the haustra themselves, have been obliterated. The patient is lying on his right side so that there are clear fluid levels in the barium sulphate suspension in the bowel.

Fig. 7.39   View of colonic epithelium at colonoscopy, revealing the inflammatory changes of ulcerative colitis.

Fig. 7.40   Colonic polyp seen at colonoscopy; this is a premalignant lesion that sometimes has a genetic basis.

aminotransferases, plasma proteins and plasma prothrombin. Serum gamma glutamyl transferase levels are especially sensitive to liver dysfunction as, for example, in alcohol related liver disease.

Smooth muscle antibodies are commonly present in the blood in chronic active hepatitis, and other autoantibody studies are used in the investigation of chronic inflammatory liver disease. Antimitochondrial antibodies are found in the blood in primary biliary cirrhosis in over 90% of cases.

Blood copper studies, with measurement of the copper-carrying capacity of serum proteins, are important in the investigation of cirrhosis of unknown cause, in order to exclude Wilson's disease, a disorder of copper transport in the blood in which copper is stored in the liver, leading to cirrhosis. Copper is also stored in the brain in this disorder, causing a progressive encephalopathy with cerebellar ataxia and extrapyramidal features. The blood copper and caeruloplasmin levels are decreased, but urinary copper excretion is increased. Excessive iron storage in the liver can also lead to cirrhosis, and detection of increased ferritin levels (an iron storage protein normally found in the liver) in the blood provide a clue to this diagnosis. Blood transferrin levels are slightly decreased, but blood iron levels are markedly increased, representing free, unbound iron in the circulation.

HEPATITIS

Antibodies to the hepatitis A, B and C viruses can be detected in the blood, and the presence of an effective immune response or of active hepatitis due to one or more of these viruses assessed. During the initial stage of infection with hepatitis B virus (HBV) HBV surface antigen (HBsAg) is present in the serum. After a few weeks or months HBsAg disappears, and levels of anti-HBs and anti-HBcAg (an antibody to a viral core antigen) rise. This is the immune state. In patients who become carriers of HBV infection HBsAg and HBeAg (a viral envelope antigen) persist, with only low levels of antibodies. Some of these patients will develop chronic persistent active HBV hepatitis. Chronic persistence of hepatitis B infection is particularly a problem in countries of the Far East and Asia, and in homosexual men in Western countries.

In patients in whom hepatocellular carcinoma develops as a complication of chronic persistent hepatitis, or in association with hepatic cirrhosis of other causation, alpha fetoprotein becomes detectable in the serum.

ULTRASOUND SCAN

A probe, emitting ultrasonic pulses, is passed across the liver and surrounding areas. Echoes detected from within the patient are received with a transducer, amplified and suitably displayed. This technique is the most commonly used method for non-invasive investigation of the liver. It can suggest the presence of cirrhosis and small metastases and is helpful in the diagnosis of fluid-filled lesions such as cysts and abscesses. It is particularly useful in identifying gallstones in the gallbladder and also in recognizing dilatation of the bile duct which may be due to malignancy or stones. Fine needles can be inserted into a suspicious lesion under direct ultrasound guidance for cytology and for drainage of fluid-filled lesions.

ISOTOPE SCAN

A radioisotope of technetium or colloidal gold is injected intravenously and taken up by the reticulo-endothelial system. A gamma camera is used to show the size and shape of the liver. Abnormal areas take up more or less isotope than normal; examples are primary or secondary hepatic tumours, abscesses and cysts. Technetium-labelled red blood cells can be used to detect the location of sources of bleeding in the gastrointestinal tract.

COMPUTED TOMOGRAPHY (CT) SCANNING

CT can be used to produce cross-sectional images of the liver and other intra-abdominal and retroperitoneal organs. This technique is of great value in the investigation of patients with disease of these organs. It is particularly helpful in staging patients with cancer of oesophagus, stomach and pancreas to assess operability. Because it can be combined with injection of vascular contrast it can be helpful in assessing intra-abdominal vascular abnormalities. It can facilitate guided biopsy of abnormalities.

ENDOSCOPIC ULTRASOUND

Endoscopic ultrasound is more sensitive in staging the mucosal depth of penetration of cancers in the oesophagus and stomach than CT scan and is frequently better at lymph node detection but is less good at detecting distant metastases. It is also valuable in assessing pancreatic abnormalities and can be used to guide biopsy.

MAGNETIC RESONANCE IMAGING (MRI)

Magnetic resonance cholangiopancreatography (MRCP) can give high quality images of the bile duct and pancreatic duct. The safety of this non-invasive technique has reduced the need for more hazardous examinations such as endoscopic retrograde cholangiopancreatography (ERCP) which is reserved for patients requiring therapeutic intervention.

NEEDLE BIOPSY OF LIVER

Percutaneous needle biopsy is the standard technique for obtaining liver tissue for histological examination. While needle biopsy can be conducted under mild sedation and local anaesthesia, it should be carried out only in hospital under supervision and blood should be available for transfusion, if necessary. Generally the method is safe and reliable but there is a tiny but definite mortality from the procedure due to leakage of bile and/or blood into the peritoneal cavity from the puncture site. This risk can be reduced by inserting a 'thrombin plug' at the puncture site in the liver capsule. The procedure should therefore always be regarded as a potentially dangerous investigation and should be performed only by those well-trained in the technique; it should generally be performed under ultrasound control. Contraindications include patients

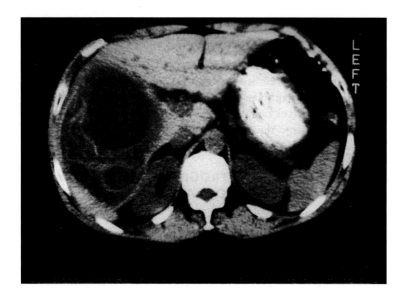

Fig. 7.41 Hydatid cyst of the liver. Several abscesses consisting of low-density lesions can be seen in the right lobe of the liver. The cyst walls are calcified in this unenhanced CT scan.

with a bleeding diathesis, deep obstructive jaundice or ascites.

EXPLORATION OF LIVER FOR LIVER ABSCESS

Liver abscesses due to *Entamoeba histolytica* are nearly always found in the right lobe (Fig. 7.41). When suspected clinically, their presence and position may be demonstrated and localized radiologically or by isotope or ultrasound scanning. Metronidazole (Flagyl) 800 mg three times a day for 10 days is now the first line of treatment and cures the great majority of cases. Where there is a lack of response to treatment after 5 days, exploration by needle aspiration for diagnostic and therapeutic purposes may be performed.

The procedure is conducted under local anaesthesia and strict asepsis. A needle of wide enough bore to admit a thick pus (a lumbar puncture needle is suitable) is selected and a piece of adhesive tape is wound around it 9 cm from its point. The needle is entered either at the site of maximum tenderness or in the right eighth, ninth or tenth intercostal space in the mid-axillary line, and passed medially in a horizontal plane to a maximum depth of 9 cm. By this means the whole of the right lobe of the liver may be explored. When pus is encountered, strong suction has to be employed to remove as much of the pus as possible and this is done with the aid of a two-way syringe. As the pus is removed, it may be replaced by a suitable volume of air (about half the volume of pus removed). The patient is then X-rayed in several positions to determine the exact site and size of the abscess, and to allow the effect of treatment to be followed.

SELECTIVE ANGIOGRAPHY OF COELIAC AXIS AND HEPATIC ARTERY

Angiography is occasionally used in the investigation of haematemesis or melaena when gastroscopy,

colonoscopy and enteroscopy fail to identify the bleeding source. It is most useful if performed when the patient is actively bleeding but may be of value if an aneurysm or abnormal tumour vasculature is present and can occasionally detect angiomas. It is an invasive technique that demands considerable skill on the part of the radiologist. A catheter is passed retrogradely up the aorta from a femoral puncture; its tip is manipulated into the coeliac axis and thus into the hepatic artery. Radiopaque contrast material may then be injected to demonstrate the bleeding source or abnormal vasculature.

GALLBLADDER AND BILE DUCTS

The main functions of the gallbladder are to concentrate and store hepatic bile and to empty this bile into the duodenum after appropriate stimuli.

ULTRASOUND

The gallbladder is most easily investigated by ultrasound. It appears as an echo-free structure. If stones are present they are usually easily seen as echo-dense with a characteristic 'acoustic shadow' behind them. Ultrasound detects 90% of gallbladder stones but only about 50% of stones in the bile ducts themselves. Ultrasound is particularly valuable in detecting dilatation of the bile duct which may be due to tumour or gallstones.

ORAL CHOLECYSTOGRAPHY

This procedure depends on the excretion of iodine-containing compounds that have been absorbed from the gut after oral ingestion, by the liver. They are concentrated in the gallbladder, making it opaque. Apart from a non-functioning gallbladder, stones, abnormalities of the wall of the gallbladder, anatomical variations and failure to contract in response to a fatty meal may be demonstrated.

INTRAVENOUS CHOLANGIOGRAPHY

Intravenous cholangiography can be used to demonstrate the bile ducts. The technique depends on the fact that an intravenously administered iodine-containing compound is excreted by the liver in the bile in such a concentration that it is radiopaque and therefore does not depend on the concentrating power of the gallbladder, as in cholecystography. As with cholecystography it cannot be performed in the jaundiced patient. It is particularly used postoperatively, after biliary tract surgery.

Of particular interest are the width of the common bile duct (usually less than 10 mm), the presence of stones seen as radiolucent filling defects, and the entry of dye into the duodenum. A dilated duct nearly always signifies an abnormality.

ENDOSCOPIC RETROGRADE CHOLANGIOPANCREATOGRAPHY (ERCP)

Using a special side-viewing duodenoscope, the duodenal papilla is identified and a cannula passed through it into the common bile duct. Radiopaque contrast fluid is then injected down the cannula and the whole of the biliary system is visualized. The technique is useful in the rapid diagnosis and localization of the different causes of jaundice due to obstruction of the main bile ducts. Needle or forceps biopsy and brush cytology may give a specific diagnosis. ERCP has an important therapeutic role in the treatment of jaundice because it allows the placement of stents which are tubes that facilitate the passage of bile into the duodenum past obstructing lesions such as tumours of the pancreas or bile duct and the removal of gallstones. It may be necessary to perform a sphincterotomy during ERCP using a cutting diathermy wire passed into the bile duct in the ampulla in a plastic catheter which can be bowed. The sphincterotomy opens the ampulla and may allow the delivery of stones in the bile duct. ERCP carries a small mortality rate and may be complicated by pancreatitis, bleeding or perforation.

PERCUTANEOUS TRANSHEPATIC CHOLANGIOGRAPHY

Percutaneous transhepatic cholangiography is a very useful investigation in patients with jaundice due to obstruction of the main bile ducts. The site of the obstruction due to tumours of the head of the pancreas, or iatrogenic and malignant bile duct strictures, can be accurately localized and differentiated. This technique is only used if ERCP fails. It also has a therapeutic function. Transhepatic drains can be placed to treat cholangitis and sepsis, stents can be placed to relieve obstruction, gallstones can be removed and wires can be passed into the duodenum to allow stenting at ERCP.

THE PANCREAS

ULTRASOUND AND CT SCANS

These are both useful methods in the diagnosis of pancreatic disease. Each method can differentiate solid from cystic lesions greater than 2.5 cm in size and the success rate in diagnosis is around 70%. Ultrasound is particularly useful in the diagnosis of true and pseudopancreatic cysts and is an essential tool for percutaneous needle biopsy. A plain X-ray is a simple and reliable method for detecting calcification in the pancreas in chronic pancreatitis.

ERCP

The ERCP procedure can display the entire pancreatic duct system. It is therefore valuable not only in the diagnosis of chronic pancreatitis but also in defining those cases which could benefit from surgery.

In patients with pancreatic carcinoma needle biopsy can be performed at ERCP, and brush cytology of the pancreatic duct may also provide histological proof of the diagnosis. A smear of fluid can be stained and examined under the microscope by the pathologist.

Pancreatic function tests are now rarely used in diagnosis, although measurement of the blood amylase level is still valuable in the diagnosis of acute pancreatitis.

8
THE ENDOCRINE SYSTEM AND METABOLIC DISORDERS

INTRODUCTION

The endocrine system comprises the classic endocrine organs:

- Hypothalamus/pituitary
- Thyroid
- Parathyroid
- Adrenal
- Pancreatic islet cells
- Gonads.

Metabolic disorders are conditions which can be attributed to:

- Biochemical abnormality
- Enzyme defect
- Abnormal receptor mechanism.

Examples of metabolic disorders include the various forms of hyperlipidaemia, abnormalities of carbohydrate metabolism and several disorders of bone integrity.

It is useful to consider disorders of the endocrine system and metabolic disorders together because the mechanisms involved in endocrine and metabolic homeostasis are closely allied in terms of functional integration. The mode of presentation of these disorders does not fit neatly into a system-based model. The symptoms are rarely specific to a particular system and, frequently, a constellation of otherwise non-specific symptoms suggests the diagnosis.

THE HISTORY

For diagnostic purposes the history consists of:

- Presenting symptoms
- History of the development of the illness
- Family history.

PRESENTING SYMPTOMS

There are a number of symptom complexes that particularly suggest an endocrine or metabolic cause. These are described below.

THIRST AND POLYURIA

Excessive thirst (*polydipsia*) and increased urine output (*polyuria*) are the most important presenting symptoms of diabetes mellitus. They are sometimes referred to as primary diabetic symptoms and they occur when the renal tubular glucose concentration is increased to the point that it exceeds the maximal tubular capacity for glucose reabsorption, causing an osmotic diuresis. Therefore, people with an increased renal threshold for glucose may be asymptomatic despite hyperglycaemia. Polydipsia and polyuria may also be due to failure of renal concentrating capacity due to deficiency of antidiuretic hormone (*cranial diabetes insipidus*) or a failure of antidiuretic hormone action (*nephrogenic diabetes insipidus*). The latter may be inherited or may occur secondary to impairment of antidiuretic hormone action by hypercalcaemia or hypokalaemia. Sometimes, apparent polydipsia and polyuria may be due to increased fluid intake, which at its most extreme may be vastly excessive (*psychogenic polydipsia*). The distinction between psychogenic polydipsia and diabetes insipidus is important. Generally, nocturnal polyuria is not a feature of psychogenic polydipsia but this is not an absolute distinction, and further investigation of urine concentrating capacity is usually required.

WEIGHT LOSS

Loss of weight is a feature of decreased food intake or increased metabolic rate. Sometimes both factors may operate to reduce body weight, as in the *cachexia* of malignant disease. Thyroid overactivity (*hyperthyroidism*) is nearly always associated with a combination of weight loss and increased appetite although, occasionally, the latter may be stimulated more than the former so that a paradoxical increase in weight occurs. Weight loss is rarely the sole presenting symptom of hyperthyroidism and other clinical features predominate, particularly in younger patients (Box 8.1). Vitiligo may be an associated feature in autoimmune thyroiditis with hyperthyroidism. In the elderly, however, hyperthyroidism may be indolent and may simulate malignant disease with a gradual weight loss. Cardiac arrhythmias are a frequent feature in the elderly. The weight loss of thyrotoxicosis must be distinguished from that due to *anorexia nervosa*. The latter is characterized by a long history of low body weight in the absence of other features of ill-health. The disorder particularly occurs in young girls. Any form of weight loss may be associated with amenorrhoea.

Other endocrine conditions in which weight loss is a major feature are listed in Box 8.2. The rapid weight loss which occurs at the onset of insulin-dependent diabetes is the single most important clinical feature in distinguishing it from the non-insulin-dependent form of the disease (type II diabetes mellitus).

WEIGHT GAIN OR REDISTRIBUTION

Increase in body weight (Box 8.3) is a predictable result of a reduction in metabolic rate. Weight gain is therefore a common feature of *primary hypothyroidism*. However, obesity is rarely a consequence of specific endocrine dysfunction, an exception being the recently described but very rare phenomenon of leptin deficiency. In the majority of patients 'simple obesity' is due to a long-standing imbalance between energy intake and expenditure; the problem frequently presents in childhood and is present in more than one family member. Glucocorticoid hormone excess (*Cushing's syndrome*) results in an increase in body fat predominantly involving abdominal, omental and interscapular fat (truncal obesity) with paradoxical thinning of the limbs due to muscle atrophy.

MUSCLE WEAKNESS

Symptomatic muscular weakness in the absence of neurological disease is a feature of several metabolic disorders, including thyrotoxicosis, Cushing's syndrome and vitamin D deficiency. In all these conditions the *metabolic myopathy* (Box 8.4) causes symmetrical proximal weakness, mainly involving the shoulder and hip girdle musculature. There is usually associated muscle wasting. The major symptom is difficulty in climbing stairs, boarding a bus or rising from a sitting position. Most patients with hyperthyroidism have proximal weakness. This may be subclinical, but can usually be demonstrated by asking the patient to rise from the squatting position. The proximal myopathy of *vitamin D deficiency* is often painful, in contrast to the other

---

BOX 8.1   Clinical features of hyperthyroidism.

- Weight loss
- Tachycardia
- Atrial fibrillation/heart failure
- Eye signs
  - lid lag
  - lid retraction
  - exophthalmos (Graves' disease)
- Sweating
- Thyroid gland enlargement and bruit (Graves' disease)
- Fine distal tremor
- Thinning of hair
- Proximal weakness; cannot rise from squat
- Chorea

BOX 8.2   Endocrine and metabolic diseases in which weight loss is a clinical feature.

- Hyperthyroidism
- Type I insulin-dependent diabetes mellitus
- Hypopituitarism
- Adrenocortical failure (Addison's disease)
- Anorexia nervosa

BOX 8.3   Conditions in which increased body weight is a feature.

- Simple obesity: energy intake/expenditure imbalance
- Primary hypothyroidism
- Cushing's syndrome
- Hypothalamic lesions
- Leptin deficiency

BOX 8.4   Conditions in which metabolic myopathy is a feature.

Painless
- Hyperthyroidism
- Cushing's syndrome, including iatrogenic steroid myopathy
- Acromegaly

Painful
- Vitamin D deficiency
- Osteomalacia
- Hypothyroidism

causes. The differential diagnosis of painful proximal muscular weakness includes polymyositis and polymyalgia rheumatica, as well as spinal root or plexus disease.

COLD INTOLERANCE

An abnormal sensation of cold which is out of proportion to that experienced by other individuals may indicate underlying hypothyroidism (Boxes 8.5 and 8.6). This symptom differs from the localized vasomotor symptoms in the hands found in Raynaud's phenomenon and is rather non-specific, especially in the elderly patient.

HEAT INTOLERANCE

The increased metabolic rate of thyrotoxicosis may be associated with heat intolerance in which, at its most extreme, the patient finds comfortable an ambient temperature which others find unpleasantly cold. This is an important symptom, highly specific for thyroid overactivity which, in part, may explain some of the seasonal variation in presentation of the condition.

INCREASED SWEATING

Some individuals experience excessive sweating (*hyperhidrosis*) as a constitutional abnormality, characterized by onset in childhood or adolescence and, sometimes, by a family history. A more recent increase in sweat secretion, on the other hand, may be an early indication of thyroid overactivity. Paroxysmal sweating is a common feature of anxiety. Increased catecholamine secretion from a phaeochromocytoma of the adrenal medulla is a rare cause of hyperhidrosis. Intermittent sweating after meals (gus-

tatory hyperhidrosis) may occur in patients with autonomic dysfunction. Growth hormone excess (acromegaly) also increases sweating, perhaps because of hypertrophy of sweat glands, and this feature can be used to assess activity of the disease in the clinic. Increased sweating should be distinguished from flushing which occurs physiologically at the time of the natural menopause. Flushing may be a presenting feature of serotonin-secreting carcinoid tumours of the gut and usually indicates extensive disease with hepatic metastases.

TREMOR

A fine rapid resting tremor is one of the cardinal clinical features of thyrotoxicosis. This must be distinguished from the coarser and more irregular tremor of anxiety which is usually associated with a cool peripheral skin temperature, in contrast to the warm skin of the thyrotoxic patient. Tremor due to neurological disease is of greater amplitude, slower rate, and may be present at rest, as in Parkinson's disease, or on movement, as in cerebellar intention tremor. It therefore rarely simulates thyrotoxic tremor.

PALPITATIONS

A sensation of increased heart rate or force of contraction may be a feature of thyrotoxicosis, but is more likely to be due to anxiety. Awareness of the heart beat while lying down is normal. Other causes of rapid heart rate include paroxysmal tachyarrhythmias. The sensation of intermittent forceful cardiac contraction, sometimes described by the patient as a missed beat, is often due to the compensatory pause following an ectopic beat, and is usually a normal phenomenon.

POSTURAL UNSTEADINESS

Dizziness, or a sensation of faintness on standing, should prompt measurement of lying and standing blood pressure. Postural hypotension, a fall of diastolic blood pressure on standing, occurs with reduced blood volume. In the absence of obvious bleeding or gastrointestinal fluid loss one should consider adrenal insufficiency as the cause. Postural hypotension is frequently due to autonomic neuropathy, especially in long-standing diabetes mellitus. It is also a common complication of any hypertensive drug therapy for essential hypertension. The drug history is particularly important in the elderly patient with dizziness.

VISUAL DISTURBANCE

Several endocrine conditions may cause visual symptoms. Decreased visual acuity may occur from space-occupying lesions compressing the optic nerve. For example, severe dysthyroid eye disease and orbital or retro-orbital tumours may present in this way. *Bitemporal hemianopia* (bilateral loss of part or all of

---

> **BOX 8.5   Conditions in which temperature intolerance is a feature.**
>
> - Intolerance to cold
>   —hypothyroidism
> - Intolerance to heat
>   —hyperthyroidism

> **BOX 8.6   Clinical features of hypothyroidism.**
>
> - Weight gain
> - Sallow complexion and dry skin
> - Thinning of scalp and lateral eyebrow hair
> - Cold intolerance
> - Deepened, gruff voice
> - Slow physical and mental activity
> - Unsteadiness and slightly slurred speech
> - Tingling in toes and fingers
> - Aching muscles with cramp
> - Mild proximal weakness
> - Slow pulse and shortness of breath

the temporal fields of vision), often asymmetrical or incongruous, is a major feature of suprasellar extension of pituitary adenomas compressing the optic chiasm, but may occur in other tumours in this location. Double vision (*diplopia*) on lateral or upward gaze, often results from medial or lateral rectus muscle tethering in dysthyroid eye disease (see Figs 12.1 and 12.2). Apparent magnification of vision (*macropsia*) can occur in hypoglycaemia.

FASTING SYMPTOMS

Tachycardia, sweating and tremor, occurring intermittently, especially when fasting, are suggestive of hypoglycaemia. These symptoms resemble those associated with the increased sympathetic drive found in states of fear or with excess secretion of noradrenaline, as in phaeochromocytoma. In severe persistent hypoglycaemia these symptoms may progress to decreased consciousness. This is a serious emergency implying neuroglycopenia sufficient to impair brain function. Spontaneous or fasting hypoglycaemia can be due to:

- Autonomous insulin production due to an insulinoma
- Glucocorticoid deficiency, with or without thyroxine and growth hormone deficiency (e.g. primary adrenal failure or hypopituitarism)
- Inappropriate insulin, or excessive sulphonylurea drug administration in a diabetic patient
- Rarer causes of hypoglycaemia, for example hepatic failure and rapidly growing malignant lesions, especially thoracic or retroperitoneal mesothelial tumours secreting pro-insulin-like growth factor II.

CRAMPS AND 'PINS AND NEEDLES'

Intermittent cramp and 'pins and needles' (*paraesthesiae*), especially if bilateral, can be due to a decreased circulating ionized calcium level. This may occur in hypoparathyroidism or be associated with a fall in the ionized component of serum calcium, due to an increased extracellular pH (*alkalosis*). The latter may occur with any alkalosis, but is particularly well-recognized in hyperventilatory states (respiratory alkalosis) and hypokalaemia (metabolic alkalosis). Refractory cramping symptoms after correction of hypocalcaemia can be due to an associated hypomagnesaemia. However, the differential diagnosis of paraesthesiae in the hands includes median nerve compression at the wrist (carpal tunnel syndrome), a syndrome that is usually accompanied by typical sensory and motor disturbance suggestive of a lesion in the median nerve (see Ch. 11).

NAUSEA

This is a rare symptom of endocrine disease. It is an important presenting feature of adrenal insufficiency in which typically it is maximal in the morning and may be associated with vomiting. Similar symptoms may occur with severe hypercalcaemia and may be the sole manifestation of this condition. These two conditions should be considered early in the differential diagnosis of a patient presenting with upper gastrointestinal symptoms in the absence of demonstrable structural disease. Occasionally, thyrotoxicosis may present with nausea and vomiting, although looseness of stools is the more common gastrointestinal manifestation of this condition.

DYSPHAGIA

Difficulty in swallowing is an unusual manifestation of endocrine disease but may be the presenting feature of multinodular thyroid enlargement with retrosternal extension. Smaller goitres only rarely result in dysphagia. Severe hyperthyroidism with generalized weakness may be associated with a reversible myopathy of the pharyngeal musculature and consequent dysphagia.

NECK PAIN AND SWELLING

Superficial discomfort in the neck may lead to the incidental finding of thyroid enlargement. However, it should be borne in mind that modest degrees of thyroid enlargement are very common, whereas pain arising from the thyroid is comparatively unusual. The most common cause of local discomfort and tenderness in the neck is inflammatory lymphadenopathy. Severe tenderness of the thyroid itself, especially when accompanied by fever and signs of thyrotoxicosis, suggests a diagnosis of viral subacute thyroiditis (de Quervain's thyroiditis). Occasionally autoimmune thyroiditis may give rise to pain and tenderness, which mimics a viral thyroiditis but is less severe. A sudden onset of localized pain and swelling in the thyroid is indicative of bleeding into a pre-existing thyroid nodule and is a recognized complication of multinodular goitre. The symptoms are self-limiting. Painless enlargement of the thyroid gland (*goitre*) presents either because of pressure effects, resulting in dysphagia progressing to tracheal compression and stridor, or cosmetic disturbance. The underlying cause of thyroid enlargement is often difficult to establish. The family history and subsequent investigation may point to autoimmune thyroiditis or dyshormonogenesis. A history of rapid enlargement of the gland, especially in an elderly patient, suggests an anaplastic thyroid carcinoma. Coexisting severe diarrhoea points towards a diagnosis of medullary carcinoma of the thyroid. In the differential diagnosis goitrogenic drugs, for example lithium, should be considered, as should residence in iodine-deficient areas. Previous exposure to neck irradiation or to radioactive iodine in childhood may also be important.

IMPOTENCE

Decreased erectile potency may be a consequence of primary abnormalities, such as:

- decreased blood supply to the penis (e.g. atherosclerosis)
- neural dysfunction (e.g. autonomic neuropathy complicating diabetes)
- testosterone deficiency (e.g. hypopituitarism and primary testicular failure)
- hyperprolactinaemia
- drug therapy (e.g. certain anti-hypertensives)
- psychological factors
- a combination of several causes.

It is often difficult to distinguish with certainty between impotence due to organic and psychological factors, although total erectile failure and the absence of nocturnal and morning erections suggest a physical cause. Impotence in a diabetic patient should not be assumed to be inevitably due to autonomic neuropathy and other causes should be considered. A reduction in testicular volume, determined by comparison with calibrated ovoids, points towards an endocrine aetiology but is not invariably found in hypopituitarism. Most importantly, it should be recognized that male impotence is often complicated by a psychological disturbance, which may serve to exacerbate the problem.

GYNAECOMASTIA

Mild breast enlargement in the male may occur as a temporary phenomenon in puberty and may persist for several years, or sometimes indefinitely. Gynaecomastia in the adult male may result from:

- Excess oestrogen stimulation
- Reduction in circulating androgen
- Antagonism of androgen action
- Androgen insensitivity (Box 8.7).

Clinical assessment of the patient with gynaecomastia should therefore include enquiry concerning any change in libido and examination of thyroid status, the genitalia, the muscles and for stigmata of chronic liver disease (Box 8.7).

AMENORRHOEA

Perhaps the most common cause of failure of onset of menses (*primary amenorrhoea*) is physiological delay of puberty, a diagnosis which can only be made with certainty in retrospect. Important pathological causes include:

- Hypothalamic–pituitary dysfunction, for example due to tumours
- Ovarian failure, for example due to failure of normal ovarian development or to cytotoxic chemotherapy
- Thyroid dysfunction
- Defects in lower genital tract development.

> **BOX 8.7   Causes of gynaecomastia.**
>
> **Increased oestrogen/testosterone ratio**
> - Chronic liver disease
> - Thyrotoxicosis
> - Phenytoin therapy
>
> **Androgen receptor antagonists**
> - Spironolactone; digoxin
>
> **Inherited androgen receptor defects**
> - Testicular feminization syndrome
>
> **Testosterone deficiency or oestrogen excess**
> - Primary and secondary hypogonadism
> - Tumour production of human chorionic gonadotrophin (HCG)
> - Oestrogen production of Leydig cell tumour of testis
>
> **Congenital and Heriditary**
> - X-linked spinal muscular atrophy (Kennedy syndrome)
> - Klinefelter's syndrome (karyotype XXY)

Important diagnostic pointers in the history include symptoms suggestive of thyroid disease, or any visible disability which might indicate compression of the optic chiasm due to a hypothalamic or pituitary tumour. Secondary amenorrhoea has similar causes. In addition, marked weight loss may lead to amenorrhoea, as in anorexia nervosa or inflammatory bowel disease. Amenorrhoea, or infrequent scanty periods, may occur in women subject to excessively rigorous physical training programmes. Clearly, normal pregnancy is the most common cause of secondary amenorrhoea.

GALACTORRHOEA

Occasionally physiological lactation may persist after breast-feeding following childbirth has ceased. Inappropriate lactation is usually bilateral. There are a number of causes which include:

- Prolactin-secreting tumours of the pituitary gland
- Idiopathic galactorrhoea, in which there is an apparent increased sensitivity to normal levels of serum prolactin
- Hyperprolactinaemia due to hypothyroidism
- Hyperprolactinaemia due to dopamine antagonist drugs
- Hyperprolactinaemia due to lactotroph-disinhibiting lesions of the hypothalamic–pituitary region.

Inappropriate secretion of breast milk should therefore always prompt enquiry for symptoms referable to the thyroid and pituitary glands, and a thorough drug history should be taken.

EXCESS HAIR GROWTH

An increase in growth of facial and body hair in adult females is a relatively common symptom which may be due to increased circulating androgens. However, it is most commonly a normal, constitutional characteristic. Pathological causes of hirsutism include:

- Polycystic ovary syndrome
- Late presentation of congenital adrenal hyperplasia
- Androgen-secreting ovarian or adrenal tumours.

The history is vital in the clinical assessment. If symptoms commenced shortly after the age of the menarche, then a tumour source of androgen is unlikely. A regular menstrual cycle is good evidence against severe androgen excess but does not exclude polycystic ovary syndrome. Increased libido on the other hand, suggests substantially increased androgen secretion, which may be either ovarian or neoplastic in origin.

BOWEL DISTURBANCE

Constipation and abdominal distension may be features of hypothyroidism or pan-hypopituitarism. Diarrhoea may occur as part of autonomic neuropathy involving the gut in diabetes mellitus. Peptic ulceration may occur in the Zollinger–Ellison syndrome, in which gastrin-secreting tumours of the gut result in increased gastric acid secretion.

SKIN CHANGES

Pallor occurs in primary testicular failure and in pan-hypopituitarism. Excessive pigmentation occurs in ACTH-dependent Cushing's syndrome, and increased sebum production causing greasy skin and acne on the face and shoulders may occur in all causes of glucocorticoid excess. In carcinoid tumours of the gut or lung increased humoral secretion results in a violaceous cyanosis-like skin discoloration. A variegate, patchy rash is a feature of porphyria, an inherited abnormality of haem metabolism. In primary hypoadrenalism there is increased pigmentation of the conjunctival membrane beneath the lids, and of the inside of the mouth, the axillae and the palmar skin creases. In hypothyroidism the skin appears dry, pale, sallow, or even slightly yellow, scalp hair is coarse and lateral eyebrow hair is thinned. In hyperthyroidism the skin is dry and hot, but often not flushed. In hypocalcaemia the nails are friable. In uraemia the skin is pale, or yellow and slightly pigmented, and in terminal uraemia a 'uraemic frost' may appear on the skin.

Vitiligo, a patchy depigmentation of the skin, is common in association with many autoimmune disorders, particularly autoimmune hypothyroidism and vitamin B_{12} deficiency.

FAMILY HISTORY

The family background of endocrine or metabolic disease may be particularly useful in the evaluation of several of the more common disorders. It is also particularly important in the assessment of less common, inherited disorders of metabolism.

DIABETES MELLITUS

In comparison with insulin-dependent diabetes, non-insulin-dependent diabetes has a strong hereditary component. Therefore a family history may be useful in the initial assessment of patients with diabetes, and also of patients with premature vascular disease in whom there may be an abnormality of glucose tolerance.

THYROID DISEASE

Autoimmune hypothyroidism and hyperthyroidism frequently show familial aggregation. Dyshormonogenetic goitre is also often inherited.

RENAL CALCULI

Primary hyperparathyroidism, an important cause of renal stones, may be familial, occurring either as an isolated disorder or as a part of the syndrome of multiple endocrine neoplasia (type I).

ATHEROMA

Large-vessel atheromatosis, particularly affecting the coronary circulation, may manifest a strong familial component. This is of considerable importance in the context of hereditary disorders of lipoprotein metabolism, especially familial hypercholesterolaemia (WHO type IIA).

THE EXAMINATION

GENERAL ASSESSMENT

This should begin with observation of the general appearance of the patient. Start by assessing the state of nutrition and with measurement of weight and height. The body mass index (BMI) is calculated from the formula:

$$BMI = \frac{Weight\ (kg)}{height\ (m)^2}.$$

The normal range for the BMI in men is 20–25 and in women is 18–24. The BMI is useful in the assessment of obesity and malnutrition (see p. 129).

The distribution of fat should be noted. Concentration of fat in the intra-abdominal, thyrocervical and interscapular regions with relative sparing of the limbs (truncal obesity) is characteristic of Cushing's syndrome and is accompanied by a typical moonfaced plethoric appearance (Fig. 8.1) due to a combination of increased subcutaneous fat and thinning of the skin.

Patients with growth hormone hypersecretion, resulting from somatotroph pituitary adenomas, also demonstrate a classic facial appearance with increased fullness and coarsening of soft tissues, including the lips and tongue, which may be accom-

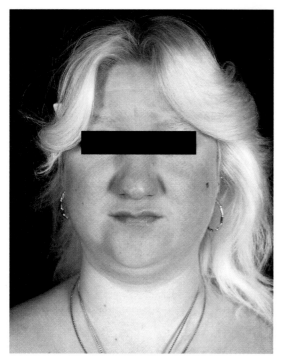

Fig. 8.1 Typical facial appearance of Cushing's syndrome. Note the increased fat deposition and plethoric appearance. The patient presented with a 2-year history of secondary infertility, easy bruising and central adiposity.

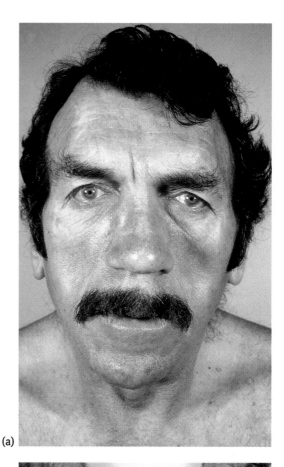

(a)

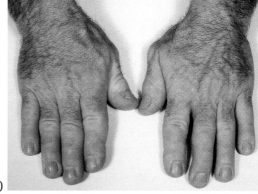

(b)

Fig. 8.2 The facial (a) and hand (b) appearance of acromegaly. There is overgrowth of the facial skeleton, coarsening of features and an increase in soft tissues most obvious in the hands. The patient had a 4-year history of excessive sweating, increased shoe size, frontal headache and 'pins and needles in fingers'.

panied by overgrowth of the zygoma, orbital ridges and mandible (prognathism) in patients with long-standing disease (Fig. 8.2). Acromegaly in young people causes continuation of growth beyond the normal time of cessation of growth at about age 16–18 years, and consequent increase in height. Increased adiposity in a child who is growing poorly suggests the possibility of growth hormone deficiency hypothyroidism or, rarely, Cushing's syndrome.

The skeletal proportions should be noted; a long-limbed appearance may indicate delayed epiphysial fusion due to hypogonadism (*eunuchoidism*) or the connective tissue abnormality Marfan's syndrome. A eunuchoid body habitus is confirmed by demonstrating that the leg length (top of symphysis pubis to ground) exceeds the sitting height or that the span exceeds the total height. Shortening of the limbs occurs with a variety of skeletal dysplasias.

The cytogenetic disorder Turner's syndrome (karyotype 45×0), which is characterized by gonadal dysgenesis and the variable presence of other visceral abnormalities, has a typical phenotypic appearance including short stature, failure of secondary sexual development, decreased or absent secondary sexual hair, an increase in the normal angulation between the humerus and the lower arm, a low posterior hair line and an exaggerated fold of skin between the neck and shoulder. It is most

important that accurate wall-mounted stadiometers be used in the assessment of normal growth and its possible disorders.

The hands should be carefully examined for evidence of finger-clubbing which, among other things, may be a rare manifestation of thyrotoxic Graves' disease (*thyroid acropachy*). Palmar erythema may also be found in thyrotoxicosis of any cause as well as in patients with chronic liver disease or rheumatoid arthritis and in pregnancy.

A unique selective shortening of the fourth and fifth metacarpals may be found as the major somatic manifestation of a group of recessively inherited disorders of parathormone action (*pseudohypoparathyroidism*; Fig. 8.3). Palmar contractures are a relatively common incidental finding and a recognized feature of chronic liver disease but also may occur in patients with long-standing diabetes mellitus. The latter is frequently associated with subtle phalangeal flexural contractions (*cheiroarthropathy*).

Subcutaneous deposits of triglyceride-rich lipoproteins in the palmar skin creases (*palmar xanthomata*) are pathognomonic of increased intermediate density lipoprotein (WHO type III hyperlipidaemia).

THE SKIN

A careful external examination may yield specific diagnostic information in addition to that evident on the initial general examination. Pigmentation, especially buccal, circumoral or palmar, may indicate the increased secretion of adrenocorticotrophic hormone which occurs with adrenal failure (*Addison's disease*; Fig. 8.4); patches of depigmentation, or vitiligo (Fig. 8.5), may also be found in Addison's disease or other organ-specific autoimmune disorders. Violaceous striae, arising as a result of stretching of thin skin with exposure of the dermal capillary circulation, suggest the possibility of glucocorticoid excess (Fig. 8.6) and abnormal dryness of the skin and coarseness of the hair are found in hypothyroidism (Fig. 8.7). Localized thickening of the dermis due to mucopolysaccharide and inflammatory cell deposition, particularly on the anterior aspects of the legs, when it is known as pretibial myxoedema, is one of the classic but relatively rare extrathyroidal manifestations of Graves' disease. An ulcerating skin lesion also demonstrating a predilection for the anterior tibial region is

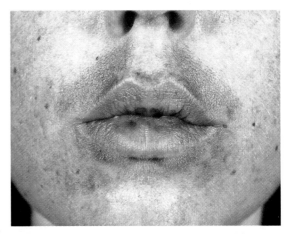

Fig. 8.4 Circumoral pigmentation in a patient with hypersecretion of adrenocorticotropic hormone (ACTH).

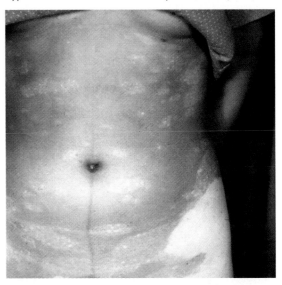

Fig. 8.5 Extensive areas of depigmentation (vitiligo) in a patient with organ-specific autoimmune disease.

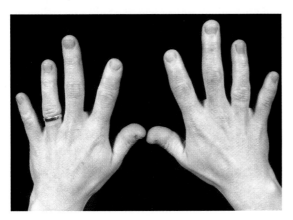

Fig. 8.3 The hands in pseudohypoparathyroidism. Note the characteristic shortening of the 4th and 5th metacarpals.

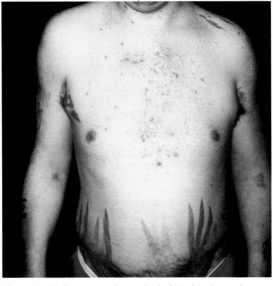

Fig. 8.6 Violaceous striae typical of Cushing's syndrome.

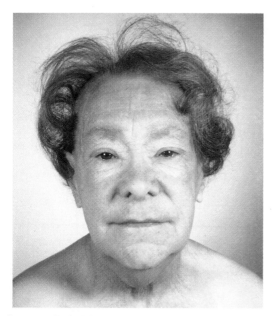

Fig. 8.7 The facial appearance of hypothyroidism. The patient demonstrates periorbital puffiness and coarsening of scalp hair. (Courtesy of Professor P.G. Kopelman.)

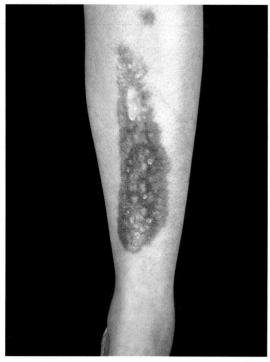

Fig. 8.8 Necrobiosis lipoidica diabeticorum. The ulceration occurs typically in atrophic skin on the anterior tibial region.

necrobiosis lipoidica diabeticorum (Fig. 8.8); this lesion is associated with marked skin atrophy and is specific to diabetes mellitus.

The examination of the skin may also demonstrate the presence of xanthelasmata, subcutaneous deposits of cholesterol just medial to the eyelids (Fig. 8.9) which are suggestive but not diagnostic of hypercho-

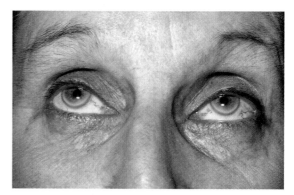

Fig. 8.9 Subcutaneous cholesterol deposition on the medial aspect of the eyelids (xanthelasma). (Courtesy of Professor G.A. Hitman.)

lesterolaemia. The latter may also be manifest by the presence of xanthomata on the Achilles or patellar tendons.

In the female, dermatological examination should also include attention to any abnormality of hair distribution, either excess hair growth in an androgen-dependent distribution (*hirsutism*) or hair loss in a male pattern, both of which may indicate increased circulating androgen and should prompt examination for evidence of virilization (see below).

THE THYROID

The neck should be examined for evidence of thyroid enlargement. Significant thyroid enlargement is usually evident on inspection. Remember that the thyroid gland always moves on swallowing. The normal thyroid may be palpable in thin patients and it should be remembered that the right lobe is slightly larger than the left; therefore diffuse thyroid enlargement, as in Graves' disease, is often apparently asymmetrical. A prominent fat pad between skin creases in the neck may easily be mistaken for thyroid enlargement.

Palpation of the thyroid gland is best carried out from behind the patient with the fingers encircling the neck; the landmarks for palpation are the laryngeal cartilage, just below which is the cricoid cartilage and the isthmus of the thyroid. The following points should be addressed:

- Is the gland diffuse and smooth as in thyroid stimulating hormone (TSH)-mediated or autoimmune thyroid enlargement? If so is it soft as in dyshormonogenesis or the diffuse goitre of puberty, or is it firm or even hard as in autoimmune thyroiditis? A bruit heard over the thyroid indicates increased blood supply and is frequently found in untreated Graves' disease; this should not be confused with a transmitted bruit from the carotid.

- Are two or more areas of nodularity palpable, suggesting a multinodular goitre (Fig. 8.10) and if

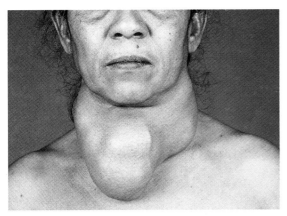

Fig. 8.10   A large multinodular goitre. Note the asymmetrical growth of the nodules.

so does it extend downward behind the sternum (*retrosternal goitre*)? Is the patient clinically thyrotoxic, indicating autonomous thyroid hormone production within one or more nodules?

- Is the palpable abnormality a single focal nodule suggesting a simple cyst, adenoma or carcinoma? Is there any lymphadenopathy which might be associated with the latter?
- Is the goitre firm and asymmetrical?
- Are there features of local pressure effects or local infiltration, for example a hoarse voice from recurrent laryngeal nerve involvement?
- Is there weight loss and debility? These features suggest lymphoma or anaplastic carcinoma.

THE CARDIOVASCULAR SYSTEM

Particular attention should be paid to any postural drop in blood pressure. This may indicate a depleted extracellular fluid volume, for example in patients with adrenal insufficiency, or autonomic dysfunction, the commonest cause of which is diabetes mellitus. Additional indicators of the latter include failure of reflex bradycardia during the Valsalva manoeuvre and loss of beat-to-beat variation in cardiac cycle length determined by ECG. A hyperdynamic circulation, sinus tachycardia or atrial fibrillation may be found in thyrotoxicosis; this may progress to cardiac decompensation and cardiac failure.

THE BREASTS AND GENITALIA

The breasts should be examined for mass lesions and, if suggested by the history, for galactorrhoea. In the male any tendency to gynaecomastia should be noted (Fig. 8.11). This may range from minor degrees of subareolar glandular enlargement to substantial breast prominence; breast enlargement associated with generalized adiposity should not be confused with true gynaecomastia.

Genital examination in the male should document testicular volume. This is particularly important in

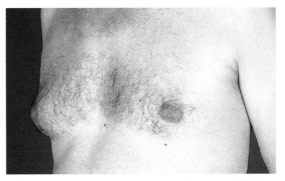

Fig. 8.11   Gynaecomastia. There is enlargement of both breasts in this man.

the assessment of pubertal development for which volume should be measured by comparison with calibrated ovoids (Prader orchidometer). Prepubertal testicular volume is less than 4 ml whereas increased volume implies pubertal gonadotrophin stimulation. Testicular atrophy in the adult male indicates hypogonadism, due either to primary testicular failure, to hypothalamic–pituitary dysfunction or to chronic liver disease. Tumours of Leydig cells are usually palpable and should be sought in any patient with gynaecomastia.

Examination of the external genitalia in the female is important when androgen hypersecretion is suspected. Enlargement of the clitoris is a feature of excess androgen secretion.

Ambiguity of the external genitalia is indicative of fetal androgen excess in the karyotypic female and testosterone or dihydrotestosterone deficiency or resistance in the male; these conditions are rare and require specialized investigation.

THE EYES

The hypercalcaemic patient should be carefully examined for corneal calcification, evident as a narrow band on the medial or lateral border of the cornea (Fig. 8.12); this usually indicates long-standing

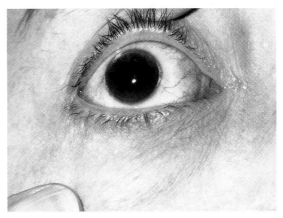

Fig. 8.12   Corneal calcification (band keratopathy) in a patient with longstanding hyperparathyroidism.

hypercalcaemia and a diagnosis of primary hyper-parathyroidism.

In patients with thyroid disease the presence of exophthalmos (*proptosis*) should be noted. This may be unilateral or bilateral and may be associated with apparent ophthalmoplegia due to tethering of the extraocular muscles, particularly the medial and inferior rectus muscles, such that diplopia occurs on upward or lateral gaze (*dysthyroid eye disease*; Fig. 8.13). These ocular signs are especially important in the diagnosis of autoimmune thyroid disease (*Graves' disease*). It must be remembered that unilateral proptosis may also occur with an orbital tumour. Lid retraction, evident as a wide-eyed staring expression, and lid lag, in which depression of the upper lid lags behind the eye in a downward gaze, are due to increased activity of the sympathetic innervation of levator palpebri superioris and are not specific to Graves' disease. Any degree of corneal exposure due to failure of complete lid apposition should be documented.

Visual acuity should be measured both with and without a pinhole to correct for any refractive error. Reduced acuity may be a feature of optic nerve compression in severe dysthyroid eye disease or of asymmetrical pressure on the optic chiasm due to hypothalamic–pituitary space-occupying lesions. In the latter, assessment of the visual fields may reveal a bitemporal hemianopia; this is frequently incomplete and incongruous reflecting the asymmetrical growth of the tumour. Examination of the optic discs with the ophthalmoscope may show pallor indicating neural atrophy resulting from long-standing pressure on the optic nerve.

In the diabetic patient retinoscopy may show characteristic microvascular changes of two main types:

- Small haemorrhages and exudates, either scattered (background retinopathy) or surrounding the macula (maculopathy), the latter being frequently associated with reduction in pinhole-corrected visual acuity
- Areas of pallor, indicating ischaemia, with or without the formation of fronds of new vessels (proliferative retinopathy).

THE NERVOUS SYSTEM

Examination of the nervous system reveals a rapid fine tremor in thyrotoxicosis. Proximal weakness with or without wasting of the shoulder and hip girdle musculature (*proximal myopathy*) is a typical feature of thyrotoxicosis, glucocorticoid excess and vitamin D deficiency. Osteomalacic myopathy is often associated with myalgia.

Hypocalcaemia is associated with increased neural excitability which may be demonstrated by gentle percussion over the proximal part of the facial nerve (as it exits from the parotid gland). The test is positive if this manoeuvre evokes involuntary facial muscular twitching (*Chvostek's sign*).

Tendon reflexes will be abnormally brisk in thyrotoxic patients and may show a slow relaxation phase in hypothyroidism. Both hypothyroidism and acromegaly may give rise to nerve entrapment syndromes particularly of the median nerve at the wrist (*carpal tunnel syndrome*).

Long-standing diabetes mellitus is frequently complicated by peripheral neuropathy with sensory loss in a stocking distribution, exaggeration of the foot arch and increased plantar prominence of the metatarsal heads due to muscle imbalance. This complication may culminate in plantar trophic ulceration.

INVESTIGATION

The investigation of endocrine and metabolic disorders usually involves: (a) the measurement of electrolytes, minerals, metabolites or hormones in plasma; and (b) isotopic, ultrasonographic, radiological or magnetic resonance imaging of specific endocrine glands. In investigating endocrine disease one is usually interested in whether a specific gland is overactive or underactive. These questions may be answered by basal hormone measurements, for example serum-free thyroxine and thyroid-stimulating hormone in thyrotoxicosis and hypothyroidism, but in many instances the lack of a clear distinction

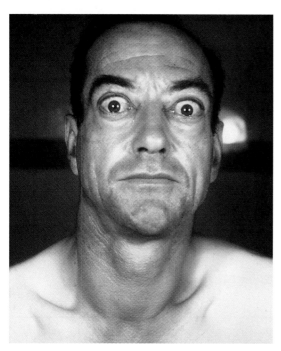

Fig. 8.13 Lid retraction and proptosis in a patient with thyrotoxic Graves' disease. There had been a 6-month history, for this patient, of effortless weight loss, tremulousness, shortness of breath on exertion and palpitations.

between basal hyposecretion, normal secretion and hypersecretion necessitates the use of stimulation tests and suppression tests.

ENDOCRINE STIMULATION TESTS

These are designed to demonstrate how much hormone a gland can secrete in response to a near maximal stimulus. Examples include:

- *Insulin tolerance testing* in which carefully controlled insulin-induced hypoglycaemia stimulates hypothalamic–pituitary secretion measured by serum growth hormone, cortisol and prolactin
- *Tetracosactrin testing* in which an injection of a synthetic adrenocorticotropic hormone (ACTH) analogue is used to assess adrenocortical reserve
- *Oral glucose tolerance test* which is an indirect test of insulin secretion and action is determined by the rise and subsequent fall in the plasma glucose level following an oral glucose load.

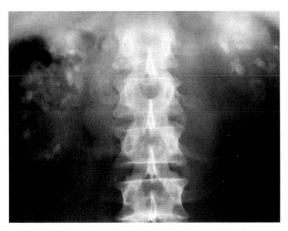

Fig. 8.14 Widespread renal calcification typical of nephrocalcinosis in a patient with longstanding hyperparathyroidism.

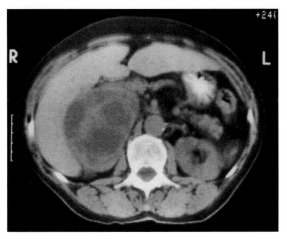

Fig. 8.15 Axial CT scan of the abdomen in a patient with a right adrenal medullary phaeochromocytoma. Note the extensive tumour mass with areas of hypodensity indicating episodes of partial tumour infarction.

ENDOCRINE SUPPRESSION TESTS

These test whether a physiological feedback mechanism is intact or if secretion of the hormone in question has become at least partly autonomous. For example, the suppression of plasma cortisol by the synthetic glucocorticoid dexamethasone is incomplete in Cushing's syndrome and suppression of serum growth hormone by an oral glucose load fails to occur in acromegaly.

ENDOCRINE IMAGING

Plain X-ray imaging is of limited value in the investigation of endocrine disorders. However, lateral and

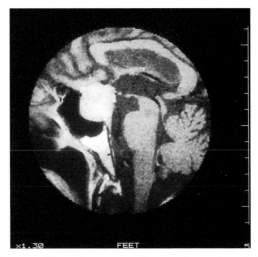

Fig. 8.16 Magnetic resonance imaging (saggital view) of the pituitary, demonstrating a large pituitary adenoma with suprasellar extension.

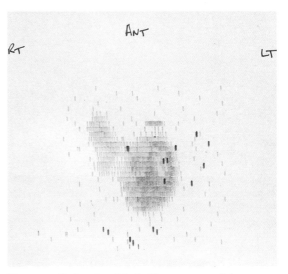

Fig. 8.17 Technetium-labelled isotope scan of the thyroid in a patient with a focal thyroid nodule. Note the focal area of uptake corresponding to the palpable lesion with surrounding inactivity indicating autonomous function within the nodule.

anteroposterior views of the pituitary fossa can be useful in demonstrating abnormal calcification in the fossa or gross expansion and erosion of the fossa due to large intrasellar or suprasellar tumours. Plain abdominal radiology may show renal calcification (*nephrocalcinosis*; Fig. 8.14) in patients with long-standing hypercalcaemia or renal tubular acidosis.

CT imaging is useful in assessing the pituitary, adrenal glands (Fig. 8.15) and thorax. However, MR imaging of the pituitary (Fig. 8.16), offers definite advantages over CT in terms of improved precision in detecting small intrasellar tumours and better definition of the lateral border of the pituitary and the cavernous sinus.

Isotopic imaging is particularly useful for demonstrating autonomous function within endocrine tumours. This technique is applicable to the thyroid gland (radio-labelled pertechnetate; Fig. 8.17), the adrenal cortex (radio-labelled selenocholesterol), the adrenal medulla (radio-labelled meta-iodobenzyl-guanidine) and parathyroids (radio-labelled thallium and sesta MIBI differential scanning).

9
THE RENAL TRACT AND UROLOGY

THE DIAGNOSTIC PROCESS IN NEPHROLOGY AND UROLOGY

These systems are more dependent than most on laboratory, histopathology and imaging techniques for completion of the diagnostic process. However, the basic principles and requirements of clinical assessment still apply—appropriate and careful history-taking and physical examination are essential, and can often lead to a diagnosis. Even if they do not, they serve the important function of directing subsequent laboratory and other technically orientated investigation.

The kidney and urinary tract, when diseased, manifest a somewhat restricted array of symptoms and signs. It is therefore helpful to adopt a syndrome-based approach—almost all patients can be categorized into one or other well defined renal and urological syndromes; keeping these in mind serves to inform the clinical diagnostic process.

In these patients there are many areas of overlap between clinical and pathological processes within a single syndrome and it is not generally helpful to create artificial distinctions between the two. Once the correct syndrome has been established, further details of assessment and management objectives become a great deal clearer. Finally, it is important to emphasize that a number of these syndromes were first described many years ago. They have stood the test of time principally because of their pragmatic value and relative ease of recognition on the basis of clinical assessment and quite simple tests.

SYMPTOMS OF RENAL AND UROLOGICAL DISEASE

PAIN

Pain arising from the urinary tract is one of the commonest symptoms and is most often due to obstruction, infection or tumour. Renal pain is usually felt in the flank region or in the loin. When renal pain arises from ureteric obstruction (e.g. a stone) discomfort may additionally radiate to the iliac fossa, the testicle or the labia, the pattern depending to a certain extent on the level of the obstruction.

Pain in the suprapubic region and the perineum usually arises from lower urinary tract infection—cystitis or urethritis. Such pain is frequently accompanied by *dysuria, frequency* or *strangury*. This constellation of symptoms constitutes the syndrome of *cystitis*. It is nearly always associated with urinary abnormalities on stick testing (protein, blood and leucocytes). In men the pain may be associated with extreme perineal or rectal discomfort, in which case prostatitis is suggested.

In young children with urinary tract infection and cystitis the symptoms may be much less obvious—cystitis should be suspected in any child who cries on micturition. Pain from the kidneys, if resulting from acute infection or abscess, may occasionally reflect tracking of pus upwards to the diaphragm or in the retroperitoneal space to the psoas muscle with, respectively, diaphragmatic pain or impairment of hip extension. Glomerulonephritis is usually painless. Large cystic kidneys or kidneys bearing a tumour may cause a dull persistent flank pain.

HAEMATURIA

This can be present with or without pain and may be continuous or intermittent. If visible to the naked eye it is termed *macroscopic or gross haematuria*; if only detected by stick tests or microscopy it is called *microscopic haematuria*. Haematuria as a result of parenchymal renal disease is usually:

- continuous
- painless
- microscopic (occasionally macroscopic)

Haematina arising from renal tumours is likely to be:

- intermittent
- associated with renal pain
- macroscopic.

Bleeding from bladder tumours is often intermittent, often with associated local symptoms suggesting cystitis.

It is important to decide early in the diagnostic process whether the haematuria originates from the kidneys or elsewhere in the urinary tract (see Box 9.1). This decision affects the order with which investigations should be conducted. For example, continuous painless microscopic haematuria with associated proteinuria in a young man or woman is most likely to be the result of glomerulonephritis or other renal pathology. However, haematuria in an older person with risk factors for urothelial malignancy (smoking) is more likely to be caused by a bladder or ureteric tumour and merits a cystoscopy early in the investigative process. It is important to remember that the commonest cause of dipstick haematuria in women is contamination from menstruation.

OLIGURIA/ANURIA

Oliguria is the passage of < 500 ml urine per day. Anuria is the complete absence of urine flow. A reduction of urine flow rate to the point of oliguria may be physiological, as in a patient whose fluid intake is low. Physiological reduction of urine flow rate implies that the glomerular filtration rate (GFR) remains normal, and that the kidney is avidly retaining sodium and water. If inadequate fluid intake leads to significant reduction in the extracellular fluid compartment (ECF), the resulting decrease in renal blood flow leads to oliguria and reduction of the GFR. Oliguria arising in this fashion is termed *prerenal* and is clearly pathological. *Renal oliguria* implies the presence of intrinsic renal disease, whereas *postrenal oliguria* results from mechanical obstruction at any level from the collecting system in the kidney to the urethra. Anuria and oliguria may be signs of renal failure.

POLYURIA

Polyuria implies no more than a high urine flow rate. There will always be an associated increase in the frequency of micturition (*frequency*) and often *nocturia* as well. Polyuria results from excessive water intake (psychogenic polydipsia or beer drinking for example), from an osmotic diuresis (glucose as in diabetes mellitus, urea as in chronic renal failure and sodium chloride as in diuretic use), and finally from abnormal renal tubular water handling as seen in pituitary diabetes insipidus or renal resistance to antidiuretic hormone—nephrogenic diabetes insipidus.

FREQUENCY

Increased frequency of micturition results from polyuria or from a decrease in the functional bladder capacity. The commonest cause of the former is excessive fluid intake whereas a decreased functional bladder capacity is seen most frequently in patients with lower urinary tract infection (cystitis) and in older men with prostatic hypertrophy and bladder outlet obstruction. Some patients with neurological diseases, in particular multiple sclerosis, also have frequency of micturition. The detrusor muscle of the bladder contracts at an inappropriately low bladder volume resulting in a low functional bladder capacity.

NOCTURIA

The term implies the need to rise during the hours of sleep to empty the bladder. In health there is a substantial diurnal variation in urine flow rate: night-time reduction in urine flow and an adequate functional bladder capacity together serve to obviate the need for night-time micturition. Thus polyuria of any cause, or any cause of reduction of functional bladder capacity, may lead to nocturia.

BOX 9.1   Causes of haematuria.

Systemic
- purpura
- sickle cell trait
- bleeding disorders, including anticoagulant drugs

Renal
- infarct/papillary necrosis
- trauma
- tuberculosis
- stones
- renal pelvis TCC, and other renal tumours
- Wilms' tumour (in children)
- acute glomerulonephritis

Post-renal
- ureteric stones
- ureteric neoplasms
- bladder tumours (transitional cell carcinoma)
- bladder tuberculosis and bilharziasis
- radiation cystitis
- drug-induced cystitis, eg cylcophosphamide
- prostatic ennlargement
- urethral neoplasms
- bacterial cystiti

DYSURIA

This is a specific form of discomfort arising from the urinary tract in which there is pain immediately before, during or immediately after micturition. The urine is often described as 'burning' or 'scalding' and there is usually an association with frequency of micturition and a decreased functional bladder capacity. Infection and neoplasia in the bladder or urethra are the most important causes. An extreme form of dysuria, *strangury*, implies an unpleasant and painful desire to void urine when the bladder is empty or nearly so.

URGENCY OF MICTURITION, INCONTINENCE AND ENURESIS

Urgency is the loss of the normal ability to postpone micturition beyond the time when the desire to pass urine is initially perceived. In extreme cases it may lead to *urge incontinence*, in which the perceived desire to void is followed immediately by voiding. In a more general sense, incontinence implies the involuntary passage of urine and almost always results from local disorders of the bladder or of its nerve supply.

SLOW STREAM, HESITANCY AND TERMINAL DRIBBLING

This triad of symptoms is most frequently seen in elderly men with prostatic hypertrophy. Here the bladder outlet is partially obstructed by the enlarging prostate gland with the result that the maximum achievable urine flow rate during micturition is reduced. Such patients often experience difficulty in initiating the process of micturition (*hesitancy*) and of completing micturition in a 'clean stop' fashion (*terminal dribbling*). The symptoms are nearly always associated with frequency of micturition and nocturia, the result of a low functional bladder capacity. In more advanced cases there may be progressive bladder enlargement with eventual *overflow incontinence* and continuous or intermittent dribbling of urine.

URETHRAL DISCHARGE

This is usually only noticed by men and always requires further investigation. There may be associated symptoms of urethral irritation and the underlying pathology is likely to be urethritis which is often infective and sexually transmitted.

PHYSICAL SIGNS IN RENAL AND UROLOGICAL DISEASE

These physical signs fall into three principal groups:

- Local signs related to the specific pathology, for example an enlarged palpable tender kidney containing a large tumour, or a palpably enlarged bladder in a patient with acute or chronic retention
- Symptoms may arise from disturbance of renal salt and water handling with resulting ECF volume expansion or contraction—to ellicit the appropriate physical signs in this category requires careful assessment of the patient's volume status
- Those signs resulting from a failure of the kidney's normal excretory and metabolic functions.

In many renal patients, particularly those with advanced chronic renal failure and uraemia, signs from all three of the above categories may be present.

GENERAL INSPECTION

Patients with chronic renal failure always look unwell. The skin is pallid, the complexion sallow and a slightly yellowish hue is often evident. The mucous membranes are pale, reflecting the normochromic, normocytic anaemia that is associated with chronic renal failure. There may be *bruises*, *purpura* and *scratch marks* due to uraemic pruritis and also an underlying disorder of platelet function and capillary fragility. The nails often appear pale and some times opaque (*leuconychia*) in patients with the nephrotic syndrome and in some patients with chronic renal failure. Intercurrent episodes of severe illness in the past may have led to the appearance of *Beau's lines* which appear as transverse ridges across the nails. *Splinter haemorrhages* in the nail beds point to underlying vasculitis which may be the cause of the renal failure or be indicative of endocarditis or other vasculitic illness; there may be an associated *purpuric rash* (Fig. 9.1). *Uraemic frost* may be seen on any part of the body and appears as a white powder which is made up of crystalline urea appearing on the skin via the sweat. The onset of chronic renal failure in childhood almost

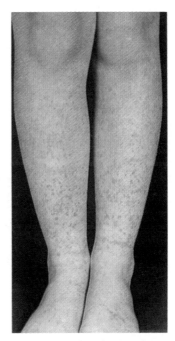

Fig. 9.1   Purpura in Henoch–Schönlein disease.

invariably results in impaired growth with resulting *short stature* in adult life. More severe bony deformity may be evident in some cases, particularly in children who may develop rickets (Fig. 9.2). Advanced uraemia is also associated with *uraemic metabolic flap*, a coarse tremor which is best seen at the wrists when in the dorsiflexed position. It is very similar to the metabolic flap seen in patients with advanced hepatic disease or respiratory failure. Metabolic acidosis, if present, leads to increased ventilation with an increased tidal volume—*Kussmaul respiration*.

THE CIRCULATION IN THE RENAL PATIENT

Of crucial importance here is the correct assessment of the patient's volume status. It is important to be able to define the patient as *euvolaemic, hypovolaemic* or *hypervolaemic*. This is a bedside diagnosis that, with practice, can be made correctly in the vast majority of patients.

Hypervolaemia is associated with some or all of the following:

- hypertension
- elevation of the jugular venous pressure
- peripheral oedema at the ankles or sacrum
- basal crackles on lung auscultation
- ascites
- pleural effusion.

In patients with *nephrotic syndrome* (see below) the oedema and salt and water retention are driven by the reduced plasma oncotic pressure. In some cases both these mechanisms are operative simultaneously. Oedema with expansion of the extracellular fluid (ECF) is often accompanied by hypertension and, particularly if the cardiac reserve is poor, may progress to pulmonary oedema and other manifestations of heart failure.

The diagnosis of *hypovolaemia* requires the absence of any signs of *hypervolaemia*. The hypovolaemic patient may have the following:

- low blood pressure, often exaggerated in the upright position—*postural hypotension*
- sinus tachycardia (exaggerated in the upright position)
- low pulse pressure (exaggerated in the upright position)
- flat neck veins even when almost supine
- poor skin turgor.

(a)

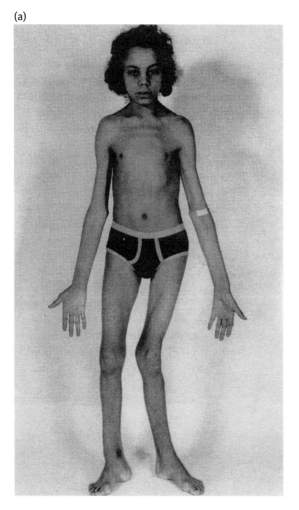

(b)

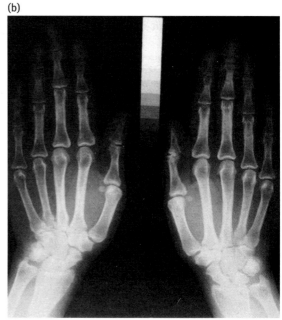

Fig. 9.2   (a) Knock knees and varus deformity of the ankles due to renal osteodystrophy. (b) X-ray of the hands of a patient with chronic renal failure and secondary hyperparathyroidism showing renal osteodystrophy. There is a loss of density of the tips of the digits (acro-osteolysis) with loss of density on either side of the interphalangeal joints and subperiosteal bone resorption. The latter is best seen in the middle phalynx of the index and middle fingers.

In the elderly, however, in whom the elastic recoil of the skin is physiologically impaired, poor skin turgor is an unreliable sign. Dry mouth and mucous membranes—though these may also result from general illness, mouth breathing and hyperventilation—are often present.

ABDOMINAL PALPATION

In slim people with relaxed abdominal muscles it is sometimes possible to feel a normal right kidney (the right kidney is situated slightly lower than the left at the level of T12–L3). More often a palpable kidney can only be felt because it is abnormally enlarged, as with hydronephrosis, multiple cysts (as in polycystic kidney disease), tumour (generally unilateral). A *distended bladder* is identified in the lower abdomen by a combination of palpation and percussion. *Rectal examination* is an important part of the clinical assessment of the renal patient; bimanual palpation of the bladder is a more reliable way of assessing bladder enlargement than is simple per abdominal examination. Rectal examination also allows evaluation of the *prostate gland*, both for benign enlargement and for the possibility of malignant change suggested by hard irregularity of the gland.

AUSCULTATION

Uraemic pericarditis and pleurisy may be suggested by pericardial and pleural friction rubs respectively. Their presence points to either advanced uraemia or a multisystem inflammatory disorder such as systemic lupus erythematosus (SLE) which may have both renal and extrarenal manifestations. Added heart sounds (S3 and S4) suggest, respectively, volume expansion and incipient heart failure, and ventricular hypertrophy, often as a consequence of hypertension. The presence of vascular bruits and/or impairment of the major arterial pulses is an important finding, raising the possibility of renal vascular disease which may underlie hypertension and/or renal failure if bilateral.

THE EYE IN URAEMIA

External inspection may reveal *corneal calcification* (*limbic calcification*), particularly in patients with long-standing hyperparathyroidism or elevation of blood calcium and phosphorous concentrations. The presence of limbic calcification should not be confused with a *corneal arcus* (*arcus senilis*)—the latter is a broader band at the edge of the cornea and merges with the sclera. Corneal arcus is usually most marked in the superior and inferior position whereas limbic calcification is seen medially and laterally or circumferentially. *Retinal changes* are extremely important in uraemic patients, many of whom have hypertension and/or diabetes. Patients with renal disease as part of systemic vasculitis may have manifestations of the latter in the retinae with haemorrhages and exudates. As a group, patients with chronic renal failure are at greatly increased risk of a range of vascular complications affecting both the macro- and the microvasculature. In the retinae, thrombosis of the central retinal artery or its branches, or of the central retinal vein and its branches, is an important manifestation of this.

THE RENAL AND UROLOGICAL SYNDROMES

These syndromes are listed in Table 9.1. Some are exclusively nephrological, others exclusively urological, while some fall into both areas. The effects of renal faliure on other organ systems are listed in Table 9.2.

THE SYNDROME OF ACUTE RENAL FAILURE

This is the abrupt onset of declining renal function occurring over a period of hours or days, usually but not always accompanied by a marked reduction of the urine flow rate—*anuria* or *oliguria*. Central to the diagnosis, however, is a rapid decline in the GFR leading to nitrogen retention and usually to sodium and water retention as well. An exception is the patient in whom the decline of GFR is not accompanied by reduction of urine flow—so called *non-oliguric acute renal failure*. The outlook depends on the cause. Many are reversible spontaneously (repair of ischaemic injury as in tubular necrosis) or as a result of therapy (removal of stone or other cause of obstruction).

THE SYNDROME OF CHRONIC RENAL FAILURE

Chronic renal failure implies that GFR has been reduced for a considerable period of time and that the reduction is largely or completely irreversible. It can

TABLE 9.1   Renal and urological syndromes.

Renal	Renal and urological	Urological
Chronic renal failure	Acute renal failure	Urinary tract infection
Acute nephritic syndrome	Asymptomatic urinary abnormality	Urinary tract obstruction
Nephrotic syndrome	Recurrent gross haematuria	Renal and urinary tract stone
Renal hypertension		
Tubular syndromes		

BOX 9.2   Effects of renal failure on other organ systems.

Disturbances of water and electrolyte balance
- Breathlessness due to salt and water overload
- Deep sighing breathing (Kussmaul respiration) due to acidosis
- Weakness and postural fainting due to hypotension caused by salt and water depletion
- Lethargy and weakness from hypokalaemia

Disturbances of the haematological system
- Lethargy and breathlessness associated with anaemia due to impaired production of erythropoietin by the kidneys
- Defective coagulation and excessive bruising (advanced renal failure)
- Haemorrhage from the gastrointestinal tract or lungs

Disturbances of the cardiovascular system
- Cardiac failure or angina associated with fluid overload, hypertension, anaemia, and impaired ventricular function (uraemic cardiomyopathy)
- Precordial chest pain due to pericarditis
- Cardiac arrhythmias associated with hyperkalaemia/hypokalaemia

Disturbances of the respiratory system
- Breathlessness and haemoptysis from fluid overload
- Chest pain due to pleurisy

Disturbances of the musculoskeletal system
- Muscular weakness and bone pain due to impairment of vitamin D activation and to excessive parathyroid gland activity
- Acute pain due to gout

Disturbances of the nervous system
- Hypertensive stroke and encephalopathy
- Clouding of consciousness, fits and coma in advanced renal failure
- Impaired sensation or paraesthesiae in the feet, due to peripheral neuropathy in long-standing uraemia
- Impaired higher mental/intellectual function

Disturbances of the eyes
- Pain from conjunctivitis caused by local deposits of calcium
- Visual blurring from hypertensive retinal damage or retinal vascular disease

result from almost any form of renal parenchymal disease, chronic renal ischaemia or unrelieved obstruction. If renal impairment is severe, there may be clinical manifestations of *uraemia*. These are usually evident when the GFR has fallen to one-third or less of normal. The implication of the term *chronic renal failure* is that the time-scale of onset and progression is rarely shorter than a few months and often much longer. A further and crucial implication is an irreversible reduction in the number of functioning nephrons with no prospect of significant recovery. These patients manifest a number of symptoms that are not attributable to specific pathophysiological changes. Lethargy, poor concentration, irritability and failure of higher mental functions and ability to handle tasks are all commonly reported. In advanced cases there may be confusion, fits and stupor. These are preterminal but also reversible if steps are taken to remove the excess amounts of uraemic toxins by dialysis. Nausea, vomiting and diarrhoea are also common in advanced uraemia and likewise improve following restoration of normal kidney function or treatment with dialysis or transplantation.

THE ACUTE NEPHRITIC SYNDROME

As in acute renal failure, the acute nephritic syndrome implies a fairly brisk onset (days, weeks or months) of reduction of GFR and retention of nitrogenous waste and usually salt and water also. *Oliguria* is, therefore, common. The underlying pathology is an acute glomerulonephritis which, as well as causing the functional abnormalities described above, also results in florid abnormalities of the urine. *Haematuria* (macroscopic or microscopic), *proteinuria* and *tubular casts* are often present. Many of the causes of acute nephritis are associated with functional abnormalities of the immune system which may be detected by laboratory tests and which may also manifest with disease in other organs, for example the skin, joints or eyes, as in systemic lupus erythematosus, Henoch–Schönlein purpura and systemic vasculitis.

THE NEPHROTIC SYNDROME

This is defined somewhat imprecisely as the presence of *heavy proteinuria* (usually >3 g/day compared with normal of <150 mg/day), *hypoalbuminaemia*, *hypercholesterolaemia* and *oedema*. It is not generally very helpful to attempt a more precise definition because the clinical response to a given level of proteinuria shows considerable variability from patient to patient. It is, however, unusual for nephrotic syndrome to occur when the proteinuria is <2 g/24 h, and conversely some patients are able to maintain a normal or near normal serum albumin concentration despite very heavy proteinuria in excess of 6 g/24 h.

Proteinuria of this magnitude implies glomerular pathology and may coexist with significant reduction of GFR. Thus a number of the pathological entities capable of causing nephrotic syndrome may also present as acute nephritic syndrome or the syndrome of chronic renal failure in other patients.

THE SYNDROME OF ASYMPTOMATIC URINARY ABNORMALITY

This is the presentation that arises in the patient who presents for a routine medical examination, often in the context of employment or life insurance. Urine testing leads to the unexpected finding of *proteinuria, haematuria* or *pyuria* in an otherwise healthy patient. Further assessment may reveal the coexistence of other renal syndromes, but nevertheless it is worth maintaining the above operational definition of the syndrome of asymptomatic urinary abnormality because this is such a frequent presentation in clinical practice. It should not be forgotten that this syndrome may not only reflect disease of the kidneys in that it can also be a manifestation of malignancy anywhere in the urinary tract, infection or stone (if asymptomatic).

THE SYNDROME OF RECURRENT GROSS HAEMATURIA

This implies intermittent, or in some cases continuous, bleeding into the urinary tract to a degree sufficient to alter the macroscopic appearance of the urine. Depending on the circumstances of the bleeding, the urine may be a rusty-brown colour, lightly tinged with red blood or more heavily bloodstained. The blood may be derived from anywhere in the urinary tract from the glomeruli at the top to the urethra at the bottom. Important causes are certain types of glomerulonephritis, renal tumours and infections (particularly tuberculosis), and tumours of the urinary tract transitional cell epithelium (urothelium) anywhere from the renal pelves to the bladder and urethra.

THE SYNDROME OF URINARY TRACT INFECTION

The normal urinary tract is sterile except at its extreme distal end. Infection in the urinary tract leads to a range of symptoms and signs that reflect the location and severity of the infection. By far the most frequent site is the bladder and the local symptoms reflect bladder irritation with *frequency of micturition, low functional bladder capacity* and pain on passing urine—*dysuria*. The presence of the syndrome of urinary tract infection is defined importantly by the presence of a significant number of infecting organisms in the urine—a working definition would be more than 10^5 colony forming units/ml urine in a carefully collected mid-stream specimen (MSU). For less common infections this definition may not be appropriate. For example, in tuberculosis of the urinary tract the number of organisms being excreted may be extremely low and formal identification on the basis of urine culture is sometimes difficult or impossible.

THE SYNDROME OF URINARY TRACT OBSTRUCTION

This syndrome may conveniently be divided into, respectively, lower and upper urinary tract obstruction. Lower urinary tract obstruction is defined by residual urine in the bladder after micturition, or in more extreme forms by urinary retention with inability to empty the bladder at all. The most common causes relate to prostatic hypertrophy (benign hyperplasia or carcinoma) and a characteristic array of symptoms and signs arises (*frequency, nocturia, poor stream, hesitancy, terminal dribbling*). All of these are a consequence of a low functional bladder capacity, inability to empty the bladder completely and impairment of the urine flow rate.

The presence of upper urinary tract obstruction is established in most cases by the demonstration of a dilated renal collecting system (renal pelvis and/or calyces), often seen to be proximal to a specific obstructing lesion. These features may be demonstrated by a number of imaging techniques, including ultrasound and intravenous urography (IVU). Both upper and lower urinary tract obstruction may coexist, most frequently when the lower urinary tract obstruction is severe and/or of long standing and leading to progressive dilatation of the upper urinary tract with consequent renal damage.

THE SYNDROME OF RENAL AND URINARY TRACT STONE

The operational definition is largely a pathological one, centering around the demonstration of one or more stones in any part of the urinary tract. Resulting symptoms and signs depend much on the location of the stone(s) and on size. For example, small stones in the kidneys are frequently asymptomatic, or they may lead to subtle urinary abnormalities with initial presentation as the syndrome of *asymptomatic urinary abnormality*. Larger stones in the kidneys frequently lead to renal pain whereas stone in the ureter is particularly likely to cause acute obstruction with very severe ureteric and renal pain. Bladder stones are usually associated with symptoms suggestive of cystitis—frequency, haematuria and pain are all common and urinary tract infection is often associated.

THE SYNDROME OF RENAL HYPERTENSION

By far the commonest cause of sustained elevation of blood pressure is essential hypertension. However, in a minority of patients with raised blood pressure renal disease will be found to be the cause and the likelihood of this is greatly increased in patients with coexisting renal disease of any kind. Hypertension may be one of the presenting features of virtually any disease of the renal parenchyma, including all forms of glomerulonephritis, many forms of tubulointerstitial disease, renal vascular disease, renal stone disease and obstruction. Renal tumours and renal infections may occasionally present with hypertension which in some cases can be the only presenting feature. Thus in any patient with newly identified hypertension the possibility of underlying renal disease as a cause should be considered. Conversely, the exclusion of renal disease as a cause of hypertension is generally straightforward, comprising the absence of symptoms and signs of renal disease, the absence of urinary abnormalities on simple stick testing and the presence of normal glomerular filtration rate as judged by serum creatinine concentration or other surrogate for GFR.

RENAL TUBULAR SYNDROMES

The majority of patients with parenchymal renal disease or obstructive renal damage manifest disordered tubular function, although in only a few of these are the tubular defects responsible for specific clinical manifestations. Tubular syndromes arising in this context are generally unobtrusive and are certainly common. Much less common is the patient in whom the tubular defect dominates the clinical picture. These defects may be inherited or acquired and are seen mainly in children. They usually require careful laboratory testing to characterize them fully. Proximal tubular abnormalities include renal phosphate wasting, aminoaciduria (of these, cystinuria with cystine stone formation is the most important) and renal tubular acidosis leading to chronic metabolic acidosis. Distal tubular defects are also associated with metabolic acidosis and with disturbances of potassium metabolism, sodium-losing nephropathy and nephrogenic diabetes insipidus with resulting failure, respectively, of salt and water conservation.

LABORATORY ASSESSMENT AND IMAGING OF THE KIDNEYS AND URINARY TRACT: ASSESSMENT OF STRUCTURE AND FUNCTION

THE URINE

The urine should be tested as part of any general medical examination—this should not be confined to patients with known renal or urinary tract disease. Not only may the testing lead to the discovery of hitherto unsuspected diseases such as diabetes or renal disease, but also documentation of normal urine often provides a very useful historical yardstick in the event of the later development of renal disease or urinary abnormalities. The urine specimen should be passed into a clean container without additives. Testing should normally be conducted as soon as possible and if delayed more than 2 hours the urine should be refrigerated (not frozen) and returned to room temperature before testing. A mid-stream urine specimen is essential for microbiological assessment and desirable for microscopic examination.

QUANTITY

Normal adults in temperate climates usually pass between 750 and 2500 ml of urine every 24 hours. The minimum daily urine output compatible with normal renal excretory function varies from person to person and also with other factors such as diet. Abnormally low urine output (oliguria or anuria) implies that the flow rate is below the minimum required to allow excretion of the daily solute load (usually < 500 ml/day in an adult). Polyuria is an imprecise term implying no more than passage of a large urine volume but not implying anything about the reasons for this.

COLOUR

Urochrome and uro-erythrin are pigments which contribute to the natural yellow tinge of urine. Darkening occurs on staining as a result of oxidation of urobilinogen to coloured urobilin. The colour of urine is also heavily influenced by the urine flow rate—high flow leads to dilute urine and hence pale colour. Bile pigments in excess colour the urine brown with a characteristic yellow froth on shaking. Small to moderate quantities of blood inpart a smoky appearance, with larger amounts leading to progressive brown or, in the case of brisk bleeding, bright red discolouration. Free haemoglobin from intravascular haemolysis (e.g. in severe malaria—blackwater fever) produces a darker red colour verging on black in severe cases. Myoglobin may appear in the urine after acute muscle necrosis (rhabdomyolysis), causing a brown-red discoloration. Certain drugs discolour the urine—examples include rifampicin (red), anthraquinone purgatives such as senna (orange), nitrofurantoin (brown) and methyldopa (grey). Urine is normally transparent when freshly passed and still warm but may be cloudy if there are large numbers of red blood cells or leucocytes, or if phosphates have precipitated in significant amounts.

SPECIFIC GRAVITY OSMOLALITY

These measurements yield similar information and, in the absence of significant glycosuria, are functions of the urinary concentrations of sodium, chloride and urea. The range of specific gravity is 1.001 to 1.035 which is equivalent to 50–1350 mosmol/kg water (Fig. 9.3). The presence of renal insufficiency

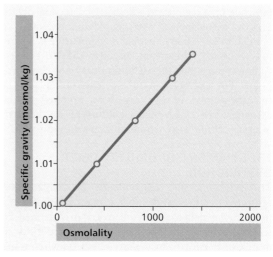

Fig. 9.3   Relationship between specific gravity and osmolality.

leads to reduction of the range of osmolality that the kidneys can generate and in advanced renal disease the osmolality becomes relatively fixed at about 300 mosmol/kg water—close to that of the glomerular filtrate (Fig. 9.4). This is termed *isosthenuria*, and predisposes the patient to sodium and water overload if intake is high, and to salt and water depletion if intake is low.

pH
This varies from pH 4–8 and can be measured crudely using paper strips impregnated with an indicator. If more accurate measurements are needed, as with suspected renal tubular acidosis, a pH electrode is used. Most people pass acid urine most of the time, exceptions being some vegetarians, certain types of renal tubular acidosis, rapid water diuresis, metabolic alkalosis and urine infection with urea-splitting organisms.

GLUCOSE
Glucose oxidase impregnated dipsticks provide a quick and semi-quantitative test for glucose in urine.

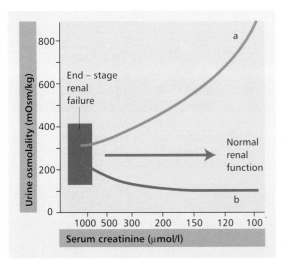

Fig. 9.4 Relationship between renal concentration and diluting capacity, and serum creatinine concentration. The serum creatinine is plotted on a logarithmic scale. This therefore represents linear changes in glomerular filtration rate, such as might occur in progressive renal failure. End in stage renal failure is shown on the left of the figure, and normal renal function on the right. Curve **(a)** represents maximum concentrating capacity, e.g. in water deprivation, when the normal kidney can maintain the serum creatinine in the normal range by increasing urine osmolality. In renal failure the urine cannot be concentrated and the serum creatinine rises. Curve **(b)** represents the maximum diluting capacity, e.g. after ingestion of large volumes of water. The normal kidney excretes urine of low osmolality. In end-stage renal failure urine osmolality cannot be reduced and the water load is not adequately handled. In end-stage renal function there is isosthenuria, i.e. the urine tends toward an iso-osmolar state (specific gravity 1.010).

By far the commonest causes of abnormal glycosuria are elevation of the plasma glucose to a point where the tubular reabsorbative capacity for glucose is exceeded (usually seen in people with diabetes) and during pregnancy, in which glycosuria occurs with normal plasma glucose concentration. Very rarely, tubular transport defects may be associated with glycosuria at normal plasma glucose concentrations and more frequently, but less predictably, patients with acquired chronic renal diseases may exhibit glycosuria at normal plasma glucose concentrations. Collectively these disorders are termed *renal glycosuria*.

PROTEIN
The normal daily urine protein output is <150 mg. Dipsticks reactive to urine albumin provide a simple semi-quantitative test. They are sensitive to 200–300 mg protein/litre and have almost completely superseded the more cumbersome sulphosalicylic acid test. The urinary protein excretion rate generally rises in the upright posture and with activity, and in some normal individuals this may lead to apparently abnormal proteinuria on spot urine specimens in ambulant patients and even in 24-hour urine collections (*orthostatic proteinuria*). Measurement of protein in an early morning urine, however reveals no protein reveals and this serves to distinguish abnormal proteinuria from orthostatic proteinuria. A further refinement is the specific measurement of urine albumin which is increasingly employed and should be <20 mg/day. Albumin excretion in the range 20–200 mg/day is termed *microalbuminuria*. Although this range is frequently too low to be detectable by stick testing, it is an important finding, particularly in diabetics in whom it predicts the later onset of overt diabetic nephropathy.

The diagnostic implications of proteinuria depend greatly on its magnitude (Table 9.2). Heavy proteinuria (in excess of 1.5 g/24 h) is nearly always of glomerular origin and albumin predominates over larger proteins such as globulins. Other proteins, rarely measured, arise from the renal tubules and include Tamm–Horsfall protein, retinol binding protein and nephrocalcin, the latter helping to prevent the formation of urinary stones.

MICROSCOPY (Figs 9.5–9.8)
This is performed after slow spinning (not more than 1000 g) of a fresh urine specimen for approximately 2 minutes. The pellet is re-suspended in 0.5 ml of urine and examined unstained on a microscope slide under a cover slip. Important findings include leucocytes (suggestive of infection), *red blood cells* and various types of *tubular casts*. The presence of tubular casts is indicative of parenchymal renal disease. They may be red cell casts or white cell casts in which Tamm–Horsfall protein matrix has solidified and is studded with red or white blood cells. Granular casts probably represent degenerate

TABLE 9.2   Proteinuria.

Mild (<500 mg/day)	Moderate (up to 3 g/day)	Heavy (>3 g/day)
Benign hypertensive nephrosclerosis	Chronic pyelonephritis	Acute glomerulonephritis
Obstructive nephropathy	Acute tubular necrosis	Chronic glomerulonephritis
Prerenal uraemia	Acute glomerulonephritis	Diabetic nephropathy
Renal tumour	Chronic glomerulonephritis	Pre-eclampsia
Fever	Obstructive nephropathy	Myeloma
Tubulointerstitial nephropathy	Accelerated phase hypertension	All causes of nephrotic syndrome
Chronic pyelonephritis	Orthostatic proteinuria	
Early diabetic nephropathy	Urinary tract infection	
Orthostatic proteinuria		

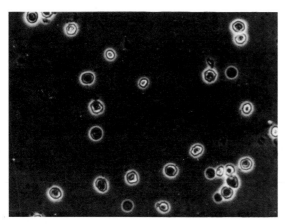

Fig. 9.5   Erythrocytes in urinary sediment.

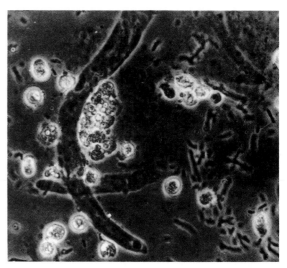

Fig. 9.7   Hyaline casts, leucocytes and bacteria in urinary sediment. Reproduced with permission from Hand Atlas of the Urinary Sediment (1971) by E.S. Spencer and I. Petersen, published by Munksgaard, Copenhagen.

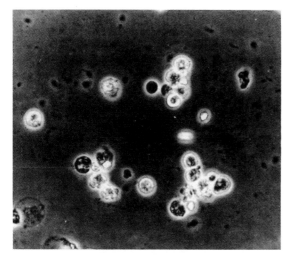

Fig. 9.6   Leucocytes in urinary sediment.

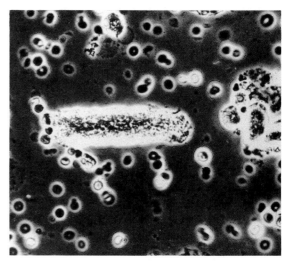

Fig. 9.8   Granular casts in urinary sediment.

cellular casts and have a grainy appearance. Haline casts contain no elements or debris and may be seen in small numbers in normal urine. It is usual to express the number of cells or casts seen per high power field. Red cell morphology may be a useful indicator to the source of bleeding. Red cells with a normal outline usually, though not always, arise from the renal collecting system or from a point downstream of that, whereas red cells arising from the glomeruli are often distorted and dysmorphic, probably as a result of movement through the glomeruli or osmotic insults during passage down the renal tubule.

MICROBIOLOGICAL EXAMINATION OF THE URINE

Mid-stream urine specimens are normally satisfactory, but are always contaminated to a certain extent during passage to the exterior. Extensive studies have shown that the finding of more than 10^5 bacteria per ml in a mid-stream specimen is usually associated with active urinary infection, especially when accompanied by leucocytes. Occasionally urine is taken directly from the bladder for diagnostic purposes. It should be sterile.

MEASUREMENT OF THE GLOMERULAR FILTRATION RATE

Accurate assessment of the glomerular filtration rate (GFR) requires measurement in blood and urine of a compound that is filtered freely at the glomerulus and neither reabsorbed nor secreted by the tubules (Table 9.3). Inulin is the best agent, but involves a continuous infusion of inulin and measurements of inulin concentration in plasma and urine—a laborious and not routinely available investigation that is generally confined to research. A number of surro-

gates for the inulin clearance method exist, however, and details of these are given in Table 9.3. The most frequently used surrogates, and also the crudest ones, are the plasma urea and plasma creatinine concentrations. Both compounds are produced endogenously (at an inconstant rate in the case of urea) and excreted by glomerular filtration. Neither is particularly accurate when used to establish the absolute level of glomerular filtration in an individual patient, although the plasma creatinine concentration is certainly very useful when used to follow changes in an individual patient's renal function, especially when the GFR is significantly reduced (Fig. 9.9). Creatinine clearance is more precise but requires a 24-hour urine collection with measurements of plasma creatinine concentration and urine creatinine excretion rate. The clearance is then calculated using the simple formula: UV/P, where U equals the urinary concentration of creatinine, V the urine flow rate (usually expressed in ml/min) and P equals the plasma creatinine concentration. This formula can be applied to urea or to any other compound subject to renal excretion. Only those compounds that are freely filtered at the glomerulus and neither secreted nor reabsorbed by the renal tubules are suitable for GFR measurement. It should be remembered that the GFR peaks at 20–25 years of age and at about 120 ml/min and declines steadily thereafter at a rate of approximately 1 ml/min/year. Appreciation of this age-related change in GFR is important in clinical practice, particularly when prescribing drugs to the elderly. The most precise measures of GFR used in clinical practice depend on measurement of the excretion of radiolabelled compounds. The most commonly used is ^{51}Cr-EDTA which gives a relatively easy and reproducible measure of GFR.

TABLE 9.3   Measurement of the glomerular filtration rate.

Method	Comments
Plasma	Poor surrogate — variable production rate — variable excretion rate
Plasma creatinine	Better than urea Poor discrimination at near-normal GFR
Creatinine clearance	Reasonable surrogate but depends on accurate timed urine collection (usually 24 hours)
^{51}Cr-EDTA practice	The best surrogate in clinical Expensive
Inulin clearance	Near perfect measurement of GFR but — needs continuous infusion — difficult urine and plasma assays — research studies only—not suited to clinical practice

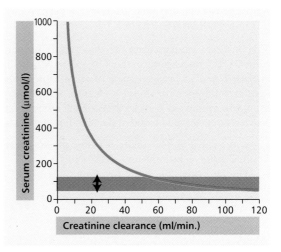

Fig. 9.9   Relationship between creatinine clearance and plasma creatinine concentrations. The normal range of serum creatinine concentration can be maintained only when the renal creatinine clearance is greater than about 60 ml/min. The red area represents the normal range of creatinine concentration.

MEASUREMENT OF RENAL TUBULAR FUNCTION

The two tests most frequently utilized are:

- tests of renal concentrating ability when probing possible causes of polyuria
- tests of renal acidification in patients with metabolic acidosis and possible underlying renal tubular acidosis.

Renal concentrating ability involves perturbing the patient in a way that should lead to the production of a concentrated urine. Water deprivation is the most common provocation and after 12 hours the urine osmolality should be at least 750 mosmol/kg (specific gravity 1.020). Failure to concentrate the urine in these circumstances indicates either impairment of vasopressin output (pituitary diabetes insipidus) or resistance of the renal tubules to the action of vasopressin (nephrogenic diabetes insipidus). These two possibilities may be distinguished by measuring the urine osmolality after an injection of vasopressin or an analogue thereof—again the urine osmolality should increase to at least 750 mosmol/kg.

Renal tubular acidification can be assumed to be adequate if the pH of a random specimen of urine is below 5.5. Urine pH > 5.5 in the presence of metabolic acidosis usually indicates renal tubular acidosis. If the patient is only minimally acidotic and the urine pH is > 5.5 a provocative test in which ammonium chloride is given at a dose of 0.1 g/kg body weight to provide an acid load and an acute mild metabolic acidosis can be performed. The pH should fall to < 5.4 if acidification is normal.

ASSESSMENT OF THE URINE IN THE STONE FORMING PATIENT

This involves measurement of the important constituents of stone whose outputs may be abnormally increased, and also measurement of at least one of the natural inhibitors of stone formation. Ideally this should be combined with analysis of the stone itself. The tests that should be undertaken in all patients are:

- plasma calcium, phosphate, alkaline phosphatase, urea, urate, creatinine and electrolytes
- 24-hour urine collection for simultaneous measurement of
  — calcium
  — uric acid
  — oxalate
  — citrate
  — creatinine
  — sodium
- nitroprusside test for cystine.

The identification of increased excretion rates of calcium, uric acid, oxalate or cystine indicates a strong predisposition to recurrent stone formation. Conversely, citrate is a natural inhibitor of stone formation and a low urine citrate is associated with increased stone risk. All patients who make radiopaque stones should be screened for cystinuria using the nitroprusside test.

KIDNEY BIOPSY

This investigation, in which one or two small cores of renal cortex are removed using a needle biopsy technique, is performed in patients in whom diffuse renal parenchymal disease is suspected. However, not everyone with renal parenchymal disease requires a biopsy. The test is invasive and carries small but definite risks of serious complication. It is important, therefore, to define the indications and contraindications carefully. The risk of the procedure can be minimized by the following preconditions:

- A cooperative patient
- Prior knowledge of the position, size and function of both kidneys (this is usually provided by a combination of ultrasound and IVU or isotope renography; a solitary functioning kidney should not be biopsied unless the diagnostic yield is deemed to be crucial)
- Absence of bleeding disorder
- Availability of blood for transfusion in the event of haemorrhage
- An appropriate indication.

Kidney biopsy is often the only way to distinguish the various forms of glomerulonephritis from one another and from tubulointerstitial diseases of the kidney.

IMAGING OF THE URINARY TRACT

PLAIN RADIOGRAPHS

In many people one or both of the kidneys can be seen outlined by perirenal fat on plain abdominal films or nephrotomograms. The information gleaned is limited, although certain types of renal stone or other calcifications may be identified.

ULTRASOUND

Ultrasound provides good images of the renal parenchyma and collecting system and in nearly all patients gives a reliable estimate of renal size as well as identifying discrete lesions within the parenchyma, hydronephrosis and stone. Doppler studies often permit assessment of blood flow in the main renal arteries and in the larger intrarenal branches. Although the upper ureter can be seen quite well in most patients, the lower ureter is not visualized adequately. Ultrasound examination of the bladder is also extremely useful, allowing calculation of the bladder capacity when full and also after micturition (emptying should be virtually complete), as well as visualization of the bladder wall and lesions projecting into the bladder itself (e.g. bladder tumours). It is sometimes combined with measurement of micturation flow rate.

INTRAVENOUS UROGRAPHY

Intravenous urography involves the injection of organic iodine compounds which are excreted and concentrated radiographically. It is an extremely good technique for examining the renal collecting system, the ureters and the bladder but gives less information than ultrasound about the renal parenchyma (Fig. 9.10). Imaging by IVU depends on renal function. This is useful in that it gives a crude measure of the symmetry or otherwise of excretory capacity but it also means that the image quality is poor in patients with renal insufficiency in whom the GFR is low (Fig. 9.11).

ANTEGRADE AND RETROGRADE UROGRAPHY

Here X-ray contrast material is instilled directly into the urinary tract via a percutaneous needle (*antegrade*) or a ureteric catheter inserted via a cystoscope (*retrograde*). These tests are invasive and are most often used in the evaluation of patients with obstruction of the urinary tract.

CYSTOGRAPHY

In cystography the bladder is filled with contrast medium via a urethral catheter and X-rays are taken before, during and after micturition. The test indicates the completeness of bladder emptying and also whether or not urine refluxes up the ureters during micturition. This also is an invasive test, the principal risk being the introduction of infection. Pressure and flow measurements may be included in more detailed studies of bladder function—urodynamics.

RADIONUCLIIDE STUDIES

^{99}Tc-DTPA (diethylenetriamine penta-acetic acid) is used to investigate the excretory function of each kidney selectively (Fig. 9.12). The test is very useful for the assessment of symmetry of function, delayed onset of excretion (as may happen in renal artery stenosis) and retention of excreted isotope (as seen in the presence of obstruction). ^{99}Tc-DMSA (dimercaptosuccinic acid) is a similar technique used to show the gross renal morphology.

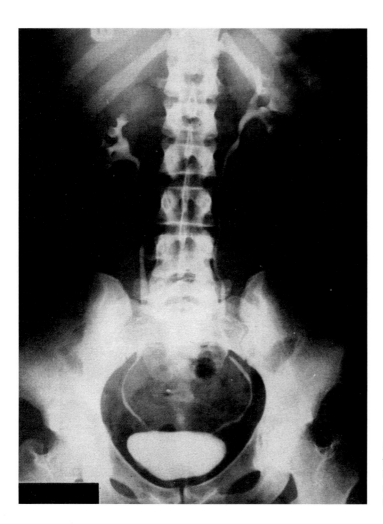

Fig. 9.10 Normal excretion urogram. In this film, taken 15 min after intravenous injection of the iodine-based contrast medium, the calyces of both kidneys, the ureters and the bladder can be seen.

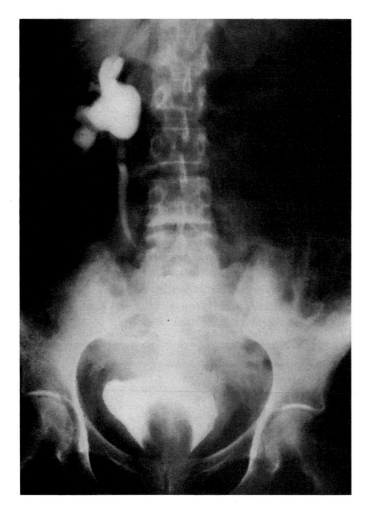

Fig. 9.11 Excretion urogram. In this film, made 30 min after injection of contrast, the left kidney fails to excrete a detectable concentration of contrast (non-functioning left kidney) and the right kidney shows dilated, hydronephrotic calyces. The right ureter is partially obstructed at the level of the body of the fifth, lumbar vertebra. The circular lucency in the bladder is the dilated balloon of a foley catheter.

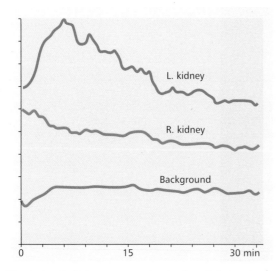

Fig. 9.12 Radioisotope excretion (ordinate) during the 30 min after intravenous injection in a patient with right renal artery stenosis and hypertension. The left kidney achieves more rapid excretion of isotope. The malfunctioning right kidney was the cause of the patient's hypertension.

COMPUTED TOMOGRAPHY AND MAGNETIC RESONANCE IMAGING

Computed tomography (CT) scanning of the kidneys sometimes complements the information gained from ultrasound and certainly yields important information about the surrounding structures in the retroperitoneum (Fig. 9.13). It is particularly useful in patients with ureteric obstruction from, for example, retroperitoneal malignancy or retroperitoneal fibrosis. In some cases, more information is obtained using magnetic resonance imaging (MRI).

ARTERIOGRAPHY AND VENOGRAPHY

These are both invasive and used in selected patients in whom detailed evaluation of the renal blood supply (arterial or venous) is required. The commonest indication is in the patient with hypertension and/or renal insufficiency in whom renal artery stenosis is suspected. *Magnetic resonance imaging* generates images of the major renal vasculature—magnetic resonance angiography (*MRA*). Although the images are generally not as good as those from conventional arteriography, the technique has the

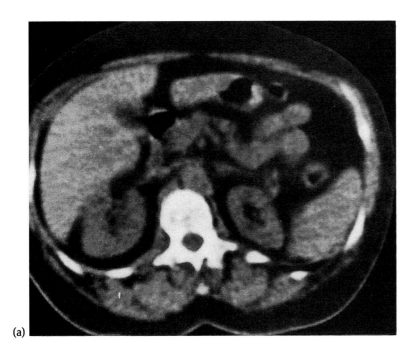

(a)

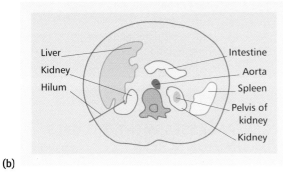

(b)

Fig. 9.13   (a) Computerized tomographic scan with (b) drawing showing normal kidneys.

advantage of being non invasive. CT imaging may also be used in this way (see p. 191).

CONCLUSIONS

From the forgoing it is evident that the detailed assessment of the patient with renal disease can be a complex and challenging process. In the vast majority of patients, however, the assessment is rel- atively straightforward, particularly if the major syndromes of renal and urological disease are kept in mind. In most cases the number of syndromes that have to be considered can be narrowed down quite quickly, and usually to one or two by the end of the physical examination. Armed with this information the doctor is then much better placed to devise an effective and efficient strategy for the laboratory investigation and imaging, and in turn make the correct diagnosis.

10
THE LOCOMOTOR SYSTEM

INTRODUCTION

Musculoskeletal symptoms are a major cause of pain and disability and patients with these disorders may account for a quarter of all general practitioner consultations. In later life, musculoskeletal diseases are the single most important factor influencing disability and so have a major impact on health and social service resources. The autoimmune connective tissue diseases, while being much less common, may still lead to significant morbidity and in some cases may be fatal if not diagnosed accurately.

The objectives of the clinician performing a musculoskeletal assessment are:

- to make a diagnosis
- to assess the impact and consequences of the condition
- to construct a clear management plan.

The clinical methods involved are largely those practised at the bedside—i.e. taking a careful, structured history and performing a thorough examination. Although musculoskeletal medicine is replete with complex imaging and immunological investigations, the majority of patients with locomotor disorders may be confidently diagnosed at the bedside using the fundamental techniques of history-taking and physical examination.

GENERAL ASSESSMENT: THE GALS LOCOMOTOR SCREEN (Figs 10.1–10.9)

Although musculoskeletal disorders are common both in general practice and in hospitals, many junior clinicians find the full detailed assessment of the locomotor system to be daunting and time-consuming. The GALS (gait, arms, legs and spine) screen has been widely adopted. It is brief and sensitive in detecting locomotor disorders that may lead to disability.

Screening history
The following three questions, if negative, make a significant musculoskeletal disorder unlikely:

- Do you have any pain or stiffness in your muscles, joints or back?
- Can you dress yourself completely without any difficulty?
- Can you walk up and down stairs without any difficulty?

Positive answers will need further assessment as detailed later in this chapter.

Screening examination
- Gait: Watch the patient walking and turning back towards you

- Spine: inspect the standing patient
  - from behind—look for abnormal spinal and paraspinal anatomy and look at the legs
  - from the side—look for abnormal spinal curves (Fig. 10.1) then ask the patient to 'bend forward and try and touch your toes'
  - from the front—ask the patient to 'try and put your ear on your left then right shoulder' and watch the neck movements (Fig. 10.2)
  - gently press the midpoint of each supraspinatus to elicit tenderness (Fig. 10.3)
- Arms: ask the patient to
  - 'put your hands behind your head, with your elbows back'; observe shoulder and elbow function (Fig. 10.4)
  - 'put your arms straight out in front of you'; observe elbow extension
  - 'put your hands and fingers out straight and turn them over'; observe pronation and supination and palmar and finger anatomy (Fig. 10.5)
  - 'make a fist with both hands' and observe power grip (Fig. 10.6)
  - gently squeeze the hand across the metacarpals to elicit tendeness (Fig. 10.7)
  - 'touch each fingertip with your thumb' and observe precision movements.

The clinician then looks for swelling and tenderness across the metacarpals by gently squeezing them (Fig. 10.6).

- Legs: with the patient still standing:
- Examine the lower limbs for swelling, deformities or limb shortening
- Then, with the patient lying on a couch
  - flex each hip and knee with a hand on the knee to feel for crepitus
  - passively rotate each hip internally and look for pain or limitation of movement (Fig. 10.8)
  - palpate each knee for warmth and swelling and press on the patella feeling for an effusion
  - squeeze gently across the metatarsals for tenderness (Fig. 10.9)
  - finally, inspect the soles of the feet for callosities, ulcers

This examination can be conducted in approximately 2 minutes, especially if the clinician performs the movements and asks the patient to follow them. The precise order of the examination is not crucial and clinicians usually develop their own pattern of examination with practice.

Recording the results

The findings of this locomotor screen can be documented with a simple method allowing the GALS screen to be performed and recorded routinely in the medical records. For example, a normal screen might noted as follows:

Screening questions: pain   0
                         dressing   ✓
                         walking   ✓

with positive answers being elaborated. Examination:

	A (Appearance)	M (Movement)
G	✓	
A	✓	✓
L	✓	✓
S	✓	✓

with abnormal findings indicated for example in rheumatoid arthritis:

	A (Appearance)	M (Movement)
G	X	
A	X	X
L	X	X
S	✓	✓

Slow painful gait
Synovitis of MCP, MTP, wrists and knee joints

The incorporation of this brief locomotor examination into the routine examination of patients is not a substitute for more detailed assessment as outlined below.

SPECIFIC LOCOMOTOR HISTORY

The full locomotor history should start with the presenting complaint and the patient should then be guided through the sequence of symptoms, associated features and events since onset. Certain characteristic points may emerge that may be diagnostic. For example, the pain from an osteoporotic vertebral fracture which is acute and self-limiting is very different from that of a spinal metastatic deposit where the pain is severe and constant with a 'gnawing' quality that keeps the patient awake and may be associated with weight loss. Similarly, the acute, severe, usually continuous throbbing pain of joint infection is easily distinguished from the mechanical pain due to osteoarthritis.

Do not forget that pain may be referred or radiate from an affected joint. There are a number of characteristic patterns of referred pain:

- Neck pain may radiate through the occiput to the vertex or to the shoulder and down the arm, with paraesthesiae if there is nerve root impingement
- Shoulder pain may radiate to the elbow and below
- Thoracic spine pain may radiate around the chest and mimic cardiac pain
- Lumbar spine pain may radiate through the buttock and leg to the knee and below with paraesthesiae in the foot with a large disc prolapse—this is called 'sciatica'
- Hip joint pain may radiate to the knee and below
- Knee pain may radiate above and below the joint.

With these patterns in mind it is prudent to examine the joints above and below the apparently affected area.

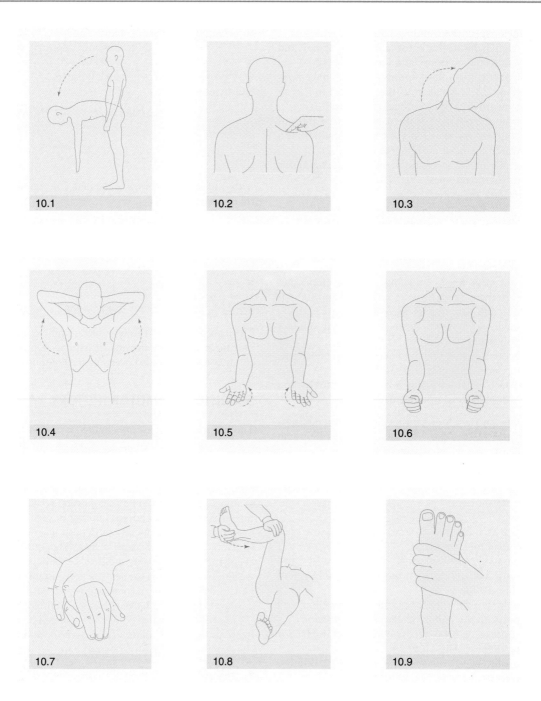

Fig. 10.1   Inspect patient from behind and side observing for normal spinal curves then ask the patient to 'bend forwards to try and touch your toes'.

Fig. 10.2   From the front, ask the patient to 'place your ear on your right then your left shoulder'.

Fig. 10.3   Gently press the mid-point of each supraspinatus to elicit the hyperalgesia of fibromyalgia.

Fig. 10.4   'Put your hands behind your head, elbows back'. Observe for pain or restricted movement.

Fig. 10.5   'Put your hands out palms down and then turn your hands over'.

Fig. 10.6   'Make a fist with both hands'.

Fig. 10.7   Look for swelling between the heads of the metacarpals and gently squeeze across the MCP joints to elicit tenderness.

Fig. 10.8   Gently flex the hips and knees feeling for crepitus at the knee during movement and look for pain and restriction of movement. Look for knee effusion.

Fig. 10.9   Squeeze across MTP joints and inspect the soles of the feet.

JOINT DISEASE

A combination of *pain* and *stiffness*, causing loss of function, is a classic feature of joint disease, but pain and swelling can occasionally occur through overuse of a normal joint. Usually one component predominates, as with stiffness in inflammation, and pain in mechanical joint problems. Therefore, specific questions will allow you to establish whether symptoms are *mechanical* (e.g. degenerative joint disease or meniscal tear) or *inflammatory* (e.g. rheumatoid arthritis or gout).

FEATURES OF MECHANICAL JOINT DISEASE

In degenerative joint disease there may be a feeling of stiffness in the affected joint after resting which disappears rapidly on activity. This *inactivity stiffness* typically lasts only a few minutes and is nearly always less than 30 minutes. Pain in the affected joint on activity, usually improving with rest, is typical. A clicking sensation in a joint, particularly in the knee, is a common complaint, but it is usually a normal phenomenon (compare with *crepitus*, p. 201). *Locking* of a joint may occur. In the knee, this means that the knee becomes locked in such a way that it will not fully extend, although it may flex. In other joints locking is less well defined and simply means that at some point through its range of motion the joint becomes stuck, usually associated with pain and often followed by swelling. Locking is due to material within the joint interfering with movement at the articular surfaces. In the knee, this is usually part of one of the menisci, or a cartilaginous loose body.

FEATURES OF INFLAMMATORY JOINT DISEASE

Early morning stiffness

Early morning joint stiffness that persists for more than 30 minutes is an important often diagnostic symptom of active inflammatory joint disease. Ask also about *redness* (rubor), *warmth* (calor), *tenderness/pain* (dolor) and *swelling* (tumor), described by Celsius as the classic features of inflammation.

Having recognized that the history suggests inflammation, and if only one joint is involved (monoarticular disease), always consider infection. Ask if there has been any fever or sweating, and if the joint is inflamed, remember that this may be due to infection and that the joint may need to be aspirated as part of the clinical examination.

Distribution of joint disease

The pattern of involvement of joints is important in diagnosis. Symmetry is useful in distinguishing various inflammatory arthropathies. There are only a few causes of an exactly symmetrical arthropathy (see Box 10.4). Other conditions have such a classic history that this is diagnostic. For example, acute inflammation in the 1st metatarsophalangeal joint (*hallux*), suggests a diagnosis of gout (Box 10.1). Another typical pattern is the pain and stiffness of the shoulder and hip girdles in polymyalgia rheumatica (Box 10.2).

Recurrent attacks of joint pain

Ask if the same joint is always involved. If not, define the patterns of involvement, the severity and duration of the episodes and any associated clinical symptoms.

Episodic joint pain

Ask if attacks of joint pain are associated with para-articular redness with the attacks lasting about 48 hours (occasionally up to 1 week) typical of *palindromic rheumatism*.

Flitting joint pains

This term is used to describe joint inflammation, beginning in one joint and then serially involving other joints, usually one at a time for about 3 days each. Gonococcal arthritis should be considered; it is characterized by typical fleeting skin lesions and urethritis, in addition to joint pain. In rheumatic fever there is associated cardiac involvement and erythema marginatum and subcutaneous nodules may occur.

The other features in the history which should be brought out are best considered under the differential diagnosis of polyarthritis (Boxes 10.3 and 10.4) as many arthropathies may have a monoarticular presentation.

BOX 10.1   Acute gout.

A 48-year-old publican presented with sudden severe pain and swelling of his left big toe. He was unable to weight bear or wear a shoe and said that he could not even bear the weight of his bedclothes on the toe at night. His past history included hypertension for which he was taking a thiazide diuretic and his alcohol intake was excessive. On examination he had tophi in the ears (Fig. 10.10) and the left 1st metatarsophalangeal joint was red, hot, swollen and exquisitely painful to touch. Aspiration of the joint revealed urate crystals.

BOX 10.2   Polymyalgia rheumatica.

A 74-year-old lady presented with a 2-month history of pain around her hips and shoulders. The key points in the history were that these regions were extremely stiff each morning for 4 hours and that there was no joint swelling. Clinically there was pain and some limitation of movements at the shoulders and hips but no synovitis. Her erythrocyte sedimentation rate was 96 mm/1st hour and she had a dramatic response within two days to a moderate dose of prednisolone.

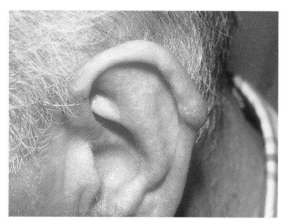

Fig. 10.10 Gouty tophus on the ear. Other sites include the elbows and fingers.

BOX 10.3 Historical pointers to the differential diagnosis of monoarticular inflammatory joint disease.

First attack
- Exclude infection by aspiration for culture and crystals
- If negative culture, but high risk group, *biopsy*, for example, tuberculosis in Asian immigrants or immunosuppressed patients

Recurrent attacks
- Flitting (gonococcal arthritis; rheumatic fever)
- Episodic (crystal arthritis; palindromic rheumatism)

Persistent synovitis with none of the above features
- Look for systemic features and check serology (e.g. latex fixation test)

BOX 10.4 Importance of distribution of joint involvement in differential diagnosis of oligo- or polyarthritis.

Typically symmetrical
- *Upper and lower limbs*
  —rheumatoid arthritis, SLE, polyarteritis nodosa
- *Especially upper limbs*
  —haemochromatosis (hand, index, middle MCP joints)

Typically asymmetrical
  —psoriatic arthritis

Typically lower limb and asymmetrical
  —spondyloarthritis (e.g. ankylosing spondylitis, Reiter's syndrome)

Define any associated features

INFLAMMATORY CONNECTIVE TISSUE DISEASES

The connective tissue diseases such as systemic lupus erythematosus (SLE), systemic sclerosis and the vas-

culitides are multisystem disorders and a careful systems enquiry (as described in Ch. 1) is needed to obtain a complete history. Important associated features of these conditions include systemic upset such as weight loss, malaise or fevers, rashes especially if they are photosensitive or vasculitic (Fig. 10.11), oral and genital ulceration, Raynaud's phenomenon (Ch. 4) and symptoms of neuropathic, cardiac, pulmonary and gastrointestinal involvement. Symptoms of dry eyes and dry mouth (sicca symptoms) are common in these conditions and may be documented with Schirmer's test (Fig. 10.12). Renal disease is an important complication of the connective tissue diseases, especially in SLE and the systemic vasculitides

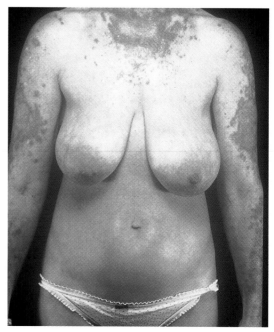

Fig. 10.11 Extensive rash in sun exposed areas in a woman with systemic lupus erythematosus and anti-Ro antibodies.

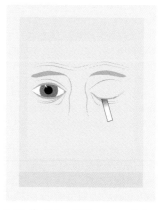

Fig. 10.12 A sterile strip of filter paper is hooked over the lower eyelid. Less than 5 mm of wetness after 5 minutes is abnormal and is associated with connective tissue disease.

and clinical assessment should always include dip-testing the urine for blood and protein and microscopy of the urine sediment if this is positive (Ch. 9) Ear, nose and throat disease with sinusitis, facial pain and deafness (Ch. 13) is common in vasculitides such as Wegener's granulomatosis and Churg–Strauss syndrome.

SOFT TISSUE SYMPTOMS

Soft tissue problems are common, usually consisting of pain, dull ache, tenderness or swelling. In the elderly such symptoms often appear spontaneously but in younger people there is usually a history of injury or overuse, either through occupation (e.g. tenosynovitis of the long flexor tendons of the hand,) or sport (e.g. Achilles tendonitis). It is important to define the exact site of the symptoms, factors that usually make them worse, and any factors inducing relief.

The localization of symptoms to specific soft tissue structures can be confirmed by careful anatomical examination (Box 10.5). The possible soft tissues involved are *joint*, *tendon*, *ligament*, *bursa* and *muscle*.

THE BONES

Bone pain is characteristically deep-seated and localized, but referred pain may confuse the clinical

---

BOX 10.5   Localization of the site of articular and extra-articular features.

Joint
- Diffuse pain and tenderness
- Generalized joint swelling
- Restriction of movement, usually in all directions of movement (specific to each joint)

Tendon
- Localized pain/tenderness at attachment (enthesis) or in the tendon substance
- Swelling, tendon sheath or paratenon
- Pain on resisted action
- Sometimes pain on stretch (e.g. Achilles)

Ligament
- Localized pain/tenderness at attachment or in ligament substance
- Pain on stretch
- Instability, if major tear

Bursa
- Localized tenderness
- Pain on stretching adjacent structures

Muscle
- Localized or diffuse pain and tenderness
- Pain on resisted action
- Pain on stretch (e.g. hamstring)

---

picture. In the case of fractures, unless pathological, there will almost always be a history of injury. In athletes, however, a fracture may be due to chronic overuse, as in stress fracture, for example, of the tibia in runners. The spontaneous onset of pain may suggest Paget's disease (with bony enlargement, e.g. skull or tibia) or metastatic deposits. Infection must also be considered, particularly in younger patients or in immunodeficiency states. Consider also congenital or familial disorders as predisposing factors, for example multiple osteochondromata or brittle bone disease (*osteogenesis imperfecta*).

EXAMINATION: GENERAL PRINCIPLES

Observe the patient entering the room (Box 10.6). Abnormalities of *gait* and *posture* may provide clues that can be pursued in history-taking. Observation of any difficulty in undressing and getting onto the examination couch will further help in assessment. The patient must always be asked to stand and walk, even when it is obvious that this may be difficult. Note how much help the patient requires from others or from sticks, crutches, etc. The locomotor system includes the muscles, bones, joints and soft tissue structures, such as tendons and ligaments. Remember that although muscle wasting may be due to primary muscle disease (e.g. polymyositis), it is more commonly secondary to disuse, perhaps because of a painful joint, or to nerve root compression or peripheral neuropathy (Fig. 10.13). Examination of the muscles is discussed further in Chapter 11.

THE BONES

The examination of the bones should always be directed by information obtained from the history.

Inspection

Look for any alterations in shape or outline and measure any shortening. In osteitis deformans (*Paget's*

BOX 10.6   Examination of the locomotor system.

General observations
- Gait
- Posture
- Mobility
- Deformity
- Independence
- Muscle wasting
- Long bones

Fractures
- Joints
- Tendons
- Skin

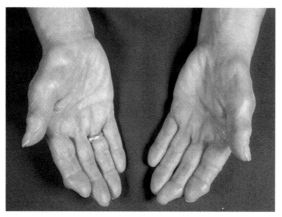

Fig. 10.13 Thenar wasting due to carpal tunnel syndrome. This is often associated with osteoarthritis—note nodal change on the terminal interphalangeal joints of the index fingers.

disease) bowing of the long bones, particularly the tibia (Fig. 10.14 (a) and (b)) and femur, is associated with bony enlargement and, usually, increased local temperature. The skull is commonly involved but this may not be apparent clinically until the disease is advanced. Early involvement of the skull bones can be detected on X-rays (Fig. 10.15 (a) and (b)). Alteration in the shape of bones also occurs in rickets due to epiphyseal enlargement. Deformity of the chest in rickets is due to osteochondral enlargement (*rickety rosary*).

Localized swellings of long bones may be caused by infections, cysts or tumours. Spontaneous fractures may occasionally be the presenting symptom in the diagnosis of secondary carcinoma, multiple myeloma, generalized osteitis fibrosa cystica (*hyperparathyroidism*), or osteogenesis imperfecta.

Palpation

On palpation bone tenderness occurs in local lesions when there is destruction, elevation or irritation of the periosteum, as in generalized osteitis fibrosa cystica, myelomatosis, bone infections, occasionally in carcinomatosis of bones and, rarely, in leukaemia. Injury is the commomest cause.

FRACTURES

Fractures are common and may involve any bone. They are painful, distressing for the patient and expensive for the community (Box 10.7). Fractures occurring in healthy bones commonly involve the long bones and are usually due to trauma. Fractures of the wrists, hips and vertebrae are more frequently complications of bone disease such as osteoporosis. Multiple rib fractures, due to falls, may be found in alcoholics, but may only be seen as healed lesions on chest X-ray. Fractures occur without apparent trauma when a bone is weakened by disease, especially with metastatic malignant deposits in bone (*pathological fractures*). Traumatic fractures invari-

(a)

(b)

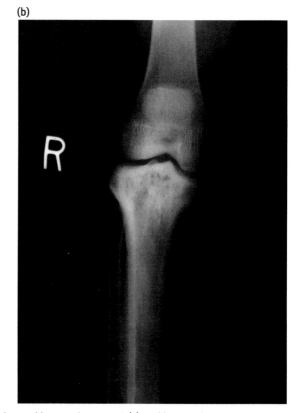

Fig. 10.14 Paget's disease of the right tibia. Note tibial bowing and bony enlargement **(a)** and bony enlargement sclerosis with some patchy porosis in the X-ray of the upper tibia **(b)**.

(a)

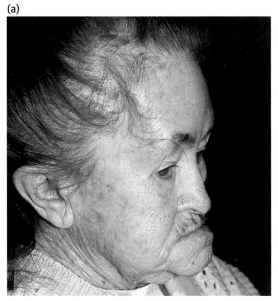

(b)

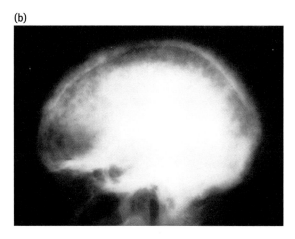

Fig. 10.15 Paget's disease, causing deformity of the skull **(a)**. Note the thickened skull vault with remodelled bone **(b)**.

BOX 10.7   Fractures: clinical features.

Type
- Closed
- Compound (open)

Complications
- Accompanying soft tissue injury (indirect)

Features
- Haemorrhage
- Deformity
- Pain
- Crepitus
- Restricted movement

Cause
- Traumatic
- Spontaneous (pathological)

---

ably present with local pain, swelling and loss of function, but pathological fractures may be relatively silent. The history will reveal the appropriate trauma, whether accidental or due to physical abuse.

Examination of suspected fracture

On examination, it is essential to establish whether the fracture is open (*compound*), or closed. In *closed fractures* the surrounding soft tissues are intact. In *open fractures* the bone communicates with the surface of the skin, either because the primary injury has broken the overlying skin or because deformation at the fracture site has caused the bone ends to penetrate the skin. There is a major risk of infection when the fracture site communicates with the open air.

Deformity is an obvious feature in the majority of fractures. It may be clinically characteristic, as in

Colles' fracture, in which there is a fracture of the distal end of the radius characterized by dorsal displacement and angulation, shortening of the wrist and rotation of the fragment, well-summarized in the description 'dinner fork deformity'. Certain fractures may show little deformity; for example, a fracture of the femoral shaft may be accompanied by only slight deformity, since there is often little separation of the bones at the fracture site and other features are disguised by the thick overlying muscle. A fracture of the neck of the femur causes deformity through external rotation of the foot and shortening of the leg.

Most fractures are characterized by local tenderness and swelling, unless the overlying muscle mass is large. Bony crepitus, due to abnormal motion at the fracture site, is a feature of fractures, but this should not be elicited unless absolutely necessary for diagnosis since it is very painful. However, if it is perceived or has been recognized by the patient it is diagnostic.

A fracture of the bone may damage the neighbouring soft tissues directly or, alternatively, a fracture may be a marker of severe injury in which direct damage to the soft tissues, such as the nerves and vessels, may have taken place. It is therefore essential to evaluate the nerve and blood supply to a limb distal to the site of the fracture. Impairment of blood supply distal to a fracture is a surgical emergency.

The presence or absence of *pulses* and *cutaneous sensation* and the colour and perfusion of the limb must always be recorded and any changes over time reported. Voluntary movement at joints distal to a fractured long bone, such as ankle movement in a fractured femur, should be noted. If this is absent, nerve injury must be suspected.

THE JOINTS

Examination of the joints can be summarized simply as 'look, feel and move' the joint (i.e. *inspection*, *palpation*, and then the *range of movement*). With practice the clinician can develop a systematic review of the joints—for example the jaw, cervical spine, shoulder girdle and upper limb, thoracic and lumbar spine, pelvis and lower limb—so that inconspicuous but important joints, such as the temporomandibular, sternoclavicular and sacroiliac, will not be overlooked. Compare the corresponding joints on the two sides of the body and always take care to avoid causing undue discomfort.

Inspection

The detection of joint inflammation is a crucial clinical skill. Inflammation is often associated with *redness* of the joint, and with *tenderness* and *warmth*. Look also for swelling or deformity of the joint. The *overall pattern* or joint involvement should be recorded. Note whether the distribution is symmetrical, as is usual in rheumatoid arthritis (Fig. 10.16), or asymmetrical, as in psoriatic arthropathy or gout (Fig. 10.17). The seronegative (non-rheumatoid) spondyloarthropathies (e.g. Reiter's disease, Fig. 10.18) tend predominantly to involve the joints of the lower limb.

Palpation

On palpation of a joint swelling, check first for tenderness. Then determine whether the swelling is due to bony enlargement or to osteophytes (e.g. *Heberden's nodes*, Fig. 10.19), to thickening of synovial tissues such as occurs in inflammatory arthritis, or to effusion into the joint space. Joint effusions usually have a characteristically smooth outline and fluctuation is usually easily demonstrable. Tenderness and enlargement of the ends of the bones, particularly the radius and ulna, can occur in hypertrophic pulmonary osteoarthropathy; a chest X-ray is essential. Gross disorganization of a joint, nearly always foot

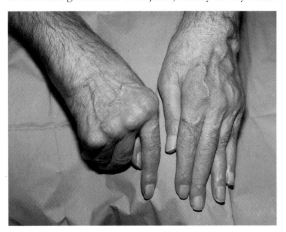

Fig. 10.16 Symmetrical joint involvement due to rheumatoid arthritis.

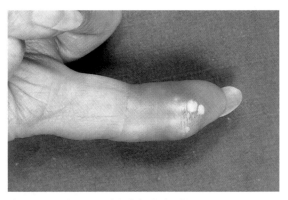

Fig. 10.17 Gouty tophi of the index finger.

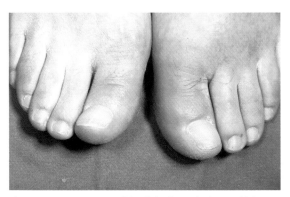

Fig. 10.18 Acute synovitis of the interphalangeal joint, due to Reiter's syndrome of the left hallux. Differential diagnosis includes gout.

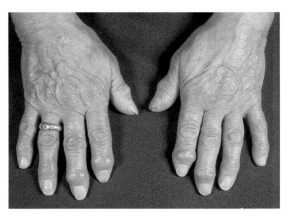

Fig. 10.19 Nodal osteoarthritis (Heberden's nodes).

and ankle joints, associated with absence of deep pain and position sense, occurs in neuropathic (*Charcot's*) joints. Charcot's joints probably arise from recurrent painless injury and overstretching of joints, and are a feature of severe chronic peripheral neuropathy, or, rarely, tabes dorsalis.

Joint tenderness may be graded depending on the patient's reaction to firm pressure of the joint between finger and thumb (Box 10.8). Grade 4 tenderness occurs only in septic arthritis, crystal arthritis and rheumatic fever. In gout, the skin overlying the affected joint is dry, whereas in septic arthritis or rheumatic fever it is usually moist.

If tenderness is present, localize it as accurately as possible and determine whether it arises in the joint or in neighbouring structures, for example in the supraspinatus or bicipital tendon rather than the shoulder joint. Other rheumatic conditions give different types of pain. For example in conditions such as complex regional pain syndrome type I (previously known as reflex sympathetic dystrophy), hyperalgesia (abnormal pain on mild pressure that is not usually painful), allodynia (abnormal sensation of pain on very light touch) and hyperpathia (a prolonged sensation of pain after repeated gentle taps on the skin) may often be seen together with altered sweating and discolouration. In fibromyalgia, there is widespread diffuse muscle and joint tenderness but no inflammation. A number of characterisitic trigger points may be tender around the neck, trunk, upper and lower limbs.

TENDON SHEATH CREPITUS

This is a grating or creaking sensation defined by palpating the tendon while the patient is asked to contract the muscle tendon complex involved. It is particularly common in the hand and is seen in rheumatoid arthritis and systemic sclerosis. In tenosynovitis of the long flexor tendons in the palm, tendon sheath crepitus may be associated with the trigger phenomenon, when the finger becomes caught in flexion and has to be pulled back into extension. Tendon sheath *effusions* can be distinguished from joint swelling by their anatomical location in association with tendons.

JOINT CREPITUS

This can be detected by feeling the joint with one hand while it is moved passively with the other. This may indicate osteoarthritis, or loose bodies (cartilaginous fragments) in the joint space, but should be differentiated from non-specific clicking of joints.

RANGE OF MOVEMENT

In examining joints for range of movement it is usually sufficient to estimate the degree of limitation based on comparison with the normal side, or on the examiner's previous experience. For accurate description the actual range of movement should be measured with a protractor (*goniometer*). Both *active* and

passive movement should be assessed. Active movement, however, may give a poor estimation of true range of movement because of muscle spasm due to pain. If pain is very severe on attempted active movement, and other findings suggest fracture, neither active nor passive movement should be attempted before X-ray examination. In testing the range of passive movement gentleness must be exercised, particularly in the case of painful joints.

Limitation of movement in a joint may be due to pain, muscle spasm, contracture, inflammation, increased thickness of the capsular or periarticular structures, effusion into the joint space, bony overgrowths, bony ankylosis, mechanical factors such as a torn meniscus, or to painful conditions quite unconnected with the joint.

EXTRA-ARTICULAR FEATURES OF JOINT DISEASE

Some of the extra-articular features of joint disease are listed in Box 10.9.

SUBCUTANEOUS NODULES

Subcutaneous nodules are associated with various conditions (Box 10.10). If gout is suspected, palpate the helix of the ear for tophi due to subcutaneous deposition of urate, which may also be found overlying joints or in the finger pulps (see Figs 10.10 and 10.17). Subcutaneous nodules in rheumatoid arthritis are firm and non-tender; they may be detected by running the examining thumb from the point of the elbow down the proximal portion of the ulna (Fig. 10.20). They can also be found at other pressure and frictional sites, such as bony prominences, including the sacrum. If an olecranon bursa swelling is found, feel also in its wall, as rheumatoid nodules, tophi or occasionally xanthomata may be found within the swelling. Subcutaneous nodules are not specific to rheumatoid arthritis, and may occur in patients with SLE, systemic sclerosis and in rheumatic fever.

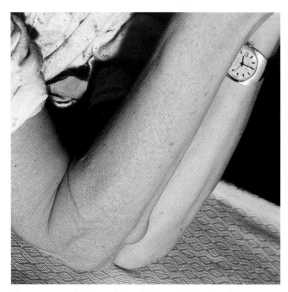

Fig. 10.20   Rheumatoid nodule overlying the olecranon of the right arm.

CUTANEOUS VASCULITIC LESIONS

These may be seen in rheumatoid arthritis, SLE and the systemic vasculitides including polyarteritis nodosa. Small vessel involvement is typically seen at the nail fold (cutaneous infarct, Fig. 10.21) but also occurs at pressure sites. Splinter haemorrhages, the classic feature of bacterial endocarditis (p. 84) may also be a feature of vasculitis.

LYMPHADENOPATHY

Lymphadenopathy may be found proximal to an inflamed joint, not only in septic arthritis but also in rheumatoid arthritis. Generalized lymphadenopathy, sometimes with splenomegaly, is a common feature of active SLE.

LOCAL OEDEMA

Local oedema is sometimes seen over inflamed joints (Fig. 10.22) but other causes of oedema must be excluded.

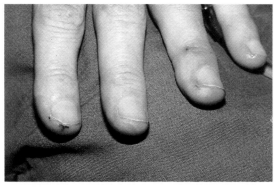

Fig. 10.21   Nail fold vasculitis in rheumatoid arthritis. This also occurs in SLE and polyarteritis nodosa.

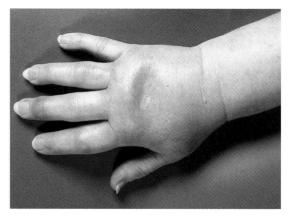

Fig. 10.22   Pitting oedema, right hand.

OTHER SOFT TISSUE SWELLINGS

Tendon sheath effusions are distinguished from joint swellings by their location in association with tendons. Enlarged subcutaneous bursae may be found over pressure areas, particularly at the olecranon surface of the elbow, due to inflammatory joint disease or secondary to friction. Deeper bursae may be defined only by finding local tenderness or by stressing adjacent tissues (e.g. greater trochanter bursitis).

EXAMINATION OF INDIVIDUAL JOINTS

The range of movement of joints is described in the scheme shown in the following pages. All motion should be measured in degrees from a neutral or zero position, which must be defined whenever possible. Some special features seen at individual joints are set out in each section.

THE SPINE

GENERAL EXAMINATION OF THE VERTEBRAL COLUMN

Inspection

Examine the patient standing and sitting in the erect posture. The normal shape of the thoracolumbar spine is an S-shaped curve. If there is an abnormality, note which vertebrae are involved and at what level any vertebral projection is most prominent. Note the presence of any local projections or angular deformity of the spine.

Palpation

The major landmarks are the spinous processes of C7 (the vertebra prominens) and the last rib, which articulates with the 12th thoracic vertebra. In many patients, however, the last rib cannot be distinctly felt and this is therefore rather untrustworthy as a guide to this level.

The neutral position of the spine is a normal upright stance with head erect and chin drawn in. Note any curvature of the spinal column, whether as a whole or of part of it. The curvature may be in an anterior, posterior or lateral direction (Fig. 10.23). Anterior curvature is termed *lordosis*. There are natural lordotic curves in the cervical and lumbar regions. Posterior curvature is termed *kyphosis*. The thoracic spine usually exhibits a slight smooth kyphosis, which increases in the elderly and especially in osteoporosis.

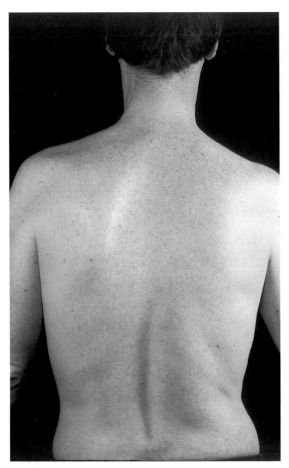

Fig. 10.23   Scoliosis of the lumbar spine, due to prolapsed intervertebral disc.

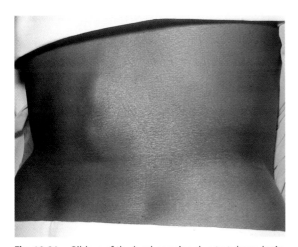

Fig. 10.24   Gibbus of the lumbar spine due to tuberculosis.

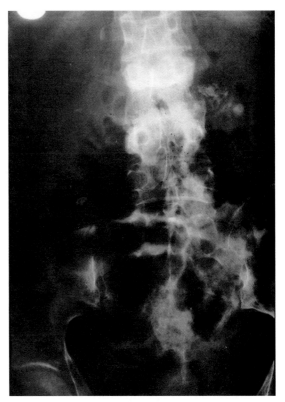

Fig. 10.25   X-ray tuberculous discitis. This shows the underlying deformity shown in Figure 10.24. There is tuberculous infection of the intervertebral disc, causing the spinal deformity.

It must be distinguished from a localized angular deformity (*gibbus*, Fig. 10.24) caused by a fracture, by Pott's disease (spinal tuberculosis, Fig. 10.25), or by a metastatic malignant deposit.

Lateral curvature is termed *scoliosis* (Fig. 10.23) and may be towards either side. It is always accompanied by rotation of the bodies of the vertebrae in such a way that the posterior spinous processes come to point towards the concavity of the curve. The curvature is always greater than appears from inspection of the posterior spinous processes. In scoliosis due to muscle spasm (e.g. with lumbosacral disc protrusion syndromes), the spinal curvature and rotational deformity decrease in flexion. When scoliosis is caused by inequality of leg length it disappears on sitting because the buttocks then become level. Scoliosis secondary to skeletal anomalies shows in spinal flexion as a 'rib hump' due to the rotation. Kyphosis and scoliosis are often combined, particularly when the cause is an idiopathic spinal curvature, beginning in adolescence.

THE CERVICAL SPINE
The following movements should be tested (Fig. 10.26):

- Rotation (ask the patient to look over one, then the other shoulder)
- Flexion (ask the patient to touch chin to chest)

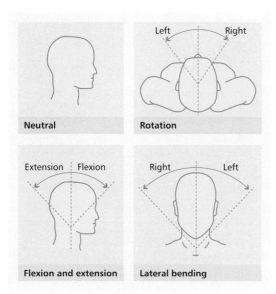

Fig. 10.26   Movements of the neck.

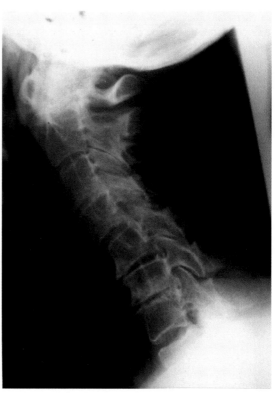

Fig. 10.27   Lateral X-ray of cervical spine showing degenerative spondylosis with narrowing of the disc spaces and reversed cervical lordosis between C4 and C6.

- Extension (ask the patient to look up to the ceiling)
- Lateral bending (ask the patient to bend the neck sideways and to try to touch the shoulder with the ear without raising the shoulder).

Note any pain or paraesthesiae in the arm reproduced by neck movement, especially on gentle sustained extension or lateral flexion, suggesting nerve root involvement. If indicated, check for any associated neurological deficit, particularly of radicular or spinal cord type.

In rheumatoid arthritis particular care is necessary in examining the neck as atlantoaxial instability may lead to damage to the spinal cord when the neck is flexed or extended. If there is any doubt about neck stability in a patient with rheumatoid arthritis arrange for lateral X-rays of the cervical spine in flexion and extension, together with a view of the odontoid peg through the mouth, and defer clinical examination.

In patients with cervical injury never try to elicit range of motion of the neck. Instead, splint the neck, take a history, look for abnormality of posture, usually in rotation, and check neurological function in the limbs including both arms and both legs. Take X-rays of the neck in the lateral (Fig. 10.27) and anteroposterior planes, *without* moving the neck. Only if the X-rays are normal should neck movements be examined.

THE THORACIC AND LUMBAR SPINE

The main movement at the thoracic spine is rotation, while the lumbar spine can flex, extend, and bend laterally. The following movements should be tested (Fig. 10.28):

- Flexion (ask the patient to try to touch their toes, without bending at the knees)

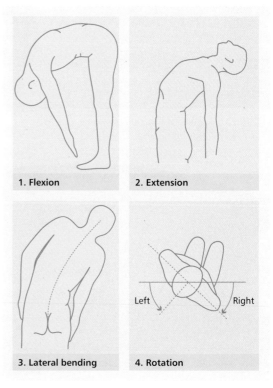

Fig. 10.28   Movements of the lumbar and dorsal spine.

- Extension (ask the patient to bend backwards)
- Lateral bending (ask the patient to run the hand down the side of the thigh as far as possible
- Thoracic rotation (ask the seated patient, with arms crossed, to twist round to the left and right as far as possible).

The normal lumbar lordosis should be abolished in flexion. The extent of lumbar flexion can be assessed more accurately by marking a vertical, 10-cm line on the skin overlying the lumbar spinous processes and the sacral dimples and measuring the increase in the line length on flexion (*modified Shober test*): this should normally be 5 cm or more. Painful restriction of spinal movement is an important sign of cervical and lumbar spondylosis, but may also be found in vertebral disc disease or other mechanical disorders of the back or neck. A useful clinical aphorism is that a rigid lumbar spine should *always* be investigated for serious pathology such as infection (e.g. staphylococcal or tuberculous discitis), malignancy or inflammation (e.g. ankylosing spondylitis). Spinal movements may be virtually absent in ankylosing spondylitis (Fig. 10.29) but, in the early stages of this condition, lateral flexion of the lumbar spine is typically affected first. In mechanical or osteoarthritic back problems flexion and extension are reduced more than lateral

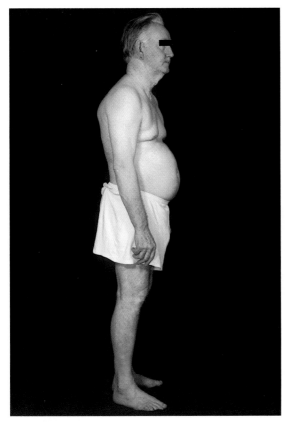

Fig. 10.29 Ankylosing spondylitis. Note dorsal kyphosis and protuberant abdomen due to poor chest expansion with abdominal breathing.

movements. In prolapsed intervertebral disc lesions, sustained gentle lumbar extension may reproduce the low back pain and sciatic radiation.

Chest expansion is a measure of costovertebral movement and should be recorded using a tape measure with the patient's hands behind the head to reduce the possibility of muscular action in the shoulder girdle giving a false reading. Reduced chest expansion is a characteristic early feature in ankylosing spondylitis. Obviously, this may also be a feature of primary pulmonary disease, such as emphysema (Ch. 5).

Examination of the back is completed by assessing straight leg raising and strength, sensation and reflex activity in the legs. Pain and limitation of *straight leg raising* (SLR) is a feature of prolapsed intervertebral disc when there is irritation or compression of one of the roots of the sciatic nerve. However, tight hamstring muscles may cause a similar picture but, if there is severe pain, it is more considerate to lower the leg to just below the limit of SLR and then to see if gentle passive dorsiflexion of the foot brings back the same pain. If in doubt, dorsiflex the foot once the limit of SLR has been reached. This further stretches the sciatic nerve (the pain increases) but does not affect the hamstrings (*Lasègue's sign*). The femoral stretch test is a useful confirmatory test and is performed with the patient lying prone: flexion at the knee will produce pain in the lower lumbar spine in a prolapsed disc at that level. Sacral sensory loss must always be carefully assessed since, if there is a central lumbosacral disc protrusion, bilateral limitation of straight leg raising may be associated with bladder dysfunction and sacral anaesthesia. This combination implies the need for immediate investigation and treatment.

THE SACROILIAC JOINTS

The surface markings of these joints are two dimples low in the lumbar region. Test for *irritability* in four ways:

- Direct pressure over each sacroiliac joint
- Firm pressure with the side of the hand over the sacrum
- Inward pressure over both iliac bones in an attempt to distort the pelvis
- Flex the hip to 90 degrees and exert firm pressure at the knee through the femoral shaft (this should only be done if the knee is not painful).

In the last three tests above, a positive test is only indicated by the patient localizing discomfort to the sacroiliac joint.

THE SHOULDER

The neutral position is with the arm to the side, elbow flexed to 90 degrees with forearm pointing forwards.

Because the scapula is mobile, true shoulder (*gleno-humeral*) movement can be assessed only when the examiner anchors the scapula between finger and thumb on the posterior chest wall. The following movements should be tested (Fig. 10.30(a) and (b)):

- Flexion
- Extension
- Abduction
- Rotation in abduction
- Rotation in neutral position
- Elevation (also involving scapular movement).

In practice *internal rotation* can best be compared by recording the height reached by each thumb up the back, representing combined glenohumeral and scapular movement. Similarly, *external rotation* can be assessed by the ability to get the hand to the back of the neck. Limitation of external rotation is a good sign of true glenohumeral disease.

Note any pain during the range of movement. In *supraspinatus tendinitis* a full passive range of move-ment is found, but there is a painful arc on abduc-tion, with pain exacerbated on resisted abduction (Fig. 10.30b). *Other tendon involvement* should also be defined by pain on resisted action.

Subacromial impingement due to a bursitis or rotator cuff abnormality may produce severe pain at the end of abduction, blocking full elevation. Acute bursitis, however, may be so painful that no abduction is allowed (grade 4 discomfort).

Acromioclavicular joint pain is always very localized and is typically felt in the last 10 degrees of elevation (170–180 degree arc).

THE ELBOW

The neutral position is with the forearm in exten-sion. The following movements should be tested (Fig. 10.31):

- Flexion
- Hyperextension.

(a)

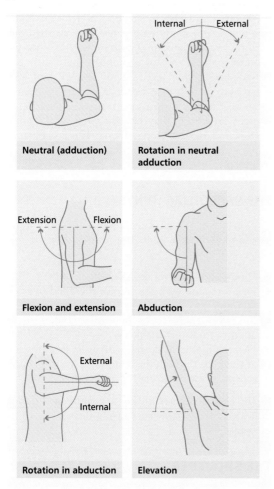

(b)

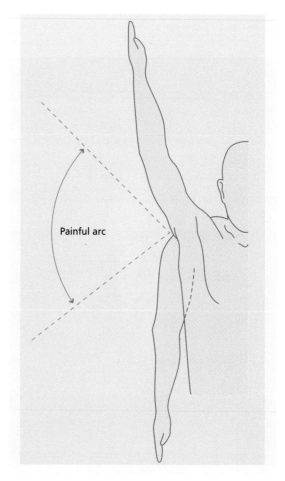

Fig. 10.30 Movements of the shoulder.

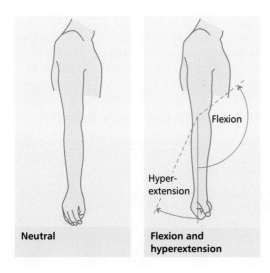

Fig. 10.31 Movements of the elbow.

Medial (golfer's elbow) and lateral (tennis elbow) epicondylitis are the most common causes of elbow pain. They are characterized by pain on active use but, if severe, may be associated with night pain.

Examination must define localized epicondylar tenderness with pain on resisted movement. Wrist extension exacerbates lateral epicondylar tenderness and wrist flexion exacerbates medial epicondylar tenderness. An elbow effusion may be palpated in the posterior triangle formed by the epicondyles and the olecranon.

THE FOREARM

The neutral position is with the arm by the side, elbow flexed to 90 degrees, and thumb uppermost. The following movements should be tested (Fig. 10.32):

- Supination
- Pronation.

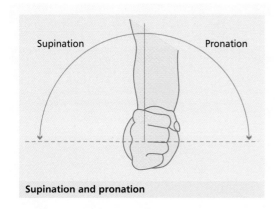

Fig. 10.32 Movements of the forearm.

THE WRIST

The neutral position is with the hand in line with the forearm, and palm down. The following movements should be tested (Fig. 10.33):

- Dorsiflexion (extension)
- Palmar flexion
- Ulnar deviation
- Radial deviation.

Even minor limitation of wrist flexion or extension can be detected by comparing movement of both wrists (Fig. 10.34). Arthritis of the wrist joints is usually due to inflammatory arthritis. Primary osteoarthritis of the wrist is rare, but secondary degenerative change is common.

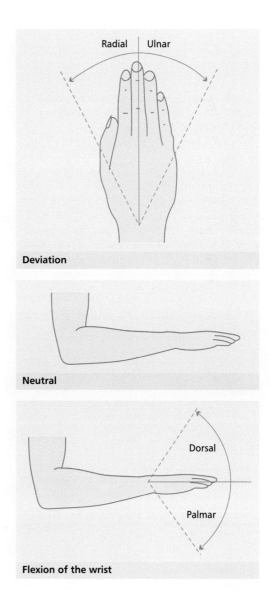

Fig. 10.33 Movements of the wrist.

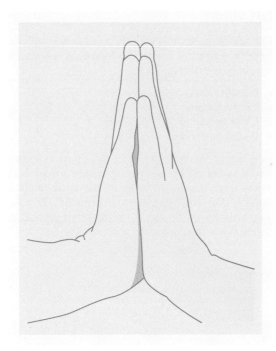

Fig. 10.34 Minor limitation of left wrist extension compared with the right. Note the slightly different angulation of the left forearm.

THE FINGERS

When identifying fingers, use the names *thumb, index, middle, ring* and *little*. Numbering tends to lead to confusion. Digit I is the thumb and digit V is the little finger. The neutral position is with the fingers in extension. Test flexion at the metacarpophalangeal (MCP), proximal interphalangeal (PIP) and distal interphalangeal (DIP) joints (Fig. 10.35).

In fractures of the fingers the commonest deformity is rotational. If the finger will flex make sure it points to the scaphoid tubercle (all the fingers will point individually in this direction). If it will not flex, look end-on at the nail and make sure it is parallel with its fellows.

THE THUMB (carpometacarpal joint)

The neutral position is with the thumb alongside the forefinger, and extended. The following movements should be tested (Fig. 10.36):

● Extension
● Flexion (measured as for the fingers)
● Opposition
● Abduction (not illustrated; movement at right angles to plane of palm).

THE HAND

DEFORMITIES IN JOINT DISEASE

Examination of the individual joints of the hand may be less informative than inspection of the hand as a whole (Fig. 10.37). The combination of Heberden's nodes and thumb carpometacarpal arthritis occurs in osteoarthritis (Fig. 10.19). A variety of patterns of deformity are characteristic of long-standing rheumatoid arthritis—for example metacarpophalangeal joint subluxation, ulnar devia-

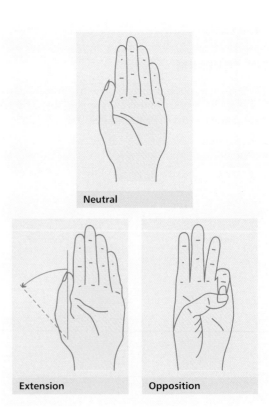

Fig. 10.36 Movements of the thumb.

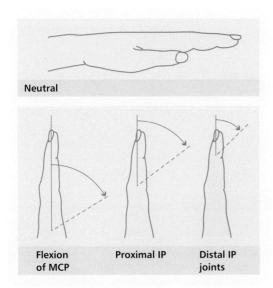

Fig. 10.35 Movements of the fingers.

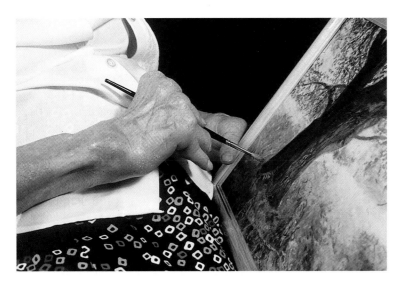

Fig. 10.37 Functional ability. Severe joint deformity due to psoriatic arthropathy, but retention of artistic ability.

tion of the fingers at the metacarpophalangeal joints, 'swan neck' deformities of the fingers (Fig. 10.38), and 'boutonnière' deformities (flexed proximal and hyperextended distal interphalangeal joints). This is due to the head of the phalanx sliding dorsally between the lateral slips of the extensor tendon, the middle slip having been damaged. In psoriatic arthritis, terminal interphalangeal joint swelling may occur with psoriatic pitting and ridging of the nail (onychopathy) on that digit.

DEFORMITIES DUE TO NEUROPATHY

The hand may adopt a posture typical of a nerve lesion (see Ch. 11). Slight hyperextension of the medial metacarpophalangeal joints with slight flexion of the interphalangeal joints is the 'ulnar claw hand' of an ulnar nerve lesion. There is wasting of the small muscles of the hypothenar eminence, with loss of sensation of the palmar and dorsal aspects of the little finger and of the ulnar half of the ring finger. In a median nerve lesion the thenar eminence (abduc-

tor pollicis brevis) will be flattened (Fig. 11.23) and sensory impairment will be found on the palmar surfaces of the thumb, index, middle and radial half of the ring fingers. Remember that carpal tunnel syndrome may be a presenting feature of wrist inflammation.

ASSESSMENT OF HAND FUNCTION

Assessment of hand function (Fig. 10.36) should include testing hand grip and pinch grip (between index and thumb). The latter may be decreased in lesions in the line of action of the thumb metacarpal, particularly scaphoid fractures.

THE HIP

The neutral position is with the hip in extension, and the patella pointing forwards. Ensure the pelvis does not tilt by placing one hand over the pelvis, while examining the hip with the other. Look for scars and wasting of the gluteal and the thigh muscles. The hip joint is too deeply placed to be accessible to palpation. The following movements should be tested (Fig. 10.39):

- Flexion: measured with knee bent. Opposite thigh must remain in neutral position. Flex the knee as the hip flexes
- Abduction: measured from a line which forms an angle of 90 degrees with a line joining the anterior superior iliac spines
- Adduction (measured in the same manner)
- Rotation in flexion
- Rotation in extension
- Extension: attempt to extend the hip with the patient lying in the lateral position.

ADDITIONAL EXAMINATION OF THE HIP JOINT

- Test for *flexion deformity*. With one hand flat between the lumbar spine and the couch, flex the normal hip fully to the point of abolishing the

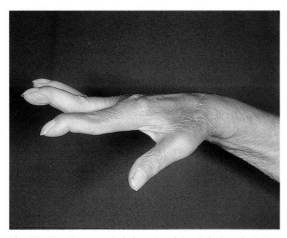

Fig. 10.38 Swan neck deformity of the right hand. Note also wasting of the small muscles of the hand due to disuse in this patient with rheumatoid arthritis.

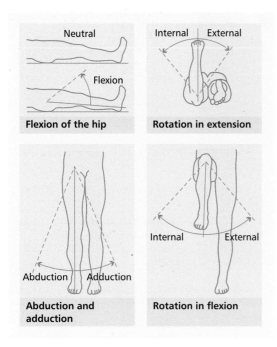

Fig. 10.39   Movements of the hip.

lumbar lordosis. The spine will come down onto the hand, pressing it on to the couch. If there is a flexion deformity on the opposite side, the leg on that side will move into a flexed position (Thomas's test).

- *Trendelenburg test.* Observe the patient from behind and ask him or her to stand on one leg. In health, the pelvis tilts upwards on the side with the leg raised. When the weight-bearing hip is abnormal, from pain or subluxation, the pelvis sags downwards due to weakness of the hip abductors on the affected side.

- *Measurement of 'true' and 'apparent' shortening.* The length of the legs is measured from the anterior superior iliac spine to the medial malleolus on the same side. Any difference is termed '*true*' shortening and may result either from disease of the hip joint or neck of the femur on the shorter side. '*Apparent*' shortening is due to tilting of the pelvis and can be measured by comparing the lengths of the two legs, measured from the umbilicus, provided that there is no true shortening of one leg. Apparent shortening is usually due to an abduction deformity of the hip.

THE KNEE

A magnetic resonance image (MRI) scan of the normal knee is illustrated in Figure 10.40. The neutral position is complete extension. Observe any valgus (lateral angulation of the tibia) or varus (medial angulation) deformity on the couch and on standing. Look for muscle wasting. The quadriceps, especially its medial part near the knee, rapidly

wastes in knee joint disease. Swelling may be obvious, particularly if it distends the suprapatellar pouch. Check the apparent height of the patella and watch to see if it deviates to one side in flexion or extension of the knee. Feel for tenderness at the joint margins, not forgetting the patellofemoral joint. Palpate the ligaments, remembering that the medial collateral ligament is attached 8 cm below the joint line. Measure the girth of the thigh muscles 10 cm above the upper pole of the patella.

JOINT SWELLING

The presence of swelling in the knee joint may be confirmed by the patellar tap test or, for small effusions, by the bulge test in which the medial parapatellar fossa is emptied by pressure of the flat of the hand sweeping proximally. It is seen to refill (the bulge) as the suprapatellar area is emptied by pressure from the flat hand. Posterior knee joint (Baker's) cysts, particularly in rheumatoid arthritis, may be palpable in the popliteal fossa. They sometimes rupture, producing calf pain and may then mimic a deep vein thrombosis. When intact, posterior knee cysts can sometimes cause venous obstruction.

The movements of the knee are flexion and extension (Fig. 10.41). Loss of flexion can be documented by loss of the angle of flexion or loss of heel-to-buttock distance in the crouch position, or on the couch. Loss of extension is detected by inability to get the back of the knee onto the flat examining couch. Hyperextension must be sought by lifting the foot with the knee extended and comparing with the normal side. Lack of full extension by comparison with the normal constitutes fixed flexion deformity. Loose bodies in the joint cause crepitus, interruption of movement (locking) and pain and effusion (Fig. 10.42).

TESTING FOR STABILITY

Test the stability of the joint by stressing the medial and lateral ligaments, first with the knee in full extension (abnormal motion is due to lax posterior structures), and then in 20 degrees of flexion. Abnormal motion in flexion is due to laxity of the collateral ligaments. With the knee flexed and the foot fixed on the couch by seating your buttock lightly against the patient's toes, check that the hamstrings are relaxed and then try to pull the tibia forward towards you. Abnormal anterior translation implies damage to the anterior cruciate ligament, provided it can be shown that the tibia has not already fallen backwards due to a torn posterior cruciate ligament. Look across both knees similarly flexed to exclude this.

THE ANKLE

The neutral position is with the outer border of the foot at an angle of 90 degrees with the leg, and

(a)

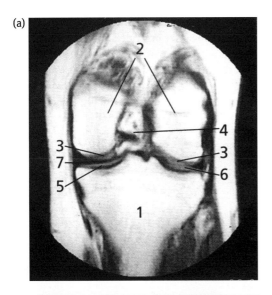

(b)

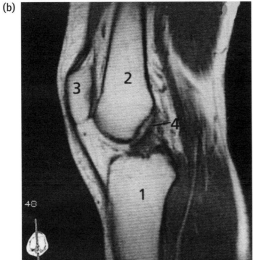

(c)

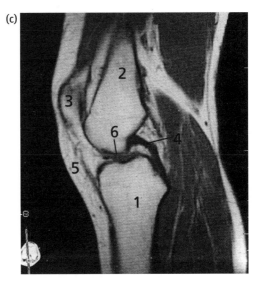

Fig. 10.40   MRI scans of the normal knee (MR image, T$_1$ weighted). **(a)** Scan to show the medial (5) and lateral (6) menisci, origin of the anterior cruciate ligament (4) and the articular cartilages (3) and synovial fluid (7). Other structures: (1) tibia, (2) articular surfaces of femur. **(b)** The anterior cruciate ligament (4). Other structures: (1) tibia, (2) femur, (3) patella. **(c)** The posterior cruciate ligament (4). Other structures: (1) tibia, (2) femur, (3) patella, (5) patellar tendon, (6) joint space.

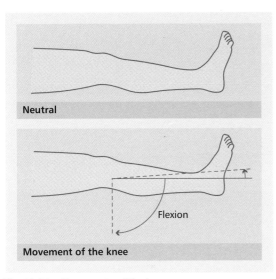

Fig. 10.41   Movements of the knee.

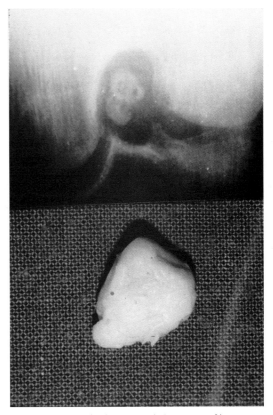

Fig. 10.42   Loose body in tunnel view X-ray of knee, showing the loose body in the intercondylar space.

midway between inversion and eversion. Observe the patient from behind in the standing position. There will be a loss of calf muscle bulk with any long-standing ankle disorder.

Look at the position of the foot with the patient standing. The heel may tilt outwards (*valgus deformity*) in subtalar joint damage. Inward (*varus deformity*) is much less common and usually not so painful. Flattening of the longitudinal arch of the foot also produces valgus at the heel but the foot curves laterally as well because the change is in the midtarsal joints in addition to the subtalar joint.

The following movements should be tested (Fig. 10.43).

- Dorsiflexion: test with the knee in flexion and extension to exclude tight calf muscles
- Plantar flexion: place a finger on the head of the talus to be sure that it is moving. A hypermobile subtalar joint can mimic movement in an arthrodesed ankle.

THE FOOT

Remember that complaints apparently relating to the foot may be features of systemic disease such as gout, or of referred vertebral problems such as a prolapsed intervertebral disc. Look for abnormalities of posture.

Callosities are areas of hard skin under points of abnormal pressure. The most common site is beneath the metatarsal heads because loss of the normal soft tissue pad allows abnormal loads. There may be abnormal spread of two adjacent toes (daylight sign, Fig. 10.44) on weight-bearing if there is a bursa between the metatarsal heads. Check for lateral deviation of the big toe (*hallux valgus*) usually associated with abnormal swelling at its base (*a bunion*). There

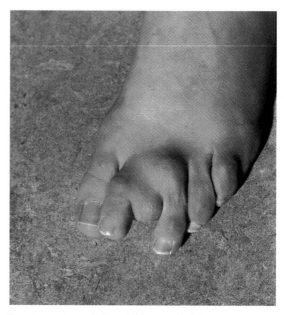

Fig. 10.44   Interphalangeal bursa of left foot. Daylight sign, due to an enlarged bursa, is usually a herald of rheumatoid arthritis.

may be deformities affecting any or all toes with abnormal curvature (*claw toes*), fixed flexion of the terminal joint (*hammer toes*) or over-riding.

The following movements should be tested (Fig. 10.45):

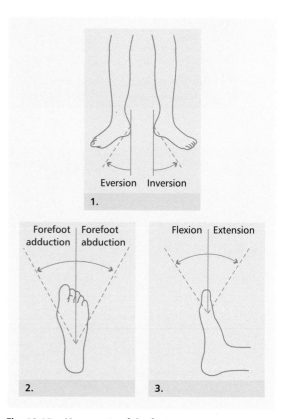

Fig. 10.45   Movements of the foot.

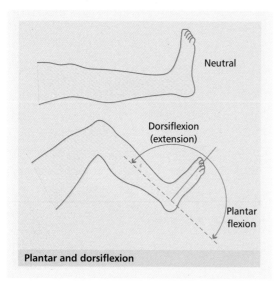

Fig. 10.43   Movements of the ankle.

- Subtalar inversion and eversion: cup the heel in the hands and move it in relation to the tibia without any up and down movement; this eliminates movement at the ankle or midtarsal joints
- Midtarsal inversion/eversion and adduction/abduction: hold the os calcis in the neutral position in one hand and grasp the forefoot in the other
- Metatarsophalangeal and interphalangeal flexion/extension.

Also look for tenderness at the Achilles tendon insertion on the back of the calcaneum and for plantar tenderness at the site of the plantar fascial insertion. Inflammation of these attachments (*enthesopathy*) is common in ankylosing spondylitis and Reiter's syndrome.

THE GAIT

It is best to study gait with the legs and feet fully exposed, and *without* shoes or slippers. Ask the patient to walk away from you, to turn around at a given point and then to walk towards you.

Abnormalities of gait are usually due either to joint problems in the legs or to neurological disorder, although alcohol or drug intoxication or malingering may occasionally cause difficulty. A full examination of the legs and feet should reveal any local cause, which may range from a painful corn to osteoarthritis of the hip. Abnormalities due to neurological disorders are described in Chapter 11.

HYPERMOBILITY

There is a wide variation in the range of normal joint movement, associated with age, sex and race. Excessive laxity or hypermobility of joints (Fig. 10.46)

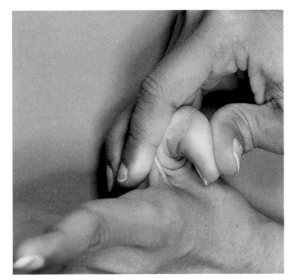

Fig. 10.46   Hyperextensibility of the digits in Ehlers–Danlos syndrome.

can be defined in about 10% of healthy subjects and is frequently familial. It is also a feature of two inherited connective tissue disorders—Marfan's syndrome and Ehlers–Danlos syndrome. Repeated trauma, haemarthrosis or dislocation may produce permanent joint damage.

INVESTIGATIONS IN THE RHEUMATIC DISEASES

When a full history and examination have been completed, investigations should be performed to support the working diagnosis, or rather to distinguish between different possible diagnoses. They can broadly be defined as:

- Tests in support of inflammatory disease
- Diagnostic tests including biopsies and radiological investigations.

TESTS IN SUPPORT OF INFLAMMATORY DISEASE

The following acute phase reactant tests are used in the assessment of inflammatory disease activity and in the subsequent monitoring of the patient.

- *Erythrocyte sedimentation rate (ESR).* This is a useful screening test though it has poor specificity, being affected by the levels of haemoglobin, globulins and fibrinogen. Higher mean values are also seen in elderly patients. Automation makes this a relatively cheap test.
- *C-reactive protein (CRP).* This is a more specific indicator of inflammation and is a good marker of the acute phase response. A high ESR with a normal CRP is a useful pointer towards connective tissue diseases especially SLE.
- *Plasma viscosity.* This is a more specific measure of the acute phase response than ESR, but may not be as widely available.
- *Serum complement.* Low levels of serum complement reflect activation due to immune complex deposition; this may be a marker of disease activity in autoimmune diseases such as systemic lupus erythematosus (SLE). Hereditary complement deficiencies are also associated with SLE.

DIAGNOSTIC TESTS

Diagnostic tests differentiate between specific diseases and are relatively specific investigations.

TESTS FOR RHEUMATOID FACTOR

Rheumatoid factors are autoantibodies in the form of immunoglobulin (Ig) directed against other IgG (immunoglobulin G) molecules. IgM rheumatoid factor can be detected by its ability to clump particles coated with human IgG (*latex test*). This test is positive in about 80% of patients with rheumatoid arthritis. Results are reported as a titre: 1 in 80 or greater being a positive result. The *Rose–Waaler haemagglutination* test uses sheep erythrocytes coated with rabbit IgG to detect IgM (titres of 1 in 32 or more are positive), but is currently being replaced by other tests. ELISA (enzyme-linked immunosorbent serum assay) techniques are much more sensitive, but produce positive results in many other conditions. Other rheumatoid factors in the IgG or IgA classes can also be detected in the sera of patients with rheumatoid arthritis, but are mainly used in research.

These rheumatoid factor screening tests are useful where a diagnosis of rheumatoid arthritis is suspected, but they are not specific. Rheumatoid factor is frequently found in patients with other connective tissue diseases, for example systemic lupus erythematosus and Sjögren's syndrome, or other inflammatory disorders such as subacute bacterial endocarditis and some viral infections.

ANTINUCLEAR ANTIBODY TESTS

Antinuclear antibody (ANA), often referred to as antinuclear factor (ANF), is a very useful screening test for SLE as it is positive in up to 95% of patients. It is, however, a non-specific test, being positive in many other connective tissue disorders, including about 20% of patients with rheumatoid arthritis. A positive test in children with arthritis may be associated with chronic iridocyclitis, which is frequently asymptomatic. Slit-lamp examination of the eye is mandatory to confirm the diagnosis.

The ANA test is carried out by incubating the patient's serum with frozen sections of normal tissue (usually rat liver). After washing, a fluorescent anti-serum to human IgG is used to detect human antibody adhering to the nuclear antigens. A titre of 1 in 80 or more is significant; adequate standardization is important.

DNA-BINDING TEST

This is a radioisotope immunochemical technique used to detect antibodies to native, double-stranded DNA. Another method is indirect immuoflourescence using the protozoa *Crithidia luciliae* where the kinetoplast at the tail containing DNA fluoresces. The test is usually reserved for patients with a positive ANA test and it is the most specific test for SLE. Occasionally it is positive in patients in whom the clinical suspicion of SLE is very high, but the ANA test is negative.

ANTIBODY TESTS TO EXTRACTABLE NUCLEAR ANTIGENS (ENA)

These tests may be suggested by a particular type of pattern of staining (*speckled*) in the routine ANA test. They can be summarized in terms of their clinical association as follows:

- *Anti-Ro (SSA) and anti-La (SSB)* typically in Sjögren's syndrome. Also seen in SLE where they are associated with photosensitivity and the neonatal lupus syndrome which may result in congenital heart block.
- *Anti-Sm* in some cases of SLE—a very specific marker if present.
- *Anti-RNP* (ribonucleoprotein) in some cases of SLE. Also picks out a group of patients who often have a mixed picture of connective tissue disorder and are therefore often diagnosed as MCTD (*mixed connective tissue disease*). The test can be considered a marker for the combination of clinical features, but the major clinical component of the condition will define management.
- *Anticentromere antibody* is found in 'CREST syndrome' (calcinosis, Raynaud's phenomenon, oesophageal symptoms, sclerodactyly and telangiectasis) and some patients with scleroderma. Often a good prognostic marker.
- *Anti-Scl 70 (DNA topoisomerase I) and anti-RNA polymerase* are found in scleroderma and often associated with severe disease.

Other antibodies used in diagnostic tests include the following:

- *Antineutrophil cytoplasmic antibodies* are a marker for vasculitic conditions. Two immuno-fluorescence staining patterns occur
  — cytoplasmic or c-ANCA with specificity for proteinase 3 (a neutrophil enzyme) is very specific for Wegener's granulomatosis (Fig. 10.47).
  — perinuclear or p-ANCA with specificity for myeloperoxidase (and some other neutrophil enzymes) occurs in other vasculitic diseases (and inflammatory bowel disease).
- *Antiphospholipid antibodies* in high titre may be associated with a syndrome characterized by

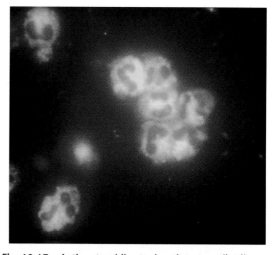

Fig. 10.47 Antineutrophil cytoplasmic autoantibodies with cytoplasmic staining (cANCA). This pattern has a high predictive value for a diagnosis of Wegener's granulomatosis.

thromboses (including cerebral infarction), thrombocytopenia and, in women, recurrent pregnancy loss (*antiphospholipid syndrome*). This antibody may be associated with SLE and called *anticardiolipin antibody* or *lupus anticoagulant*, despite the association with thromboses. A false positive VDRL may also be found in these patients.

- *Anti-Jo 1 (histidyl t-RNA synthetase)* is a marker for the idiopathic inflammatory myopathies such as dermatomyositis and polymyositis, especially when complicated by interstitial lung disease.
- *Human leucocyte antigen (HLA) typing*: there is a strong association of the tissue antigen HLA-B27 with ankylosing spondylitis, but it is of limited diagnostic value. Although about 95% of ankylosing spondylitis patients in the UK possess the B27 antigen, it is also found in 8% of the normal population. Ankylosing spondylitis therefore remains a clinical diagnosis, supported by typical radiographic findings. HLA-B27 typing is, however, of some value in the differential diagnosis of seronegative (latex negative) peripheral arthritis, particularly in children.
- *Antistreptolysin-O (ASO) test*: the presence in the serum of this antibody in a titre greater than 1/200, rising on repeat testing after about 2 weeks, indicates a recent haemolytic streptococcal infection.

URIC ACID

A consistently normal plasma uric acid level (< 375 μmol/litre in women, < 425 μmol/litre in men) usually excludes the diagnosis of untreated gout. Raised levels occur in many circumstances and do not establish in themselves the diagnosis of gout (see below). On a low purine diet, the 24-hour urinary urate excretion should not exceed 600 mg. Higher levels indicate 'overproduction' of urate and a risk of renal stone formation.

SYNOVIAL FLUID EXAMINATION

Synovial fluid may be obtained for examination from any joint in which it is clinically detectable. The knee is the most convenient source: after infiltration with a 1% local anaesthetic, a 21-gauge needle is inserted into the joint on its medial aspect between the patella and the femoral condyle. The aspirated fluid should be placed in a plain sterile container; if a cell count is required, some of the fluid should be mixed with ethylenediaminetetraacetic acid (EDTA) anticoagulant.

An injured joint can also be aspirated (Box 10.11). The swollen joint after injury may reveal clear pink fluid suggesting a *meniscal lesion*, or show frank blood. The latter is usually indicative of a *torn anterior cruciate ligament*. If blood is aspirated look at its surface for globules of fat. This is derived from the marrow and confirms an intra-articular fracture. Synovial fluid examination is diagnostic in two conditions—*bacterial infections* and *crystal synovitis*—and every effort should be made to obtain fluid when

> **BOX 10.11   Findings in synovial fluid after aspiration of the knee joint.**
>
> - Cloudy fluid or pus: bacterial infection (see text).
> - Urate or pyrophosphate crystals: gout or pseudo-gout
> - Pink fluid: torn meniscus
> - Blood: trauma, haemophilia, villonodular synovitis

either of these is suspected. Polarized light microscopy can differentiate between the crystals of urate in gout and those of calcium pyrophosphate dihydrate in pseudo-gout. Outside these conditions, synovial fluid examination is unlikely to be diagnostic. Frank blood may point to trauma, haemophilia or villonodular synovitis, while inflammatory (as opposed to degenerative) arthritis is suggested by opaque fluid of low viscosity, with a total white cell count > 1000 cells/μl, neutrophils $> 50\%$, protein content > 35 g/litre, and the presence of a firm clot. Culture of this fluid may produce a bacterial growth, usually of staphylococci, but occasionally *Mycobacterium tuberculosis* or other organisms.

BIOPSIES USEFUL IN DIFFERENTIAL DIAGNOSIS

The following biopsies may be useful in differential diagnosis of rheumatic diseases:

- *Synovial biopsy* is of little value in the differential diagnosis of inflammatory polyarthritis, but should be considered in any unusual monoarthritis to exclude infection, particularly tuberculous, or rare conditions such as sarcoid or amyloid arthropathy, or villonodular synocitis.
- *Rectal biopsy* can be useful in the diagnosis of amyloidosis secondary to chronic inflammatory disease, but renal biopsy may still be necessary if the cause of renal impairment is not clear.
- *Renal biopsy* is essential in the vasculitides or SLE where active glomerulonephritis is suspected. Vasculitis may also be confirmed on renal biopsy but, in general, tissues found to be abnormal on clinical examination or by further investigation (e.g. skin, muscle, sural nerve or liver) should be considered first for diagnostic biopsy in undifferentiated systemic vasculitis.
- *Biopsy of the lip* may be useful to confirm Sjögren's syndrome.
- *Temporal artery biopsy* is often diagnostic in patients with clinical features of temporal (giant cell) endarteritis. This is the investigation of choice.

RADIOLOGICAL EXAMINATION

Only radiographs likely to yield specific information should be requested. However, in unilateral joint disease it is useful to examine both sides for comparison (Fig. 10.48(a) and (b)). In patients with inflammatory polyarthritis three routine films are helpful in the diagnosis and assessment of progression: *both hands and wrists* on one plate, *both feet* on another, to compare bone density and to look for periosteal reaction or erosive change, and one of the full *pelvis* (Fig. 10.49), to show the sacroiliac and hip joints.

Radiographs taken to confirm or exclude a fracture must be taken in two planes. It is essential that either the whole limb is turned or the imaging equipment rotated. The limb must not be twisted at the fracture site. When looking for a fracture in a bone, run a pen tip or its equivalent around the cortex of the bone as seen on the film (without leaving marks). Any break in continuity will reveal itself; do not confuse an epiphysis with a fracture. Note soft tissue swelling and distension of joints.

ARTHROGRAPHY

Injection of contrast medium into the knee joint can be used to confirm the diagnosis of a ruptured popliteal cyst although utrasonography will demonstrate this non-invasively as well as demonstrating patency of the popliteal venous system when distinguishing a popliteal cyst from deep venous thrombosis. A double-contrast technique is useful in

demonstrating abnormalities of the menisci in the knee.

SPECIALIZED RADIOLOGY

The following imaging techniques can provide precise information about localized pathology but are dependent on the clinician making a clear diagnostic request:

- *High resolution ultrasound* is of value in defining soft tissue structures, including muscles and tendons, and provides an excellent means for guiding aspiration and biopsy procedures.
- *Computed tomography (CT).* The combination of superior tissue contrast and tomographic technique permits definition of soft tissue structures obscured by overlapping structures, including the intervertebral disc, and other joints normally difficult to visualize, such as sacroiliac (Fig. 10.50), sternoclavicular and subtalar.
- *MRI* provides unique advantages in evaluation of the musculoskeletal system, but it is vital that the clinician defines the pathology suspected, as correct positioning and sequence selection (T weighting) are vital in optimizing image quality. It is of particular value in the non-invasive investigation of disc disease (Fig. 10.51) including spinal infection, and is generally felt to be the most sensitive technique for diagnosis of avascu-

(a)

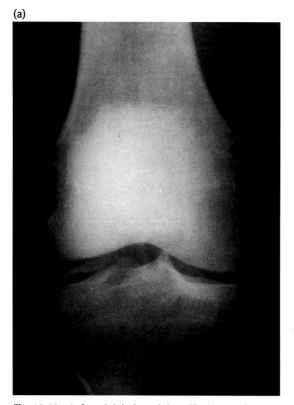

(b)

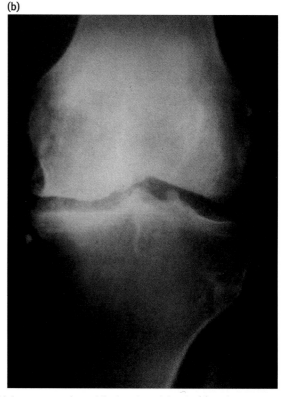

Fig. 10.48   Left and right knee joints. The X-rays show normal joint anatomy but with chondrocalcinosis **(a)** and osteoarthritic change **(b)** on the opposite side. Note the increased **bone** density and narrowing of the joint space.

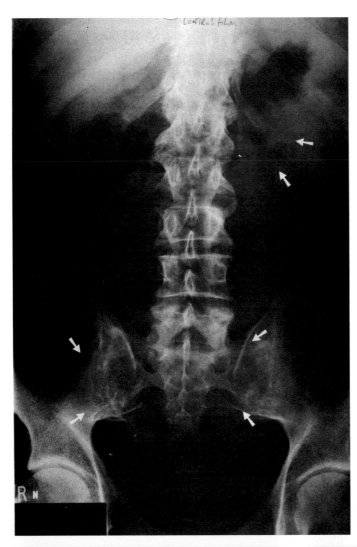

Fig. 10.49   X-ray of lumbosacral spine and upper pelvis. There is fusion of several vertebrae, and of the sacroiliac joints (arrows) from ankylosing spondylitis. The renal papillae on the left are calcified, evidence of previous papillary necrosis from analgesic abuse.

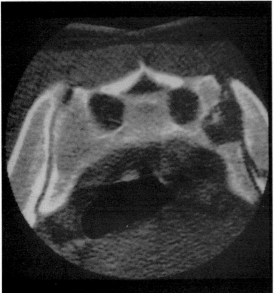

Fig. 10.50   CT scan of sacroiliac joints, showing distinctive lesion on the left side with a sequestrum due to tuberculosis.

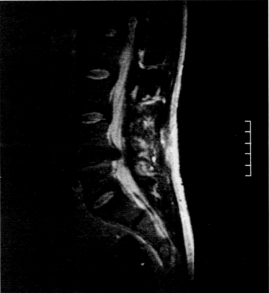

Fig. 10.51   There is a disc protrusion at L4–5, with degeneration of the disc itself, shown by the less bright signal in the intervertebral disc at this level.

lar necrosis. Enhancement by the use of intra-venous paramagnetic contrast (e.g. gadolinium) has further improved definition in spinal imaging. MRI is increasingly used in imaging of major joints in the limbs, especially the knee (Fig. 10.40), hip, shoulder and elbow.

- *Isotopic scanning* (scintigraphy) can be used in the diagnosis of acute (e.g. infection or stress fracture) or multiple (e.g. metastases) bone lesions by use of the first 2-minute (dynamic blood flow) phase, second 10-minute (blood pool) and third 3-hour late phase (osteoblastic) (Fig. 10.52) following intravenous injection of diphosphonate compounds. Tomographic scinti-graphy can further refine definition of the isotope uptake (e.g. in stress fracture of the pars interarticularis).

- *DEXA (dual energy X-ray absorptiometry)* is widely used to assess bone mineral density in metabolic bone disease and osteoporosis. Interval scans may be used to assess the effects of therapy.

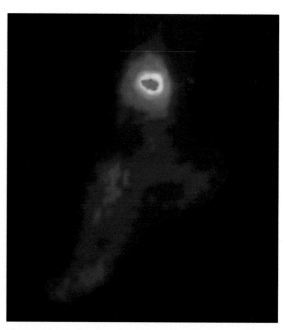

Fig. 10.52 Technetium bone scan in a distance runner, showing focally increased uptake in the lower tibia owing to a stress fracture.

11
THE NERVOUS SYSTEM

INTRODUCTION

The aim of the neurological assessment is to assess the patient's illness in both functional and anatomical terms. A detailed and complete neurological examination is an ordeal for ill patients and a test of concentration and cooperation for those in good general health. Over-long examination may defeat its own ends, especially when sensation is investigated, by leading to variable and incongruous findings. The examination should therefore be planned in relation to the problems posed by the information acquired from the patient's history. Like other specialists, the neurologist looks for patterns of functional abnormality (Box 11.1). These patterns represent features consistent either with *lesions in neuronal systems*, including nuclei and their interconnecting pathways, or with *disease syndromes*. *Negative* features reflect loss of function due to a lesion in the nervous system (e.g. weakness). *Positive* features also develop, for example seizures in disease of the cerebral cortex and involuntary movements or tremor in disease of the basal ganglia. While it is important to understand the scientific basis for any given symptom, in order to be able to advise how best to deal with it, most neurological diagnoses are made on the basis of pattern recognition. As always in medical practice, the history sets the scene.

THE NEUROLOGICAL HISTORY

The history gives information about the onset and course of the disorder. This may in itself be diagnostic. The neurological examination should be based on the information provided by the history, to assess the extent of the disabilities described, and to evaluate

BOX 11.1 Patterns of neurological disease, defined by onset and course.

Onset	Course	Symptoms and signs	Diagnosis
Gradual	Progressive	Hemiparesis	Cerebral tumour
		Focal seizures	Cerebral tumour
		Paraplegia	Spinal cord disease
	Rapid course	Seizures, coma	CNS infection
		Generalized weakness	Polyneuritis
			Muscle disease
	Step-wise	Pain in the arm	Brachial neuritis
		Painful and weak limb	Root lesion
		Weak, unsteady limb	Multiple sclerosis
Sudden	Recovery	Unilateral visual loss	Optic neuritis
		Recurrent seizures	Epilepsy
		Transient focal weakness	Transient ischaemic attack (TIA)
	Residual disability	Hemiparesis, ataxia, etc.	Stroke
	Partial recovery	Headache, stiff neck, vomiting	Subarachnoid haemorrhage
	Recurrent	Headache, blurred vision	Migraine

the presence or absence of any features that might extend or modify the diagnosis suggested by the history.

Find out how the symptom developed or extended during the course of the illness:

● Was the clinical course step-wise, with several exacerbations and partial remissions (a feature of demyelinating disease, stroke and some remittent peripheral neuropathies)?
● Was the clinical course steadily progressive?
● Is the illness more rapidly worsening now than at the onset?
● Is the patient now improving?

Consider whether there are features characteristic of a particular diagnosis, such as a history of previous visual disturbance in one eye in suspected multiple sclerosis. If there is doubt about the sequence of events or about the nature of an episode, especially if the patient's conscious state was disturbed during an episode (e.g. in a seizure), *talk to an observer or family member to find out more*. If the patient appears vague, or the story is inconsistent, talk to someone else who knows the patient to find out whether there has been any deterioration in thought, memory or behaviour that might suggest a progressive dementia or progressive focal higher level brain disturbance such as aphasia.

Spend time on the history; it is especially important and revealing in neurological diagnosis. Remember, however, that the patient is trying to describe the effects of damage to the nervous system. It is especially difficult for a person with a damaged nervous system to understand the nature of the symptoms with which he or she is confronted since these features are outside ordinary experience as well as being frightening. Headache is a particularly common symptom and can be used to illustrate the kind of information required in relation to symptom type, temporal factors, causation, treatments and other health-related factors (Box 11.2).

THE NEUROLOGICAL EXAMINATION

Try always to conduct your examination in a logical fashion, and plan it in relation to the history. For example, if a patient is complaining of sciatic pain, begin with the lower limbs and lumbar spine. This flexibility means that your technique should be skilled—this requires practice and confidence. *Observation* of ordinary activity—for example the way the patient walks into the room and undresses for examination—is often very helpful. In hospital, people are often found lying in bed, so make a point of seeing what activity the patient is able to undertake, even if this is difficult. Keep in mind the main points of the guidelines in Box 11.3. Look for patterns of abnormality (see Box 11.1) that support or refute a diagnosis suggested by the history. Thus,

---

> **BOX 11.2   Assessment of headache: an example of the analysis of a common neurological symptom. (This can be used as a generic system of enquiry into other problems.)**
>
> 1. What *clinical types* of headache does the patient describe? (There may be more than one.)
> 2. *Temporal* aspects of the headache.
>   —when did it begin?
>   —why ask for help now?
>   —temporal features—is it cyclic? daily? unremitting?
>   —duration of each headache?
> 3. *Character* of the headache as a symptom.
>   —intensity?
>   —nature and quality?
>   —site and spread?
>   —associated symptoms?
> 4. *Causative* factors:
>   —precipitating features?
>   —aggravating and relieving factors?
> 5. *Responsiveness* to environment:
>   —what are the limitations imposed by headache as a symptom?
>   —what medications and other treatments are used, and with what benefit?
> 6. *Health* between attacks:
>   —completely well, or with persistent symptoms?
>   —depression? anxieties? fears?
>   —social and work-related consequences?
> 7. What does the patient *believe* is the cause?

> **BOX 11.3   Guidelines for a brief, but comprehensive, neurological assessment.**
>
> **Mental state**
> Much useful information can be obtained during history-taking:
>
> ● Is the history given *accurately, concisely* and *with insight*? Or is the patient *concrete, circumlocutory* or *vague*?
> ● Is the patient's *memory* normal?
> ● Is the patient *neatly dressed* and *well-cared for*?
> ● Is the patient's *behaviour* normal?
> ● Is the patient *aphasic* or *dysarthric*?
> ● Is the patient *confused*?
> ● Can the patient *find the way* in and out of the room?
> ● Can the patient *dress* and *undress* without help?
>
> **Gait**
>
> ● Is the patient's gait *spastic, hemiparetic, ataxic* or *parkinsonian*?
> ● Does the patient have *foot drop*?
>
> **Cranial nerves**
>
> ● Test *ocular movements* and look for nystagmus
> ● Test *facial movements*
> ● Test *tongue protrusion* and *palatal movement*

Visual fields

Aphasia, and abnormal visual fields are proof of disease above the tentorium cerebelli:

- Is there a *hemianopia*?
- If so, is it *homonymous, bitemporal, unilateral* or something else?
- Is the patient's *central vision* normal? (This is crudely assessed by testing the visual acuity)
- Can the patient read small print with or without glasses?

Fundi

- Is there *papilloedema*?
- Is there *optic atrophy*?
- Are there *hypertensive, uraemic* or *diabetic* changes?

Motor

- Is there any *weakness* of the outstretched upper limbs?
- Is there *distal* or *proximal weakness* or *wasting*?
- Is the patient's *muscular tone* normal, spastic or extrapyramidal in type?
- Look for *cerebellar ataxia* in the limbs
- Assess the *tendon reflexes* and *plantar responses*
- Assess *gait* and the patient's *ability to get up from a low chair*

Sensory

- Test *position sense* in the patient's fingers and toes and vibration sense in the feet (*posterior columns*)
- Test *pinprick* in the patient's four limbs and on the face (*lateral spinothalamic tracts*)
- *Light touch* need only be tested if the patient complains of numbness

General

- Examine the patient's *skull, spinal movements* and posture
- Look for *cutaneous naevi*
- Listen for *bruits in the neck*

neck rigidity in a patient with headache and fever is consistent with meningitis, and an extensor plantar response in a patient complaining of a previous episode of hemiparesis is consistent with, but not necessarily diagnostic of, cerebral infarction. A careful history is more likely to yield useful information than a routine examination.

BASIC CONCEPTS

The nervous system is made up of central and peripheral motor and sensory pathways, the cerebellar system, and the cerebral hemispheres. The spinal cord is a distinct anatomical structure in which motor and sensory pathways are in close juxtaposition. The central nervous system (CNS) is protected by the skull, and the bones of the spine. These neural structures receive blood from the carotid, vertebral and spinal arteries. The patterns of abnormality in neurological disease (Box 11.1) represent the effects of dysfunction in neural systems and pathways. These cause *negative symptoms and signs*, such as weakness, loss of vision, sensory loss or difficulty walking, or *positive abnormalities*, such as seizures, pain or involuntary movements.

THE MOTOR SYSTEM

There are two basic patterns of motor abnormality—the *lower* and the *upper motor neurone syndromes*.

The lower motor neurones consist of:

- Anterior horn cells and motor nerve cells in motor nuclei in the brainstem
- Efferent motor nerve fibres which pass via the anterior spinal nerve roots and peripheral nerves to the muscles
- Motor endplates on muscle fibres that excite the muscle fibres
- Muscle fibres innervated by these nerve fibres and their terminal axonal branches.

The upper motor neurone consists of the motor cortex, the corticospinal (pyramidal) tracts that synapse on the motor nuclei in the brainstem, and the anterior horn cells in the spinal cord. The corticospinal tracts contain these fibres and also fibres which arise from the post-central cortex and from subcortical structures. The motor area of the cortex occupies the anterior aspect of the central sulcus (Rolandic fissure) and the adjacent parts of the pre-central gyrus. In the motor cortex those parts of the body involved in the most skilled movements, for example the fingers and thumb and the lips and tongue, have the largest areas of cortical representation. The areas for tongue, jaw and facial movements lie in the inferior part of the motor cortex, those for the arm, trunk and leg are arranged in sequence in the motor area, which extends to the vertex and on to the medial surface of the cerebral hemisphere (Fig. 11.1).

The corticospinal tracts project through the anterior two-thirds of the posterior limb of the internal capsule. Here the order of representation of the body is face, shoulder, elbow, hand, trunk and lower limb from before backwards. The corticospinal fibres then pass through the middle three-fifths of the cerebral peduncles in the mid-brain. In the pons, the corticospinal tract becomes broken into scattered bundles by the transverse pontine fibres and nuclei pontis. In the upper part of the medulla the corticospinal fibres occupy the pyramids, on the anterior aspect of the brainstem. In the lower part of the medulla most of the corticospinal fibres decussate with those of the opposite side, pass posteriorly into the spinal cord, and form the crossed lateral corticospinal tracts.

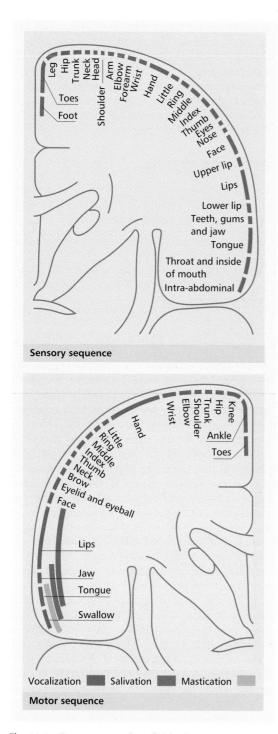

Sensory sequence

Vocalization ▮ Salivation ▮ Mastication ▮

Motor sequence

Fig. 11.1 Rasmussen and Penfield's diagram of localization in the sensory (top) and motor (bottom) cortex.

Lower motor neurone lesion

Lower motor neurone lesions cause weakness, with characteristic signs, especially absence of appropriate tendon reflexes (Box 11.4). The distribution of the abnormality depends on the causative process. Focal neurogenic weakness occurs with single nerve or nerve root lesions. Distal neurogenic weakness occurs

---

BOX 11.4   Main clinical features of motor disorders.

Lower motor neurone syndrome
- Weakness
- Decreased muscle tone
- Absent tendon reflexes
- Muscle wasting, often severe
- Fasciculation in affected muscles
- Distribution of weakness and wasting consistent with lesion in spinal segments, nerve root or peripheral nerve

Upper motor neurone syndrome
- Weakness in corticospinal distribution: shoulder abduction and finger movements, hip flexion and toe dorsiflexion
- Spastic increase in muscle tone
- Increased tendon reflexes
- Extensor plantar response
- Little or no atrophy

Dystonia and extrapyramidal disorders
- Plastic or spastic increase in muscle tone
- Abnormal postures
- Involuntary movements and tremor
- Loss of postural reflexes
- Normal or increased tendon reflexes
- Plantar responses normal or extensor

---

in peripheral neuropathy. Generalized neurogenic weakness occurs in anterior horn cell disease, such as motor neurone disease (amyotrophic lateral sclerosis) or spinal muscular atrophy.

Upper motor neurone lesion

The corticospinal system initiates voluntary and skilled motor acts, particularly fine distal movements. The syndrome resulting from a small internal capsular infarct, affecting corticospinal fibres *alone*, consists initially of weakness of the contralateral side of the body. Rapid improvement usually occurs. The residual impairment in 'pure' corticospinal tract lesion consists of:

- Loss of fine, rapid, distal movements of the hand and fingers, as in picking up a small object
- Weakness of shoulder abduction
- Weakness of hip flexion
- Weakness of dorsiflexion of the foot
- Weakness of the lower part of the face.

The more familiar syndrome of severe paralysis of one side of the body (*hemiplegia*), with a flexed upper limb posture, or of a single limb (*monoplegia*), is usually the result of a more extensive lesion affecting extrapyramidal or other subcortical structures in addition to the corticospinal fibres themselves. Even in a dense hemiplegia, movements of the head and trunk (axial movements) are virtually uninvolved. The pathways for such postural movements are predominantly under subcortical control and are represented bilaterally. In fact, most lesions of the corticospinal system also damage neighbouring extrapyramidal nuclei and pathways, and all such cases are loosely grouped as *corticospinal lesions*. The classic signs of *upper motor neurone lesion* should always include *weakness, increased tendon reflexes*, and an *extensor plantar response* (Box 11.4).

When the corticospinal system is suddenly damaged or destroyed, as by haemorrhage or injury, there is a temporary depressant effect on the anterior horn cells (*neuronal shock*). Paralysis is accompanied at first by loss of muscle tone and absent or reduced tendon reflexes. The characteristic hypertonia and increased reflexes of a corticospinal lesion appear after a few hours or days.

THE EXTRAPYRAMIDAL SYSTEM

The extrapyramidal system consists of the basal ganglia, the subthalamic nuclei, the substantia nigra and other structures in the brainstem concerned with movement and posture. The extrapyramidal system is complex and includes fibres from the cerebral cortex and the thalamus. There are no direct pathways from the basal ganglia to the spinal cord; extrapyramidal connections with the lower motor neurones are indirect, through pathways arising in the brainstem. These include the dentatorubrospinal, reticulospinal, vestibulospinal and olivospinal tracts. The extrapyramidal system is important in the control of posture and in the initiation of movement, especially *postural mechanisms*, in functions such as sitting, standing, turning over in the lying position, walking and running. Complex movements such as reaching for an object require both postural adjustments and fine distal movements, which are under corticospinal control.

Extrapyramidal lesion
Lesions of the extrapyramidal system (Box 11.4) cause difficulty in initiating voluntary movement, impairment of orienting and balancing reflexes (*negative features*), and alterations in muscle tone and involuntary movements (*positive, or released features*). Strength is usually unaffected.

THE CEREBELLUM
The cerebellum receives afferent fibres from the spinal cord, vestibular system, basal ganglia and cerebral cortex. It modulates movement mainly through its connections, via the thalamus, with the basal ganglia and cerebral cortex.

Cerebellar lesions
Lesions of the cerebellum cause incoordination (*ataxia*). Muscle tone may be reduced. Disease of the cerebellar vermis causes a characteristic ataxia of the trunk, so that there is difficulty sitting up or standing,

but with little or no incoordination of the limbs. Paralysis is not a feature of cerebellar disease. Tendon reflexes are not increased, although they may be 'pendular'.

THE SENSORY SYSTEM

Sensory input reaches the nervous system from:

- Specialized receptors and free nerve endings in the skin and superficial tissues
- Other receptors, such as muscle spindles, Golgi tendon organs, pacinian corpuscles and free nerve endings in muscles
- Other specialized receptors in the joints.

Sensory information from internal organs and viscera enters the nervous system via autonomic afferent systems. All afferent nerve fibres enter the central nervous system through the posterior root ganglia and the posterior roots. Disease of these 'first sensory neurones' may thus affect all modalities of sensation. Much sensory input is concerned with the reflex control of posture and movement and is not consciously perceived. For example, the conscious recognition of posture, movement, and position of a limb (*kinaesthesia*) is primarily dependent on input from muscle spindles, with contributions from cutaneous and joint receptors. However, the major role of muscle spindles and tendon organs is probably in the monitoring of voluntary and reflex movements, through 'efference copy'. Spindle and Golgi afferents travel rostrally in the ventral and dorsal spinocerebellar tracts to enter the cerebellum, and cerebral hemispheres.

CUTANEOUS SENSATION
After entering the spinal cord, cutaneous sensory nerve fibres are ordered and grouped for projection rostrally to the brain. There are two groups of sensory nerve fibres. One group projects to cells in the posterior horn of the spinal grey matter at or near the level at which they enter. Second sensory neurone fibres arise from these cells in the posterior horn. Some of these cross immediately, or within a few segments, to the opposite lateral and anterior columns of the cord and so ascend to the brainstem as the *anterior and lateral spinothalamic tracts*. The lateral spinothalamic tracts modulate the sensations of pain and temperature. The fibres from the lower part of the body are arranged in the lateral portion of this pathway, and those from the upper parts of the body more medially.

The afferent fibres in the second group do not synapse in the grey matter of the posterior horns of the spinal cord, but ascend in the ipsilateral posterior columns. These *posterior column fibres* carry impulses which determine the appreciation of position, movement, size, shape, discrimination and texture, and vibration (which should be regarded only as touch rapidly applied). The medial of the two posterior columns, the *fasciculus gracilis*, contains fibres originating in the lower part of the body, whereas the lateral, the *fasciculus cuneatus*, carries fibres predominantly from the upper limbs. *The uncrossed somatotopic lamination of fibres in the posterior columns is thus the converse of that in the crossed lateral spinothalamic tracts.*

Brainstem sensory pathways

In the upper part of the spinal cord the posterior column fibres terminate in the gracile and cuneate nuclei. The fibres of the second sensory neurone originate in these nuclei and immediately cross to the opposite side of the medulla in the sensory decussation. In the medulla, therefore, all sensory impulses are carried in sensory tracts situated on the opposite side to that from which they arise. But even here they are not arranged in a single pathway: spinothalamic fibres pass through the lateral part of the medulla, while the posterior columns enter the medial lemniscus. Higher in the brainstem the two sensory pathways are joined by the second sensory neurone fibres from cranial nerve nuclei. The fibres of the medial lemniscus and spinothalamic tract synapse in the thalamus. From this level a third system of sensory fibres conveys sensory input through the internal capsule to the cerebral cortex.

The anatomy and physiology of the sensory pathways is important in understanding certain pain syndromes. The two major pathways themselves are important in their interactions. Different patterns of impulses in different-sized fibres of differing conduction velocity determine the sensations perceived at the highest levels of the nervous system. The importance of spinal mechanisms in the dorsal horn in the control of the flow of afferent information has been emphasized in the 'gate control' theory of sensation. This concept has underlined, furthermore, the pre-eminent role of the dorsal columns in exploratory, movement-directed behaviour, rather than in the passive reception of sensory input, and the importance of small thinly myelinated or unmyelinated fibres in the generation of the sensation of pain.

THE SPINAL CORD

The spinal cord extends from the foramen magnum caudally to the interspace between the twelfth thoracic and first lumbar spines; the thecal membranes continue down as far as the body of the second sacral

		Cervical			Dorsal
	5	6	7	8	1
Shoulder	Supraspinatus				
	Teres minor				
	Deltoid				
	Infraspinatus				
	Subscapularis				
	Teres major				
Arm	Biceps				
	Triceps				
Forearm	Brachio-radialis				
	Supinator				
	Extensor carpi radial.				
	Pronator teres				
	Flexor carpi radial.				
	Flexor pollic. long				
	Abduct. poll. long.				
	Extens. poll. brev.				
	Extens. poll. long.				
	Extens. digitor.				
	Extens. indicis.				
	Extens. carpi. uln.				
	Extens. digitor. min.				
	Flexor digitor. sublimis				
	Flexor digitor. profund.				
	Pronator quadratus				
	Flex. carpi. uln.				
	Palmaris long.				
Hand	Abductor poll. brev.				
	Flexor poll. brev.				
	Opponens poll.				
	Flexor digit. min.				
	Opponens digit. min.				
	Adduct. poll.				
	Palmaris brev.				
	Abductor digit. min.				
	Lumbricales				
	Interossei				

Table 11.1 Segmental innervation of the muscles of the upper limbs.

vertebra. The cervical enlargement reaches to the seventh cervical spine. Its largest part is at the level of the fifth cervical vertebra. The lumbar segments lie opposite the tenth and eleventh thoracic spines and the next interspinous space.

The spinal segments do not correspond exactly with the vertebrae overlying them. This is important in assessing patients with spinal cord compression due to vertebral disease. To determine which spinal segment is related to a given vertebral body:

- For the cervical vertebrae, add one level
- For thoracic 1–6, add two levels
- For thoracic 7–9, add three levels
- The tenth thoracic arch overlies lumbar 1 and 2 segments
- The eleventh thoracic arch overlies lumbar 3 and 4 segments
- The twelfth thoracic arch overlies lumbar 5
- The first lumbar arch overlies the sacral and coccygeal segments
- In the lower thoracic region the tip of a spinous process marks the level of the body of the vertebra below.

The spinal cord is organized in segments, from each of which a pair of anterior (motor) and posterior (sensory) nerve roots arise. The *myotomes* and *dermatomes* supplied by the pairs of nerve roots are shown in Tables 11.1 and 11.2 and in Figures 11.2 and 11.3. Knowledge of these is important since it provides the basis for clinical recognition of nerve root and peripheral nerve lesions. The distribution of sensory loss found after some common peripheral nerve lesions is shown in Figures 11.4 and 11.5. Compare these with the patterns of sensory loss due to root lesions, shown in Figures 11.2 and 11.3. These patterns of motor and sensory disturbance are particularly important in the hand because of the common clinical problems posed by the distinction between ulnar, radial and median nerve lesions and lower cervical root problems and, in the foot, between lumbosacral root lesions and common peroneal nerve palsies. The clinical features of mononeuropathies are listed in Box 11.5, and the common causes of brachial plexus lesions in Box 11.6.

Note that C8 and C6 sensory loss extends to the elbow on both ventral and dorsal surfaces of the forearm, but that median nerve sensory loss predominantly affects the palmar surface of the hand. In both ulnar and median nerve lesions sensory loss extends no further proximally than the wrist. On the body itself there is a line of demarcation between the T2 and C4 segments at the clavicle. The level of the

Region	Muscle	D12	L1	L2	L3	L4	L5	S1	S2
Hip	Ilio–psoas		■						
Hip	Tensor fasciæ					■	■		
Hip	Gluteus medius					■	■	■	
Hip	Gluteus minimus					■	■	■	
Hip	Quadratus femoris					■	■	■	
Hip	Gluteus maximus						■	■	■
Hip	Obturator intern.						■	■	■
Thigh	Sartorius			■	■				
Thigh	Adduct. long.			■	■				
Thigh	Quadriceps			■	■	■			
Thigh	Gracilis			■	■				
Thigh	Adductor brevis			■	■				
Thigh	Obturator ext.				■	■			
Thigh	Adduct. magn.				■	■			
Thigh	Adduct. minim.				■	■			
Thigh	Semitendinosus					■	■	■	
Thigh	Semimembranosus					■	■	■	
Thigh	Biceps femoris						■	■	■
Leg	Tibialis ant.					■	■		
Leg	Extens. hall. long.					■	■		
Leg	Extens. digit. long.					■	■		
Leg	Soleus						■	■	■
Leg	Gastrocnemius						■	■	■
Leg	Peroneus long.						■	■	
Leg	Peroneus brev.						■	■	
Leg	Tibialis post.						■	■	
Leg	Flexor digitor. long.						■	■	
Leg	Flexor halluc. long.							■	■
Foot	Extens. hall. brev.					■	■	■	
Foot	Extens. digit. brevis					■	■	■	
Foot	Intrinsic muscles of the foot						■	■	■
Foot	Interossei							■	■

Table 11.2 Segmental innervation of the muscles of the lower limbs.

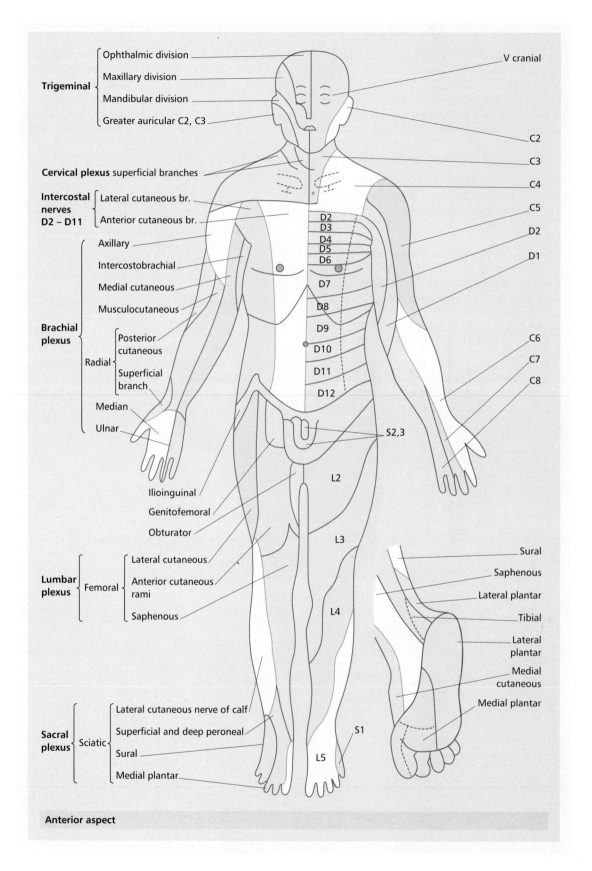

Trigeminal {
- Ophthalmic division
- Maxillary division
- Mandibular division
- Greater auricular C2, C3

Cervical plexus superficial branches

Intercostal nerves D2 – D11 {
- Lateral cutaneous br.
- Anterior cutaneous br.

Brachial plexus {
- Axillary
- Intercostobrachial
- Medial cutaneous
- Musculocutaneous
- Radial {
  - Posterior cutaneous
  - Superficial branch
- Median
- Ulnar

Lumbar plexus {
- Ilioinguinal
- Genitofemoral
- Obturator
- Femoral {
  - Lateral cutaneous
  - Anterior cutaneous rami
  - Saphenous

Sacral plexus {
- Sciatic {
  - Lateral cutaneous nerve of calf
  - Superficial and deep peroneal
  - Sural
  - Medial plantar

V cranial

C2
C3
C4
C5
D2
D1

C6
C7
C8

D2
D3
D4
D5
D6
D7
D8
D9
D10
D11
D12

S2,3

L2

L3

L4

L5

S1

Sural
Saphenous
Lateral plantar
Tibial
Lateral plantar
Medial cutaneous
Medial plantar

Anterior aspect

Fig. 11.2   Anterior view to show the segmental innervation of skin (left), and peripheral nerve supply (right).

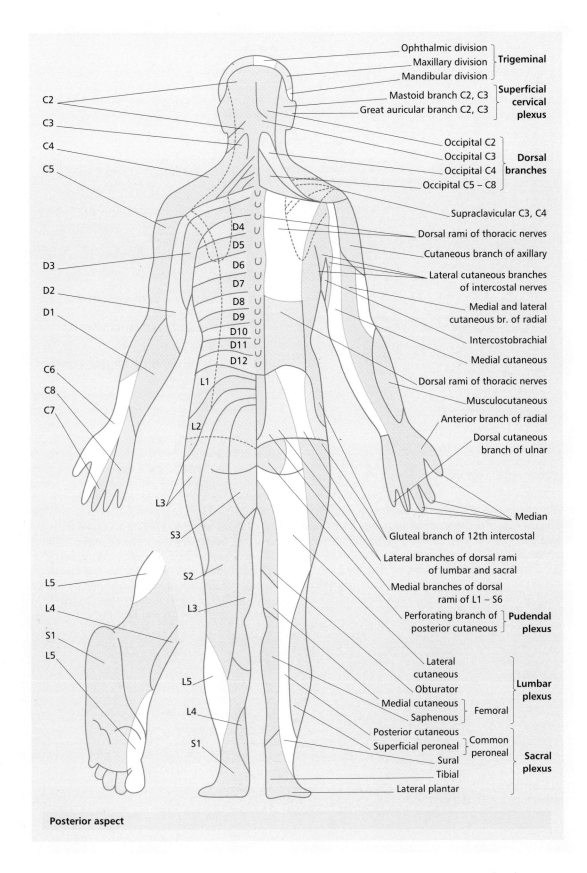

Fig. 11.3   Posterior view to show the segmental innervation of skin (left), and peripheral nerve supply (right).

(a)

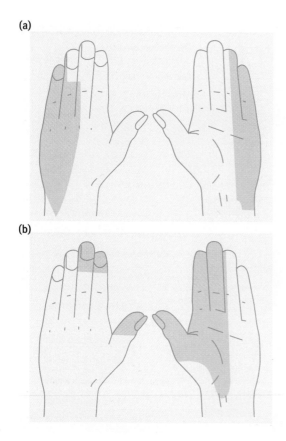

(b)

Fig. 11.4 Cutaneous sensory loss: **(a)** after the division of the ulnar nerve above the elbow; **(b)** after division of the median nerve in the arm.

nipple represents T6, the xiphisternum T8, the umbilicus T10 and the inguinal ligament T12. The deltoid area represents C5. The patella and antero-medial shin represent L4. Sensory impairment in an L5/S1 distribution closely resembles that found in a common peroneal nerve lesion, except that the medial borders of the forefoot and large toe are involved in the former but not in the latter.

BOX 11.5   Mononeuropathies; disorders of single nerves.

- Motor and sensory involvement in distribution of affected nerve
- Acute mononeuropathies are often painful
- Multiple nerves may be affected (mononeuritis multiplex)

BOX 11.6   Causes of brachial plexus lesions.

- Brachial neuritis
- Infiltration by tumour, e.g. carcinoma of breast may infiltrate the brachial plexus, lymphoma may infiltrate nerve roots
- Radiation plexopathy, rarely follows radiotherapy for breast cancer
- Vasculitis
- Trauma, especially in traffic accidents or at work, direct or stretch injuries
- Compression, e.g. by cervical rib or tumour

CLINICAL SYNDROMES OF SPINAL CORD DISEASE

At any level of the spinal cord, therefore, there are two major groups of sensory fibres conveying sensory information towards the brain: one in the anterolateral columns carrying pain and temperature from the opposite half of the body, and a second in the posterior columns, conveying the appreciation of posture, weight, size, shape and other qualities of sensation from the same side of the body. A unilateral lesion of the spinal cord thus results in loss of pain and thermal sensibility below the level of the lesion on the opposite side of the body, while on the side of the lesion there is, in addition to spastic paralysis, disturbance of the sense of position and of movement and loss of recognition of weight, size, shape, touch and vibration. This group of clinical signs is called the *Brown–Séquard syndrome* (see Fig. 11.6 and Box 11.7).

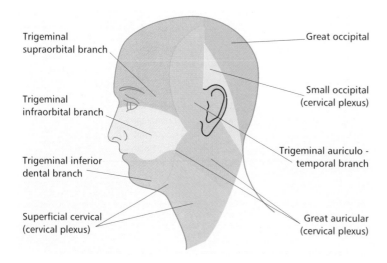

Trigeminal supraorbital branch

Trigeminal infraorbital branch

Trigeminal inferior dental branch

Superficial cervical (cervical plexus)

Great occipital

Small occipital (cervical plexus)

Trigeminal auriculo - temporal branch

Great auricular (cervical plexus)

Fig. 11.5 The distribution of the sensory nerves of the head. Compare with the sensory distribution shown in Figures 11.2 and 11.3.

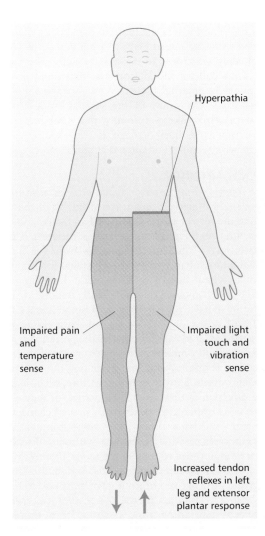

Hyperpathia

Impaired pain and temperature sense

Impaired light touch and vibration sense

Increased tendon reflexes in left leg and extensor plantar response

Fig. 11.6 Brown–Séquard syndrome (see Box 11.7). Note the distribution of corticospinal, posterior column and lateral spinothalamic tract signs. The cord lesion is on the left side.

In progressive spinal cord disease a characteristic sequence of clinical events occurs during the course of the untreated illness. The early involvement of sphincter function seen in intrinsic cord syndromes develops because these nerve fibres are situated deeply in the white matter, deep to the corticospinal fibres. Conversely, these fibres are involved relatively late in cord compression (Box 11.8). *The sequence of clinical events resulting from intrinsic spinal cord disease (e.g. syringomyelia) is different from that occurring in progressive extrinsic cord disease (e.g. compression of the cord by tumour).*

VASCULAR SUPPLY OF THE BRAIN AND SPINAL CORD

The brain is supplied by the internal carotid and vertebral arteries (Fig. 11.7). Embolism from the heart

---

BOX 11.7   Clinical features of the Brown–Séquard syndrome.

This is a clinical syndrome usually due to extrinsic compression of the cord, but it may also arise with intrinsic cord lesions.

Below the level of the lesion
Features ipsilateral to the lesion
- Impaired light touch
- Impaired vibration sense
- Corticospinal tract signs

Features contralateral to the lesion
- Impaired pain sensation
- Impaired temperature sensation

At the level of the lesion
Features ipsilateral to the lesion
- Segmental zone of hyperpathia (and spontaneous pain), representing irritation of the compressed segment
- Sometimes lower motor neurone signs at this level (e.g. in arm)

BOX 11.8   Features of progressive intrinsic and extrinsic spinal cord disease, in their order of development.

This sequence is particularly characteristic of tumours arising within the spinal cord, or compressing it from without.

Intrinsic disease
- Urge incontinence/retention of urine
- Dissociated sensory loss
- Spinothalamic pain
- Bilateral corticospinal tract signs
- Paraplegia and sensory level

Extrinsic disease
- Root pain, worsened by movement
- Progressive asymmetrical paraparesis
- Brown–Séquard syndrome
- Paraplegia with sensory level
- Incontinence/retention of urine and faeces

---

more frequently affects the left than the right carotid circulation. The two vertebral arteries unite at the lower border of the pons to form the basilar artery, which runs up the anterior surface of the pons in the midline, before dividing into the two posterior cerebral arteries. It gives off paramedian and short and long circumferential branches, which supply the pons and parts of the mid-brain and cerebellum. The *posterior cerebral artery* supplies the occipital lobe, the lower part of the temporal lobe and the uncus, the inner part of the crus and the corpora quadrigemina, and the posterior part of the posterior limb of the internal capsule. Occlusion of this artery

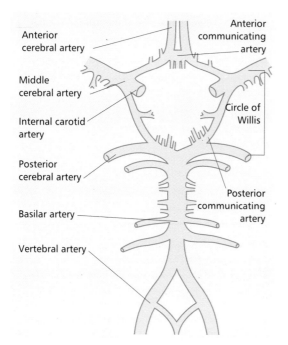

Fig. 11.7 The blood supply to the brain and the circle of Willis.

at its origin causes infarction of the occipital visual cortex and the sensory fibres in the internal capsule fibres; sometimes the calcarine artery, and hence the visual cortex, is affected in isolation.

The *internal carotid artery* gives off the *anterior cerebral artery*, which curves round the anterior end of the corpus callosum, and supplies the inner surface of the cerebral hemisphere as far back as the parieto-occipital fissure. It also supplies the superior frontal gyrus, and gives a branch to the anterior part of the internal capsule and to the basal ganglia.

The *middle cerebral artery*, which lies in the Sylvian fissure, is the main branch of the internal carotid artery. Embolism from the internal carotid artery or from the heart often involves the middle cerebral artery. The middle cerebral artery gives off *cortical branches*, which supply the frontal lobes, including the motor cortex, and the superior parts of the parietal and temporal lobes. These branches anastomose with those of the adjoining anterior cerebral and posterior cerebral arteries so that occlusion of one of them may sometimes be largely compensated by the establishment of a collateral circulation. The middle cerebral artery also gives off *central branches*, which penetrate into the brain substance and supply the central white matter and the basal ganglia. There are two main groups of these central branches: an anterior group called the *lenticulostriate*, and a posterior group, the *lenticulo-optic*. The lenticulostriate arteries are particularly associated with *hypertensive intracerebral haemorrhage*. These central arteries also anastomose with one another.

VENOUS DRAINAGE OF THE BRAIN

Venous blood leaves the brain in the *venous sinuses*. Blood from the interior of the brain enters the cerebral veins, which end in the straight sinus. The sagittal sinus collects blood from the brain and drains through the internal jugular veins into the superior vena cava. Occlusion of the sagittal sinus causes bilateral stroke-like symptoms with a combination of infarction and haemorrhage in the hemispheres, often with seizures and altered consciousness.

SPINAL ARTERIES

The *anterior and posterior spinal arteries* arise from the vertebral arteries and travel caudally in the pia mater, the former in the anteromedian fissure and the two latter on the posterior surface of the cord. These vessels receive radicular tributaries from the intercostal and lumbar arteries at each spinal level. In the lumbar region one of these radicular branches, the artery of Adamkiewicz, is particularly important. The anterior spinal artery supplies most of the spinal cord; only the posterior parts of the posterior horns and posterior columns are supplied by the posterior spinal arteries. Both anterior and posterior spinal arteries function as anastomotic vessels linking the radicular feeding vessels. Flow does not, therefore, occur in any one direction in these vessels but varies, or may even reverse, in response to local factors such as changes in posture and variations in intra-abdominal and intrathoracic pressure. There are two zones of *watershed flow* in the cord, one in the *upper thoracic cord* between flow descending from the vertebral circulation and flow derived from thoracic radicular feeding vessels, and another in the *lower thoracic region* between descending flow derived from thoracic feeding vessels and ascending flow from the artery of Adamkiewicz. These are sites of predilection for infarction of the spinal cord in, for example, aortic dissection.

SPINAL VEINS

The main veins of the spinal cord are situated dorsally and ventrally in the midline. Like the arteries, they communicate by radicular branches with the lumbar and intercostal veins, and empty into the vertebral veins. The blood in the spinal veins flows upwards; hence in compression of the spinal cord (e.g. by tumour) there is venous engorgement below the level of compression. This may be seen during myelography or magnetic resonance imaging of the spinal cord.

CLINICAL EXAMINATION OF THE NERVOUS SYSTEM

MENTAL FUNCTIONS

The neurologist is especially interested in the mental state in relation to features suggestive of organic disease of the brain. Nonetheless, the neurological approach to the mental state examination is similar to that taken by the psychiatrist, although with a difference in emphasis that reflects the different symptom complexes of organic and functional brain syndromes.

Analyse the mental state early in the examination, even if this analysis is limited to a subjective assessment of personality, memory, education and abstractional ability formed during the process of history-taking. This assessment is helpful in understanding symptoms. For example, if the patient's memory is impaired, his or her description of the illness will be limited. If the patient is comatose (see Ch. 15), confused, or unable to understand speech, any attempt to undertake a detailed examination is likely to be futile. If in doubt, talk to relatives or friends. Rapid bedside protocols for mental state testing which can be scored and used to quantify roughly the deficit are available (see Tables 3.1 and 3.2).

APPEARANCE, BEHAVIOUR AND COMMUNICATION

The patient's general bearing is important. A rough estimate of the level of intelligence can be made from the patient's vocabulary, and of the educational level from the occupational history. Note whether there is any disturbance of consciousness, such as confusion, stupor or coma:

- What is the patient's level of intelligence and education?
- Is the person disturbed, agitated or confused? Or apathetic?
- Is attention easily held, or fleeting?
- Does the patient show a reasonable degree of interest in his or her surroundings?
- What reaction is there to your approach and greeting?
- Is the patient well-groomed or unkempt?
- Are there any unusual features (e.g. facial tics or inappropriate behaviour)?
- Does conversation flow easily or not?
- Is the patient silent, monosyllabic or over-talkative?
- Is the content of speech and conversation appropriate and consistent?
- Are there features of *flight of ideas* (a rushing stream or ideas with some connection) or of *thought disorder*, when one remark follows another without logical connection?
- Does the patient keep on repeating your questions or their own remarks (*perseveration*)?
- Is there a disorder of language (*aphasia*)? Are strange words (*neologisms*) used or are real words strung together oddly (*word salad*)?

EMOTIONAL STATE

Make an assessment of the patient's *mood*. As a rough guide, consider your own reactions—do you feel sad or cheerful after talking with the patient?

- Is there a general impression of happiness, distress or depression?
- Does the patient enjoy life?
- Does the patient feel fed up with life, even perhaps to the extent that there is a risk of suicide?
- Does the play of facial features suggest preoccupation with a private world?
- Is the patient perplexed at their own mental state?
- Is there insight and understanding of the disorder and its implications?
- Note whether the patient seems irritable or resentful, or whether your words are received with suspicion.

Emotionally distressed or disturbed people (for example those with an anxiety state, depression or mania) often note *abnormal sleep*. Ask:

- Is sleep too long or too brief?
- If too long, is any particular action likely to precipitate this *hypersomnia*?
- If too little, is the difficulty in getting to sleep, waking frequently, or waking early in the morning and being unable to go to sleep again?
- Is there a physical cause for insomnia, such as pain, cough, asthma?

DELUSIONS AND HALLUCINATIONS

Delusions are false beliefs that continue to be held despite evidence to the contrary (see Ch. 3). Delusions are usually due to non-organic psychoses. *Hallucinations* are false impressions referred to the special senses (hearing, seeing, smelling, etc.) for which no cause can be found and which the patient knows to be imagined or unreal events. Hallucinatory experiences are often not volunteered and should be enquired for in patients suspected of suffering degenerative or paroxysmal disorders of the brain. Hallucinations of taste and smell are especially characteristic of temporal lobe epilepsy (*partial seizures*), and may be accompanied by a stereotyped visual hallucination of a half-remembered, unidentified scene perhaps experienced many years previously. Voices may be heard as part of this temporal lobe seizure. Hallucinations of small animals or insects crawling through the room, or on the walls or bed, are particularly associated with *delirium tremens* during withdrawal from alcohol. They are often accompanied by terror.

In *migraine*, an evolving scintillating patch (*scotoma*) in the visual field, with a hard ragged edge, often precedes the development of headache. In occipitoparietal lesions, complex visual hallucinations may occur.

ORIENTATION IN PLACE AND TIME

Test this with questions from the Mini-mental State Examination (see Table 3.2). Note down the patient's answers.

CLOUDING OF CONSCIOUSNESS

States of clouded or altered consciousness are important, particularly in patients with head injury or raised intracranial pressure who may gradually deteriorate during a period of observation. *Coma* is a state in which the patient makes no psychologically meaningful response to external stimulus or to inner need. In stupor the patient, although inaccessible, does show some response, for instance to painful stimuli. Above these levels various degrees of altered consciousness and lethargy can be recognized, which may be accompanied by confusion (see Ch. 3). The examiner must be alert to any minor defects in the patient's capacity to grasp what has happened. Such defects will usually be manifest in the patient's responses to tests for orientation, recent memory and appreciation of environment. The assessment of coma and altered consciousness is described in Chapter 15. In *dementia* (Box 11.9) the patient is awake and alert, but muddled in time, place and person (*confusion*), and has impaired memory and mental processing; in *delirium* the patient is similarly confused but alertness is impaired (i.e. the patient is *drowsy*). Thus, the demented patient may or may not also be delirious, and delirium—sometimes called an *acute confusional state*—can occur as an acute abnormality without underlying dementia. Dementia is not necessarily irreversible; it is a clinical syndrome which has a number of different causes.

MEMORY

Memory consists of the ability to grasp and retain new information. Memory therefore requires adequate processing of input, followed by registration and then appropriate recall. Memory is modality-specific, that is it can be related to auditory, visual, sensory or olfactory stimuli, or may be related to abstract or internalized experience (e.g. imagined material).

The degree to which recent memory is lost is an index of the severity of organic brain disorder (not necessarily permanent). Enquire about the day of the week and date in the month, and the names of prominent national and international public figures. Ask the patient to recall information recently read in the paper or seen on television. In formulating these questions, attention should be paid to the person's educational background and likely personal interests. Bring up a subject discussed a few minutes previously, or give the patient a simple story or address to remember, and note how much is remembered after a short interval or after distraction.

Short-term memory is memory for events of a few seconds or minutes past. It is characteristically impaired in Wernicke–Korsakoff syndrome, and in many patients with Alzheimer-type dementia. It is usually tested by assessing whether the patient can repeat seven digits backwards, with or without distraction, and by asking the patient to spell 'world' backwards. Working memory, consisting of memory for tasks involving mental manipulations, such as remembering a telephone number while dialling it, is usually spared in patients with disturbances of recent memory, for example in Wernicke–Korsakoff syndrome. *Long-term memory* is relatively resistant to the effects of neurological or psychiatric disease.

OTHER MENTAL TESTS

Tests of *reasoning* can be given at the bedside or in the clinic (Ch. 3). The most commonly used and robust tests are serial (100 – 7, etc.), spelling 'world' forwards and backwards—a test of memory as well as educational level—and questions such as asking which month precedes May and which precedes October, etc. Tests in which the patient is asked the meaning of rare words or asked to interpret common proverbs or sayings are commonly used as an index of *abstractional abilities. Judgement* may similarly be assessed: 'What would you do if you saw a house on fire?' or 'What would you do if you found a stamped and addressed envelope lying in the road?' In dementia these questions often provoke *concrete* answers or a confused reply. *Constructional* and *drawing* tests may also be useful (see below).

RELEASED REFLEXES IN DEMENTIA AND CONFUSIONAL STATES

In dementia and some organic confusional states, certain *'higher level' reflexes* may be elicited. Some may also be found in patients with large focal lesions; for example, the grasp reflex is characteristically released in patients with contralateral frontal lobe disease. In infancy the presence or absence of these reflexes is used as part of the developmental assessment (p. 394). The most important of these higher level reflexes are the *grasping and avoiding*

BOX 11.9   Clinical features of dementia.

Frontal lobe features
- Impaired judgement
- Altered, blunted personality
- Loss of emotional control
- Loss of mental inhibition
- Failure to plan ahead
- Impairment of language production

Temporal lobe features
- Loss of memory for recent events
- Impaired immediate recall
- Language disorder (Wernicke-type aphasia)
- Formed visual or auditory hallucinosis

Parietal lobe features
- Impaired sensory integration
- Disorientation in visual space
- Impaired visual recognition
- Receptive aphasia
- Disturbed body image

responses, the *palmomental reflex*, the *glabellar tap reflex*, and released oral responses such as the *snout response*, and tactilely and visually evoked *sucking reflexes*.

Grasping and avoiding responses

Grasping is elicited by stroking the palmar surface of the patient's hand on its radial aspect, preferably using a firm, distally moving stimulus between the patient's thumb and forefinger. The patient's hand grasps the examiner's. This grasp is not easily inhibited even if the patient is distracted, for example by being asked his or her address. If traction is applied by lightly pulling against the patient's flexed fingers, the patient tends to oppose with an equivalent force. Grasping is typically associated with contralateral frontal lobe disease. The *palmar avoiding response*, consisting of withdrawal of the patient's hand from dorsal, and sometimes from palmar contact is found in patients with contralateral parietal lobe disease or lesions in its connections. It is best evoked by lightly stroking the ulnar side or dorsum of the hand.

Palmomental reflex

The *palmomental reflex* consists of a brief contraction of the ipsilateral mentalis muscle, causing puckering of the chin, in response to scratching the skin near the thenar eminence with a key or pin.

Glabellar tap reflex

A series of sharp finger taps to the glabella normally elicits only two or three blinks before this response is inhibited, but in patients with diffuse degenerative disorders, especially senile dementia, and also in Parkinson's disease, the response is disinhibited and a blink follows each of a rapid train of stimuli.

Snout and sucking reflexes

Gentle pressure of the examiner's knuckle against the patient's lips causes reflex puckering of the orbicularis oris. This is usually associated with similar contraction of the facial musculature evoked by very light taps to the lips with a tendon hammer or with the fingers. Anticipatory opening of the mouth as part of released sucking may be elicited by approaching visual stimuli (e.g. the shining metal end of a tuning fork), or by light contact with the cheeks near the corners of the mouth.

SPEECH AND LANGUAGE

The distinction between defects of articulation and enunciation of speech (called *dysarthria*) and disturbances of the structure and organization of language itself (*aphasia*) is the first step in analysing speech.

DYSARTHRIA

With practice, defective *articulation* of speech can usually be identified reliably, even when the speech shows regional or foreign accents. *Stammering* is a developmental disorder, more common in boys than in girls. It is not usually due to acquired organic brain disease. In lalling, or 'baby speech', all the difficult consonants are dropped; the patient speaks like a baby. In adults this is usually the result of congenital or infantile deafness. Speech is usually louder than normal in the congenitally deaf. Certain constant features of different types of dysarthria can be recognized. There are four main types of dysarthria: *cerebellar, pseudobulbar, bulbar and cortical dysarthria*.

Cerebellar dysarthria

The patient speaks slowly and deliberately, syllable by syllable, as if scanning a line of poetry. The normal flowing, *prosodic* rhythm of syllable, word and sentence production is lost and in extreme forms each syllable is given equal emphasis. Ask the patient to say 'rhinoceros': it will be pronounced 'rhi-noc-er-os'. This scanning or staccato disturbance of speech rhythm is the classic form of severe cerebellar dysarthria. It is important to recognize minor, less obvious forms since its presence indicates bilateral disease of the cerebellum or of its brainstem connections. Minor cerebellar dysarthria causes slowing and slurring of speech.

Pseudobulbar (spastic) dysarthria

Individual syllables are slurred, and the precision of consonant pronunciation is lost. Thus 'British Constitution' becomes 'Brizh Conshishushon'. This form of dysarthria is due to bilateral lesions in the corticospinal fibres supplying the muscles of the face, larynx, tongue and respiration, i.e. the lesion is *supranuclear* to, or above the level of, these brainstem nuclei. It is therefore a feature of *pseudobulbar palsy*: the jaw jerk is brisk and, in most patients, examination of the limbs reveals evidence of bilateral corticospinal tract lesions (e.g. bilateral extensor plantar responses). Pseudobulbar dysarthria is a feature of an upper motor neurone lesion.

Dysphagia may be a prominent associated feature, with particular difficulty in swallowing liquids, including saliva. There is often *emotional incontinence*, the inappropriate production of released laughter or, more commonly, crying in response to an attempt to communicate. Sometimes a patient with a profound pseudobulbar palsy may be unable to make a sound, although comprehension is normal. This is called *aphonia*. In hysterical aphonia phonation occurs during spontaneous or voluntary coughing, or in singing, but in pseudobulbar aphonia coughing is silent.

Bulbar dysarthria

Bulbar palsy, due to lower motor neurone lesions affecting the speech musculature, results in non-specific slurring of speech. This is usually readily separated from other forms of dysarthria. There are usually other features of bulbar palsy, particularly *dysphagia*; fluids tend to be regurgitated through the nose and solid foods are difficult to swallow. Palatal air escape may be audible during phonation.

Cortical dysarthria

There is an irregular hesitancy in word production, associated with difficulties in abstract, volitional movements of the lips and tongue (*orofacial apraxia*). Cortical dysarthria is associated with aphasia due to left frontal and temporal lesions. It never occurs as an isolated abnormality and the term 'cortical dysarthria' should therefore be used with caution.

Formal tests for dysarthria

Nonsense syllables that test the lips and jaw—for example 'papapapa' and 'tatatata', the tip of the tongue 'sasasa', and the body of the tongue 'kakaka'—are useful. They can be combined into repetitive tasks as 'patakapataka' and 'fasaxafasaxa' to evaluate rhythm and prosody more objectively. The repetition rate is slowed in patients with dysarthria of any cause.

APHASIA

The term '*aphasia*' means a disturbance of the ability to use language, whether in speaking, writing or comprehending. In assessing an aphasic patient it is important to relate the functional defect in language to the patient's disability as a whole: how does it affect him or her? Formal analysis of the aphasia can then be attempted. This will help in understanding the patient's problem and in localizing the causative lesion (Fig. 11.8). Aphasia is an important neurological sign, even when it is only a very slight deficit, because it implies disease in restricted parts of the dominant hemisphere, almost always the left hemisphere (Fig. 11.9). No other clinical sign is specific for this localization. A common error is to fail to recognize a language disorder in a patient with fluent aphasia, and to erroneously diagnose a confusional state, which implies diffuse rather than focal brain disease.

Everyday use of language includes the following:

- The ability to *use words* in spoken speech. This includes *articulation, fluency* (the ability to put words together into phrases and sentences of varying complexity, in various grammatical constructions, without hesitations and errors), *naming* and the accurate *repetition* of complex statements and concepts.
- The ability to *comprehend* spoken speech.
- The ability to *read to oneself* (not aloud).
- The ability to *write*.
- The ability to comprehend *other symbols*, e.g. mathematical or musical symbols.

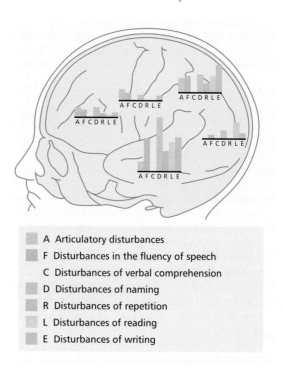

A Articulatory disturbances
F Disturbances in the fluency of speech
C Disturbances of verbal comprehension
D Disturbances of naming
R Disturbances of repetition
L Disturbances of reading
E Disturbances of writing

Fig. 11.8   The average degree of disturbance of various language modalities which occurs when there is an isolated lesion of various lobes (frontal, Rolandic, parietal, temporal and occipital).

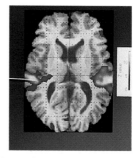

Fig. 11.9   PET scanning. Listening to words-fMRI. When the subject listens to words, both temporal lobes are activated, but the dominant left temporal lobe (to the right of the picture) is the more active.

Speech defects can be analysed, therefore, as disturbances of *articulation, fluency, verbal comprehension, naming, repetition, reading and writing* (Fig. 11.8). Disturbances of fluency, verbal comprehension, repetition and writing are all prominent in left anterior temporal lobe lesions (*amnestic or Wernicke's aphasia*). Left frontal lesions affect articulation and fluency more than the other categories of language. Left parieto-occipital lesions impair reading (visual language functions); left parietal lesions impair several other associative functions, but particularly writing. Generally, the lateralization of speech corresponds to handedness, but most left-handed people have left hemisphere dominance rather than right.

Assessment of articulation and fluency on the one hand and of reading and writing on the other enables recognition of lesions in front of and behind the central sulcus (Rolandic fissure). This is a useful clinical concept—'anterior' and 'posterior' aphasic syndromes. The terms 'expressive' and 'receptive' aphasia are more or less synonymous but they ignore the equally important functions of reading, writing, repetition, articulation and fluency. When examining an aphasic patient, assess spoken and written speech separately.

Assessment of spoken speech

First assure yourself that the patient's hearing is adequate. *Fluency* is best assessed in spontaneous conversational speech. Begin by assessing speech in the context of an ordinary conversation about everyday things or about the patient's illness itself. Note the presence of hesitations, the searching for a forgotten word, and its compensation by the use of a descriptive phrase (*paraphasia*). Note any *neologisms* (invented or nonsense words), or inappropriately used words or phrases. Note also any articulatory disturbances, particularly clumsiness and difficulty in coordinating movements of lips and tongue (*orofacial apraxia*). Orofacial apraxia is a *bilateral* disturbance of lip and tongue movement that can occur with *unilateral*, left frontal lesions. It is usually very pronounced when the patient is asked to put out the tongue or close the eyes and these movements should not, therefore, be used to establish comprehension of speech or the patient's cooperation.

The aphasic patient can often use only a few words. Note these, and any words or phrases repeated again and again (*perseveration* or *repetitive utterances*). If the patient has a considerable vocabulary, note whether speech is slurred, and consider whether the disorder is only a disturbance of *articulation* rather than aphasia. Test speech articulation with such words and phrases as 'British Constitution', 'West Register Street', 'biblical criticism', 'artillery', and the nonsense syllables described above. Then show some common objects—a knife, a pen, a matchbox, etc.—and ask the patient to *name* them. Sometimes patients with aphasia have a general idea of the word they want to use, but cannot exactly pronounce it; they may omit some syllables or substitute others, so that the listener can hardly make out the word intended. In anterior aphasias patients are often well aware of the difficulty, since they can monitor their speech; this is distressing. These are signs of *amnestic* or *nominal* aphasia.

Patients with left posterior lesions, whether in addition to a frontal lesion or occurring alone, show defective ability to monitor their own speech. Their speech not only shows syllabic and word substitutions but it may contain *neologisms*. Mistakes in the use of words, such as calling a knife a pen, are examples of *word substitution*, a more marked abnormality than *syllabic substitution*. In extreme examples of this disorder, characteristic of left posterior temporal lesions, speech consists of syllabic neologisms making no sense at all—*jargon aphasia*. Patients with jargon aphasia tend to talk incessantly, often in relation to inappropriate sounds in their environment, for example, in response to a voice on the radio or in another part of the room. Thus patients with left frontal lesions speak hesitantly, with poor fluency, and those with left temporoparietal lesions speak fluently, but their speech is often devoid of meaning. A further point of difference between these two types of speech defect is that patients with more posteriorly placed lesions show marked difficulties in comprehension of spoken speech. Indeed, this is a marked feature of patients with *fluent aphasia*, since it is an underlying defect in the adequate monitoring of these patients' own spoken speech.

Speech repetition is a useful test. Patients with left frontal lesions can repeat words and simple phrases, although they may introduce syllabic or other errors, but those with more posterior lesions may be unable even to approach the task. The patient should be asked to repeat a simple sentence, clearly stated by the examiner, such as: 'Today is Wednesday June 4th, and this is the Royal London Hospital'. Remember never to shout at an aphasic patient: hearing is normal. If the patient is able to repeat what you say, endeavour to find out whether or not what you have said has been heard and understood. Finally, ask the patient to read aloud, note whether they can find their way about the page, and whether speech errors appear.

Assessment of written language

Reading and writing tests are important in the assessment of aphasia.

Reading

Reading aloud tests the visual comprehension of language and spoken speech. Reading silently tests comprehension of language through the visual system; this is best tested by asking the patient to obey simple written commands without reading aloud, for example 'Touch your nose with your left hand'. When the patient reads aloud, errors in spoken speech can be readily detected since the intended speech pattern is known from the written material. Disturbances of reading are called *dyslexia*. Functional magnetic resonance imaging (MRI), and positron emission brain imaging (PET) studies have shown that words and non-word sounds are handled differently in the brain (Fig. 11.9), and that people with congenital dyslexia show abnormal processing of words (Fig. 11.10).

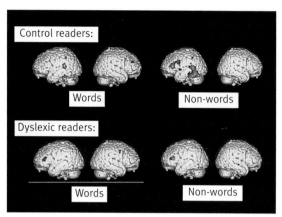

Fig. 11.10   PET scanning. Normal and dyslexic readers. Note that the language part of the temporal lobe is more active in normal readers than in congenitally dyslexic subjects, who are unable to process language normally.

Writing

A specific central impairment of writing is called *dysgraphia*. Ask the patient to write his or her name. Ask for a written reply to a simple question such as 'What is your address?' If verbal comprehension is poor, put your question in writing. If the right hand is paralysed, ask the patient to write or print with the left. Note whether the patient uses a wrong word at times, or whether there is repeated use (*perseveration*) of any particular word. Can the patient write to dictation or copy words and sentences? Try, using a newspaper.

Comprehension of other symbols

Write down some simple calculations, such as:

$$
\begin{array}{ccc}
2 & 2 & 2 \\
+2 & +2 & +2 \\
\hline
4 & 5 & 6
\end{array}
$$

and ask the patient to point out which is correct. Inability to understand and manipulate mathematical symbols, *acalculia*, may occur in posterior parietal lesions affecting the dominant hemisphere.

Gesture

Many aphasic patients make attempts to use gesture to communicate, but gestural language may be impaired in patients with anterior lesions. Furthermore, many aphasic patients, especially those with Wernicke's (temporal) aphasia, or with posterior fluent aphasias, do not fully understand complex gestural instructions.

APRAXIA

The term '*apraxia*' means the inability to perform certain acts or movements, even though there is no sensory defect, weakness, or ataxia. The underlying components of the movement can be performed sep-

arately. The apraxic patient is unable to use objects, though their use can be recognized and described. Apraxia results from damage to the left parietal cortex or to parietal white matter of the left or of both hemispheres, or from disease of the connections between the two hemispheres through the corpus callosum. Rarely, when the corpus callosum is damaged, apraxia may affect only the left side, since the dominant left hemisphere is then disconnected from the right hemisphere. However, apraxia is more commonly a bilateral disorder.

Apraxia can be formally tested for by asking the patient to use objects or to make or imitate certain movements. For instance, when given a box of matches and asked to strike a match the apractic patient may fail to open the box, or to take a match from it, or to strike the match, or may show an inability to recognize which end to strike against the box. It is, of course, important to be sure that the patient understands the request. In *ideational apraxia* the patient has no concept of the use of the object, in *ideomotor apraxia*, the concept is present but the motor programme for the usage is not accessible.

THE CRANIAL NERVES

Examination of the functions of the cranial nerves is an important part of the neurological assessment. The third to twelfth cranial nerves arise from the brainstem and innervate facial, cranial and cervical tissues. The first and second cranial nerves actually consist of central nervous tissue rather than peripheral nerve. All the cranial nerves may be involved in disease processes in their intracranial and extracranial courses, and at their sites of origin within the brain and brainstem.

THE OLFACTORY (FIRST) NERVE

The central processes of the bipolar sensory cells in the olfactory epithelium pass through the cribriform plate to the second olfactory neurones in the olfactory bulb. The olfactory bulb neurones project to the olfactory centres in the uncus and parahippocampal gyrus.

Testing smell

Have three small bottles containing pungent odours, such as oil of cloves, oil of peppermint, or tincture of asafoetida. Common bedside substances such as soap, fruit or scent may also be used. Present these to each nostril separately and ask the patient to name them. Avoid the use of irritating substances such as ammonia, since these partially stimulate the trigeminal nerve. In *anosmia* (Box 11.10) the sense of smell is absent. Before concluding that this is due to neurological disease exclude local changes in the nose itself, such as catarrh. *Parosmia* is a rare abnormality of olfaction in which pleasant odours seem offensive. *Hallucinations of smell* may occur as an aura of a temporal lobe seizure.

- Closed head injury
- Subfrontal meningioma
- Previous bacterial meningitis
- HIV infection
- Sinusitis
- Other local nasal disorders
- Drugs (e.g. copper-chelating agents, antibiotics)

THE OPTIC (SECOND) NERVE

From the retina, the fibres of the *optic nerve* (Figs 11.11 and 11.12) project to the *optic chiasm*, where fibres from the inner nasal half of each retina, representing the temporal field, decussate. Those from the outer temporal half, representing the nasal field, remain on the same side. The *optic tracts*, formed by this decussation, consisting of fibres from the outer half of the retina on the same side, and from the inner half of the retina on the opposite side, project to the *lateral geniculate bodies*; some pregeniculate fibres project to the superior colliculi. The *optic radiation* projects from the lateral geniculate body through the posterior limb of the internal capsule to the striate *calcarine cortex of the occipital lobe* (Fig. 11.13). The input from homologous fields of the two eyes is represented in the geniculate bodies and in the striate visual cortex in adjacent columns of neurones.

Fibres subserving the upper visual fields pass through the white matter of the temporal lobe; those from the lower field pass through the parietal lobe. The left half of the visual field is represented in the right calcarine visual cortex and vice versa (Fig. 11.12). The most peripheral part of the visual field is represented anteriorly in the calcarine fissure and the most medial part, the macular field, is represented at the occipital pole (Fig. 11.12).

TESTING VISION

Always examine the *visual acuity* and the *visual fields*. Colour vision, visual localization, visual recognition and other aspects of vision, such as motion perception, may also be tested, if appropriate. Ensure that any refractive error is corrected and that ocular disease that might impair the visual acuity or the visual fields is recognized. Test each eye separately. Test the visual acuity before testing the visual fields. The visual acuity is a measure of central visual sensitivity. Vision better than 6/60 in the metric system, (20/200 in Imperial feet) implies that some macular function is present.

Visual acuity

For technique of testing, see Chapter 12.

Visual fields

The visual field is the whole extent of the field of vision in each eye. It is limited by the size of the retina and by the margins of the orbit, nose and cheek. The visual field is larger to large than to small objects, or to bright than to dim objects. *Colour* vision is mainly confined to the central or macular field, corresponding to the central part of the retina rich in *cone cells*. The *rod cells*, sensitive to white light, are more uniformly distributed across the whole area of the retina. Moving stimuli are best perceived in the peripheral field since specialized movement-sensitive receptor cells are located mainly in the peripheral parts of the retina, especially in the *unpaired temporal crescent*. This part of the retina is also particularly responsive to the sudden appear-

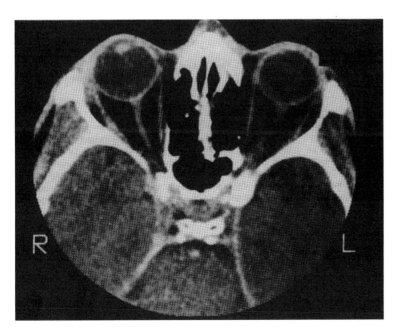

Fig. 11.11 Computerized tomographic (CT) scan of the head in a normal subject. This CT image is oriented in the plane of the orbits. Both eyes are visible. In the right eye the lens appears as a relatively high-attenuation zone. In the orbits the medial and lateral rectus muscle and the optic nerves can be seen forming a cone with its apex at the posterior margin of the orbits. The temporal lobes are situated on either side of the pituitary fossa and optic chiasm. The two orbits are separated by the nose and ethmoid sinuses.

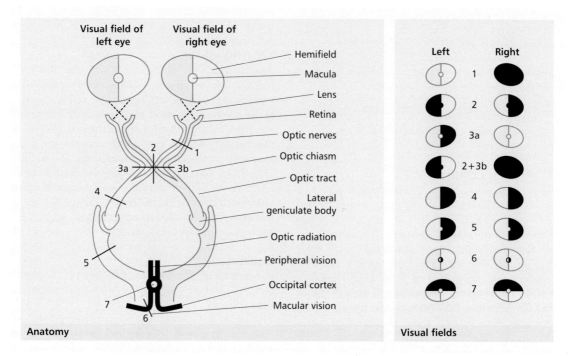

Anatomy

Visual fields

Fig. 11.12 The visual pathways. Lesion at 1 produces blindness in the right eye with loss of the direct light reflex. Lesion at 2 produces bitemporal hemianopia often beginning in the central fields as a bitemporal scotomatous defect. Lesions at 3a and 3b produce binasal hemianopia (a rare disorder). Lesions at 2 and 3b produce blindness of the right eye with temporal hemianopia of the left visual field. Lesion at 4 produces right homonymous hemianopia with macular (splitting) involvement. Lesion at 5 produces right homonymous hemianopia with sparing of the macular field. Lesion at 6 produces right homonymous central (macular) hemiscotoma.

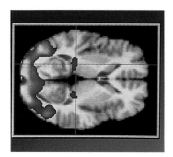

Fig. 11.13 PET scanning. Functional segregation in the visual system. Activation of the visual system during a visual task. The occipital cortex and its association cortex, and the lateral geniculate bodies are visible.

ance or disappearance of stationary visual stimuli, but appreciation of the form of an object is poorly developed in this part of the field. Form and detail are best perceived in the central field; it is this aspect of visual function that is tested by assessment of the *visual acuity*.

The visual cortex contains columns of neurones that are responsive to precise visual stimuli, for example, dark surrounds, linear dark–light junctions oriented in particular planes, and specialized colour-receptive cells. This cortical organization enables the matrix of cells in the retina to function as a precise transducer of visual information in terms of position, shape, size, colour and movement. The higher level

cortex related to vision contains groups of cells, and even individual cells, responsive to environmental recognition, visual memory (modality-specific memory) and facial recognition. Colour vision itself is processed in a particular part of the visual-related cerebral cortex.

Plotting the visual fields

There are several methods for assessing the *visual fields*. The simplest and most practical is *confrontation testing*—comparing the extent of the patient's visual field with your own. Both eyes should be tested together first (*binocular testing*), and then each must be tested separately (*monocular testing*) to exclude a field defect limited to part of the visual field of one eye only.

Confrontation test using a finger

This test maps the whole field. Sit opposite the patient, at a distance of about 1 metre. To test the field in the right eye, ask the patient to cover the left eye with the left hand, and to look steadily at your left eye. Cover your right eye with your right hand and gaze steadily at the patient's right eye. In this way slight movements of the patient's eye, which cause errors in the test, can be detected. Hold up the index finger of your left hand in a plane midway between the patient's face and your own, at first at almost a full arm's length to the side. Test the four quadrants of the field separately. Keep moving your finger and bring it nearer to the midline until you yourself first perceive moving fingers. Ask the patient to say when first they see the movement, making sure all the time that he or she steadily fixes gaze on your eye. If the patient fails to see the fingers, keep bringing your hand nearer until he or she does see them. Test the field *in each eye separately* in every direction—upwards, downwards, to right and to left—using the extent of your own field for comparison.

Red pin confrontation test

This is a sensitive test of the *central field*. Instead of using your finger, use a red-headed pin, held up as in the finger confrontation test. It is sometimes useful to mount the pin on the rubber eraser of a pencil, in order to be sure your hand is out of the patient's visual field. This method allows the patient's field, including the size of the physiological blind spot (see below), to be compared precisely with the examiner's field. *A good rough and ready preliminary test is to ask the patient to compare the contour and colour of the palm of your hand held up separately in the fields of each eye.* When there is disturbed central vision the patient will notice a difference in colour intensity in the two eyes; however, disease in the lens (e.g. cataract) and other ocular diseases also cause this abnormality.

The central, macular field of vision extends about 20 degrees from the fixation point. This central visual field may be relatively intact when the peripheral fields are markedly restricted (Fig. 11.12). The central field is often abnormal when there is disease of the anterior visual pathways, for example optic neuritis. A central area of impaired vision (*central scotoma*) can be recognized by this method because the red pin-head cannot be perceived in the scotoma or, in less severe examples, because the intensity of the red colour is reduced (desaturated) in this part of the field.

The *physiological blind spot* is situated to the temporal side of the central point of fixation of the visual field. It corresponds to the point of entry of the optic nerve into the retina; this is the *optic disc*, found slightly to the nasal side of the macula when visual-ized with the ophthalmoscope. At the optic disc there are no retinal receptor cells and there is thus a small blind spot in the field corresponding to this region. It should always be possible to identify this blind spot when testing the visual field to confrontation with a red pin, and its size should correspond exactly with the examiner's own blind spot when the red pin is held equidistant between the examiner's eye and the patient's eye. The blind spot sometimes appears to be absent in an uncooperative patient, or if the patient is attempting to mislead the examiner. Less reliance can be placed on visual field testing in such patients.

Perimetry

The visual field can be quantitatively mapped using a *perimeter*. There are many different types of perimeter but all use the same principles, adapted for testing peripheral or central vision. Automated perimeters, commonly used in eye departments, allow the patient to sit comfortably with the chin resting on a chin rest adjusted so that the eye to be tested is oriented at the centre of a hemispherical, illuminated field, upon which spots of light of various intensities, colours or sizes may be projected (*static perimetry*), or moved (*kinetic perimetry*), in order to detect the limits of the field and its sensitivity in various parts. In the more elaborate perimeters, the examiner can observe the patient's eye through a small telescopic eyepiece in the centre of the hemisphere, in order to detect any movement of the patient's eye away from fixation on this central point. Simpler, portable perimeters can also be used with good results. These consist only of a hemispheric arm along which a small white or coloured disc of varying size may be moved by a simple mechanical system.

The area within 30 degrees from fixation (that includes the 20 degrees of macular vision) is best examined either with an automated perimeter, having first corrected any refractive errors with lenses, or by using a *Bjerrum screen*. The Bjerrum method is simple, easy to use, and does not require complex or expensive equipment. The patient sits with the head steadied by a chin- and head-rest 1 or 2 metres from a 2-m^2 wall-mounted black screen. A white object, 10 mm in diameter, is fixed to the centre of the screen on a level with the patient's eye to act as a fixation point. The blind spot is mapped first, using another white object 10 mm in diameter. The peripheral field is then mapped with the same 10-mm object: at a distance of 2 metres the field should be circular and extend to about 25 degrees, that is, to the edge of the 2-m^2 screen. With a smaller white or red object areas of blindness or defective perception are sought around the blind spot, especially between this area and the macula (the *centrocaecal* area), and in the horizontal meridian on the nasal side of the fixation spot (Fig. 11.14). The limits of the fields for each test object are marked on the screen with black pins, and subsequently transferred to a chart for recording in the patient's case notes. Each test object is

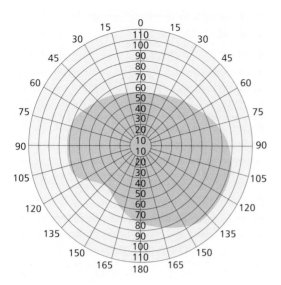

Fig. 11.14 The extent of the right field of vision with a white target of 20 mm diameter mapped on a perimeter at a distance of 330 mm.

to define an area bounded by an isopter—a line joining points of equal acuity (Fig. 11.14).

Since the fixation point of the *monocular field* is not exactly central, and the field is not a circle, but an irregular ovoid, the outer and inner parts of the field are unequally divided. With a test object of 5 mm diameter the average field of vision is 100 degrees laterally, 60 degrees superiorly, 60 degrees medially and 75 degrees inferiorly. The slightly larger field charted with a 20-mm object is shown in Fig. 11.14; note the restriction of the lower nasal field by the bridge of the nose. The *binocular field* extends 200 degrees in the lateral plane and about 140 degrees vertically. Most of the visual field is binocular. On each side of the area of binocular vision is a lateral semilunar area which is unpaired (i.e. it is monocular) and which accounts for the remainder of the field. This is called the *temporal crescent*. Since the visual acuity is much lower at the periphery than at the point of fixation, it is possible, by using a graduated series of objects, to plot out a series of isopters, each of which corresponds to the field for a known size of object, at a known distance from the eye and at a constant illumination.

ABNORMALITIES IN THE FIELD OF VISION

A zone of loss of vision in the centre of the field is called a *central scotoma*. A unilateral central scotoma is a common feature of demyelination in the optic nerve (*optic neuritis*), a common feature in *multiple sclerosis*. *Paracentral scotomas* are due to disease of the choroid or retina near the macula. When unilateral paracentral scotoma is often due to *vascular disease*, such as retinal embolism or *retinal artery branch occlusion*. When bilateral, paracentral scotomata may be due to toxic causes, especially alcoholism or vitamin B_{12} deficiency. *Glaucoma* can

cause a paracentral *'arcuate' scotoma*; this has a characteristic comma-like shape and is due to damage to a nerve fibre bundle in the retina or optic nerve. Bilateral paracentral scotoma can also result from a lesion in the posterior part of the visual cortex, but this is very rare (see Fig. 11.12).

Hemianopia means loss of sight in one-half of the visual field. When the same half of both fields of vision is lost, the hemianopia is described as *homonymous*—for example right homonymous hemianopia when the right half of the field of each eye is affected (see Fig. 11.12). Blindness limited to one quadrant of a field is termed a *quadrantanopia*. When the visual loss in the homonymous fields of the two eyes is similar (*congruous hemianopia*) the lesion is likely to be post-geniculate. *Incongruous hemianopa* is more likely to be due to a lesion in the optic tracts or chiasm. *Superior or inferior altitudinal hemianopia* means loss of the upper or lower halves of the visual field respectively. This may occur with damage to an optic nerve by ischaemia or trauma. Bilateral altitudinal field defects are uncommon; they are usually due to occipital lesions. *Bitemporal hemianopia* is loss of vision in the temporal (outer) halves of both fields. It is due to loss of function of the nasal half of each retina. It can only be produced by a lesion of the optic chiasm, involving those fibres of the optic nerves, derived from the nasal parts of the retina, which decussate at this site. The most common causes are pituitary tumours or perichiasmal inflammatory or traumatic lesions extending out of the sella turcica to involve the optic chiasm (Fig. 11.15). The bitemporal loss in these disorders may not involve the whole temporal field, but is often restricted to the central fields, indicating clinical importance of testing the central visual fields. *Binasal hemianopia* means loss of the nasal or inner half of each field, indicating loss of function of the temporal half of each retina. It is very rare, but results from bilateral lesions confined to the uncrossed optic fibres on each side of the optic chiasm. It may also occur in open-angle glaucoma. Bitemporal and binasal hemianopias are sometimes described as *heteronymous*, in contradistinction to the homonymous variety.

Concentric constriction of the visual fields sometimes occurs in long-standing papilloedema, in bilateral lesions of the striate (visual) cortex and in some retinal disorders (e.g. retinitis pigmentosa). It is also found in frightened patients. *Tunnel vision*, in which the concentric constriction is of the same extent even when tested at a distance, is a classic feature of simulated disease, and of hysterical conversion. The normal field is 'cone shaped', so that it is larger in area when the patient is tested at 2 metres than at 1 metre.

Colour vision

For methods of testing, see Chapter 12.

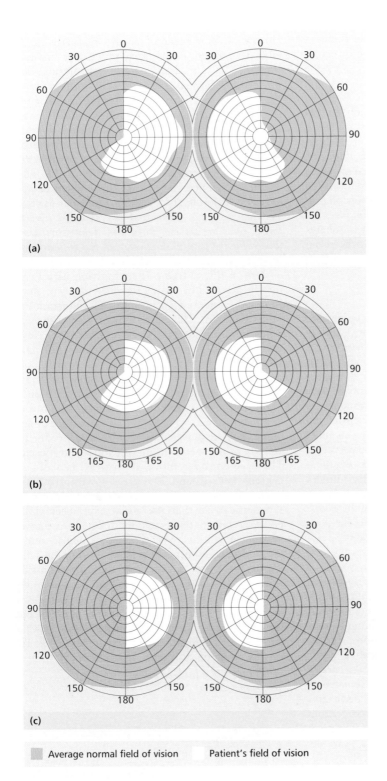

(a)

(b)

(c)

| Average normal field of vision | Patient's field of vision |

Fig. 11.15 Fields of vision in a patient with a pituitary tumour (chromophobe adenoma) showing the development of bitemporal hemaniopa. These fields were plotted many years ago; in the modern era of safe neurosurgery, operative decompression of the optic chiasm by hypophysectomy would have been carried out at the time of initial diagnosis in May. **(a)** May: VA (visual acuity) Lt 6/12 Rt 6/18.
(b) August: VA Lt 6/12 Rt 6/12.
(c) October: VA Lt 6/12 Rt 6/12. The fields were plotted on a Bjerrum's screen at a distance of 2 m from the eye to the point of fixation at the centre of the screen, using a 10-mm white object. The coloured areas show the average normal field of vision and the white areas show the patient's field.

Subjective visual sensations

Floaters (muscae volitantes)—little grey specks seen floating before the eyes, especially on looking at a white surface or up to the sky—are a common normal phenomenon due to awareness of parts of the retinal blood vessels seen reflected from the posterior surface of the lens, or to vitreous opacities. In *migraine*, zigzag lines, known as 'fortification figures' or *teichopsia* are a characteristic feature at the beginning of the attack. *Visual hallucinations* occur in a number of neurological diseases, notably in delirium tremens and in temporal and occipitoparietal disorders; they may also form part of the aura in epilepsy. *Photopsias*, tiny white flashes seen in the visual field, may occur in acute optic neuritis. They are often induced by ocular movement.

Visual agnosia and cortical blindness

Complex disturbances of visual perception and of visually directed behaviour result from lesions in the parietal connections of the occipital cortex, especially inattention to visual stimuli in the abnormal field. In *visual agnosia* (*Anton's syndrome*), due to lesions in the central parietal connections of the striate cortex, the patient is unaware or uncomprehending of the visual deficit. In *cortical blindness* the lesions are in the striate cortex of both hemispheres and the patient is aware and distressed by the visual disorder. The pupillary light reflexes are normal in both of these cortical disorders.

OCULAR MOVEMENTS AND PUPILS

The external ocular movements, and the pupils, are controlled by the *third* (oculomotor), *fourth* (trochlear) and *sixth* (abducens) nerves. These nerves arise from nuclei in the brainstem, and function as a physiological unit. They are located in the brainstem close to the Sylvian aqueduct at the level of the superior corpora quadrigemina, and extend caudally to the floor of the fourth ventricle. The nucleus of the *third nerve* is the most rostral of the three; its most rostral neurones supply parasympathetic innervation to the ciliary muscle and iris (*Edinger–Westphal nucleus*); neurones innervating extraocular muscles are located in the more caudal part of the oculomotor nucleus. Caudal to this is the nucleus of the *fourth nerve*. The *sixth nerve nucleus* is situated in the floor of the fourth ventricle at the level of the pons.

The *third nerve* emerges on the inner aspect of the cerebral peduncles, between the *superior cerebellar and posterior cerebral arteries*, and passes forward in close relation to the *posterior communicating artery* before entering the lateral wall of the *cavernous sinus*. It is thus at risk in patients with brain herniation associated with cerebral mass lesions, and in aneurysms of the posterior communicating arteries. The fourth nerve emerges on the rostral part of the roof of the *fourth ventricle*. The *fourth nerve* is, uniquely, the only cranial nerve that decussates between its nucleus and its point of emergence from the brainstem, and that emerges dorsally. The *sixth nerve* emerges between the medulla and pons. Its long intracranial course renders it particularly vulnerable to the effects of pressure.

The sixth nerve innervates the external rectus muscle and the fourth nerve innervates the superior oblique muscle. All the other extraocular muscles, the sphincter pupillae (the muscle that causes pupillary constriction during accommodation) and the levator palpebrae superioris, are supplied by the third nerve.

Ocular movements

Horizontal movement of an eye outwards (laterally) is termed *abduction*, movement inwards (medially) is termed *adduction*; vertical movement upwards is termed *elevation* and downwards is *depression*. The eye is also capable of *diagonal* movements (*version*) at any intermediate angle. *Rotary* movements—the eye rolling like a wheel towards the nose (internal rotation) or away from the nose (external rotation)—are not possible voluntarily, but occur normally as part of the reflex compensation necessary to adjust for slight degrees of head tilt during tasks involving macular fixation, as when reading. Note that *the superior and inferior recti act as elevators and depressors alone when the eye is in abduction, and the superior and inferior obliques act similarly when the eye is in adduction* (Fig. 11.16). Their function may therefore be assessed by testing the movements of elevation and of depression in both full abduction and full adduction. This test of ocular movement is much more informative than simply testing elevation and depression in the mid-position of gaze. Lateral gaze, however, must always be tested along the horizontal meridian. Vertical and horizontal ocular movements made from the mid-position of gaze are called *cardinal movements*. The medial and lateral recti always act directly in a single plane, but all movements require the coordinated activity of the whole group of extraocular muscles. The eyes normally move 50 degrees medially, 30 degrees upwards and 50 degrees downwards.

The movements of the two eyes are normally symmetrical, so that the visual axes meet at the point at which the eyes are directed—*conjugate* movement of the eyes. Conjugate ocular movements depend on brainstem integration of the activity of the third, fourth and sixth nerve nuclei. *Infranuclear* (lower motor neurone) lesions of the third, fourth and sixth nerves lead to weakness of individual eye muscles or groups of muscles, and *supranuclear* (upper motor neurone) lesions lead to paralysis of conjugate movements of the eyes. The classification of disorders of ocular movement is shown in Box 11.11.

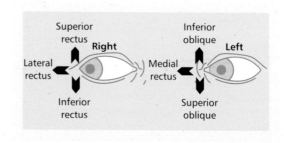

Fig. 11.16　The action of the external ocular muscles with the patient confronting the examiner.

Lower motor neurone (infranuclear) lesions

Infranuclear lesions of the sixth, fourth and third nerves lead to the following abnormalities:

Sixth nerve

- Inability to move the eye outwards (laterally) with *diplopia* (double vision)
- Sometimes *convergent squint*—because of the unopposed action of the medial rectus, innervated by the ipsilateral third nerve.

Fourth nerve

- Impaired downward movement
- On downward gaze in mid-position the eyeball is rotated outwards by the unopposed action of the inferior rectus (Fig. 11.16).

- Diplopia only below the horizontal plane, with the images uncrossed, but the false one tilted. Rarely, a visible squint.

Third nerve

- Downward and lateral displacement of the eye
- Movement only laterally and a little downwards
- Dilated pupil, due to unopposed action of the cervical sympathetic innervation of the dilator pupillae muscle
- Loss of reflex pupillary constriction on accommodation.

These are the features of a complete oculomotor nerve palsy (Fig. 11.17). However, third nerve palsy is often partial, and in some cases, particularly diabetic third nerve palsy, the pupil is spared. The pupillary abnormalities found in third nerve palsy must not be confused with those of sympathetic lesions (Horner's syndrome), in which there is no abnormality of ocular motility.

In summary, lesions involving one or more of the three nerves controlling ocular movement cause:

- Defective movement of the eye
- Squint
- Double vision (*diplopia*)
- Pupillary abnormalities.

Of these signs, diplopia and pupillary abnormalities are the most consistent.

STRABISMUS

A squint or strabismus is an abnormality of ocular movement such that the visual axes do not meet at the point of fixation. Strabismus is not necessarily accompanied by diplopia. There are two types: *paralytic* and *non-paralytic*.

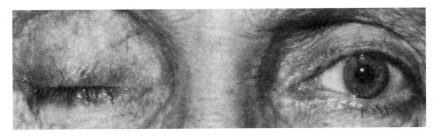
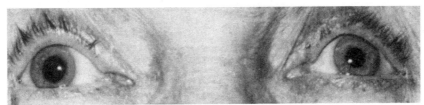

Fig. 11.17   Right third nerve palsy. Note the right ptosis, the dilated pupil, and the external strabismus. This was due to a berry aneurysm of the right posterior communicating artery.

Paralytic strabismus (squint)

Paralytic strabismus is due to weakness of one or more of the extraocular muscles. The following clinical features occur:

Limitation of movement

In paralytic strabismus weakness of one or more extraocular muscles causes impairment of ocular movement in the direction of action of the muscle(s) affected. Although this weakness is usually obvious it is sometimes so slight, or the unaffected muscles mask it so much, that the defective movement of the eye is hardly apparent.

When an eye fails to move at all, or fails to move through its normal angular excursion, the angle of deviation of this eye, compared with the observed movement of the normal eye, is the *squint* or *primary deviation*. This is the angle which a line from the object to the nodal point of the eye makes with the visual axis. If the unaffected eye is covered, so that the patient fixates with the affected eye (cover test, see below), the covered normal eye will deviate still more than the primary deviation of the affected eye. This deviation of the healthy eye is called the *secondary deviation* and occurs because of the disparity between the progammed neural activity of the brain and the lack of actual movement caused by the weakened muscle. The difference between the primary and secondary deviations in paralytic strabismus is the most important feature differentiating it from concomitant, non-paralytic strabismus.

False orientation of the field of vision

A patient with paralysis of the right lateral rectus muscle who closes the left eye and attempts to touch an object held in the horizontal plane on the right side will point wide, to the right side of the object. This results from information reaching the brain from the retina due to the weakness of action of the affected lateral rectus muscle failing to match the position expected to result from the execution of the motor programme for that movement. This is a form of sensory mismatch.

Dizziness or instability

Dizziness may occur in paralytic strabismus when both eyes are open. It is due to the confusing experience of double vision and to false orientation.

Diplopia

Patients with paralytic strabismus complain of double vision. This occurs because defective movement of one eye results in the images from the two eyes arising from different points on the two retinae. Binocular fusion cannot therefore occur in the visual cortex and two separate or overlapping images are perceived. In paralytic strabismus, the image from the macula of the healthy eye is seen distinctly (the *true image*), whereas the image on the affected side is derived from the retina outside the macula. This latter image is indistinct and blurred; it is called the *false image*. Most patients can clearly recognize which of the two images is the true and which the false image. The false image is projected into that part of the field of vision into which the paralysed muscle should move the eye if it were normal; it is perceived *in the direction of action of the weak muscle*. Doubt as to which is the false image can usually be resolved by covering one eye with a red glass and asking the patient whether the red or the normally coloured image is the real one (*red glass test*, see below).

In order to overcome diplopia, the head may be involuntarily turned in the direction of action of the paralysed muscle. This *head tilt* gives information as to which muscle is involved.

Diplopia should always be assessed in the nine cardinal directions of gaze (Fig. 11.16 and Box 11.12). The objective of this formal analysis is to *decide to which eye the furthest displaced of the two images, i.e. the false image, belongs*. Move the test object in the cardinal directions until the position of maximal displacement of the two images is ascertained.

Red glass test

Examine the patient seated, with a red glass over the right eye and a clear glass over the left. At a distance of about 0.5 m move a light in the directions indicated in Box 11.12. Each of the lateral squares corresponds to a pair of associated muscles. Thus maximal vertical diplopia produced when the patient looks up and to the right, into the right superior square, shows that either the right superior rectus or the left inferior oblique muscle is the affected muscle. In this example, the higher of the two images, the false image, indicates the affected eye.

Remember that in *paralytic strabismus* the angular deviation of the two visual axes varies with different

---

> **BOX 11.12   Charting diplopia in the nine cardinal directions of gaze in paralytic diplopia (see also Fig. 11.16).**
>
> The muscles used in each direction of gaze are listed
>
> | Upwards to the left | Upwards | Upwards to the right |
> |---|---|---|
> | left SR | left and right SR | right SR |
> | right IO | left and right IO | left IO |
> | | | |
> | *To the left* | *Straight ahead* | *To the right* |
> | left LR | contraction of all | right LR |
> | right MR | extraocular muscles | left MR |
> | | | |
> | *Downwards to the left* | *Downwards* | *Downwards to the right* |
> | left IR | left and right IR | right IR |
> | right SO | left and right SO | left SO |
>
> SR = superior rectus; IR = inferior rectus;
> LR = lateral rectus; MR = medial rectus;
> SO = superior oblique; IO = inferior oblique.

positions of the two eyes, and the secondary deviation is always greater than the primary deviation.

Non-paralytic strabismus

In *non-paralytic (concomitant) strabismus*, the angular deviation of the visual axes is the same in whatever position the eyes move, so that the primary and secondary deviations are always equal. *Thus, the ocular axes are misaligned, but there is no weakness of the external ocular muscles.* This is common in 'congenital strabismus'.

Use the *cover test* to assess the primary and secondary deviations. Ask the patient to look at an object immediately in front of him or her. Suddenly cover the apparently fixing eye. If the uncovered eye makes any movement in taking up fixation, it must have previously been deviating, indicating that a squint is present. If the eye now behind the cover (which was previously fixing) is now tested by uncovering it, it will deviate in the same relative direction as was the other eye, and *to the same angular amount*, that is, the primary and secondary deviations are equal.

The *clinical features* of non-paralytic strabismus are as follows:

- It begins in early childhood, usually before the fifth year and almost always before 3 years of age
- The movements of the eyes, tested individually, are full in all directions
- Diplopia is almost never a symptom
- The primary and secondary deviations are equal
- The deviating eye usually has defective vision (amblyopia ex anopsia).

A squint may be *intermittent* or *constant* and, if constant, *monocular* when only one eye deviates whilst the other usually fixes, or *alternating* when either eye fixes independently. An *esophoria* is a medial deviation of the eye under cover, with the eye moving outwards to fix gaze when the cover is removed. An *exophoria* is an external deviation under cover with medial movement when the cover is removed.

SUPRANUCLEAR GAZE PALSIES

These are upper motor neurone palsies of gaze movements, such impairment or paralysis of the movement of *both* eyes in one direction (*conjugate gaze palsy*). The patient may be unable to look to either side, or upwards or downwards; or convergence alone may be lost. Paralysis of *lateral conjugate gaze* is characteristically found with lesions in the pons. The lesion is in the pontine paramedian reticular formation (PPRF) near the abducens and vestibular nuclei. *Bilateral paralysis of lateral conjugate gaze* may occur with centrally placed pontine lesions above the level of the abducens nuclei. Weakness of lateral conjugate movement also occurs in hemiplegia due to cerebral lesions, when there is disruption of the connections from the frontal eye fields, especially in the acute stage of a stroke. Palsies of *conjugate upward gaze* indicate disease of the central parts of the mid-brain or inferior thalamic region, often near the oculomotor nuclei. Impaired *downward gaze* is very rare, but occurs with brainstem lesions at a lower, usually medullar, level.

Tonic conjugate deviation of the eyes is an abnormality in which both eyes are kept persistently turned in one direction, usually in the lateral plane. It is usually due to a lesion causing weakness of conjugate gaze, but may also occur in irritate cortical lesions. In the former, the eyes (and usually also the head) are turned towards the side of the lesion, if the lesion is in the cerebral hemisphere, as in a patient with acute hemiplegia, i.e. the patient 'looks towards his lesion'. An *irritative cortical lesion* causes deviation towards the healthy side, usually accompanied by nystagmoid jerks of the eye toward this side. This is a form of *focal epilepsy*. If the lesion is in the pons, these rules are reversed, the deviation being towards the sound side in a paralytic lesion. Irritative lesions in the brainstem, however, are exceptional. *Skew deviation of the eyes*—in which one eye is directed upwards and the other downwards—occurs in lesions of the labyrinth and in cerebellar disease. Other abnormal ocular movements, such as *ocular bobbing*, *opsoclonus* and *ocular dysmetria*, also associated with acute cerebellar lesions, are rare.

Saccadic movements are rapid, programmed, conjugate, fixation movements that normally arise for visual or auditory stimuli. *Pursuit* movements are slower conjugate following movements, determined by visual fixation, that involve macular reflexes. Assessment of *saccadic* and *pursuit* gaze movements is useful in practice. Ask the patient to move the eyes rapidly from fixation on one finger to another held about 30 degrees away in the horizontal plane; then ask the patient to follow a slowly moving finger across visual space in the same horizontal plane, or in the vertical plane. In Parkinson's disease, pursuit movements are slowed, or interrupted by slowed saccades. In Huntington's disease, an inherited dementia with chorea; upward and lateral saccades are slow, but downward saccades are usually of normal velocity. In higher level disturbances of visual perception (e.g. parieto-occipital lesions causing agnosia or misperceptions of visual space to one side) saccadic movements may be impaired toward the midline in the affected field.

Internuclear ophthalmoplegia is due to a lesion in one medial longitudinal fasciculus in the mid-brain or upper pons. On attempted lateral gaze there is rhythmic nystagmus of the abducting eye with impaired medial deviation of the adducting eye. The latter may cause diplopia. In addition, the adducting eye moves more slowly than the contralateral abducting eye, especially during attempted saccadic movements. The abnormality is less obvious if tested only during slow ocular following movement. Movements in all other planes, and the pupils, are normal. The lesion is on the side of the impaired adduction, not on the side of the nystagmus (Fig. 11.18). This sign is important because it is common in multiple sclerosis, when it is often bilateral.

In the '*one-and-a-half syndrome*' a lesion in the parapontine region involves both the pontine paramedian reticular formation (PPRF) and the medial longitudinal fasciculus (MLF) (Fig. 11.18) on the same side. There is failure of lateral conjugate gaze to one side (the side of the lesion), together with impairment of adduction of the eye on that side and nystagmus on abduction (lateral movement) of the opposite eye. The latter is the only horizontal movement possible; one eye will not move at all horizontally and the other only in abduction—one-and-a-half lateral movements are paralysed. Vertical gaze movements and the pupillary reactions are normal.

NYSTAGMUS

Nystagmus is a disturbance of ocular movement characterized by involuntary, conjugate, often rhyth- mical oscillations of the eyes. These movements may be horizontal, vertical or rotary. In any given direction of gaze the speed of the movement is quicker in one direction than the other; the *quicker movement*, representing reflex correction of a slower deviation in the opposite direction, conventionally describes the direction of the nystagmus, and indicates the side of the lesion in the cerebellum or brainstem.

Ask the patient to look straight ahead and note whether the eyes remain steady. Then ask the patient to look to the extreme right, then to the left, and then upwards and downwards. It is best to ask the patient to look at your finger in each of these positions. Observe the rate, amplitude and rhythm of any nystagmus in each direction of gaze and whether or not it is sustained.

Nystagmus is graded as follows:

- *Grade 1.* Nystagmus with fast phase to left, looking toward the left.
- *Grade 2.* Nystagmus with fast phase to left, looking straight ahead.
- *Grade 3.* Nystagmus with fast phase to left, looking toward the right.

Nystagmus occurs in disorders of the vestibular system, either central or peripheral, and with lesions of the central pathways concerned in ocular movements (e.g. *the vestibulocerebellar connections in brainstem or cerebellum* or *the medial longitudinal fasciculus*), or with weakness of the ocular muscles (e.g. myasthenia gravis). *Vestibular nucleus nystagmus* is jerk-type, often with a rotary component, and not worsened by positional stimuli. *Labyrinthine nystagmus* is also jerk-type, with a rotary component, but is induced by positional changes. *Gaze-evoked nystagmus* is irregular and conjugate. *Convergence-retraction nystagmus* is due to high brainstem lesions, and is often associated with impaired conjugate upward gaze. Nystagmus is often induced by *drugs*, especially benzodiazepines, phenytoin and other anticonvulsant drugs, and barbiturates. Nystagmus due to long-standing visual impairment (e.g. 'miner's nystagmus') is pendular and often rotary on central fixation of the eyes. *Congenital nystagmus* also shows this pendular quality. Some forms of vestibular nystagmus, particularly that associated with benign epidemic vertigo, and with posterior fossa neoplasms, may be induced only by certain movements of the head (*positional nystagmus*). A few irregular jerks of the eyes are often seen in full lateral deviation in normal subjects. The brief duration and irregularity of these normal ocular movements distinguish them from true nystagmus.

Optokinetic nystagmus is a physiological phenomenon that occurs when the patient follows a rapidly moving scene (*railway train nystagmus*). The eyes fixate and follow the moving stimulus and then refixate by making a rapid saccade back to the

(a)

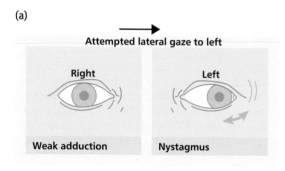

(b)

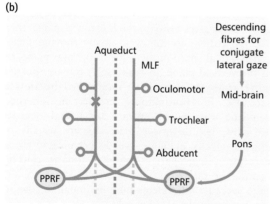

Fig. 11.18   **(a)** Right internuclear ophthalmoplegia. This abnormality is a frequent clinical feature in patients with multiple sclerosis. **(b)** Diagrammatic representation of interconnection of oculomotor, trochlear and abducent nerve nuclei with the pontine paramedian reticular formation (PPRF) via the medial longitudinal fasciculus (MLF). A lesion (X) in the right NLF will cause impaired adduction of the right eye with nystagmus of the abducting left eye during attempted lateral gaze to the left. A lesion in or near the PPRF causes impaired conjugate lateral gaze to the same side.

primary position of gaze. There is thus a slow component in the direction of the moving stimulus and a fast phase in the opposite direction. This phenomenon has been used in a crude test of visual acuity by utilizing a striped drum or tape with stripes of varying width, but testing for optokinetic nystagmus is used mainly to assess patients with hemianopia or brainstem lesions. In *parietal hemianopia* there may be neglect of the visual environment on the hemianopic side, even with a very mild degree of visual impairment; this is accompanied by suppression of the fast phase of optokinetic nystagmus when the stimulus is moving from the abnormal visual field toward the normal field. The fast phase is replaced by a slow tonic deviation of the eyes in the direction of movement of the stimulus. In *brainstem lesions* optokinetic testing is useful in establishing the presence of conjugate gaze palsies, internuclear ophthalmoplegia and abnormalities of the velocity of saccadic eye movements.

EXAMINATION OF THE PUPILS
Always note the size, shape and reactivity of the pupils to light and accommodation.

Size
Compare the size of the two pupils, first in ordinary illumination and then in a bright light, such as a flashlight. Note whether the pupils are large or small at rest, and whether any irregularity is present. The size of the pupil in healthy subjects is variable. As a rule, the pupils are larger in dark eyes than in light eyes. They tend to be small in elderly subjects. Slight inequality of the pupils may be present in perfectly healthy subjects. If one pupil is larger than the other, which is the abnormal? This is not always easily decided, but the pupil which is less mobile is usually the abnormal one.

Shape
Note whether the pupil is circular in outline, as it should be, or whether its contour is irregular. Irregularities are usually due to adhesion of the iris to the lens, as a result of an old iritis.

Mobility
The pupillary reaction to light is a reflex. The afferent fibres travel in the optic nerve, leaving it before the synapse in the lateral geniculate bodies, and entering the brainstem in the pretectal region. These afferent fibres synapse in the oculomotor nuclei. The efferent fibres, which are parasympathetic, reach the pupillary sphincters in the oculomotor nerve after synapsing again in the ciliary ganglion in the orbit.

Testing the light reflex
Use a shady, indirectly illuminated room, and examine each eye separately. Ask the patient to look into the distance, for example across the room, to be sure accommodation is relaxed. Shine a bright light into one eye; the pupil should contract almost immediately, then dilate again a little and, after undergoing a few slight oscillations, settle down to a smaller size. When the light is switched off the pupil will rapidly dilate to its previous diameter.

Swinging light test
This is a test for an afferent (optic nerve) pupillary abnormality. Because some of the fibres in the optic nerves decussate in the optic chiasm, light shone into one eye stimulates the brainstem oculomotor nuclei concerned with pupillary constriction bilaterally. When a bright light is shone into one eye, *both pupils contract*. This is the *consensual pupillary reaction*. To test the consensual light response keep one eye shaded while shining a bright light into the other. Observe the pupil of the unilluminated eye. The pupillary constriction may be brisk and well-sustained in the stimulated eye but, when the light is shone immediately into the other eye, this pupil may slowly dilate a little, and then oscillate (*hippus*), indicating that the consensually mediated light reaction of the second eye is more active than its direct reaction. On this second side there must therefore be an *afferent defect* (Gunn pupil), i.e. a lesion in the optic nerve. This is a particularly useful sign in *optic neuritis* and in ischaemic or compressive lesions of the optic nerve. In some patients with post-chiasmal but pregeniculate hemianopia, the pupillary light reaction is less active when a narrow beam of light is shone from the hemianopic side than when shone from the normal side. However, this *hemianopic pupillary reaction* sign (Wernicke pupil reaction) is difficult to elicit.

Accommodation reaction
The pupils become smaller on accommodating for a near object (*miosis*). Convergence of the eyes, accommodation and miosis are closely related reflexes. Hold up one finger close to the patient's nose. Ask the patient to look away at a distant object. Then ask him or her to look quickly at your finger. As the eyes converge the pupils become smaller. If vision is defective ask the patient to hold his or her own finger about 30 cm in front of the face, and then to 'look at the finger'. Accommodation is rarely lost in brainstem lesions but may be impaired with lesions of the oculomotor nerve and in autonomic neuropathies.

The *Argyll Robertson pupil* is the classic pupillary abnormality of neurosyphilis. The pupil is small and irregular, reacts briskly to accommodation, but does not react to light directly or consensually. The pupil dilates slowly and irregularly to conjunctival atropine instillation. The abnormality is typically bilateral but it is usually more marked on one side. The lesion is in the pretectal region of the mesencephalon.

The *tonic or Adie pupil* is characterized by absent or delayed pupillary constriction to light or to accommodation/convergence. Once constricted the pupil dilates only very slowly, either in response to darkness or to far gaze. The pupil may thus appear small or large (more usually larger) and this sometimes leads to confusion with the Argyll Robertson syndrome. The pupil in Adie's syndrome varies in size from day to day but *never* reacts promptly to light. The abnormality is frequently unilateral so that it may cause unequal pupils (*anisocoria*). It is sometimes associated with absent tendon reflexes, often on the same side as the pupillary abnormality (Holmes–Adie syndrome). The distinction between the Argyll Robertson and Adie pupillary abnormalities is important since the latter, probably due to partial parasympathetic denervation, is of little clinical significance. The distinction may be made by instillation of sterile 2% methacholine into the conjunctival sac; the Adie pupil constricts but the Argyll Robertson pupil does not.

Horner's syndrome is due to paralysis of the cervical sympathetic nerve. The sympathetic nerve fibres supplying the pupil originate in the lower cervical and upper thoracic regions of the spinal cord (C8 and T1), from which they emerge in the first thoracic nerve roots and pass to the sympathetic ganglia by the rami communicantes. From the cervical sympathetic chain the sympathetic nerve fibres pass along the internal carotid to the cavernous plexus, and thence via the ophthalmic division of the trigeminal nerve to the eye. Sympathetic nervous activity causes pupillary dilatation and elevation of the upper lid, the latter through contraction of the smooth muscle fibres in the levator palpebrae superioris.

In Horner's syndrome the pupil is small, due to the unopposed action of the parasympathetic fibres in the third nerve. In the upper eyelid there is smooth muscle as well as striated muscle. This smooth muscle is innervated by the cervical sympathetic nerves. Slight ptosis therefore occurs after a lesion of the cervical sympathetic but the pupil is then small (see Fig. 12.16), rather than large as in third nerve palsy. There is a slight degree of enopthalmos (apparent retraction of the eye into the orbit). There may be loss of sweating on the forehead, the face and neck, both in front and behind, extending as low as the third rib and third thoracic spine, and over the whole of the upper limb on the same side. Lesions in the cervical sympathetic have different causes on the two sides because of the different course of the cervical sympathetic within the chest.

Horner's syndrome consists of the following:

- Slight drooping of the upper lid (ptosis)
- Pupillary constriction
- Absence of pupillary dilatation on shading the eye or on instillation of cocaine
- Loss of the ciliospinal reflex.
- Impaired sweating on the ipsilateral face.

Ciliospinal reflex
Dilatation of the normal pupil when the skin of the neck is pinched is due to reflex excitation of the pupil-dilating fibres in the cervical sympathetic. The response is abolished by lesions of the cervical sympathetic and, sometimes, by medullary, cervical and upper thoracic cord lesions.

THE FIFTH (TRIGEMINAL) NERVE
The *sensory root* of the fifth nerve originates from nerve cells in the trigeminal (Gasserian) ganglion and enters the lateral surface of the pons at about its middle. Fibres which subserve light touch terminate in a large nucleus in the pons, situated lateral to the motor nucleus near the floor of the fourth ventricle, while the fibres for pain and thermal sensation enter the descending bulbospinal tract, which extends as low as the second cervical segment of the cord before ascending in the medial lemniscus. Immediately distal to the trigeminal ganglion the nerve separates into its three divisions (Fig. 11.19). The *first or ophthalmic division* supplies the conjunctiva and the conjunctival surface of the upper but not of the lower lid, the lacrimal gland, the mesial part of the skin of the nose as far as its tip, the upper eyelids, the forehead, and the scalp as far as the vertex. Lesions of the ophthalmic division result in loss of cutaneous and corneal sensibility in the areas described above. Trophic changes in the cornea (*neuropathic keratitis*) may occur. The corneal reflex is abolished.

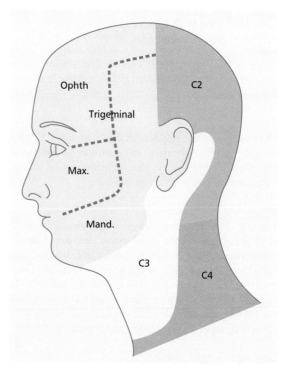

Fig. 11.19 Lateral view of the skin area supplied by the trigeminal (fifth) nerve and the second, third and fourth cervical segments.

The *second or maxillary division* supplies the cheek, the front of the temple, the lower eyelid and its conjunctival surface, the side of the nose, the upper lip, the upper teeth, the mucous membrane of the nose, the upper part of the pharynx, the roof of the mouth, part of the soft palate, the tonsils, and the medial inferior quadrant of the cornea. Lesions of the maxillary division lead to loss of sensation in the above areas and occasionally to loss of the palatal reflex.

The *third or mandibular division* supplies the lower part of the face, the lower lip, the ear, the tongue, and the lower teeth. It also supplies parasympathetic innervation to the salivary glands. The mandibular division is joined by the motor root and this innervates the muscles of mastication. The *motor root* originates from a small nucleus, medial to the main sensory nucleus, and partly also from nerve cells scattered around the cerebral aqueduct. It emerges at the side of the pons, just anterior to the sensory division, passes inferior to the trigeminal ganglion, and joins the mandibular division.

Lesions of the whole trigeminal nerve lead to loss of sensation in the skin and mucous membrane of the face and nasopharynx (see Fig. 11.19). The salivary, buccal and lacrimal secretions may be diminished and trophic ulcers may develop in the mouth, nose and cornea. Taste is spared, but lack of oral secretions may result in its subjective impairment. Weakness of the muscles of mastication is often a prominent feature.

Testing motor functions of the fifth nerve

Ask the patient to clench the teeth: the temporal and masseter muscles should stand out with equal prominence on each side (this is better checked by palpation than by inspection). If there is paralysis on one side, the muscles on that side will fail to become prominent and, on opening the mouth, the *jaw will deviate towards the paralysed side*, being pushed over by the healthy lateral pterygoid muscles.

Testing the sensory functions

Test sensory acuity in the trigeminal innervation (Fig. 11.19) to light touch, cold and pin prick.

Testing the corneal reflex

Twist a light wisp of cotton into a fine hair and lightly touch the lateral edge of the cornea at its conjunctival margin with the wisp, having asked the patient to gaze into the distance or at the ceiling. If the reflex is present the patient blinks. It is helpful to steady your hand by gently resting the little finger on the patient's cheek. The two sides should be compared. The corneal reflex can sometimes be tested more easily by lightly blowing a puff of air into each cornea in turn. The cornea should *never* be touched or wiped with the cotton wisp, since in the presence of corneal anaesthesia there is a risk of corneal ulceration.

THE SEVENTH (FACIAL) NERVE

The facial nucleus is situated in the pons lateral to the nucleus of the abducens nerve. On leaving the facial nucleus the axons wind round the abducens nucleus and emerge medial to the vestibulocochlear nerve, between the olive and the restiform bodies. The facial nerve enters the internal auditory meatus. In the temporal bone, in close proximity to the aditus of the tympanic antrum, it gives off a branch to the stapedius muscle. The nerve fibres subserving taste from the anterior two-thirds of the tongue pass from the lingual nerve into the chorda tympani, joining the facial nerve in its course through the temporal bone, and pass through the geniculate ganglion of the facial nerve and the nervus intermedius into the medulla oblongata. The intra-temporal part of the nerve is vulnerable to trauma and oedema, since it is enclosed in a bony canal. It emerges at a point opposite the junction of the anterior border of the mastoid process with the ear, and spreads out on the side of the face to supply the facial muscles. The facial nerve is almost entirely a motor nerve. It supplies all the muscles of the face and scalp, except the levator palpebrae superioris. It also supplies the platysma. In facial palsy due to intratemporal lesions there is sometimes a small area of altered cutaneous sensation at the auricle, representing the somatic afferent component of the facial nerve.

Taste

The sense of taste should always be examined when a facial nerve lesion is suspected. Taste in the anterior two-thirds of the tongue is subserved by the facial nerve, but the taste fibres from the posterior third of the tongue enter the brainstem in the glossopharyngeal nerve. All the taste fibres enter the tractus solitarius and relay in the nucleus of this tract. The ascending fibres pass via the thalamus to the temporal part of the post-central gyrus and to the amygdala. *Ageusia* or loss of taste occurs with lesions of the peripheral pathways or with centrally placed pontine lesions, which may involve the gustatory lemnisci. Loss of taste may result from lesions in any part of the peripheral and central course of the taste fibres.

In addition to asking about loss of taste, ask whether there have been any abnormal taste sensations or hallucinations of taste. These may form the aura of an epileptic fit, especially in temporal lobe epilepsy. Test the sense of taste using strong solutions of sugar and common salt, and weak solutions of citric acid and quinine, as tests of '*sweet*', '*salt*', '*sour*' and '*bitter*' respectively. Apply these solutions to the surface of the protruded tongue with a small swab on a spatula. The patient should be asked to indicate perception of the taste *before* the tongue is withdrawn in order to decide whether taste is disturbed anteriorly or posteriorly. After each test the mouth must be rinsed. The bitter quinine test should be applied last, as its effect is more lasting than that of the others.

Motor effects of facial nerve lesions

These are usually obvious. The affected side of the face has lost its expression. The nasolàbial fold is less pronounced, the furrows of the brow are smoothed out, the eye is more widely open than on the normal side. *Bilateral* facial weakness can be difficult to recognize.

Testing the facial nerve

The following five tests can be used to test for facial nerve lesions:

- Ask the patient to shut their eyes as tightly as possible. Note that the affected eye is either not closed at all or, if the eye is closed, the eyelashes are not so deeply buried in the face as on the healthy side. Try to open the eyes while the patient attempts to keep them closed. If the orbicularis oculi is acting normally, it should be almost impossible to open them against the patient's effort. The effect of screwing the eyes tightly shut causes the corners of the mouth to be drawn upwards. In paralysis of the lower part of the face, the corner on the affected side is either not drawn up at all, or not so much as on the healthy side. Food fragments collect between teeth and gums. Saliva, and any fluid that has been drunk, may escape from the affected angle of the mouth.
- *Bell's phenomenon*, in which the eyeball rolls upwards during attempted forced eye closure, is a normal phenomenon which is preserved in facial palsies of lower motor neurone type. It is thus particularly obvious when eye closure is impossible in a patient with facial nerve palsy.
- Ask the patient to whistle—this is impossible in facial palsy.
- Ask the patient to smile or show the upper teeth. The mouth is then drawn to the healthy side.
- Ask the patient to inflate their mouth with air and blow out the cheeks. Tap with the finger on each inflated cheek in turn. Air can be made to escape from the mouth more easily on the weak or paralysed side.
- Finally, test the sense of taste on the anterior part of the tongue.

Localizing facial weakness

Lesions situated above the facial nucleus, in the nucleus, or distal to it, result in different types of facial weakness. Lesions above the facial nucleus cause *upper motor neurone* or *supranuclear facial palsies*, lesions in the nucleus cause *nuclear facial palsy*, and lesions distal to the nucleus cause *lower motor neurone* or infranuclear paralysis.

In *supranuclear facial paralysis* the lower part of the face is chiefly affected. This is because the parts of the facial nuclei innervating the upper face are bilaterally innervated. A unilateral lesion, therefore, will cause only partial paralysis of the upper part of the face, including eye closure, on the one side, but movements of the mouth on that side will appear much more severely affected. Sometimes a supranuclear lesion, usually thalamic in location, affects only the fibres concerned in emotional movement; this function should be assessed separately from voluntary movement. Taste is not affected in supranuclear lesions. Facial reflexes, elicited by lightly tapping the facial muscles around the mouth, are often increased in supranuclear lesions. Supranuclear lesions do not produce facial muscle atrophy.

In *infranuclear facial paralysis* at the level of the whole facial nerve (e.g. in the temporal bone) both the upper and lower parts of the face are equally involved, because the final common pathway is damaged. Infranuclear facial paralysis may be produced by a lesion of the nucleus or of the facial nerve itself. A lesion inside the facial canal—unless it is towards the outer end—involves the fibres of the chorda tympani and therefore also causes loss of taste sensation in the anterior two-thirds of the tongue. Because the stapedius muscle is paralysed, sounds on the side of the facial palsy may seem unusually loud (*hyperacusis*). A lower motor neurone lesion, whether nuclear or infranuclear, causes atrophy of the facial muscles. Partial facial nerve lesions occur with peripheral lesions (e.g. in parotid cancer) which may cause weakness of the lower face but not the upper.

Abnormal facial movements

The muscles supplied by the facial nerve are frequently affected by spasmodic (*synkinetic*) movements. These may involve all the facial muscles, or only groups of them. They occur most commonly as a result of aberrant regeneration of facial nerve fibres during partial recovery from an infranuclear (e.g. Bell's) lesion. Facial spasms of a different type occur in some patients with dystonia and in other extrapyramidal disorders, especially tardive dyskinesias following phenothiazine medication. They may also occur in multiple sclerosis and in hemifacial spasm.

THE EIGHTH (VESTIBULOCOCHLEAR) NERVE

This special sensory nerve consists of two components. One innervates the cochlea and subserves hearing; the other supplies the labyrinth and semicircular canals and subserves equilibration, balance and sensations of bodily displacement.

The *auditory* fibres, which arise from the cochlear ganglion, enter the brainstem at the lower border of the pons and are distributed to the dorsal and ventral cochlear nuclei. The secondary auditory tracts, after partial decussation, terminate in the inferior colliculi and the medial geniculate bodies, and another system that takes origin from these passes through the internal capsule to the cortical centre for hearing in the first and second temporosphenoidal gyri.

Sounds received in one ear reach the opposite hemisphere of the brain, but owing to the partial decussation of the secondary auditory tracts neither unilateral cerebral nor brainstem lesions produce unilateral deafness.

The *vestibular* fibres originate in the vestibular ganglion, and terminate in a group of nuclei in the pons and medulla. The vestibular nerve is closely connected with the cerebellum. It also has a cerebral projection to the temporal lobe.

Abnormal auditory sensations

Tinnitus is a persistent 'ringing in the ears'. The character of the sound varies. It may be humming, buzzing, hammering or whistling. Although common, it is almost never due to neurological disease. *Hyperacusis*, a disorder in which even slight sounds are heard with painful intensity, sometimes occurs when there is paralysis of the stapedius muscle due to a facial nerve palsy. *Recruitment*, occurs in patients with sensorineural deafness due to damage to the cochlea, as in Ménière's syndrome (Ch. 13). *Auditory hallucinations* and *delusions of voices* are common in the non-organic psychoses (e.g. schizophrenia), but may also occur in organic psychoses. Other complex auditory hallucinations, for example music, sometimes arise as epileptic auras when there is a lesion in the temporal lobe.

Tests of hearing

See Chapter 13.

Vertigo

The patient will usually describe this as *giddiness, dizziness* or *unsteadiness*. In vertigo, external objects seem to move round the patient. Ask about this and, if so, in what direction the environment seem to move. Ask also whether the vertigo or giddiness causes loss of balance. The distinction between vertigo and giddiness is rarely important. Both may occur in disease of the vestibular system, i.e. the ear, vestibulocochlear nerve, brainstem, or temporal lobe. The examination is described in Chapter 13.

Positional vertigo

In some patients vertigo is induced by certain head postures, or by sudden changes in head posture. The subjective sensation of rotational disequilibrium is accompanied by a rotary nystagmus in the primary position, often enhanced by gaze to one or other side. If this posture is reproduced during examination, for example by suddenly lying the patient in the supine position, the nystagmus and vertigo will develop either after a short delay (*benign positional vertigo*, associated with labyrinthine disease) or immediately (an indication of serious *brainstem disease*). It usually continues for only a few seconds. Benign positional vertigo can often be elicited only once or twice in an examination (p. 309).

THE NINTH (GLOSSOPHARYNGEAL), TENTH (VAGUS) AND ELEVENTH (ACCESSORY) NERVES

The glossopharyngeal, vagus and accessory nerves arise in an elongated nucleus in the floor of the fourth ventricle. They emerge by several roots along the lateral aspect of the medulla, beginning rostrally in the groove between the olive and restiform bodies. The spinal part of the accessory nerve emerges from the lateral column of the cord, perhaps beginning as low as the sixth cervical root. It passes up through the foramen magnum to join its medullary part, and emerges with it through the jugular foramen. After emerging, its two divisions separate, the medullary or accessory portion joining the vagus nerve and supplying motor fibres to the larynx and pharynx. The spinal portion supplies the sternomastoid and the upper part of the trapezius muscle.

The glossopharyneal nerve

The ninth nerve is sensory from the posterior third of the tongue and the mucous membrane of the pharynx. It supplies motor fibres to the middle pharyngeal sphincter and the stylopharyngeus muscle. It contains taste fibres from the posterior third of the tongue.

The glossopharyngeal nerve is rarely damaged alone, but damage can best be diagnosed by examining the nerve's sensory and reflex functions. Loss of taste in the posterior part of the tongue may occur with a lesion of the trunk of the glossopharyngeal nerve.

Tickle the back of the pharynx, and note if reflex contraction occurs (*palatal reflex*). This is also a test of the vagus (below).

The vagus nerve

Motor and sensory vagal axons originate in the nucleus ambiguus, emerge in the upper roots of the accessory nerve, pass through the pharyngeal plexus, and innervate the muscles of the palate, pharynx, and larynx through the *recurrent and superior laryngeal nerves*. Visceromotor and the cardio-inhibitory parasympathetic fibres originate in the dorsal nucleus of the vagus in the floor of the fourth ventricle. Damage to the vagus is obvious clinically only through its *palatine* and *laryngeal* branches.

The palate

Ask if there has been *regurgitation of fluids* through the nose during swallowing. This is a common symptom in total paralysis of the soft palate, due to defective elevation of the palate during swallowing. In addition, in palatal palsy the patient is unable to pronounce words that require complete closure of the nasopharynx (*palatal dysarthria*). Thus 'egg' is sounded as 'eng', 'rub' becomes 'rum', and so on. In unilateral paralysis these symptoms are not so severe, or may even not be apparent. Difficulty in swallowing (*dysphagia*) particularly affects solids in lower motor neurone lesions, but is more marked for fluids in upper motor neurone lesions.

For direct examination of the soft palate, place the patient facing the light with the mouth open and introduce a tongue depressor. The position of the uvula at rest is variable even in health. Watch the movements of the palate during phonation. Ask the patient to say 'ah' and observe whether both sides of the palate arch upwards. If one side is paralysed, it will remain flat and immobile and the median raphe will be pulled towards the other side. In bilateral paralysis the whole palate remains motionless. Minor degrees of asymmetry of the palate and of the tongue occur as part of a hemiparesis due to an upper motor neurone lesion; this is not a palatal palsy.

The vagus nerve and the larynx

The *superior laryngeal* branch of the vagus contains sensory nerve fibres from the larynx above the level of the vocal cords, and motor fibres which innervate the cricothyroid muscle. Unilateral damage to the nerve is usually symptomless. Bilateral paralysis causes the vocal cords to be relaxed. The voice is therefore hoarse and deep and high notes are impossible. The *recurrent laryngeal* branch supplies sensation to the larynx below the level of the vocal cords and motor fibres to all the laryngeal muscles *except* the cricothyroid. Paralysis of the vocal cords leads to characteristic laryngoscopic features, *speech is characteristically blurred and ineffectual*, and the patient cannot cough clearly ('bovine cough'). Bilateral paralysis may cause stridor or even respiratory obstruction because the paralysed cords lie in partial adduction, thus partially blocking the airway.

The accessory nerve

The accessory nerve is purely motor, contributing to the innervation of the laryngeal, and pharyngeal muscles, as well as the sternomastoid and trapezius muscles. The spinal part of the nerve dips below the sternomastoid muscle about 2 cm below the tip of the mastoid process and re-emerges from underneath that muscle about the middle of its posterior border. Paralysis of the upper part of the *trapezius* is demonstrated by asking the patient to shrug the shoulders while the examiner presses downward on them. Paralysis of the *sternomastoid* causes weakness of rotation of the chin towards the opposite side.

THE TWELFTH (HYPOGLOSSAL) NERVE

The hypoglossal nerve arises from its nucleus in the lower part of the floor of the fourth ventricle, close to the midline. It emerges between the anterior pyramid and the olive. It is a purely motor nerve, supplying the tongue and the depressors of the hyoid bone.

Ask the patient to put out their tongue as far as possible. With unilateral hypoglossal lesion, the tongue is pushed over to the paralysed side instead of being protruded straight. Be careful not to mistake an apparent deviation of the tongue, really due to the mouth being twisted to one side, for a real deviation. Such an apparent deviation occurs in facial paralysis. Ask the patient to move the tongue from side to side, and to lick each cheek with it; observe whether this can be done freely. Strength may also be assessed by pressing against the tongue with a finger as the patient protrudes it into each cheek in turn. Note whether there is any *wasting* of the tongue (Fig. 11.20), and whether there is any *tremor or fasciculation* of it. The presence of wasting indicates that the lesion is either nuclear or infranuclear (lower motor neurone).

Fasciculation should be assessed with the tongue relaxed in the mouth, not when protruded. Bilateral fasciculation of the tongue is almost pathognomic of *motor neurone disease (amyotrophic lateral sclerosis)*. *Tremor* of the tongue is common in Parkinson's disease, either when the tongue is at rest or when it is protruded.

THE MOTOR SYSTEM

The motor system should be examined with the following aspects of motor function in mind:

- Movement and strength
- Bulk of muscles
- Tone of muscles
- Reflexes
- Gait
- Involuntary movements.

MUSCLE STRENGTH TESTING

Much the most reliable method of making a quick assessment is to watch the patient walking, standing up from lying and sitting positions, dressing or undressing, and lightly jumping or hopping. Try to

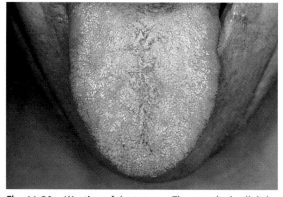

Fig. 11.20 Wasting of the tongue. The atrophy is slightly more marked on the right than the left in this patient with motor neurone disease. The tongue was fasciculating.

test these functions with the patient barefoot. These movements require proximal and distal strength and coordination and much can be learned by observing them carefully. The strength of individual muscle groups should then be assessed more formally.

Each movement made during this assessment is tested by comparison with the examiner's own strength or by comparison with what the examiner judges to be normal in a person of comparable build to the patient. It therefore requires practice and experience. Very simple requests produce better results than long explanations: a demonstration or gesture is often more effective than any verbal explanation. Remember that most patients have no knowledge of anatomy. Certain muscles and muscle groups are more important than others, because they are representative of particular functions, such as the corticospinal tract, or certain peripheral nerves, for example the median nerve, or nerve roots, for example S1.

Testing the muscles of the upper limb

Abductor pollicis brevis

This muscle (see Fig. 11.21(a) and (b)) is supplied by the median nerve, which is often damaged by compression in the carpal tunnel at the wrist (*carpal tunnel syndrome*). Ask the patient to abduct the thumb in a plane at right angles to the palmar aspect of the index finger, against the resistance of your own thumb. The muscle can be seen and felt to contract (see Fig. 11.22). Atrophy of the thenar eminence (Fig. 11.23) is often evident.

Opponens pollicis

Ask the patient to touch the tip of the little finger with the point of the thumb. Oppose the movement with your thumb or index finger (see Fig. 11.24).

First dorsal interosseous

Ask the patient to abduct the index finger against your resistance (see Figs 11.25–11.27).

Interossei and lumbricals

Test the patient's ability to flex the metacarpophalangeal joints and to extend the distal interphalangeal joints (see Fig. 11.28). The interossei also

(a)

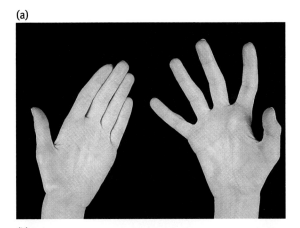

(b)

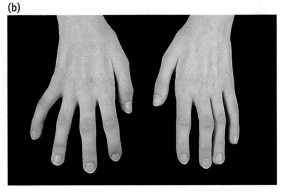

Fig. 11.21   Wasting of the small hand muscles in a chronic neuropathy. **(a)** There is marked wasting of the abductor pollicis brevis and **(b)** guttering of the dorsal surface of the hand indicating atrophy of the dorsal interossei.

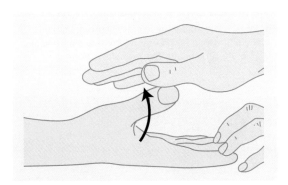

Fig. 11.22   Testing the abductor pollicis brevis.

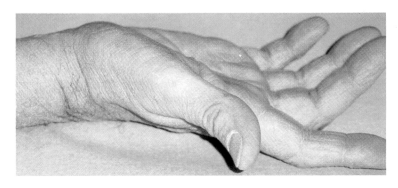

Fig. 11.23   Atrophy of the thenar eminence.

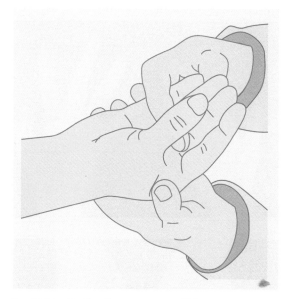

Fig. 11.24　Testing the opponens pollicis.

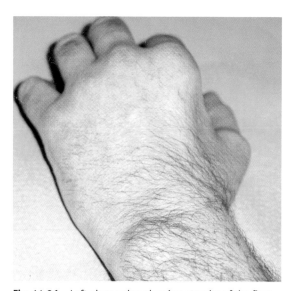

Fig. 11.25　Right ulnar nerve palsy showing marked atrophy of the right first dorsal interosseous muscle and flexion of the little finger. The left hand is normal.

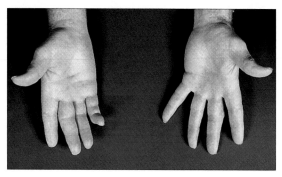

Fig. 11.26　Left ulnar palsy, showing atrophy of the first dorsal interosseous muscle with the hand at rest, often the best posture in which to recognize the abnormality.

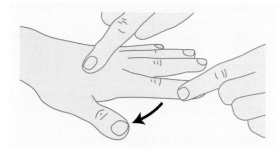

Fig. 11.27　Testing the first dorsal interosseous muscle.

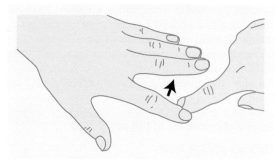

Fig. 11.28　Testing the first palmar interosseous muscle.

adduct and abduct the fingers. When these muscles are paralysed and power is retained in the long flexors and extensors of the two fingers, as in ulnar nerve palsy, a 'claw-hand' deformity is produced. The proximal phalanges are overextended and the distal two are flexed. The fingers are slightly separated (see Fig. 11.21).

Flexors of the fingers

Ask the patient to squeeze your fingers. Allow the patient to squeeze only your index and middle fingers—this is sufficient to assess strength of grip without having your fingers painfully crushed (see Fig. 29(a)–(d)).

Extensors of the wrist

Get the patient to make a fist, a movement which results in firm contraction of both the flexors and extensors of the wrist, and try forcibly to flex the wrist against the patient's effort to maintain the posture. It should be almost impossible to overcome the wrist extensors of a healthy man or woman. The wrist flexors can be similarly tested (see Fig. 11.30). Slight weakness of the extensors of the wrist may be elicited by asking the patient to grasp something firmly in their hand. If the extensors are weak the wrist becomes flexed as they do so, because the flexor muscles are then stronger than the extensors. Weakness or paralysis of the extensors of the wrist, as in radial nerve palsy, leads to *wrist-drop*.

(a)

(c)

(b)

(d)

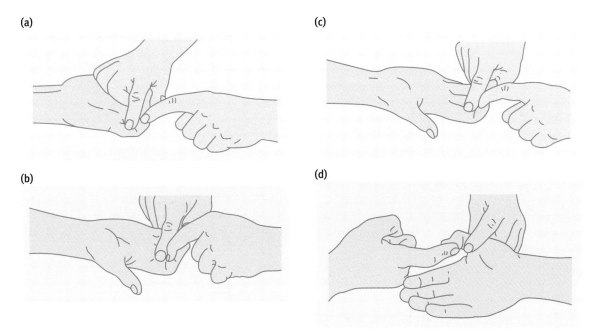

Fig. 11.29   Testing **(a)** flexor digitorum profundus III and IV; **(b)** flexor digitorum sublimis; **(c)** flexor digitorum profundus I and II; **(d)** flexor pollicis longus.

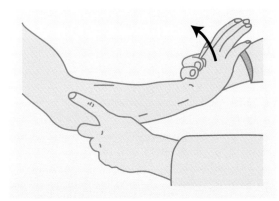

Fig. 11.30   Testing the extensor carpi radialis longus.

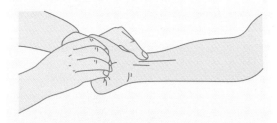

Fig. 11.31   Testing the flexor carpi radialis.

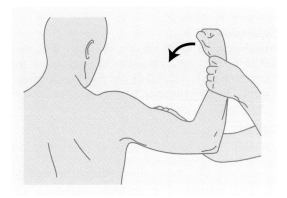

Fig. 11.32   Testing the biceps.

Flexors of the wrist
Ask the patient to squeeze your fingers. Allow the patient to make a fist, and try to overcome wrist flexion (see Fig. 11.31).

Brachioradialis
Place the arm midway between the prone and supine positions; then ask the patient to bend up the forearm, while you oppose the movement by grasping the hand. The muscle, if healthy, will be seen and felt to stand out prominently at its upper part.

Biceps
Ask the patient to bend up the forearm against resistance, with the forearm in full supination. The muscle will stand out clearly (see Fig. 11.32).

Triceps
Ask the patient to straighten out the forearm against your resistance (see Fig. 11.33(a) and (b)).

(a)

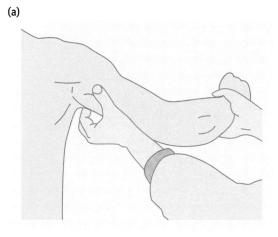

(b)

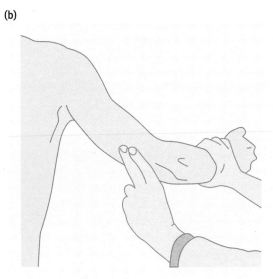

Fig. 11.33   Testing the triceps: **(a)** long head; **(b)** whole muscle.

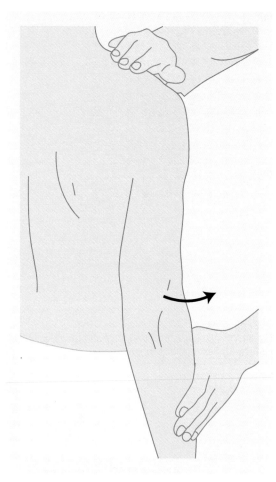

Fig. 11.34   Testing the supraspinatus.

Supraspinatus

Ask the patient to lift the arm straight out at right angles to the side. The first 30 degrees of this movement is carried out by the supraspinatus (see Fig. 11.34). The remaining 60 degrees is produced by the *deltoid*.

Deltoid

The anterior and posterior fibres of the deltoid help to draw the abducted arm forwards and backwards respectively. The middle fibres abduct the shoulder (see supraspinatus, above) (see Fig. 11.35).

Infraspinatus

Ask the patient to tuck the elbow into the side with the forearm flexed to a right angle. Then ask the patient to rotate the limb outwards against your resistance, the elbow being held against the side throughout. The muscle can be seen and felt to contract (see Fig. 11.36).

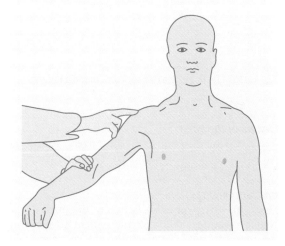

Fig. 11.35   Testing the deltoid.

Pectorals

Ask the patient to stretch the arms out in front, and then to clasp the hands together while you endeavour to hold them apart (see Fig. 11.37).

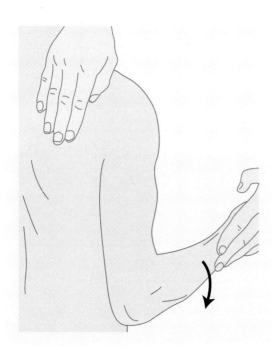

Fig. 11.36   Testing the infraspinatus.

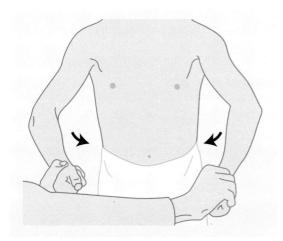

Fig. 11.37   Testing the pectoralis major.

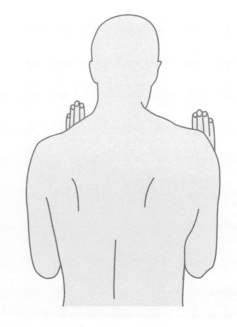

Fig. 11.38   Testing the serratus anterior.

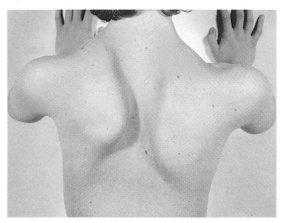

Fig. 11.39   Testing for winging of the scapulae.

Serratus anterior

When this muscle is paralysed the scapula is 'winged', with the vertebral border projecting posteriorly. The patient is unable to elevate the arm above a right angle, the deformity becoming more apparent as they try to do so. Pushing forwards with the hands against resistance, such as a wall, also brings out the deformity (see Figs 11.38 and 11.39).

Latissimus dorsi

Ask the patient to clasp the hands behind their back while you, standing behind the patient, offer passive resistance to the downward and backward movement. Alternatively, the two posterior axillary folds can be felt as the patient coughs (see Fig. 11.40).

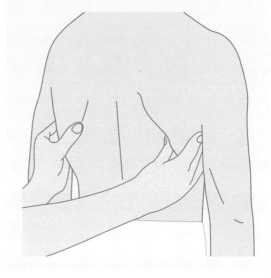

Fig. 11.40   Testing the latissimus dorsi.

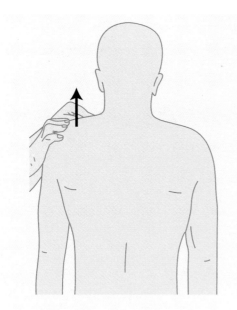

Fig. 11.41   Testing the trapezius.

Trapezius

The upper part of the *trapezius* is tested by asking the patient to shrug their shoulders while you try to press them down from behind. The muscle's lower part can be tested by asking the patient to approximate the shoulder blades (see Fig. 11.41).

Testing the muscles of the trunk

Beevor's sign and abdominal weakness

Paralysis of a portion of the anterior abdominal wall can be detected by the displacement of the umbilicus that occurs when the patient attempts to lift up the head from the pillow against resistance. With paralysis of the lower segment the umbilicus moves upwards (Beevor's sign), but when the upper segment is affected the umbilicus is pulled downwards. This sign is useful since it may indicate the level of a lesion in the thoracic region in spinal cord disease. Severe weakness of the muscles of the abdomen and of the hip flexors is usually obvious because the patient is unable to sit up in bed from the supine position without the aid of the arms. *Babinski's 'rising up sign'* is shown by getting the patient to lie supine with the legs extended and then to sit up without using the hands. In *spastic paralysis* of a leg the affected limb will rise first, but in *hysterical paralysis* this does not occur.

Diaphragm

The diaphragm is innervated by the upper cervical segments but it is usually spared in cervical cord disease, except in motor neurone disease (amyotrophic lateral sclerosis), certain muscle diseases and sometimes in brachial neuritis. A simple bedside test is to ask the patient to take a deep breath and to count slowly—most people can easily get to 20 or more with a single breath. *Diaphragmatic weakness*

prevents a brisk sniff—a respiratory movement that requires a sudden maximal diaphragmatic contraction. A major feature of a weak diaphragm is inability of the patient to breathe easily when lying flat. This sometimes presents as difficulty sleeping, which is found to be due to oxygen desaturation in the supine posture. Weakness of the diaphragm is often not noticed unless actively sought for.

Spinal extensors

To test the *erector spinae* and muscles of the back, ask the patient to lie prone, and then to try to extend the head from the bed by extending the neck and back. If the back muscles are healthy, they will be seen to stand out prominently during this effort.

Testing the muscles of the lower limb

Intrinsic muscles of the foot

These are difficult to examine (see Fig 11.43). When the interossei are weakened or paralysed a foot deformity may develop. A similar deformity in patients with spastic hemiparesis of very long duration is due to spastic dystonia and not primarily to muscular weakness. In familial peripheral neuropathies a hollow wasted foot deformity (*pes cavus*) is characteristic (Fig. 11.42).

Dorsiflexion and plantarflexion of the feet and toes

These functions are tested by asking the patient to elevate or depress the distal foot against resistance.

Extensors of the knee

Bend up the knee, and then, pressing with your hand against the shin, ask the patient to try to straighten it

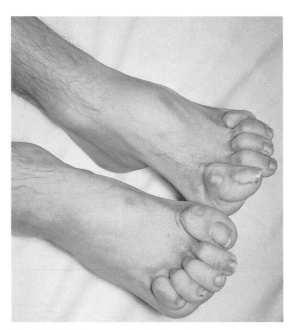

Fig. 11.42   Pes cavus, with clawing of the toes in a patient with familial neuropathy. This patient had Refsum's disease and the peripheral nerves were slightly enlarged.

(a)

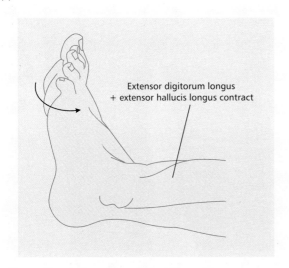

Extensor digitorum longus + extensor hallucis longus contract

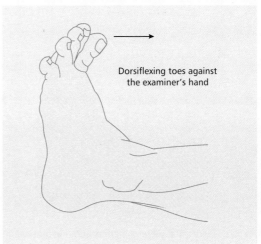

Dorsiflexing toes against the examiner's hand

(b)

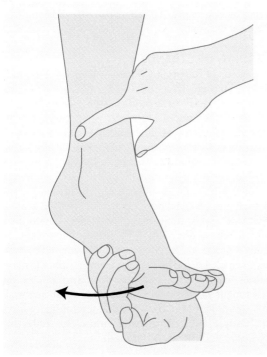

(c)

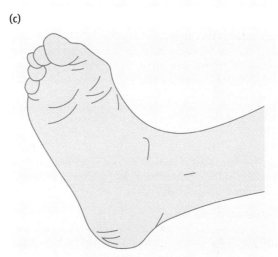

Fig. 11.43 Testing (a) extensor digitorum longus and extensor halucis longus; (b) peroneus longus and brevis; (c) small muscles of the foot.

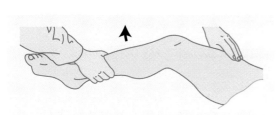

Fig. 11.44 Testing the quadriceps femoris.

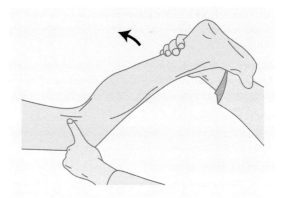

Fig. 4.45 Testing the hamstring muscles – knee flexion.

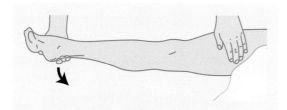

Fig. 11.46   Testing the adductors of the thigh.

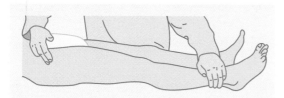

Fig. 11.47   Testing the gluteus medius and minimus, and tensor fasciae latae.

out again. This muscle is stronger than your arm, and is more easily tested by asking the patient to stand up from a low chair, or to hop on either leg. Look for atrophy of the quadriceps musculature (Fig. 11.44).

Flexors of the knee
Raise a leg up from the bed, supporting the thigh with your left hand and holding the ankle with your right. Then ask the patient to bend the knee against your resistance. You should not be able to overcome this muscle (Fig. 11.45).

Extensors of the hip
With the patient's knee extended, lift his or her foot off the bed; then ask the patient to push it down against your resistance. This is normally a very strong movement and should be impossible to overcome. As for the other leg extensors, a better functional test is to observe the patient standing from a low chair and hopping.

Flexors of the hip
With the patient's leg extended, ask him or her to raise the leg off the bed against resistance. Alternatively, the related movement of flexion of the thigh, with the thigh already flexed to a right angle, can be tested.

Adductors of the thigh
Abduct the limb and then ask the patient to bring it back to the midline against resistance (Fig. 11.46).

Abductors of the thigh
Place the patient's legs together and ask him or her to separate them against resistance (Fig. 11.47).

Rotators of the thigh
With the patient's lower limb extended on the bed, ask him or her to roll it outwards or inwards against resistance.

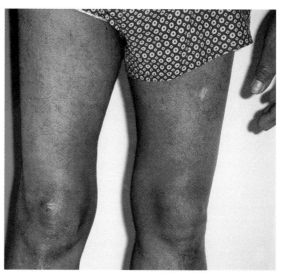

Fig. 11.48   There is wasting of the thigh extensor muscles, particularly evident in the medial component of the quadriceps group. The small scar on the left side is from a muscle biopsy. The patient had limb girdle muscular dystrophy.

GRADING OF STRENGTH
The Medical Research Council Scale is used to grade muscle strength (see Box 11.13). This scale is clinically based, easy to reproduce, but essentially non-linear. It requires practice in order to be reproducible. Grades 1, 2 and 3 assess quite small differences in very weak muscles, but Grade 4 contains a wide variation in strength. Grade 5 is normal, a subjective interpretation of widely varying strength in different muscles in people of different ages, gender, and physical development. The MRC scale is therefore highly subjective. Nonetheless, it has been shown repeatedly to be both useful and reliable in clinical practice. The MRC scale was devised to evaluate muscles during recovery from peripheral nerve palsies in wartime, and therefore emphasizes the assessment of very weak muscles. Several quantitative techniques are now available that measure force or torque in contracting muscles, reflecting *isometric* and *isokinetic* strength.

BOX 11.13	The Medical Research Council Scale for grading muscle function.
Grade 0	Complete paralysis
Grade 1	A flicker of contraction only
Grade 2	Power detectable only when gravity is excluded by appropriate postural adjustment
Grade 3	The limb can be held against the force of gravity, but not against the examiner's resistance
Grade 4	There is some degree of weakness, usually described as poor, fair or moderate strength
Grade 5	Normal power is present

PATTERNS OF WEAKNESS

The pattern of weakness and disability described by the patient and observed on examination is of great help in considering diagnosis. Try to work out the pattern of weakness when watching the patient coming into your consulting room, or by formally observing the gait and posture, and the capacity for movement of the upper limbs. This is important in determining the emphasis of your physical examination.

Hemiplegia is paralysis of one side of the body involving the arm and leg, and usually also of the face (*facio-brachio-crural hemiparesis*). It is virtually always due to a lesion in the corticospinal pathway, and is therefore an upper motor neurone syndrome. *Crossed paralysis* is weakness in an ipsilateral cranial muscle group with a contralateral hemiparesis; it is a sign of brainstem disease. A *paraplegia* is a paralysis of both legs, nearly always due to a spinal cord lesion, and so upper motor neurone in type. *Monoplegia* is a paralysis of one limb, which may be the arm (*brachial monoplegia*) or the leg (*crural monoplegia*); this may be due to root or plexus disease. In *quadriplegia*, a feature of cervical cord disease, all four limbs are weak.

In weakness due to a *corticospinal lesion*, as in spastic hemiparesis, there is weakness, in the leg, in hip flexion and in dorsiflexion of the foot and, in the arm, in abduction/extension of the shoulder and in dorsiflexion of the wrist. There is a supranuclear (UMN) facial palsy. The face and arm, or the leg, may be particularly involved, depending on the location of the lesion in the hemisphere. Slowness and clumsiness of rapid fine finger movement is a feature of spastic hemiplegia. The gait is characteristically affected, with a slow, dragging, rolling gait on the affected side, the hip and foot not being lifted up to clear the ground, so that the toe of the shoe wears quickly. Antagonistic movements, such as hip extension and plantarflexion of the foot, are strikingly less involved than extensor muscles in the early stages. This characteristic pattern of weakness is important in diagnosis.

The detection of hemiplegia in a patient who is comatose may be difficult. However, if the paralysis is of recent onset, hypotonia may be detected in the paralysed limbs. If the arm, for example, is raised from the side and allowed to drop, it falls, if it is paralysed, as if it did not belong to the patient; the sound arm also falls, but not in such an utterly limp fashion. The face is asymmetrical, the angle of the mouth more open on the paralysed side, and the affected cheek moves loosely outwards and inwards with respiration. The abdominal and tendon reflexes may be absent on both sides, but an extensor plantar response can usually be obtained on the hemiplegic side (see section on reflexes, p. 265).

Myasthenic weakness

In *myasthenia gravis* (Fig. 11.49), weakness, which usually affects the external ocular and bulbar muscles

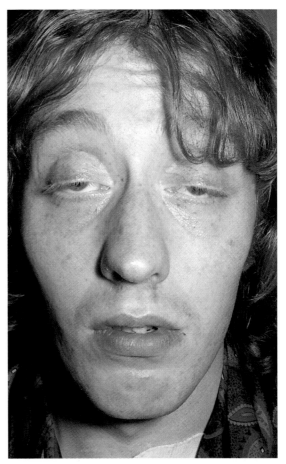

Fig. 11.49   Myasthenia gravis. There is bilateral ptosis with resting divergence of the eyes and lower facial weakness, so that the mouth and jaw hang open. There is compensatory overactivity of the frontalis muscles in an effort to open the eyelids.

more than the rest of the skeletal musculature, is worsened or provoked by repeated contraction of the affected muscles (*myasthenic fatigue*). The degree of detectable weakness therefore varies during the course of the day. In the *Lambert–Eaton myasthenic syndrome (LEMS)* there is weakness initially, but during continued contraction of a muscle or continued exertion strength improves at first, followed by weakness if exertion is continued. During the phase of increased strength the tendon reflexes, which are often difficult to elicit in this condition, become quite brisk. These features are quite difficult to detect without experience of the condition, and the diagnosis is usually made by electromyography (EMG). Lambert–Eaton syndrome was first described in association with small cell carcinoma of the bronchus, but in about half the people with the syndrome it occurs as an idiopathic autoimmune disorder.

Neurogenic weakness

In lower motor neurone lesions weakness is associated with muscular atrophy, reduced tone and absent

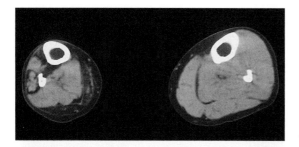

Fig. 11.50 Old poliomyelitis. CT scan. Wasting of the muscles of the right leg (to the left of the picture). Note that all the muscles are wasted compared with the normal left side. Also the tibia and fibula are smaller, indicating that the wasting must have been present since childhood.

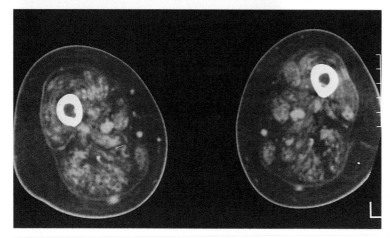

Fig. 11.51 Type 3 spinal muscular atrophy. CT scan. There is atrophy, fibrosis and fat replacement of most of the muscles of the thighs and the abnormality is symmetrical. The patient is immobile and has become obese.

tendon reflexes. These are the features of *lower motor neurone lesion*. The distribution of the weakness and atrophy is important in diagnosis (Figs 11.50 and 11.51) since it may be *localized*, as in peripheral nerve (see Figs 11.21 and 11.25) or root disease, or *generalized*, as in anterior horn cell disease, for example motor neurone disease. In the latter and, to a lesser extent in other types of neurogenic weakness, *fasciculations* may occur. These are spontaneous contractions of groups of muscle fibres, probably representing enlarged, re-innervated motor units, or parts of such motor units. Fasciculations vary in distribution and frequency, and may also occur in fatigued normal subjects. They mostly originate from abnormal generator sites in the peripheral nervous system, although some have their origin more proximally. In chronic neurogenic weakness *action fasciculation* may be noted. This occurs during initial contraction of a muscle; the muscle is seen to undergo rhythmic fasciculation-like contraction as motor units are recruited into the muscular effort. Fatigue is a common feature of neurogenic weakness, but also occurs in some myopathies.

Peripheral neuropathy

When there is a generalized disease of the peripheral nerves (Box 11.14), whether affecting axons or myelin sheaths, a distinctive pattern of weakness and, often, of sensory disturbance is found (see Fig. 11.60). Distal tendon reflexes are diminished in axonal neuropathies, and in demyelinating neuropathies there may be areflexia. In disease of individual peripheral nerves (*mononeuropathies*) the

clinical features are restricted to the distribution of the affected nerve (Box 11.5), and in brachial plexus lesions (Box 11.6) to the wider motor and sensory distribution of the cervical roots.

Myopathic weakness

In myopathies (Fig. 11.52), dystrophies (Fig. 11.53) and polymyositis, muscle weakness is strikingly proximal, usually symmetrical and often affects the pelvifemoral muscles more severely than the pectoral girdle muscles. Affected muscles are atrophic and may feel firmer than normal. In Duchenne muscular dystrophy pseudohypertrophy of some weak muscles develops (Fig. 11.54). In inflammatory muscle disease the muscles are tender to palpation, and may

---

BOX 11.14 Peripheral neuropathy; major clinical features of polyneuropathies.

- Symmetrical distal weakness and wasting
- Symmetrical distal sensory impairment
- Loss of tendon reflexes
  — generalized loss in demyelinating neuropathies
  — distal loss in axonal (dying back) neuropathies
- Tremor of outstretched fingers in chronic neuropathies
- Pes cavus in early-onset, familial neuropathies
- Enlargement of peripheral nerves in chronic demyelinating neuropathies, and in leprosy (Hansen's disease)
- Distal burning pain in small fibre neuropathies, e.g. diabetes mellitus

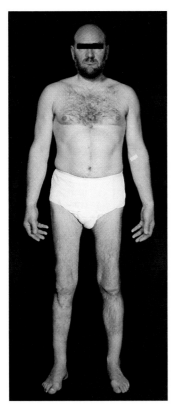

Fig. 11.52 Myopathy due to adult onset acid maltase deficiency (type III glycogenosis). There is atrophy of proximal muscles, usually involving the pelvic femoral and pectoral girdle muscles, e.g. thighs and deltoids. In this disease the diaphram is particularly affected.

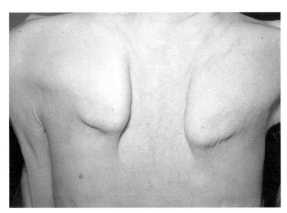

Fig. 11.53 Fascioscapulohumeral (FSH) muscular dystrophy. Note the wasted, winged scapulae and the severe wasting of the left upper arm musculature.

be swollen. Fasciculations do not occur in myopathic weakness.

Myotonia

In certain inherited muscular disorders, of which *myotonic dystrophy* is the commonest, relaxation is impaired following contraction of a muscle. In some myotonic disorders affected muscles may be weak. The phenomenon of *myotonia* is most evident when

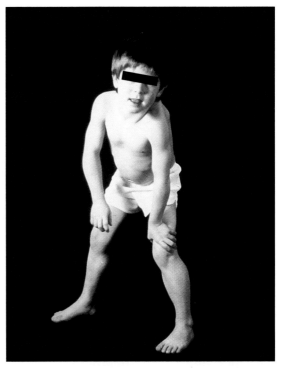

Fig. 11.54 Duchenne muscular dystrophy (Xp21 dystrophy). there is pseudohypertrophy of the weak muscles, e.g. the calves and deltoids. The child is 'climbing up himself' with legs widely placed as he gets up from the sitting position to the standing position. This is Gowers' sign.

the muscles are cold and it is therefore often best demonstrated in the hand. Ask the patient to grip your hand firmly and then to let go suddenly. The grasp is maintained for a moment and then is slowly and gradually released. Myotonia can be demonstrated in the tongue and in other muscles (e.g. the thenar eminence) by lightly striking the muscle with a small patellar hammer. A dimple of contraction appears that relaxes only slowly.

BULK OF MUSCLES

Muscle bulk (Fig. 11.55) is best assessed clinically by inspection and palpation. Wasted or atrophic muscles are not only smaller, but also softer and more flabby than normal when they are contracted. When muscular wasting is accompanied by fibrosis, as in muscular dystrophy or polymyositis, the muscles feel hard and inelastic. They may become shortened so that it is difficult to stretch them passively to a normal degree—*contractures*. Contractures may also occur as a result of prolonged hypertonia in a group of muscles.

Muscular atrophy is not caused only by neurological disorders. Generalized muscular wasting is seen in cachexia of any cause. It is a normal feature of ageing. Localized muscle atrophy may be due to injury or disease of a joint—*disuse atrophy*; this occurs, for example, in the quadriceps in patients with diseases of the knee. In disuse atrophy strength

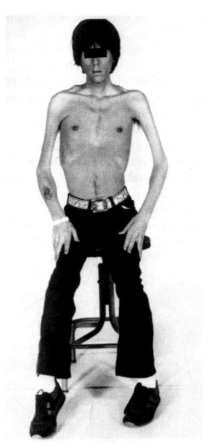

Fig. 11.55   Muscular atrophy due to fascioscapulohumeral muscular dystrophy. Note the atrophy of the limb and shoulder muscles, especially the biceps and deltoids. Thinning of the thigh musculature can be recognized even through the trousers.

is comparatively well-preserved in relation to the degree of muscular wasting. Some patients, especially boys with Duchenne muscular dystrophy (Fig. 11.54), develop large muscles (*pseudohypertrophy*) due to fibrosis and fatty replacement in the affected muscles. The calves, buttocks and infraspinati are particularly affected in Duchenne disease. These enlarged muscles are weak in spite of their size. True hypertrophy of muscles occurs in response to continued excessive workloads as in certain occupations, or following athletic training. It may also occur in certain myotonic disorders. Hypertrophy and atrophy can be quantitatively assessed by transverse CT or MR imaging of muscles (Fig. 11.50), or by ultrasound studies.

TONE OF MUSCLES

Muscular tone is a state of tension or contraction found in healthy muscles. An increase in tone is called *hypertonia* and a reduction *hypotonia*.

   Hypotonia occurs in:

- Lower motor neurone lesions
- Lesions of the afferent sensory pathways (e.g.

sensory neuropathies, tabes dorsalis)
- Cerebellar disease (due to abnormal suprasegmental mechanisms)
- Sleep
- Drug effects (e.g. hypnotics, anti-spasticity agents).

Hypertonia occurs in:

- Spasticity, due to upper motor neurone lesions
- Dystonia, due to basal ganglia disease
- Parkinson's disease, when tone is increased in a 'cogwheel' pattern
- Dementia, when tone is increased in all passive movements ('*gegenhalten*')
- In muscles acting across a painful joint.

The degree of tone is estimated by handling the limbs and moving them passively at their various joints. The maintenance of tone is dependent on a spinal reflex arc. Afferent fibres from the primary and secondary endings of the muscle spindles enter the spinal cord and synapse with the anterior horn cells, from which efferent fibres arise and pass to the muscles. Tone is diminished or lost if this reflex arc is damaged. Muscle tone is mainly regulated by corticospinal and extrapyramidal pathways.

Spasticity

Hypertonia following lesions of the corticospinal system (upper motor neurone lesions) is termed *spasticity*, a term which has a precise meaning. It describes a state of increased tone which is of 'clasp-knife' type when the limb is fairly rapidly flexed or extended. The resistance to stretch increases during the applied stretch, and then suddenly gives way, like opening a pen-knife. These are the lengthening and shortening reactions described by Sherrington. Spasticity is therefore a form of rigidity which is *stretch-sensitive*. Moreover the degree of increased tone developed during any passive stretch is *velocity-dependent*, i.e. it is proportional to the speed of the applied stretch.

   Spasticity due to *cerebral or brainstem lesions* has a characteristic distribution shown by the typical posture of the limbs in such patients. The upper limbs are held in flexion and the lower limbs in extension with the feet in plantarflexion (physiological extension). Thus in the arms the flexor muscles are mainly involved, but in the legs the extensor muscles are predominantly affected. This distribution is most evident in the erect posture, and may even be reversed if the patient is placed head down, showing that it is driven by labyrinthine/vestibular afferent activity.

Rigidity

Extrapyramidal rigidity is a form of hypertonia due to disease of the basal ganglia. The resistance to passive movement in this disorder is regularly or irregularly variable and is aptly described as like a lever engaging on the teeth of a cogwheel (*cogwheel rigidity*). It can usually be enhanced by asking the patient to contract another muscle, e.g. to clench the fist on the opposite side (*Jendrassik manoeuvre*). In the commonest extrapyramidal disorder, *Parkinson's disease*, the hypertonia is accompanied by a general attitude of flexion of the limbs and trunk. This type of rigidity is often accompanied by *akinesia*, a tendency for the patient not to spontaneously move the affected limb or part of the body. Parkinson himself termed this 'a peculiar disinclination to move' (Fig. 11.56). Sometimes a plastic type of rigidity is found in which the resistance developed to passive movement is uniform during all phases of the applied movement. This is *paratonic rigidity* or *gegenhalten* (literally: 'go-stop'). It is found in catatonic states and in patients with clouded or confused consciousness from any cause, especially dementia. It is not simply evidence of lack of cooperation. Its physiological basis is unknown. In *hysterical rigidity* the resistance to passive movement increases in proportion to the effort applied by the examiner. The increased resistance in simulated rigidity has an irregular, jerky character.

When the muscles are *hypotonic*, there is little or no resistance to passive movement of the limb; when handled or shaken the unsupported part flops about inertly. Hypotonic muscles are abnormally soft to palpation. The outstretched hypotonic upper limb may assume an abnormal posture, as in cerebellar disease or chorea, hyperextension at the elbow, overpronation of the forearm, wrist flexion and finger hyperextension.

REFLEXES

When the tendon of a lightly stretched muscle is struck a single sharp blow with a soft rubber hammer (thus suddenly stretching the muscle and exciting a synchronous volley of afferent impulses from the primary sensory endings of the muscle spindles in the stretched muscle), the muscle contracts briefly. This is the *monosynaptic stretch reflex* or

tendon reflex. It is a test of the integrity of the afferent and efferent pathways, and of the excitability of the anterior horn cells in the spinal segment of the stretched muscle. Properly performed, examination of the tendon reflexes is a reliable and reproducible method for assessing this system of neurones and their higher connections. It is important to become skilled in the technique for eliciting these reflexes (Fig. 11.57):

- Put the patient at ease
- Always make sure the patient is warm and comfortable
- Always use the same type of tendon hammer
- Always examine tendon reflexes in the same manner, standing on the same side of the bed—*standardise your technique*
- Reassure the patient that the hammer is soft
- Repeat the test several times if necessary.

When examining the tendon reflexes in the legs, care taken to allow the patient's genitalia to be properly covered is repaid by more easily elicitable reflexes. The patient should be asked to relax or to 'let the muscles go to sleep'. Some neurologists prefer to assess the tendon reflexes with the patient sitting on the edge of the couch facing the examiner. However, they are more usually tested with the patient supine on a couch.

Knee jerk

The patella hammer is named from its invention as an instrument for eliciting the patellar reflex, the first tendon reflex to become a regular part of the neurological examination. The knee jerk consists of contraction of the quadriceps when the patellar tendon is tapped. The spinal segments concerned are the second, third and fourth lumbar. It is best tested with the patient supine. Pass your hand under the knee to be tested; the knee rests in the observer's palm or on the dorsum of the observer's wrist. The patellar tendon is struck midway between its origin and insertion. Following the blow there will be a brief extension of the knee due to contraction of the

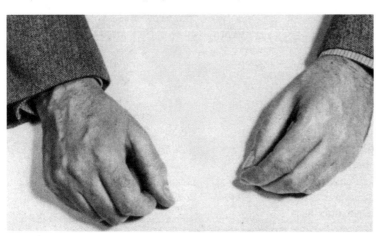

Fig. 11.56 Parkinson's disease. The left hand is held partially flexed and immobile. This has resulted in slight oedema of the skin of the hand causing the joints and tendons to appear indistinct. Since the hand is not used, its venous return is not as prominent as on the other side.

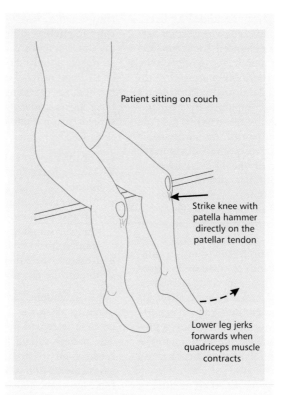

Patient sitting on couch

Strike knee with patella hammer directly on the patellar tendon

Lower leg jerks forwards when quadriceps muscle contracts

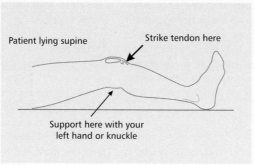

Patient lying supine

Strike tendon here

Support here with your left hand or knuckle

(a)

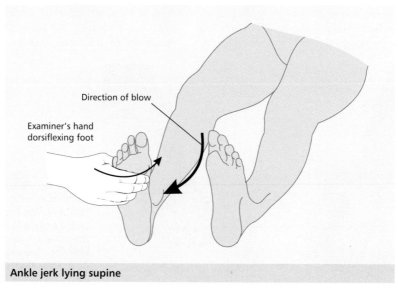

Direction of blow

Examiner's hand dorsiflexing foot

(b)   **Ankle jerk lying supine**

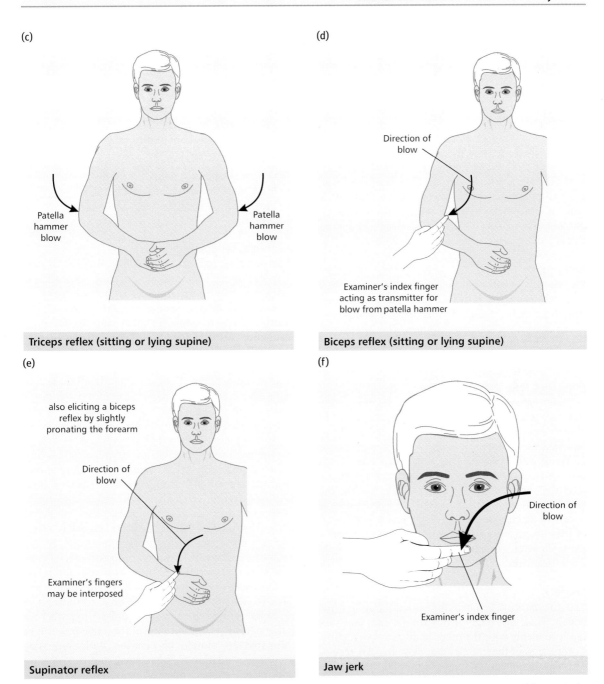

(c)

Patella hammer blow

Patella hammer blow

Triceps reflex (sitting or lying supine)

(d)

Direction of blow

Examiner's index finger acting as transmitter for blow from patella hammer

Biceps reflex (sitting or lying supine)

(e)

also eliciting a biceps reflex by slightly pronating the forearm

Direction of blow

Examiner's fingers may be interposed

Supinator reflex

(f)

Direction of blow

Examiner's index finger

Jaw jerk

Fig. 11.57 Methods for testing tendon reflexes (see text). The words 'jerk' and 'reflex' are interchangeable. **(a)** Knee jerk; **(b)** ankle jerk; **(c)** triceps reflex; **(d)** biceps reflex; **(e)** supinator reflex; (f) jaw jerk.

quadriceps. The reflex can sometimes be more easily elicited with the patient sitting up, the legs dangling freely over the edge of the bed.

The briskness of the knee jerk varies in different individuals. In health it is hardly ever entirely absent. Sometimes, as in the case of the other tendon reflexes, it cannot be elicited without applying *reinforcement* (Jendrassik's manoeuvre). This is done by asking the patient to make a strong voluntary muscular effort with the upper limbs; for example, to hook the fingers of the two hands together and then to pull them against one another as hard as possible,

or to make a fist with the ipsilateral hand. While the patient is doing this, a further attempt is made to elicit the knee jerk. Reinforcement acts by increasing the excitability of the anterior horn cells and by increasing the sensitivity of the muscle spindle primary sensory endings to stretch (by increased gamma fusimotor drive).

Ankle jerk

Place the lower limb on the bed so that it lies everted and slightly flexed. Then with one hand, slightly dorsiflex the foot so as to stretch the Achilles tendon and, with the other hand, strike the tendon on its posterior surface. A quick contraction of the calf muscles results. This reflex can also be conveniently elicited when the patient is kneeling on a chair. It is a test of the first and second sacral segments.

Triceps jerk
Flex the elbow and allow the forearm to rest across the patient's chest. Tap the triceps tendon just above the olecranon. The triceps contracts. The reflex depends upon the sixth and seventh cervical segments. Care must be taken to strike the triceps *tendon* and not the belly of the muscle itself. All muscles show a certain amount of irritability to direct mechanical stimuli, but this is a direct response, not a stretch reflex.

Biceps jerk
Flex the elbow to a right angle and place the forearm in a semipronated position; then place your own thumb or index finger on the biceps tendon and strike it with the patellar hammer. The biceps contracts. The fifth and sixth cervical segments are tested with this reflex.

Supinator jerk
A blow upon the styloid process of the radius stretches the supinator causing supination of the elbow. The elbow should be placed slightly flexed and slightly pronated, in order to avoid contraction of the brachioradialis. This reflex depends on the fifth and six cervical segments. With lesions at this level the supinator or biceps jerks may be lost but brisk flexion of the fingers is seen. This phenomenon is known as *inversion* of the reflex and it is evidence of hyperexcitability of the anterior horn cells below the C5/6 level. The responsible lesion is in the C5/6 spinal segments.

Jaw jerk
Ask the patient to open the mouth, but not too widely. Place one finger firmly on the chin and then tap it suddenly with the other hand as in percussion. Contraction of the muscles that close the jaw results. This jerk is sometimes absent in normal subjects and is increased in upper motor neurone lesions at a level *above* the trigeminal nerve nuclei.

Clonus
When the tendon reflexes are exaggerated as a result of a corticospinal lesion there may be clonus. To test for *ankle clonus* bend the patient's knee slightly and support it with one hand, grasp the forepart of the foot with the other hand and suddenly dorsiflex the foot. The sudden stretch causes a brief reflex contraction of the calf muscles, which then relax; continued steady stretch causes a regular oscillation of contraction and relaxation which is called *clonus*. *Sustained clonus* is abnormal, and is evidence of an upper motor neurone lesion. It is always associated with increased tendon reflexes and an extensor plantar response.

Unsustained clonus may occur in healthy persons, particularly in those who are very tense or anxious; in these subjects the plantar responses are flexor.

Grading the reflexes
The tendon reflexes are graded as follows:

0 Absent
1 Present (as a normal ankle jerk)
2 Brisk (as a normal knee jerk)
3 Very brisk
4 Clonus.

Abnormal tendon reflexes
The tendon reflexes are *diminished or absent (hyporeflexia)* with lesions affecting the afferent pathways, the anterior horn cells themselves, or the efferent pathways (lesions of the lower motor neurone). For example, in tabes dorsalis the posterior roots are affected; in poliomyelitis the anterior horn cells are diseased; and in most peripheral neuropathies both the efferent (motor) and afferent (sensory) nerve fibres are abnormal. In all these conditions tendon reflexes may be absent. *Hyperreflexia* occurs with upper motor neurone lesions. It is also found in anxious or nervous people, in thyrotoxicosis and in tetanus. Hyperreflexia is therefore only of pathological significance if it is asymmetrical or if it is associated with other signs of an upper motor neurone lesion, for example an extensor plantar response. In cerebellar disease the reflexes may have a characteristic *pendular* quality. This is clearly evident only when there is a severe cerebellar ataxia and it is not a sign of diagnostic importance. It may be considered a manifestation of hypotonia.

In hypothyroidism both the contraction and relaxation phases of the tendon reflex may be prolonged. This is sometimes called, somewhat confusingly, a *myotonic reflex*. It is also found in hypothermic patients. The relaxation time of the ankle jerk can be estimated by simple observation with surprising accuracy in relation to the normal, and is a sensitive and reliable clinical index of hypothyroidism.

Superficial reflexes (Table 11.3)

The plantar reflex
Assessment of the plantar reflex (the Babinski response) is of great clinical importance; it is an objective response which can easily be compared by various observers. To elicit it the muscles of the lower limb should be relaxed. The *outer edge of the sole of the foot* is stimulated by firmly scratching a key or a stick along it from the heel towards the little toe. A medial movement across the sole of the metatarsus was not used by Babinski. In healthy adults even a slight stimulus produces contraction of the tensor fascia lata, often accompanied by a slighter contrac-

TABLE 11.3 Superficial spinal reflexes.

Reflex	How excited	Clinical result	Level of cord
Anal	Stroking or scratching skin near anus	Contraction of anal sphincter	3rd and 4th sacral segments
Bulbocavernosus	Pinching dorsum of glans penis	Contraction of bulbocavernosus	3rd and 4th sacral segments
Plantar response	Stroking sole of foot and toes, or leg	Flexion of toes, and of foot	5th lumbar and 1st sacral segments
Cremasteric	Stroking skin at upper and inner part of thigh*	Upward movement of testicle	1st and 2nd lumbar segments
Abdominal	Stroking abdominal wall below costal margin and in iliac fossa	Contraction of abdominal muscles	7th and 12th thoracic segments
Scapular	Stroking skin in interscapular region	Contraction of scapular muscles	5th cervical to 1st thoracic segment

* The cremasteric reflex can often be more easily elicited by pressing over the sartorius in the lower third of Hunter's canal.

tion of the adductors of the thigh and of the sartorius. With a slightly stronger stimulus, flexion of the four outer toes appears, which increases with the strength of the stimulus until all the toes are flexed on the metatarsus and drawn together, the ankle being dorsiflexed and inverted. This is called the *flexor plantar response*. With still stronger stimuli withdrawal of the limb occurs. The plantar reflex is never completely absent in healthy subjects.

An abnormality in the plantar response in lesions of the corticospinal system was first described by Babinski. This abnormal response, *Babinski's extensor plantar response*, replaces the normal flexor plantar response; it is found only in patients with corticospinal tract lesions and is thus a pathognomonic feature of an upper motor neurone lesion. In the extensor plantar response dorsiflexion (extension) of the great toe precedes all other movement (Fig. 11.58). It is followed by spreading out and extension of the other toes, by dorsiflexion of the ankle and by flexion of the hip and knee. This abnormal response is called

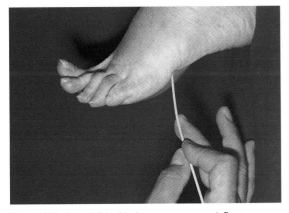

Fig. 11.58 The Babinski plantar response. A firm stroking stimulus to the outer edge of the sole of the foot evokes dorsiflexion (extension) of the large toe and fanning of the other toes.

the *extensor* plantar response because the movement of the toes is in extension according to anatomical terminology. However, the extensor plantar response is, in reality, part of the nociceptive flexion withdrawal response described in the decerebrate preparation by Sherrington. Like the normal flexor plantar response, the extensor plantar response is best elicited from the outer edge of the sole of the foot; more medial stimuli usually elicit flexion as part of the *grasp response*, a different phenomenon. In major corticospinal lesions the area from which the extensor plantar reflex can be elicited (receptive field) enlarges, spreading first inwards and over the sole of the foot, and then upwards along the leg to the knee or even higher. For this reason extension of the great toe, generally associated with some dorsiflexion of the foot, can sometimes also be obtained by squeezing the calf or pressing heavily along the inner border of the tibia (*Oppenheim's sign*), or by pinching the calcaneus tendon (*Gordon's reflex*). In adults, the extensor plantar response occurs with disease involving corticospinal pathways, but in children below the age of 1 year the extensor response is the normal response. The flexor response appears in the subsequent 6–12 months as myelination of the corticospinal pathways is completed.

Flexor spasms may occur during testing of the plantar reflex. These consist of an exaggerated extensor plantar response, the whole limb being suddenly drawn up into flexion and the large toe extended. This is the fully developed human counterpart of Sherrington's nociceptive flexion withdrawal response. It is common in spinal cord disease and in some patients with bilateral upper motor neurone lesions at a higher level. Flexor spasms are often particularly severe in the presence of posterior column disease (as in multiple sclerosis or subacute combined degeneration), or when there is a constant barrage of small unmyelinated fibre input to the spinal cord, as in the presence of bedsores or urinary tract infection in a patient with a cord lesion. *Extensor spasms*, conversely, are more likely to occur in patients with corticospinal tract lesions when posterior column function is normal.

Superficial abdominal reflexes

These are elicited with the patient lying relaxed and supine, with the abdomen uncovered. A light stimulus, such as a key or a thin wooden stick, is passed across the abdominal skin in the plane of the dermatome from the outer aspect towards the midline. A ripple of contraction of the underlying abdominal musculature follows the stimulus. These reflexes are absent in upper motor neurone lesions above their spinal level. In disease of the thoracic spine they may indicate the segmental level of the lesion by their absence below this level. It is often impossible to elicit abdominal reflexes in anxious patients, in the elderly or obese, and in multiparous women.

Corneal reflex

See page 249.

Palatal reflex

See pages 251.

Sphincteric reflexes

These are the reflexes concerned with swallowing, micturition and defecation. They depend upon complex muscular movements excited by increased tension in the wall of the viscus concerned, and involve both unstriated and striated muscles.

Swallowing. Ascertain whether there is any difficulty in swallowing (dysphagia), noting especially whether there is any regurgitation of food through the nose. Patients with neurological dysphagia usually note difficulty in swallowing liquids, whereas those with mechanical obstruction to the oesophagus or pharynx cannot swallow solids.

Defecation. Ask if there is any difficulty with defecation or continence, both to formed and liquid stool, and to flatus. Is anorectal sensation normal? The reflex action of the voluntary anal sphincter may be tested by introducing the lubricated gloved finger into the anus and noting whether contraction of the sphincter occurs with normal force, whether the sphincter is weak or paralysed, or whether any spasm is excited. The activity of the reflex may also be tested by gently pricking the skin on either side near the anus. A brisk contraction of the sphincter should immediately occur—the *anal reflex*. In addition, the anal sphincter normally contracts briskly in reflex response to a sudden cough—the *cough reflex*. The degree of tension in the anal sphincter during a voluntary sphincter squeeze—'tighten up'—should be noted. In patients with weakness of the pelvic floor, usually due to damage to the innervation of the pelvic floor musculature, coughing is accompanied by descent of the pelvic floor a distance of several centimetres onto the examiner's finger.

This is often associated with stress incontinence of faeces or of urine.

Micturition. Always ask whether there is any difficulty in controlling or initiating micturition and whether bladder and urethral sensation are normal. Retention, incontinence or urgency of micturition should be noted. *Urinary incontinence* in neurological disorders may be due to *overflow* from an atonic distended bladder in which sensation has been lost. In this case the bladder will be enlarged to palpation or percussion and suprapubic pressure may result in the expulsion of urine from the urethra (*stress incontinence*). Incontinence may also be due to *reflex micturition*, occurring either at regular intervals as the bladder partially fills, or precipitately and unexpectedly in response to a sudden noise, to movement or to exposure to cold (*unstable bladder; urge incontinence*). Urge incontinence is frequently idiopathic but may be an early feature of intrinsic disease of the spinal cord.

Sexual function. When there is incontinence associated with neurological disease, difficulty with penile erection, ejaculation or, in both sexes, orgasm, may be noted.

COORDINATION OF MOVEMENT

The smooth recruitment, interaction and cooperation of separate muscles or groups of muscles is necessary to perform motor acts. If coordination is impaired (*ataxia*), motor performance becomes difficult or even impossible. The coordination of groups of muscles is a function of various factors, such as afferent impulses coming from the muscle and joint receptors, cerebellar function, and corticospinal tract function. When ataxia is present it is not always easy to say which of these factors is at fault. Movements can be monitored by vision, but vision is not a factor in the coordination of most normal movements. However, when there is loss of the sense of position of a limb or joint, the sensory defect may be compensated for by vision, and the disturbance of movement may become apparent only when the eyes are closed or the patient is in the dark (Fig. 11.59). *Sensory ataxia* occurs typically in sensory neuropathies or posterior column lesions, when position sense is impaired in the legs. Before ataxia can be ascribed solely to cerebellar disease, therefore, it is important to ascertain whether joint position sense is impaired or not. Proximal weakness may mimic cerebellar ataxia, but this can usually be recognized easily by testing muscular strength.

Testing coordination in the upper limbs

Ask the patient to touch the point of their own nose then your forefinger, held in front of their face, with their index finger. If this movement is performed naturally and without random errors, coordination is normal. The patient should then be asked to perform the same actions with the eyes closed; any additional irregularity indicates that there may be impairment

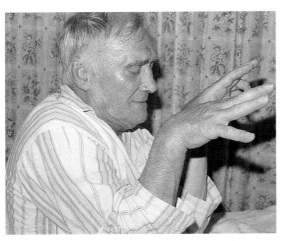

Fig. 11.59 Paraneoplastic sensory neuropathy due to small cell carcinoma of the lung. With the eyes closed the patients outstretched arms become flexed and abnormal postures develop in the fingers.

of position sense in the limb. Coordination of the fingers in rapid movements (e.g. rapidly touching each finger in turn with the thumb, or the thumb and index) are specially useful tests. In *cerebellar ataxia* the errors of movement tend to occur *at right angles to the intended direction of movement*. In *anxious subjects* errors tend to occur in the direction of the movement itself.

Dysdiadochokinesis, consisting of impaired ability to execute rapidly repeated movements, is a useful sign of cerebellar ataxia. Ask the patient to flex the elbow to a right angle and then alternately to supinate and pronate the forearm as rapidly as possible 'as though screwing in a light bulb'. All normal persons can do this very rapidly but usually slightly less rapidly with the non-dominant than with the dominant arm. When dysdiadochokinesia is present the movements are slow, awkward, irregular and incomplete, and often become impossible after a few attempts. The sign can also be elicited by asking the patient to tap the examiner's palm with the tips of the fingers, alternately in pronation and supination, as fast as possible. Minor degrees of ataxia can then be both felt and heard.

Watch the patient dressing or undressing, handling a book or picking up pins. These complex and practised everyday movements offer a very sensitive way of assessing coordination.

Testing coordination in the lower limbs
Several formalized observations are important in testing for ataxia in the legs:

Heel shin–ankle test
The patient lies supine on the bed. Ask the patient to lift one leg straight up in the air, then to bend the knee and place the heel of this leg on the opposite knee and to slide the heel down the shin towards the ankle. In *cerebellar ataxia* a characteristic, irregular,

side-to-side series of errors in the speed and direction of movement occurs. The test should be performed *with the eyes open*. Also, watch the patient draw a large circle in the air with the toe. The circle should be drawn smoothly and accurately, but in cerebellar ataxia it is 'squared off' irregularly.

Romberg's sign
This is a test for *loss of position sense* (sensory ataxia) in the legs, not of cerebellar function. Ask the patient to stand with feet close together, then to continue in this posture with the eyes closed. If Romberg's sign is present, as soon as the eyes are closed the patient begins to sway about, or may even fall. *The essential feature of the sign is therefore that the patient is more unsteady standing with the eyes closed than with them open.* When there is defective position sense in the legs, as in sensory neuropathy or tabes dorsalis, standing cannot be maintained steadily without visual fixation. The test is also more difficult with labyrinthine lesions or with cerebellar ataxia, but with loss of position sense it is grossly abnormal. In labyrinthine lesions there is positional nystagmus, and in cerebellar ataxia there is ataxia of the limbs examined on the couch. A useful additional test when considering whether Rombergism is due to labyrinthine disease is to ask the patient to jump quickly up and down on both feet with legs together, hands outstretched, and eyes closed (*Unterberger's test*). In labyrinthine disease the patient will gradually progress across the floor, or fall to one side, the side of the labyrinthine lesion.

Walking
Always test walking when assessing ataxia (see below). When there is incoordination (*ataxia*) the patient will deviate off the straight line. Watch particularly for unsteadiness as the patient turns to walk back towards you. The test is made more difficult by asking the patient to '*tandem walk*' along a line, like a tightrope walker, placing the heel of one foot immediately adjacent to the toe of the one behind.

GAIT
Analysis of a patient's gait is of major importance in diagnosis (Box 11.15). The legs should be adequately exposed and, as far as possible, free of constricting clothing (e.g. a dressing gown). If possible the feet should be bare. Ask the patient to walk freely up and down the room, and then along a straight line. Choose a line between floor tiles, or in the pattern on the carpet. Get into the habit of using the same marks on the floor each time you carry out the test.

Consider the following:

- Can the patient walk at all?
- How much help is needed?
- Can the patient walk in a straight line or is there deviation to one side or the other?

BOX 11.15   Gait disorders.

Upper motor neurone
- *Hemiplegia.* Circumduction of leg with inability to flex hip and dorsiflex foot against resistance (or gravity). Triple flexion posture of upper limb
- *Paraplegia and quadriplegia.* Scissoring, stiff-legged gait and flexed posture

Lower motor neurone
- *Foot drop.* Weakness of dorsiflexion and eversion of the foot leads to excessive hip flexion to compensate; due to common peroneal nerve palsy or L5/S1 root lesion, or to peripheral neuropathy
- *Quadriceps weakness.* Knee extension weak, leading to sudden falls, difficulty rising from chair or descending stairs
- *Proximal weakness.* Rolling gait, with difficulty climbing stairs. Arms cannot be lifted above shoulder height. Axial weakness may be present
- *Peripheral neuropathy.* Distal weakness and sensory loss

Cerebellar syndrome
- *Ataxia.* Unsteadiness and inability to walk on a narrow base, or to turn quickly

Extrapyramidal syndromes
- *Parkinson's disease.* Shuffling festinant gait, with flexed posture, tremor of hand and face
- *Dystonia.* Involuntary movements and rigid postures
- *Involuntary movements.* Chorea, athetosis, ballismus

Sensory ataxia
Cerebellar-like ataxia associated with distal loss of position sense:

Apraxic gait
- Loss of concept of walking, often associated with tiny rapid steps

Hysteria
- Bizarre, 'functional' gait disorder; miraculously the patient does not fall

- Does the patient tend to fall? In what direction?
- Can the patient turn quickly through 180 degrees without unbalancing?
- Is there a recognizable gait disorder?

In investigating the underlying cause of an abnormal gait, begin by excluding local causes, such as osteoarthritis of the hip, an old knee injury or local pain in the leg or pelvis.

In a *spastic gait* the patient walks on a narrow base, has difficulty in bending the knees and drags the feet along as if they were glued to the floor. This can be heard as well as seen. The foot is raised from the ground by tilting the pelvis, and the leg is then swung forwards so that the foot tends to describe an arc, the toe scraping along the floor—*circumduction*

of the leg. A spastic gait is a characteristic feature of corticospinal lesions, especially spinal cord disease. The *hemiplegic gait* is essentially a spastic gait in which only one leg is affected.

The gait in *sensory ataxia* may be described as 'stamping'. The patient raises the foot very suddenly, often abnormally high, and then jerks it forward, bringing it to the ground again with a stamp, and often heel first. By using the eyes in place of position sense the patient may succeed in walking fairly steadily, but when walking in the dark, or with the eyes closed, there is severe ataxia. Other signs of loss of postural sense will be present. When there is weakness of the extensor muscles of the feet, as, for example, in common peroneal nerve palsy, the gait is *high-stepping* in order to avoid tripping as a result of the toes catching the ground.

The gait of *cerebellar ataxia* appears 'drunken' or 'reeling'. Patients with this gait disorder walk on a broad base, the feet planted widely apart and placed irregularly. The ataxia is equally severe whether the eyes are open or closed. Other signs of cerebellar disease are usually present (Box 11.16).

A *festinant gait* is characteristic of Parkinson's disease (Box 11.17). The patient is bent forwards (*flexion dystonia*) and advances with rapid, short, shuffling steps, so that the gait appears as though the patient is trying to catch up with the centre of gravity. The arms do not swing. So patients, if gently pulled backwards, begin to walk backwards and are unable to stop (*retropulsion*). With bilateral lesions

---

BOX 11.16   Clinical signs of cerebellar lesions.

- Cerebellar ataxia
- Intention tremor
- Involvement of limbs, trunk and external ocular movement (nystagmus)
- Past-pointing
- Rebound
- Impaired ability to generate alternating rhythmic movements

---

BOX 11.17   Parkinson's disease: main clinical features.

- Distal pill-rolling tremor (about 5 Hz)
- Tremor mainly involves hands
- Often unilateral predominance
- Cogwheel rigidity
- Akinesia of face and limbs
- Impassive facies
- Drooling
- Flexed posture
- Loss of righting reflexes, and impaired balance, with postural instability
- Autonomic features; e.g. incontinence, postural hypotension

in the deep frontal white matter a rather similar short-stepped but rapid, tapping gait occurs, called *marche à Petipas* (the Russian ballet master of 100 years ago) to describe its resemblance to the rapid steps of a ballet dancer on points. In *dystonia and chorea* involuntary movements are usually exaggerated during walking, and unusual foot placement responses may occur so that the toes may extend away from the floor (*avoiding response*) or the feet may appear glued to the floor (*grasping response*).

A *waddling gait* is a feature of proximal pelvic girdle muscular weakness, especially of myopathies and muscular dystrophies. The body is often tilted backwards, with an increased lumbar lordosis; the feet are planted rather widely apart and the body sways from side to side as each step is taken. Weakness of the glutei, especially gluteus medius, causes the hip to drop when the affected leg is held off the ground in the erect posture (*Trendelenburg's sign*). This also occurs with disease of the hip joint (Ch. 10).

INVOLUNTARY MOVEMENTS

In a number of different diseases of the nervous system, involuntary, unintended movements occur, either at rest or superimposed on voluntary movement. The different kinds of involuntary movement are not specific disease entities, but represent clinical phenomena. Most are due to diseases of the basal ganglia and extrapyramidal system, but epilepsy can also cause non-voluntary movement.

Epilepsy

Involuntary movement of one side of the body, or one limb, may be due to focal epilepsy. Very rarely, such an attack may continue for hours or even days (*epilepsia partialis continua*). Focal seizures cause complex, repetitive, brief movements which are exacerbated by arousal or by handling the limb and which can usually be relieved by anticonvulsant drug therapy. Stereotyped repetitiveness of the movement is characteristic. A classification of epilepsy is given in Box 11.18, and of the causes of epilepsy in Box 11.19.

BOX 11.18   Seizures: a basic clinical classification.

Generalized epilepsy
- Major generalized seizures: grand mal epilepsy
- Minor generalized seizures: petit mal epilepsy, myoclonic seizures

Partial epilepsy
- Simple partial seizures: temporal lobe epilepsy
- Complex partial seizures: with secondary generalization
- Focal motor seizures of childhood
- Myoclonus epilepsy

BOX 11.19   Causes of epilepsy.

Idiopathic epilepsy has no evident cause, may have a genetic basis (low seizure threshold), and usually begins before age 20 years.

Symptomatic epilepsy may arise with any cortical or subcortical lesion, e.g. tumour, infection, infarction or degenerative disease of the brain. Epilepsy is less common with white matter disease, and does not complicate disease in the cerebellum or brainstem.

Idiopathic epilepsy
- Major and minor generalized seizures of childhood or adolescent onset
- Myoclonic seizures
- Focal motor seizures of childhood
- Simple partial epilepsy

Symptomatic epilepsy
- Late-onset major generalized seizures
- Late-onset simple and complex partial epilepsy
- Drug-induced epilepsy
- Epilepsy following a brain injury, e.g. trauma, tumour or infection

---

Myoclonus

Myoclonus is a rapid, usually irregular, jerking movement of a group of muscles in a limb, or even of the whole body, often occurring in response to an extraneous stimulus such as a sudden loud noise. A sudden start when surprised, or bodily jerks on falling asleep or waking, are common varieties of myoclonus experienced by most people. *Flexion myoclonus* may occur as a manifestation of major epilepsy or with degenerative disorders of the cerebellum, and in certain types of encephalitis, when it often exhibits *periodicity*. Less commonly, irregular myoclonic jerks may occur in a single limb, or a ripple of jerky irregular contraction may pass through the muscles of a limb—*segmental myoclonus*. Myoclonus can occur with lesions at many levels in the central nervous system; it does not have localizing value.

Tremor

Regular or irregular distal movements having an *oscillatory character* are classified as tremors (Box 11.20). The tremor of *anxiety* is usually fine and rapid at rest,

---

BOX 11.20   Common causes of tremors.

- Anxiety
- Essential tremor
- Physiological tremor
- Thyrotoxicosis
- Parkinson's disease
- Heavy metal poisoning, e.g. mercury, manganese, thallium

sometimes with a coarse irregularity during voluntary movement. *Thyrotoxic* tremor is characteristically fine and rapid, but may be complicated by choreiform involuntary movement. In *essential tremor* the tremor is coarse and distal, and often exaggerated in awkward postures, as when the outstretched fingers are held pointing at each other, in full inversion, in front of the patient's nose. The head and neck are frequently affected by a nodding tremor. Essential tremor is usually relieved to some extent during movement. It is often familial. *Cerebellar tremor* is present only during movement (*intention tremor*). *Extrapyramidal tremor* (e.g. Parkinson's disease) is accompanied by signs of extrapyramidal disease. *Senile tremor* is similar to benign essential tremor. *Hysterical tremor* tends to involve a limb or the whole body and it is characteristically worsened by the physician's attempt to control it.

The tremor of *Parkinsonism* is usually easily recognized. There is a rapid, rhythmic, alternating tremor, predominantly in flexion/extension but often with a prominent rotary component between finger and thumb (*pill-rolling tremor*). Proximal muscles may be involved, and the lips and tongue are frequently involved. The tremor is almost always more severe in the arm than in the leg. It is usually asymmetrical and is associated with other symptoms and signs of this extrapyramidal disease (Fig. 11.53), such as hypokinesia, cogwheel rigidity, postural abnormalities, gait disorder and an expressionless, quiet voice.

Athetosis

Athetosis is a complex, writhing involuntary movement, usually more pronounced in distal than in proximal muscles. It seems to consist of an interaction between various postures of the hand or foot, especially *grasping* and *avoiding* (see p. 233). The fingers are alternately widely extended, the arm following into an extended, abducted and externally rotated posture, and then the fingers clench, often trapping the thumb in the palm, and the limb flexes slightly and rotates internally. Athetosis may be unilateral or generalized. In very severe generalized athetosis, for example *torsion dystonia*, the trunk and axial musculature is affected and the patient may scarcely be able to stand. Marked, fixed torsional and flexion deformities may develop. Rarely, it may occur as a paroxysmal phenomenon.

Chorea

The word *chorea* means 'a dance'. The involuntary movements are brief, fluid and at first often difficult to discern. Ordinary voluntary movements, such as walking or picking up a cup and saucer, may be embellished with rapid extra little flourishes of movement. Muscular tone is often decreased. The outstretched upper limbs may assume a hyperpronated posture and little flicks of movement of the digits or

wrist, or of the face and tongue, may occur. At rest the patient appears 'fidgety' and 'unable to sit still'. The movements often appear less obvious during voluntary movement, and are increased by anxiety.

Chorea occurs as part of a dominantly inherited presenile dementia (*Huntington's disease*), with rheumatic fever (*Sydenham's chorea*) and after certain drugs (e.g. phenothiazines). It may also occur with other systemic diseases (e.g. *thyrotoxicosis* and *systemic lupus erythematosus*) and in old age (*senile chorea*), and in *pregnancy*. Unilateral chorea may occur with deeply placed lesions in one hemisphere, which may be violent, consisting of ballistic, flinging movements of the limbs (*hemiballismus or hemichorea*).

Dyskinesias

The word '*dyskinesia*' is particularly used to describe *phenothiazine-induced* involuntary movements, which predominantly affect the pharyngeal and facial perioral musculature, and *levodopa-induced* axial torsional movements, although similar movements occur in choreo-athetoid and dystonic patients not previously treated with these drugs. Levodopa-induced involuntary movements tend to develop at times of peak plasma levels of dopamine (*peak-dose dyskinesias*), or at low levels (*end-dose dyskinesias*).

Dystonia

This is an *abnormally maintained posture*, often associated with continuous, plastic rigidity. The dystonias are closely related to choreo-athetosis; indeed the expression '*dystonic movements*' is sometimes used, but the term can also be used to describe the flexed posture of Parkinson's disease (*flexion dystonia*) or the fixed hemiplegic flexed posture (*hemiplegic dystonia*). The abnormal postures of dystonia vary in relation to different circumstances: for example, dystonic posturing in torsion dystonia may be relieved by lying supine or by standing in contact with a wall. The term dystonia is sometimes used to include all involuntary movements that are accompanied by abnormal postures.

Torticollis

Spasmodic torticollis consists of a jerky or maintained *rotational and abducted posture of the neck*. It is a form of dystonia. It can often be partially self-modified by certain postural adjustments, for example touching the chin with the index finger. It may precede more generalized torsion dystonia, but often occurs in isolation from other movement disorders.

Tics

These are simple, normal movements which become *repeated* unnecessarily to the point that they become an embarrassment. They often occur in the context of psychiatric disorders. In contrast to the other involuntary movement disorders, they can be readily imitated. Head-nodding is a common example. Tics may be difficult to separate from other involuntary movements, but an important feature is their inconsistency, for example they may disappear when the patient is reassured or apparently unobserved.

Myokymia

This is a persistent twitchy, often rhythmical movement usually affecting the periorbital muscles. It may occur as a benign phenomenon in fatigued or anxious people. It is sometimes due to lesions in the facial nerve or its nucleus. Myokymia is rarely a generalized disorder of autoimmune origin (*Isaac's syndrome*).

Asterixis

An irregular, abrupt, brief loss of posture, especially evident in the outstretched hands or tongue, occurs in decompensated hepatic failure (*hepatic flap*) and in other metabolic disorders (e.g. uraemia, poisoning with hypnotic drugs), and in respiratory failure.

Tetany

In tetany, commonly due to hypocalcaemia or alkalosis, there is a characteristic posture of the affected hand (see Fig. 1.3b). The fingers and thumbs are held stiffly adducted and the hand is partially flexed at the metacarpophalangeal joints; the toes may be similarly affected (*carpopedal spasm*). Ischaemia of the affected limb, produced by a sphygmomanometer cuff inflated above the arterial pressure for 2 or 3 minutes, will augment this sign or produce it if it is not already present (*Trousseau's sign*). Another useful test is to tap lightly with a patellar hammer in the region of exit of the facial nerve from the skull, about 3–5 cm below and in front of the ear. The facial muscles twitch briefly with each tap (*Chvostek's sign*).

Cramps

Spontaneous contraction of part or whole of a muscle, especially of the calf muscles, is common in normal people. It is a frequent feature in chronic or progressive neurogenic muscle weakness, motor neurone disease, and in metabolic disorders, e.g. hyponatraemia (as in *heat stroke*) and hypomagnesaemia. It is due to hypercontraction of muscle fibres, and is relieved by passive stretch of the affected muscle.

THE SENSORY SYSTEM

A sensory modality is a sensory experience recognized by individuals as unique. This practical psychophysical definition accords with general experience. There are six main sensory modalities that can be tested at the bedside:

- Tactile sensibility (this includes light touch and pressure, and tactile localization and discrimination)
- Position sense; the appreciation of passive movement
- Recognition of the size, shape, weight and form of objects
- Vibration
- Pain
- Temperature.

Perception depends on the physiological interaction of afferent inputs at different levels in the nervous system. In some instances, as in the recognition and naming of objects, it depends also on the ability to manipulate the object felt. The perception of vibration, therefore, does not depend on a special set of nerve fibres responsible only for transmitting vibration sense to the central nervous system, but rather is a form of sensation subjectively similar to rapidly applied light touch which, in clinical practice, is found to be disturbed when there is a lesion of the large-diameter afferent fibres in the peripheral nerves, posterior columns or, sometimes, at a higher level. There is a long-standing classification of sensory modalities into epicritic and nociceptive modalities—indicating light cutaneous discriminatory sensibilities and pain-directed responses—that is broadly related to activity in large myelinated and small, thinly myelinated nerve fibres in the peripheral nerves. There are receptors in the skin and tissues that are sensitive to touch, pain and other physical stimuli, especially warm and cold. These are found at different density in different portions of the skin. For example, the fingertips are very sensitive to minor skin deformation, and therefore to light touch and discrimination.

TECHNIQUE OF SENSORY EXAMINATION

The important tests are light touch, vibration, position sense, and pin-prick (surface pain). Begin testing sensation with touch and position sense (use a pin later, when you have gained the patient's confidence). Always apply the sensory stimulus first to an area of sensation that you know from the history or suspect to be abnormal and mark out its borders *from the abnormal to the normal*. The patient will point out the sudden change to normality. Areas of diminished sensation should be carefully, *but quickly*, mapped out so that their distribution in relation to root lesions, peripheral nerve lesions or lesions in the central nervous system can be studied (Fig. 11.60). It is important to do this quickly, accurately and, as far as possible, *without repetition*. The longer the time taken to test sensation, the more confusing will be the result: the test requires concentration and cooperation by both patient and examiner.

Inconsistency in the patient's responses may be due to fatigue, poor cooperation, lack of understanding or suggestibility. If there is inconsistency, simplify the test. Ask the patient to say 'now' whenever the stim-

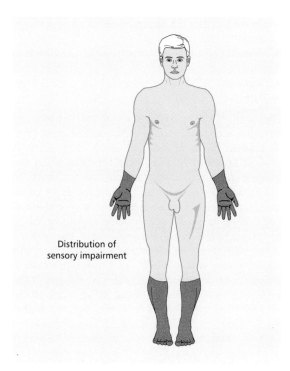

Distribution of sensory impairment

Fig. 11.60 Pattern of sensory loss in peripheral neuropathy.

ulus is felt, and test with the eyes shut and then with them open. It may be useful to test a related form of sensation, for example temperature sense in the case of pinprick or position or vibration sense in the case of light touch. Always encourage the patient to be very careful to make the correct response. Never make much of small differences. Remember that it is normal to experience changes in the sharpness of a pin between the nailbed and the dorsum of the finger, or at about the level of the clavicle when the stimulus ascends the anterior chest wall. The pulp of the fingers is rather insensitive to pain but very sensitive to light touch and to discriminative tests such as two-point discrimination. Vibration sense is best perceived over a bony prominence.

It is generally better to test sensation with the patient's eyes open, although it is obviously necessary to prevent the patient seeing the fingers and toes when testing position sense. People are usually more alert and attentive with their eyes open than with them shut, and alertness is crucial in sensory testing. Except in testing position sense it will not affect the result to have the patient actually watching the procedure. It can be a frightening experience to be suddenly pricked with a pin when one's eyes are closed. Such surprises, which destroy a patient's confidence in the examiner, should be avoided. Compare the findings with the abnormalities, if any, described by the patient as part of the neurological history. Most people are very aware of sensory abnormality, except perhaps in the case of temperature sense which may be lost without the patient being aware of it, especially if the area

affected is around the shoulders, as in syringomyelia, rather than involving the hands or feet.

TACTILE SENSIBILITY (LIGHT TOUCH)

Use a wisp of cotton wool or the tip of your index finger. Ask the patient to indicate whether the touch is felt, and if it feels normal. *How* is it abnormal? It may be abolished or reduced (*hypoaesthesia*), misperceived as a painful, irritating or tingling sensation (*hyperaesthesia*) or mislocalized. Very rarely there may be a delay between the stimulus and its recognition by the patient. Areas of diminished sensation should be carefully delineated and recorded.

The ability to discriminate between two points is a useful quantitative sensory measurement. Use a pair of blunt dividers (*two-point discriminator*). The patient is asked whether one or both points can be felt. Normally 2 mm of separation of the points can be recognized as two separate stimuli on the fingertips, and rather wider separation—about 1 cm—on the pulps of the toes. This is an excellent objective sensory test which is particularly useful in cases of posterior column or parietal cortical lesions and in some peripheral nerve lesions (such as the carpal tunnel syndrome) that involve large afferent fibres and impair discriminatory sensation.

POSITION SENSE

Ask the patient to look away or shield the eyes with clothing or a bedsheet. Explain that you will move a finger (or toe or elbow) up or down and ask the patient to tell you which way it has been moved. Normal people can recognize movements of a few degrees at all joints, including knee, ankle, elbow and wrist, in addition to the more commonly tested fingers and toes. It is sometimes helpful to ask the patient to imitate with the opposite limb or digit the position of the limb or digit being tested. It is essential that the patient should be relaxed sufficiently to allow the limb to be moved *passively*. The *appreciation of movement* is closely related to the sense of position and can be tested at the same time. Gradually move a digit or limb into a new position, with the patient's eyes closed. Ask them to say 'now' as soon as movement is perceived. Note the angle through which the limb was moved. If the appreciation of movement is diminished, this angle is many times greater than that in a normal limb. Movements of less than 10 degrees can be appreciated at all normal joints.

When position sense is disturbed in the upper limbs, the outstretched fingers may twist, rise and fall when held out with the eyes closed. These involuntary movements (*pseudoathetosis*) occur unknown to the patient and disappear almost completely when the patient watches the position of the fingers. Patients with defective position sense may be unable to manipulate small objects, fasten buttons and so on without visually observing their movements (*sensory ataxia*).

RECOGNITION OF SIZE, SHAPE, WEIGHT AND FORM

These faculties can be tested in the hands with the eyes closed. To test *size appreciation*, place objects of the same shape, but of different sizes, for example small rods or matches of different length, one after the other, in the patient's palm. Ask which is the larger. To test *weight* ask which is the heavier. To test *recognition of shape* familiar objects such as coins, a pencil, a penknife, scissors, etc., are placed in the hand, and the patient is asked to identify them or to describe their form. *Astereognosis*, loss of shape appreciation, occurs with *parietal lesions*, when position sense and light touch are normal, although there is usually some associated defect in these modalities. It also occurs with *posterior column lesions*, when position sense, vibration sense and light touch are profoundly disturbed.

APPRECIATION OF VIBRATION

Place the foot of a vibrating tuning-fork on a bony prominence, such as the dorsum of the large toe, the lateral malleolus, the dorsum of a finger, or the tip of the shoulder. Vibration can be felt. As it gradually fades in intensity, ask the patient to say when he or she ceases to feel it. If the examiner can still perceive it, the patient's perception of vibration is impaired. There is often some loss of vibration sense in the feet and legs in old age. This is a valuable semi-quantitative test, as the ability to appreciate vibration may be lost in various diseases, for example in peripheral neuropathies and in posterior column disorders. A tuning fork of 128 Hz (lower C) should be used. Vibrations of higher frequency are more difficult to perceive.

PAIN

Pain may be evoked by a cutaneous stimulus (e.g. a light pin prick) or by pressure on deeper structures (e.g. muscles or bones). Superficial and pressure pain should be tested separately.

Superficial pain

The point of a pin should be used as the stimulus. Care must be taken that the patient distinguishes between the *sharpness* of the point (that is, its relative size) and the *pain* which the prick evokes; even when sensibility to pain is abolished, the patient may recognize that the stimulus is pointed, and thus confuse the observer by calling it 'sharp'. Always test from an area of abnormality toward normal skin. The pin used should be an ordinary domestic pin, rather than a hypodermic needle: the latter is designed to cut skin relatively painlessly and is not suitable for sensory testing. Pins used to test sensation should be adequately sterilized before re-use, or destroyed, because of the possibility, however remote, of transmission of hepatitis B or human immunodeficiency virus (HIV) infection. Disposable test pins are available, and these should be used whenever possible.

Pressure pain

This is examined by squeezing a distal muscle or the Achilles tendon. This sensation is particularly disturbed in tabes dorsalis.

Abnormal responses to superficial pain testing

Absence of sensibility to pain is termed *analgesia*; partial loss of pain sensibility is called *hypoalgesia*; an exaggerated sensibility, so that even a mild stimulus causes an unnatural intensity of painful sensation, is *hyperalgesia*. This occurs in some patients with spinal cord disease, for example in spinothalamic lesions and in tabes dorsalis—now a rare disorder—and also in certain patients with deep-seated parietal or thalamic lesions (*thalamic pain*). The pain experienced has a peculiar, ill-localized and persistent character. It often has a burning quality and it may occur as an intractable spontaneous phenomenon or only in response to cutaneous stimuli. *Allodynia* is an abnormal sensory experience, usually painful, to a normal stimulus. *Paraesthesiae* are tingling sensations that are sometimes so intense as to be painful; they may occur spontaneously or in response to light cutaneous stimuli. They may result from overactivity of sensory neurones when stimulated, or from cross-talk between adjacent damaged axons in the peripheral nerve fibre bundle that is active after stimulation of the skin.

TEMPERATURE SENSE

Temperature sense can be tested by using test tubes containing warm and cold water. The part to be tested is touched with each in turn, and the patient says whether each tube feels hot or cold. At the bedside, however, it is often sufficient to use the cold metallic sensation of the touch of the end of an ophthalmoscope or tuning-fork for rough assessment of temperature sensation. Quantitative thermal threshold testing apparatus is available that allows more accurate testing of thermal sensory function, but this is a research method not routinely applicable to clinical practice.

OTHER DISTURBANCES OF SENSATION

Sensory inattention is an important feature of lesions of the parietal lobe. Ask the patient to close the eyes. Simultaneously stimulate homologous points on opposite sides of the body by touch or by pin prick, then ask the patient to indicate which side (or sides) was touched. In sensory inattention the stimulus on the abnormal side is not perceived even though there is no subjective difference between left and right to conventional comparative testing. This is also called *sensory extinction* or *sensory neglect*. *Bilateral simultaneous sensory stimuli* can also be used when testing vision and hearing; a similar defect may be found. In the presence of fixed hemisensory loss, of course, the sign is invalid. Some patients with parietal lesions will also show *spatial summation* in which a stimulus is perceived only if an area of skin larger than a certain critical area is stimulated, or *temporal summation* in which an ill-localized and often perverted or painful sensation is felt after rapidly repeated stimuli applied to the same point. Single stimuli will be missed.

These abnormalities are part of a perceptual defect related to *agnosia*, a disorder in which the patient is unaware of the nature or the severity of a sensory disorder. In its most extreme form there may even be denial of illness (*anosognosia*). In patients with higher perceptual defects of this type a number of other bedside tests may be useful. These include *constructional tests*, such as the patient's ability to draw a map of their surroundings, to copy a complex figure (for example, two interlocking irregular pentagons), to draw a clock face or a human face, or to draw more complex figures, for example a house. Visual and tactile memory can be tested by variations of these tests. Constructional ability is particularly impaired with right parietal lesions (*constructional apraxia*). Specific sensory disorders, such as inability to recognize faces (*prosopagnosia*), visual and tactile perseveration and *synaesthesias* (sensations perceived in a different modality than that applied) are some features of parietal cortical lesions.

THE AUTONOMIC NERVOUS SYSTEM

The autonomic nervous system consists of afferent and efferent, post-ganglionic, sympathetic and parasympathetic neurones in the periphery, together with the central preganglionic components of these systems in the intermediolateral cell columns in the spinal cord, and rostral connections in the brainstem and cerebral hemispheres. These neuronal systems are autonomous, but not free from voluntary control. They are concerned with modulation of function in the cardiovascular and gastrointestinal systems, with temperature regulation, sexual reflexes, bladder and bowel detrusor and sphincter activity, and pupillary and respiratory reflex control mechanisms. Thus, patients with disturbances of the autonomic nervous system may show complex clinical abnormalities. The clinical presentation will be determined by the distribution of abnormality in the central or peripheral components of this neuronal system (Box 11.21).

In the rare syndrome of *progressive autonomic failure* there is degeneration of both preganglionic and post-ganglionic neurones, leading to several *autonomic abnormalities*:

- Inability to maintain the blood pressure in the erect position (*orthostatic hypotension*)
- Constipation and other disorders of gastrointestinal motility
- Incontinence of urine
- Impotence
- Pupillary areflexia

> **BOX 11.21   Features of autonomic disorders.**
>
> - Postural hypotension
> - Impotence and erectile failure
> - Retention or incontinence of urine
> - Poor urine stream (detrusor failure)
> - Constipation, and faecal incontinence
> - Oesophageal and GI dysmotility
> - Pupillary immobility
> - Impaired sweating
> - Snoring and sleep apnoea

- Disturbances of sweating
- Orthostatic hypotension, causing syncope in the erect posture
- Loss of cardiovascular reflexes.

Loss of cardiovascular reflexes causes:

- Tachycardia at rest
- Absence of the normal slowing of the pulse in response to the Valsalva manoeuvre
- Absence of the normal slight increase in the pulse rate and blood pressure on standing
- Absence of the normal increase in blood pressure during hand grip
- Absence of the blood pressure increase with stressful tasks such as mental arithmetic.

These autonomic abnormalities may also develop in peripheral neuropathies, especially in diabetic neuropathy, when the post-ganglionic neurones of the sympathetic and parasympathetic nervous system in the periphery are involved.

BEDSIDE ASSESSMENT OF AUTONOMIC FUNCTION

- Check the pupillary responses to light and accommodation
- Is the skin normal? If dry, suspect absence of sweating
- Is there a resting tachycardia?
- Does the pulse rate slow with deep inspiration?
- Are there trophic changes in distal skin, e.g. absence of hair growth?

Standing test for orthostatic hypotension

Have the patient lying quietly on a couch for 15 minutes, with sphygmomanometer and cardiac rate meter or lead 1 ECG attached. Check the resting blood pressure. Then ask the patient to stand. *Note the pulse rate from the R–R interval at the 15th and 30th beats* after standing, and measure the blood pressure 1 and 3 minutes after standing. In normal subjects the systolic blood pressure should not decrease by more than 10 mmHg. In patients with autonomic dysfunction the systolic blood pressure falls more than 30 mmHg. The 30th:15th pulse ratio is >1.03 in normal subjects, and ≤ 1.0 when there is autonomic disturbance.

Deep breaths test

Lie the patient flat. When the pulse has steadied, record the pulse rate during six *maximal* deep breaths. In normal subjects the pulse rate should fall by >15 beats/min; with autonomic disturbances the pulse rate slows <10 beats/min.

Handgrip test

With the patient lying flat, measure the maximal hand grip force by having the patient grip a sphygmomanometer cuff as hard as possible. Then measure the rise in diastolic blood pressure after a 30% handgrip sustained for 5 minutes. The diastolic pressure should rise >16 mmHg; in autonomic disorders the diastolic pressure will rise <10 mmHg.

Valsalva test

The patient blows into a sphygmomanometer, maintaining a pressure of 40 mmHg for 15 seconds. The ratio of the highest pulse rate in the preliminary rest period to the lowest pulse rate during the test is >1.5 in normal subjects and <1.1 in patients with autonomic disturbances. The test may be repeated up to three times if the initial result is equivocal.

Other tests

Tests of bowel motility and of bladder and urethral function using cystometry are also useful in evaluating the extent of autonomic dysfunction. Quantitative pupillometry, and the response to conjunctival application of parasympathomimetic and sympathomimetic drugs can also be used (see Ch. 12).

SIGNS OF MENINGEAL IRRITATION

The main feature is neck stiffness, or increased resistance to passive flexion of the neck. It should be tested formally whenever there is a clinical possibility of meningeal irritation. It is a more sensitive test than Kernig's sign. These signs are not always due to *meningitis* (Figs 11.61 and 15.1) or to *sub-arachnoid haemorrhage*, although these are the most frequent causes. These two tests depend upon the fact that stretching the spinal nerve roots in meningeal irritation causes reflex muscular spasm in the paraspinal and sacral muscles.

NECK STIFFNESS

Ask the patient to flex the neck as fully as possible to ascertain the degree of movement possible, and then to relax. Then passively flex the neck. The chin should normally touch the chest without pain. In meningeal irritation neck flexion causes pain in the posterior part of the neck, sometimes radiating down the back, and the *movement is resisted* by spasm in the extensor muscles of the neck. In addition to meningeal irritation, neck rigidity is also caused by diseases of the cervical spine, and by raised intracranial pressure due especially to a posterior fossa tumour, with rostral-caudal displacement of the vermis in the foramen magnum, leading to local dural irritation. *Head retraction*, now rare, represents an extreme degree of neck rigidity. It was formerly a feature of untreated tuberculous meningitis.

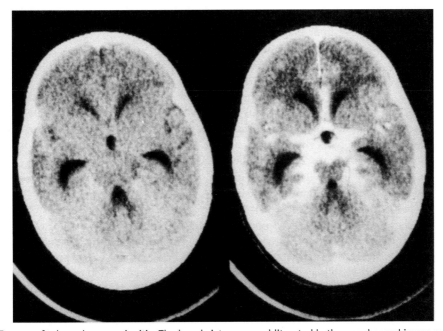

Fig. 11.61 CT scans of tuberculous meningitis. The basal cisterns are obliterated in the unenhanced image on the left. On the right the inflamed meninges and the inflammatory exudate have been visualized (enhanced) following intravenous injection of iodine-based contrast. The white central areas represent the abnormality. The clinical sign of neck stiffness represents reflex spasm in the neck extensors caused by inflammation of the basal meninges.

KERNIG'S SIGN

Kernig's sign is elicited with the patient supine on the bed. Passively extend the patient's knee on either side when the hip is fully flexed. In patients with meningeal irritation affecting the lower part of the spinal subarachnoid space this movement causes pain and spasm of the hamstrings.

NERVE ROOT ENTRAPMENT

When nerve roots are damaged by entrapment at intervertebral foramina, or by compression with disc prolapse, pain occurs spontaneously and in response to movement, particularly when the root is stretched. Thus, flexion and rotary movements of the lumbar spine in lumbosacral nerve root syndromes, rotation of the trunk or coughing in thoracic disc lesions, and stretching of the arms and neck in cervical root disease will cause a shooting pain radiating into the territory of the sensory innervation of the affected root.

STRAIGHT LEG RAISING

This test is useful in patients with sciatica. The sciatic nerve and its roots are stretched by passively elevating the patient's extended leg with the hand, which is placed behind the heel. The movement is restricted by sciatic pain when a lumbosacral spinal root is entrapped, as in lumbosacral intervertebral disc protrusion. This is not a sign of meningeal irritation, but of nerve root entrapment.

TRUNK ROTATION AND COUGHING

This, with coughing, is a useful test in suspected thoracic disc lesions since it may replicate sudden stabbing pain in a root distribution.

ARM ELEVATION AND MOVEMENT

Elevation of the arm may induce root pain in people with cervical root entrapments due to disc herniation. The patient will usually know which movement is likely to induce the symptom.

BRIEF EXAMINATION OF THE NERVOUS SYSTEM

A detailed examination of the whole nervous system is time-consuming and something of an ordeal for the patient. A scheme for a quick routine examination is therefore useful in the examination of patients *not suspected of neurological disease*, in order to exclude major neurological disability. Follow the plan in Box 11.3. Always have some idea of what abnormalities are likely to be present before starting to examine the nervous system. Think in terms of patterns of abnormality, as outlined in Box 11.22.

BOX 11.22   Clinical patterns of neurological disease.

Stroke
Sudden hemiparesis, with recovery in hours, days or weeks (see Figs 11.71 and 11.77)

Multiple sclerosis
Previous painful, monocular loss of vision; subsequent relapsing and remitting neurological illness, with weakness, diplopia, sensory symptoms, and bladder dysfunction (see Fig. 11.70)

Idiopathic epilepsy
Infantile febrile convulsions; repeated partial or generalized convulsions

Spinal cord compression (see Boxes 11.7 and 11.8)
Progression of spastic paraparesis, with local signs, including root pain, at the level of compression; Brown–Séquard features may be present

Parkinson's disease
Insidious onset of resting tremor; impassive facies; loss of equilibrum, difficulty with posture and balance; poor, small handwriting; quiet voice; slowness of movement (see Fig. 11.56)

Motor neurone disease (ALS)
Progressive wasting and weakness, with focal onset; cramp and muscular twitching, slurred speech and difficulty swallowing; normal bladder; normal intellect (see Fig. 11.20)

Diabetic neuropathy
Painful, burning legs with skin redness distally; absent ankle jerks and distally impaired vibration sense; weight loss

Meningitis
Rapid onset of progressive headache, vomiting, fever, lassitude and drowsiness; petechial rash; neck stiffness (see Fig. 11.61, Table 11.4))

Acoustic neuroma
Intermittent dizziness for months or years; progressive unilateral deafness; lateralized Grade 1 or 2 nystagmus

Muscular dystrophy
Progressive proximal muscular weakness and atrophy; calf hypertrophy and male childhood onset suggest Duchenne disease (see Figs 11.52–11.55)

Migraine
Episodic unilateral headache preceded by flickering visual blurring or spots of light in vision, and vomiting; duration minutes or hours (see Box 11.2)

Tension headache
Continuous headache like a band around head, with anxiety and background of social stress or fear of illness (see Box 11.2)

Peripheral neuropathy

Gradual or rapid onset of distal or proximal and distal weakness in all four limbs, with distal sensory loss, absent distal reflexes or generalized areflexia (see Fig. 11.60)

Lumbosacral disc disease

Low back pain after lifting; sciatic radiation; sensory impairment on lateral aspect of ankle/foot; weak ankle eversion; painful straight leg raising; absent ankle jerk (Fig. 11.75)

SPECIAL INVESTIGATIONS

There are many methods for clinical investigation of neurological disorders. Investigation must be planned to yield relevant results at reasonable clinical risk and financial cost.

LUMBAR PUNCTURE

This procedure is used for obtaining samples of cerebrospinal fluid (CSF). The lumbar meninges are punctured using a long hollow needle inserted between the spines of two lumbar vertebrae, below the level of the termination of the conus medullaris.

Technique for lumbar puncture

First, examine the fundi to exclude raised intracranial pressure. Lumbar puncture is almost always contraindicated in the presence of raised intracranial pressure because of the risk of consequent transtentorial or tonsillar herniation.

Locate the third and fourth lumbar spines. The fourth lumbar spine usually lies in the transverse plane of the iliac crests. The puncture may be made through either the L3/4 or L4/5 interspace. Lie the patient on their left side on a firm couch or on the firm edge of a bed, with the trunk flexed so that the knees and chin are as nearly approximated as possible. The patient's back should be on the edge of the couch, and *its transverse axis*—i.e. a line passing through the posterior superior iliac spines—*should be vertical*. Local anaesthesia may be produced by injecting 1% or 2% sterile procaine at the chosen site, first raising a bleb under the skin, and, when this is insensitive, anaesthetizing the whole dermis. It is not necessary to inject procaine into the deep ligaments; this usually causes more pain than it relieves. A special disposable needle, about 8 cm in length, with a withdrawable stylet should be used. The stylet should fit accurately and should not protrude through the bevelled cutting edge of the needle.

Push the needle firmly through the skin in the midline or just to one side of it and press it steadily *forwards and slightly towards the patient's head*, with the bevel pointing towards the side on which the patient is lying. When the needle is felt to enter the spinal cavity, withdraw the stylet. CSF will drip slowly from the needle end. Collect CSF in three sterilized stoppered test tubes. If any blood is present, a marked difference in the amount in the first and subsequent tubes indicates that the blood is due to trauma from the puncture. The patient should lie flat for 8–24 hours afterwards, in order to reduce the chance of post-lumbar puncture headache developing.

The CSF pressure can be measured at the time of lumbar puncture with a manometer. For this measurement, the patient should be lying with the head on a pillow, at the same level as the sacrum, breathing quietly and with muscles relaxed. The neck and legs should *not* be too intensely flexed. The normal CSF pressure is 60–150 mm of CSF. The pressure rises and falls a centimetre or two with respiration. The pulse is also reflected in pressure fluctuations in the CSF. A slight cough will cause a sudden rise and fall, indicating that the needle is well placed in the subarachnoid space.

Queckenstedt's test is a crude method to detect a block in the circulation of CSF in the spinal canal, for example, in spinal tumours. The diagnosis of spinal tumour, if suspected, is nowadays made by magnetic resonance (MR) imaging, *without previous lumbar puncture*, since lumbar puncture may cause clinical deterioration. With the needle and manometer in position and the patient breathing quietly as described above, an assistant compresses one or other, but not both, jugular veins. This causes a sudden increase in intracranial pressure, which is immediately seen in the manometer as a sudden rise of CSF pressure, followed by an equally rapid fall when the pressure on the vein is released.

Difficulties with lumbar puncture

The commonest cause of a 'dry-tap'—the failure to obtain CSF—is an incorrectly performed puncture. This is usually because the patient is not in the correct position. The needle is therefore not introduced at right angles to the transverse axis of the back, and misses the spinal canal. Frequently, the needle is introduced too deeply so that it traverses the spinal canal and wedges against the posterior margin of the intervertebral disc; if the needle is withdrawn slightly, CSF will begin to flow. Occasionally, however, a 'dry-tap' is due to a complete block to the flow of CSF through the spinal canal. In this circumstance urgent MRI or other imaging of the spinal canal is required. Contrast myelography using cisternal or lateral cervical puncture is an outmoded technique that should only be carried out under radiological control by an experienced physician.

Abnormalities of the CSF

Normal CSF is clear and colourless, like water.

Yellow coloration

Any yellowness (*xanthochromia*) is pathological and is due either to old haemorrhage, to jaundice, or to excess of protein. In *Froin's syndrome* a pronounced yellow colour is associated with great excess of protein and the formation of a coagulum. It is now a very rare phenomenon. Even slight increases in CSF protein, however, cause a noticeable increase in viscosity of the fluid and an excessive frothiness of its surface when it is gently shaken.

Turbidity

Turbidity of the fluid may be due to the presence of white blood cells, either as a result of infection or following subarachnoid haemorrhage. If it does not clear on standing it is due to microorganisms.

Bloodstaining

The presence of *blood* may be due to injury to a vessel by the needle or to subarachnoid haemorrhage. In the latter case the blood is more uniformly mixed with the fluid, and the supernatant fluid remains yellow after centrifugation. A traumatic tap causes initial pink coloration, often streaky, that gradually clears in the later of the three or more tubes of CSF taken.

Cytology

Cytological examination of a turbid fluid is of great importance. A centrifugal deposit should be examined with Leishman's stain in order to obtain an idea of the character of the cells present; and by Gram's and Ziehl–Neelsen's methods for bacteria (Fig. 11.62). Cell counts are performed with a counting chamber and must be done immediately the fluid has been collected. Counts done some hours later give inaccurate results because the leucocytes stick together and to the sides of the tube, and endothelial cells break up in a short time. If any clot has formed, an accurate cell count cannot be obtained but the cells in the clot can be stained and examined. Normal fluid contains 2–5 lymphocytes/µl.

An increased cell count may consist of polymorphonuclear cells or lymphocytes. In a *polymorphonuclear* CSF more than 75% of the cells are polys;

in a *lymphocytic* CSF more than 98% are lymphocytes. Bacterial meningitis is associated with a polymorphonuclear pleocytosis, viral meningitis and syphilis with a lymphocytic CSF, and tuberculous meningitis with either a lymphocytic or a mixed type. The latter is termed *pleocytosis*. In TB meningitis the CSF sugar is very low, and the CSF protein very high (Table 11.4). Cytological examination of the centrifugal deposit may reveal malignant cells in patients with secondary neoplastic invasion of the meninges from lymphoma or carcinoma (see Fig. 11.63).

The CSF should also be examined bacteriologically and chemically. Normal CSF contains only a trace of albumin and hardly any globulin, the *total protein* being not more than 40 mg/dl. In some neurological diseases, particularly in multiple sclerosis, and in many acute and subacute virus infections, the globulin fractions in the CSF are increased. *The CSF IgG concentration* can be directly measured by immunoelectrophoresis. It is compared with the blood IgG and albumin levels in order to show whether a raised CSF IgG level is due to endogenous IgG synthesis within the central nervous system. Techniques are available to study the various components of IgG found in the CSF; in multiple sclerosis the abnormal IgG may be *oligoclonal*.

Glucose is present in normal CSF in a concentration of 2.5–4.2 mmol/l, which is about a half to two thirds of the blood glucose concentration. In purulent tuberculous or fungal meningitis and rarely in carcinomatous meningitis the CSF sugar is *reduced to less than half of the blood glucose*. It is also low if the patient is hypoglycaemic.

One or more of the tests for syphilis are often performed on the CSF.

The typical changes in the CSF in various neurological diseases are summarized in Table 11.4.

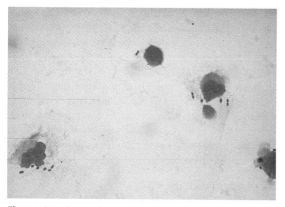

Fig. 11.62   Smear from cellular deposit in CSF from a patient with acute meningitis showing Gram-positive diplococci, many located intracellullarly in polymorphonuclear leucocytes.

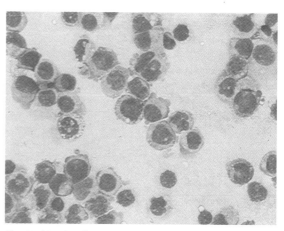

Fig. 11.63   Cerebrospinal fluid cytology. Cell deposit from cerebrospinal fluid almost exclusively comprising carcinoma cells shed from the leptomeninges. Metastasis to meninges from primary carcinoma of the breast. May–Grünwald–Giemsa stain. X 160.

TABLE 11.4   Typical changes in the cerebrospinal fluid (CSF) in various diseases.

Disease	Physical characteristics	Cytology (cells/μl)	Protein (g/l)	Glucose* (mmol/l)	Stained deposit	Culture
Normal	*Clear and colourless*	*Lymphocytes 0–5*	*0.1–0.4*	*2.5–4.2*	*No organisms*	*Sterile*
Bacterial meningitis	Yellowish and turbid Lymphocytes 5–50	Polymorphs 200–2000	0.5–2.0	< 2.0	Bacteria	Positive
Tuberculous meningitis	Colourless, sometimes viscous or yellow	Polymorphs 0–100 Lymphocytes 100–300	May be 5.0–15	< 2.0	Tubercle bacilli in CSF in most cases	Usually positive
Viral meningitis	Usually clear	10–100 mixed cells at first, becoming lymphocytic in 36 hours	0.1–0.6	2.5–4.2	No organisms	Sterile
Multiple sclerosis	Clear and colourless	Rarely 5–20 lymphocytes IgG level raised with monoclonal bands	0.1–0.6	2.5–4.2	No organisms	Sterile
Neoplastic meningitis (infiltration)	Clear or yellowish	5–1000 cells of mixed type	0.5–2.0	< 3.0	Inflammatory and malignant cells	Sterile

* CSF glucose is usually more than half the blood glucose. Simultaneous blood and CSF glucose measurements should always be performed.

THE ELECTROENCEPHALOGRAM (EEG)

Electrodes applied to the patient's scalp pick up small changes of electrical potential, which after amplification are recorded on paper or displayed on a video monitor and recorded electronically. The EEG is of particular value in the investigation of epilepsy; it is also used in the diagnosis of encephalitis and, sometimes, in the assessment of patients with dementia.

THE ELECTROMYOGRAM (EMG)

Electrical activity occurring in muscle during voluntary contraction, or in denervated muscles at rest, can be recorded with needle electrodes inserted percutaneously into the belly of the muscle, or with surface electrodes (silver discs attached to the skin overlying the muscle with a salty paste). This electrical activity is amplified and displayed as an auditory signal through a suitable loudspeaker and as a visual signal on an oscilloscope. It may be recorded on magnetic tape or selected potentials may be printed. On-line quantitative analysis of the EMG is useful in the diagnosis of primary diseases of muscle (*myopathies* and *dystrophies*) and of lower motor neurone lesions (*denervation*).

The speed of conduction of afferent impulses (*sensory nerve conduction velocity*) and efferent impulses (*motor nerve conduction velocity*) in peripheral nerves can be calculated using an electrical nerve stimulation technique and suitable recording electrodes with amplifying or digital averaging equipment. These methods are useful in the diagnosis of peripheral nerve disorders, particularly those due to local compressive lesions such as, for example, carpal tunnel syndrome, and in the clinical assessment of nerve plexus or radicular disease. Similar investigations of sensory conduction in the central nervous system can be achieved by averaging signals recorded from the head (*somatosensory evoked potentials*), and *visual and auditory evoked potential* measurements can be used to study visual and auditory pathways in the brain. It is also possible to study *motor evoked potentials* in the brain, using a special magnetic brain stimulator.

NEUROIMAGING

Routine radiographs of the skull and spine are now used relatively rarely. *Myelography*, a technique for visualizing the spinal subarachnoid space following the instillation of radio-opaque contrast by lumbar puncture, has been replaced by newer, more sensitive neuro-imaging methods, especially CT and MR imaging.

Computed tomography scanning (see Ch. 22)

Computed tomography (CT) scanning provides tomographic images of the brain of high resolution, without the need for invasive procedures. A crystallographic X-ray detection device is used instead of conventional X-ray film and a photographic image is produced by computerized averaging techniques. The resulting pictures are displayed as sections of the head in the coronal or basal plane (Figs 11.64 and 11.65). Intravenous or subarachnoid iodine-based contrast is sometimes used to enhance the vascular or spinal CSF compartments respectively. CT scanning of the nervous system is a rapid, widely available, high-resolution technique that is particularly useful in the assessment of trauma (Fig. 11.66), stroke (Fig. 11.67), suspected haemorrhage or tumours (Fig. 11.68) of the nervous system. Tuberculomas are well demonstrated by this technique (Fig. 11.69).

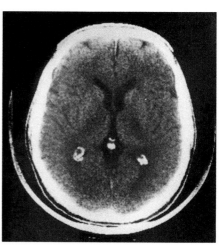

Fig. 11.64   Normal CT scan showing the cerebral ventricles, the sulci at the surface of the brain, the central calcified pineal gland and the two calcified parts of the choroid plexus. In the posterior parts of the skull there is a linear artefact resulting from the computer processing required to produce the image.

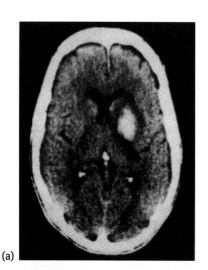

(a)

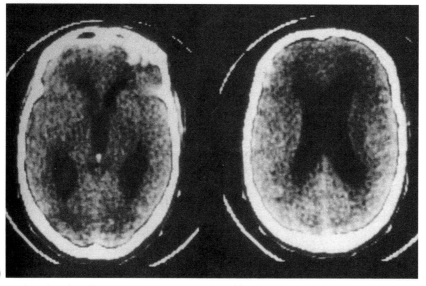

(b)

Fig. 11.65   CT scans illustrating lesions in the brain. **(a)** Left capsular haemorrhage. The haemorrhage appears relatively dense; it is surrounded by a zone of oedema and has caused displacement of the midline structures to the opposite side, The haemorrhage is in the typical location associated with hypertensive haemorrhage. **(b)** Hydrocephalus. The ventricular system is enlarged and there are periventricular lucent zones, due to oedema or seepage of CSF into the cerebral white matter in these regions indicating that the hydrocephalus is progressing (decompensated hydrocephalus).

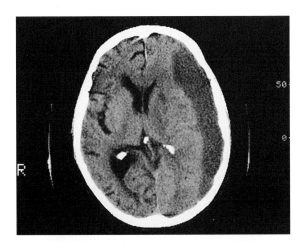

Fig. 11.66 CT scan in a patient presenting with confusion. There is chronic left subdural haematoma with midline shift. The patient had been involved in a fight a few weeks previously.

(a)

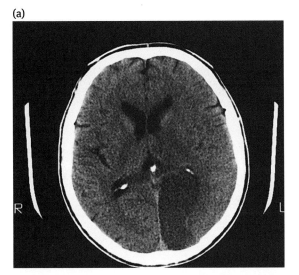

(b)

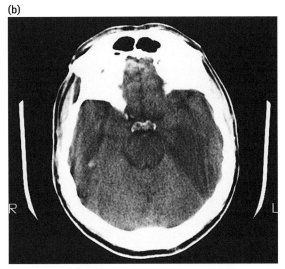

Fig. 11.67 CT scan. **(a)** infarction in a left posterior cerebral artery territory involves the occipital lobe and its deep white matter. The infarct extends anteriorly into the posterior part of the temporal lobe **(b)**. There is a slight mass effect with swelling of the left hemisphere causing herniation of the midline to the right. The sagittal sinus is clearly seen in **(a)**.

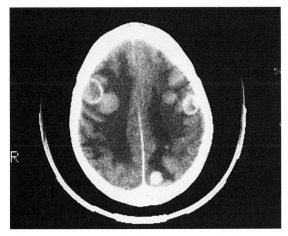

Fig. 11.68 CT scan. Multiple metastases in the brain from primary carcinoma of the breast. There is marked oedema of the white matter.

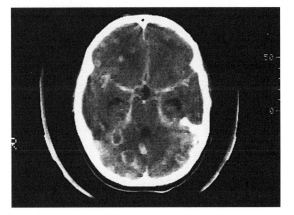

Fig. 11.69 Enhanced CT scan. Multiple tuberculomas in the brain. The lesions show enhancement of their capsules. They vary in size. Note that there is effacement of the cortical pattern suggesting widespread meningeal inflammation.

Magnetic resonance imaging

For magnetic resonance imaging (MRI) the patient is placed in a uniform, high magnetic field (0.5–1.5 tesla). Radiofrequency current is used to interpose brief pulses into the field causing changing magnetization of protons, and a signal recorded from the coil surrounding the magnet. Computerized reconstruction of this pattern of signals allows a proton-based image of the tissue, of high resolution, to be generated. Lesions such as multiple sclerosis (Fig. 11.70), infections, infarction (Fig. 11.71) and infiltrative tumours (Fig. 11.72) can be detected readily. MRI is particularly useful in the investigation of spinal cord disease (Figs 11.73 and 11.74), and intervertebral disc problems (Fig. 11.75).

Angiography

This is a method for studying the intracranial and extracranial vessels. A water-soluble radiopaque contrast medium is injected percutaneously into a

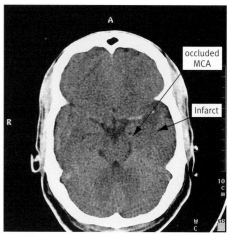

Fig. 11.71   CT scan. Early cerebral infarction. There is occlusion of the left middle cerebral artery due to embolism from traumatic dissection of the wall of the left carotid artery, causing infarction in the left middle cerebral artery territory (MCA).

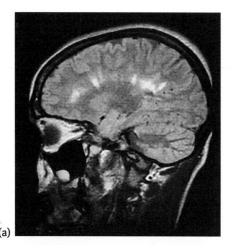

(a)

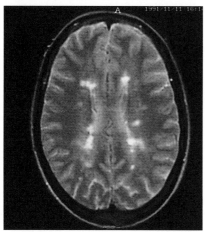

(b)

Fig. 11.70   MRI scan. Multiple sclerosis. T_2-weighted of a woman aged 45 showing **(a)** sagittal and **(b)** axial images. There are bright lesions in the periventricular white matter. In the sagittal image the abnormal signals have a finger-like form pointing towards the lateral ventricle (Dawson's fingers).

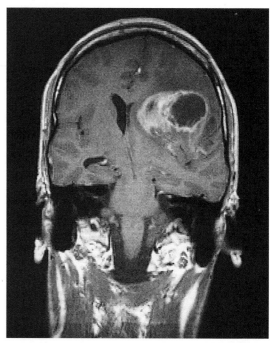

Fig. 11.72   MRI scan. T_1-weighted coronal slice. There is a large cystic malignant glioma in the left hemisphere which is causing subfalcine herniation of the brain to the right with compression of the lateral ventricle, and pressure on the mid-brain.

carotid artery in the neck, or into a vertebral artery, usually by catheterization of a major vessel such as the femoral, axillary, brachial or subclavian arteries. Digital X-ray images are made in various planes in the following few seconds as the contrast medium traverses the cerebral circulation. The arterial, capillary and venous circulations can be studied and abnormalities of the distribution, size, position and lumen of these vessels can be seen. Angiography is

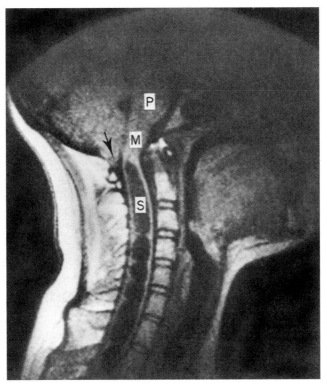

Fig. 11.73   MRI scan of the brain. Sagittal view of the craniocervical junction in a patient with syringomyelia. The neck and chin can be recognized to the left and right in the picture. Note the normal density (representing the water content) of the central parts of the intervertebral discs. The tongue, pharynx and larynx, and soft tissues of the neck are recognizable. Note the pons (P) and medulla (M). There is tonsullar herniation (arrow) into the foramen magnum and a long irregular cyst (syrinx) has caused enlargement of the cervical spinal cord (S).

(a)

(b)

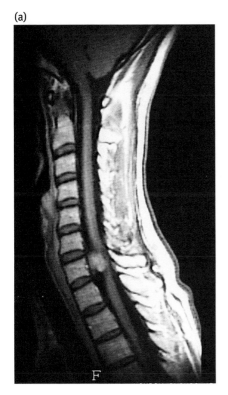

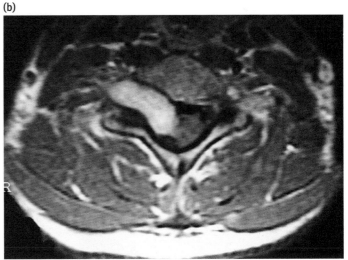

Fig. 11.74   **(a)** MRI scan with gadolinium enhancement. There is a neurofibroma at the C6 spinal level which is compressing the spinal cord, causing progressive paraparesis. **(b)** The tumour enhances slightly and can be seen as a sausage-shaped mass arising in the intervertebral foramen and compressing the spinal cord in the axial view.

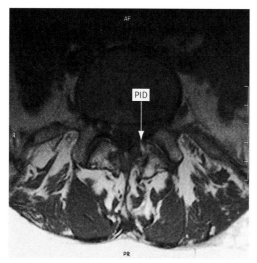

Fig. 11.75   MRI scan. Left L4/5 lumbosacral disc protrusion (PID) presenting with sciatica and sensory disturbance in left L4 distribution. There was spontaneous resolution of the clinical signs and symptoms over several weeks.

used especially for diagnosis of aneurysms (Fig. 11.76), arteriovenous malformations and cerebral tumours. It is also useful in cerebral vascular disease (Fig. 11.77). CT and MR methods—in the latter case not involving the use of contrast agents—are rapidly replacing contrast angiography in some clinical situations (Fig. 11.78).

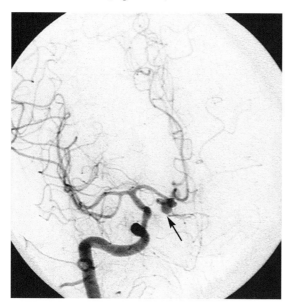

Fig. 11.76   Oblique right carotid angiogram with digital subtraction showing a multiloculated anterior communicating artery aneurysm (arrow).

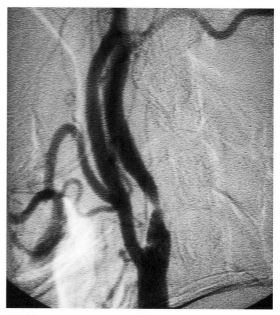

Fig. 11.77   Carotid artery stenosis, presenting with transient ischaemic attacks (hemiparesis).

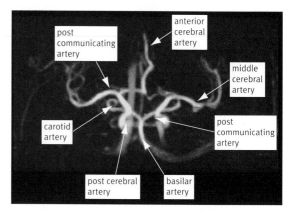

Fig. 11.78   Magnetic resonance angiography—non-invasive technique for visualization of the neck and intracranial vessels. This is a normal study.

12
THE EYE

Before examining the patient with an ocular problem, a detailed history of the presenting complaint and associated visual symptoms must be obtained.

HISTORY

Disturbances of vision may be sudden or gradual, and involve one or both eyes. The patient may complain of haloes around bright lights, floaters, flashes, or experience visual hallucinations (formed and unformed). Objects may appear smaller (*microureia*), larger (*macropsia*) or distorted (*metamorphopsia*). Disorders of ocular movement may manifest themselves as diplopia or just blurring.

Pain in the eye may be described as a gritty (foreign body) sensation on the surface, often exacerbated by blinking, or as a deeper ache within the eye; in both types of pain there may be associated photophobia. Severe ocular pain with vomiting may indicate an acute glaucoma. Migraine often presents with visual symptoms and headache. Pain may be referred to the eye from neighbouring disease.

There may be abnormal secretions from the eye such as mucus or pus. In tear insufficiency the eye feels dry. Excessive tear production associated with discomfort (*lacrimation*) may indicate local ocular disease, while painless overflow of tears (*epiphora*) indicates a defect of the lacrimal drainage system.

Lastly, the patient may complain of an abnormal appearance such as red eye, abnormal position of the lids, protrusion of the globe or pupillary abnormality.

In addition to the ocular history a routine general medical and surgical history is necessary. Particular note should be made of the past ophthalmic history such as the presence of a squint in childhood, a previous injury, or the wearing of glasses at any time. The family history may reveal a history of glaucoma, conditions affecting visual acuity, colour vision or squint, or the presence of neurological disease associated with visual loss.

VISUAL ACUITY

TESTS FOR DISTANT VISION

Visual acuity is measured with *Snellen's test types*, a series of letters of varying sizes constructed so that the top letter is visible to the normal eye at 60 m, and the subsequent lines at 36, 24, 18, 12, 9, 6 and 5 m respectively. Visual acuity (VA) is recorded according to the ratio

$$d/D,$$

where d is the distance at which the letters are read by the patient, and D the distance at which they can be read by a normal eye. The patient is usually placed at a distance of 6 m (20 feet) from the test types ($d = 6$) and each eye is tested separately. The patient reads down the chart as far as he or she can. If only the top letter is visible, the visual acuity is 6/60. A normal eye can read down to at least the seventh line, i.e. a visual acuity of 6/6 (20/20 in US nomenclature). If the visual acuity is less than 6/60, the patient is moved toward the test types until they can read the top letter. If the top letter is visible at 2 m, the visual acuity is 2/60. Visual acuities of less than 1/60 are recorded as *counting-fingers* (CF), *hand movements* (HM), *perception of light* (PL) or *no perception of light* (no PL). A person with an uncorrected refractive error may have reduced visual acuity, and a rough estimate of their corrected visual acuity may be obtained by asking them to view the chart through a pin-hole aperture.

If the patient wears glasses, the type of lens being worn should be determined. Hold the lens up and look at an object through it. Then move the lens from side to side and watch the object. If the object appears magnified and seems to move in the opposite direction to the lens, the lens is convex; if the object appears smaller and seems to move in the same direction, it is concave. Patients with *myopia*, or short sight, use concave ('minus' or diverging) lenses and those with *hypermetropia* or long sight, have convex ('plus' or converging) lenses.

In order to tell whether a lens is spherical or cylindrical, look at a straight object through it and then slowly twist the lens round. If the lens is cylindrical, the object will appear to rotate. Cylindrical lenses are used to correct *astigmatic* errors.

TESTS FOR NEAR VISION

Visual acuity at the ordinary reading distance is assessed by using reading test types of varying sizes, the notation being based on the printers' point system. The smallest print is N5. The near vision is recorded as the smallest type which the patient can read comfortably.

COLOUR SENSE

Colour sense is tested by the use of pseudo-isochromatic plates consisting of multi-coloured dots outlining certain digits, the best known being those of Ishihara. People with defective colour vision confuse certain colours. Ishihara pseudo-isochromatic plates are so constructed that a person with abnormal colour vision will not see a number or will read a different number from a normal person.

The most common anomalies of colour vision are various types of red–green deficiency, inherited as sex-linked recessive conditions, which occur in about 8% of men and 0.5% of women in the UK. People with congenital blue–yellow deficiencies and with total colour-blindness are rare. Acquired defects of colour vision occur in macular and optic nerve disease.

VISUAL FIELDS

The methods for testing the visual fields are described in Chapter 11.

EXAMINATION

After the vision has been tested, the eyes should be examined systematically.

THE EYELIDS

The shape and position of the eyelids should be noted. People of Asiatic origin have a long narrow palpebral aperture with an upward and outward obliquity and a characteristic fold of skin along the upper lid. The highest point of the aperture is at the junction of its middle and inner thirds. In Down's syndrome the palpebral fissure is also oblique. However, in addition, it is short and wide, with its highest point at the centre of the lid.

Abnormalities in the eyelids include the following:

Ptosis (drooping of the upper lid)
This may be congenital or acquired—these may be distinguishable by examination of old photographs. Ptosis may be unilateral if due to paralysis of the oculomotor nerve or the sympathetic supply to the eye (Horner's syndrome), but is more usually bilateral when due to ocular myopathy.

Lid retraction (Fig. 12.1)
If the upper lid is abnormally retracted, a band of white sclera is visible above the iris when the eyes are looking straight ahead. The commonest cause is dysthyroid eye disease, which may be accompanied by other signs such as infrequent blinking and *lid lag*, in which movement of the upper lid seems to lag behind that of the eyeball when the patient looks downwards. In addition, patients with dysthyroid eye disease frequently have a degree of forward displacement of the eyeball (*proptosis* (Fig. 12.2) when unilateral, or *exophthalmos* when bilateral). In severe cases of dysthyroid eye disease, marked exophthalmos leads to corneal exposure and ulceration; optic

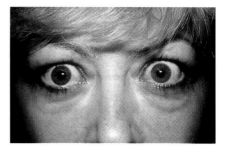

Fig. 12.1   Dysthyroid retraction. There is a slight exophthalmos (bilateral proptosis).

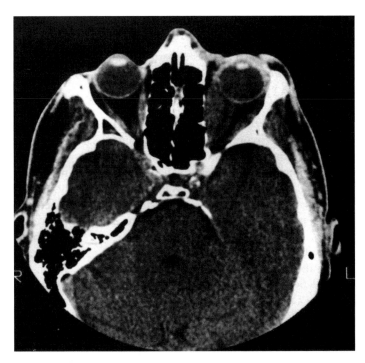

Fig. 12.2   Left-sided thyroid eye disease with exophthalmos and marked hypertrophy (inflammation) of the medial and lateral rectus muscles on that side. These muscles in the other eye are also slightly enlarged. The optic nerve can be seen clearly between the enlarged muscles on the left hand side.

nerve compression may also occur, even in cases with minimal proptosis. Both these complications require urgent medical or surgical orbital decompression. The differential diagnosis of proptosis includes space-occupying lesions in the orbit, and apparent ('pseudo') proptosis where a myopic eye is longer than normal.

Entropion
This is inversion of the lid margin with associated malposition of the lashes which may rub on the cornea.

Ectropion
This is eversion of the lid margin, often associated with watering (*epiphora*).

Blepharitis
Inflammation of the lids or blepharitis presents as redness and scaling of the lid margins around the base of the lashes.

Xanthelasma palpebrarum
These are fatty deposits which develop in the upper and lower eyelids in patients with long-standing hypercholesterolaemia (see Fig. 8.9).

THE LACRIMAL GLAND

The lacrimal gland is examined by pulling up the outer part of the upper lid while asking the patient to look downwards and inwards. Acute inflammation (*dacroadenitis*) results in a tender swollen gland, with oedema of the upper lid and localized conjunctival injection. Chronic dacroadenitis, a painless enlargement of the lacrimal gland which is frequently bilat-

eral, occurs in sarcoidosis and lymphoproliferative disorders. Tumours of the lacrimal gland produce a hard swelling of the gland associated with displacement of the globe.

Involvement of the lacrimal gland by any disease process may produce symptoms of a dry eye.

THE CONJUNCTIVA

The conjunctiva lining the eyeball (bulbar conjunctiva) and that lining the inner surface of the eyelids (palpebral conjunctiva) should be examined. To examine the palpebral conjunctiva of the lower lid, the lower lid should be pulled down and the patient asked to look upwards. To expose the palpebral conjunctiva of the upper lid, ask the patient to look downwards, then place the right thumb at the upper part of the upper lid and pull it up so as to evert the eyelashes. Grasp the lashes between the forefinger and thumb of the left hand and evert the lid by rotating it round the right thumb.

The conjunctiva may be pale in anaemia, yellow in jaundice, or red (injected) in conjunctivitis and other inflammatory eye disorders.

CONJUNCTIVITIS
Marked injection of the bulbar conjunctiva with a mucopurulent discharge suggests a bacterial infection; marked injection with a serous discharge and tender pre-auricular lymphadenopathy is indicative of a viral infection; puffy lids, conjunctival oedema (*chemosis*) and a history of itchiness suggest an allergic condition. Follicles in the upper palpebral conjunctiva occur in trachoma, whereas their presence in the lower palpebral conjunctiva suggests a viral conjunctivitis.

Distinction must be made between other causes of red eye such as keratitis, iritis and acute glaucoma (see p. 298).

THE CORNEA

INFLAMMATION OF THE CORNEA (KERATITIS)

This may be superficial or deep (interstitial); it is accompanied by circumcorneal injection. Superficial keratitis and corneal ulceration can be shown by staining the cornea with the dye fluorescein. A drop of fluorescein is instilled into the conjunctival sac and the excess dye is then washed out with normal saline. Corneal ulcers are stained green.

Interstitial keratitis causes a hazy cornea, often with an intact epithelium; it is usually caused by a viral infection but can also occur in syphilis. There is growth of capillaries into the cornea. Both keratitis and trauma to the cornea may result in corneal opacities; small opacities are described as *nebulae*, larger ones as *leucomata*.

Severe corneal infections, particularly bacterial, may result in a massive inflammatory response, with pus in the anterior chamber (*hypopyon*). This will progress to a sight-threatening *endophthalmitis* if not treated.

ARCUS SENILIS

Arcus senilis is a crescentic opacity near the periphery of the cornea. It usually starts at the lower part of the cornea, extending to form a complete circle. It is common in old people, but may occur in the young (arcus juvenilis) in association with type IV hyperlipoproteinaemia.

THE IRIS

Note should be made of any difference in the colour of the two irides (*heterochromia*), abnormality in the shape or size of the pupils, or signs of iritis.

IRITIS (ANTERIOR UVEITIS, IRIDOCYCLITIS)

In iritis circumcorneal injection occurs (but also in keratitis and acute glaucoma). In addition, there may be white specks visible on the posterior surface of the cornea (*keratitic precipitates*), or an exudate in the anterior chamber. The pupil may be constricted and irregular due to the formation of adhesions (*posterior synechiae*) between the edge of the pupil and the anterior surface of the lens. Other abnormalities of the pupils are described on page 299 and in Chapter 11.

OCULAR TENSION

The intraocular pressure (IOP) may be assessed by palpating the eyeball, although only gross variations from normal can be appreciated. The sclera is palpated with the two forefingers through the upper lid with the patient looking downwards and the other fingers resting on the patient's forehead. The degree of fluctuation gives an indication of the IOP. More accurate measurements of the IOP can be made with Schiötz or applanation tonometers. A diminished IOP occurs in diabetic coma and in severe dehydration from any cause. An increased IOP is a characteristic feature of glaucoma.

THE LENS

The presence of lens opacities (*cataract*) is suggested by loss of the normally bright red reflex. The commonest cause is ageing, but they are also seen in association with diabetes mellitus, after injury, and as a side-effect of corticosteroids and many other conditions. They are also a feature of certain hereditary diseases, for example myotonic dystrophy.

THE FUNDUS (Fig. 12.3)

Examination of the fundus of the eye with an ophthalmoscope is an essential part of all complete medical examinations. Valuable information may be obtained about the state of the optic nerve head, the arteries and veins of the retina, and a number of disorders of the retina, pigment epithelium and choroid.

In routine medical examinations it is usually possible, with practice, to examine the optic disc and surrounding retina without dilating the pupil, but for a complete examination of the fundus the pupils should be dilated by instilling a few drops of 1% cyclopentolate (Mydrilate) or 1% tropicamide (Mydriacyl) into the conjunctival sacs. In patients with a predisposition to closed-angle glaucoma, an acute attack of glaucoma may be precipitated when the pupils are dilated. Risk factors for angle closure include old age and hypermetropia. Any such patient should therefore be asked whether they ever see

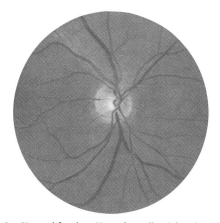

Fig. 12.3   Normal fundus. Note the yellowish colour of the optic disc and the retinal veins (the larger, darker vessels) and arteries leaving the centre of the disc superiorly and inferiorly. A single arterial branch passes laterally to supply the macular part of the retina.

haloes (coloured rings) around lights, and the anterior chamber should be examined (preferably with a slitlamp): patients with a shallow anterior chamber should have their pupils dilated only under the supervision of an ophthalmologist.

The patient should be examined either sitting or lying down in a darkened room. Ask the patient to look straight ahead keeping the eyes still. With the ophthalmoscope held at arms length from the patient's eyes, opacities in the media of the eye (cornea, anterior chamber, lens, vitreous) will appear as black specks or lines against the red reflex of the fundus.

The ophthalmoscope should then be brought as close as possible to the patient's eye (observer's right eye to patient's right eye) and the light directed slightly nasally. In this way the optic disc can be found and the light will not shine directly on the macula. If the patient's pupils are not pharmacologically dilated, shining a light on the macula will make the pupils constrict and the examination of the fundus difficult or impossible. If the optic disc is not in focus, the lenses of the ophthalmoscope should be gradually adjusted until the disc becomes sharply focused. If the observer's eye is emmetropic and his or her accommodation is relaxed, the strength of the lens necessary to bring the fundus into focus gives an indication of the refractive error of the patient's eye. Plus lenses indicate hypermetropia and minus lenses myopia. The optic disc, retinal blood vessels, macula and retinal periphery should be examined in turn.

THE OPTIC DISC

SHAPE

The normal disc is round or slightly oval (Fig. 12.3). If astigmatism is present, the disc may appear more oval than normal (Fig. 12.3).

COLOUR

The normal disc is a pale pink colour, distinctly paler than the surrounding fundus. The temporal side of the disc is usually paler than the nasal side.

An abnormally pale disc suggests *optic atrophy*. In oedema of the optic nerve head, resulting from raised intracranial pressure (*papilloedema*) or from inflammation (*papillitis*), the disc is pinker than normal (hyperaemic) and may approach the colour of the surrounding retina (Fig. 12.4).

PHYSIOLOGICAL CUP

In its central part there is usually a depression in the disc—the physiological cup. This cup is paler than the surrounding rim of the disc, and from it the retinal vessels enter and leave the eye. In glaucoma the cup may be greatly increased in size and the retinal vessels will kink as they cross the edge of the rim. When the cup is deep, as in advanced glaucoma, retinal vessels disappear as they climb from the floor

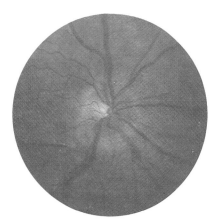

Fig. 12.4   Papilloedema.

to the rim, and reappear as they bend sharply over the edge of the rim; in less advanced cases a vertically oval cup extending to the edge of the disc may be seen (Fig. 12.5).

EDGE OF THE DISC

This is normally well-defined. In normal eyes there is sometimes a ring of dark pigment or white sclera surrounding the optic disc. These signs are most commonly seen in highly myopic eyes.

THE RETINAL BLOOD VESSELS

These radiate from the disc, dividing dichotomously into many branches as they pass towards the periphery of the retina. The retinal arteries are narrower than the veins, brighter red in colour, and have a brighter longitudinal streak where light is reflected from their convex walls. *Spontaneous retinal artery pulsation* is an abnormal finding, which may occur if the intraocular pressure is very high or if the central retinal artery pressure is very low. *Spontaneous venous pulsation* is frequently seen in normal eyes but is often absent in papilloedema. It is important to study the points where arteries and veins cross. Most

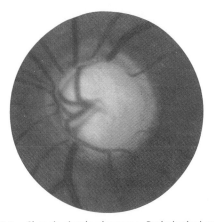

Fig. 12.5   Chronic simple glaucoma. Pathological cupping of the disc. The cup is oval in the vertical plane and appears pale. The retinal vessels are displaced nasally because of the angulation of the optic cup.

frequently it is the artery that crosses the vein, and in normal eyes neither vessel shows any change in colour, diameter or direction.

THE MACULAR REGION

This is defined anatomically as that portion of the posterior retina containing xanthophilic pigment (hence, macula lutea), and two or more layers of ganglion cells. At the centre of the macula (measuring approximately 5.5 mm in diameter) is the fovea. The fovea has a darker, glistening appearance and is devoid of blood vessels. Pathological changes in the macular region are important as they produce a greater reduction in vision than similar changes in any other part of the fundus.

THE PERIPHERY OF THE FUNDUS

This area can be examined only if the pupil is dilated with a mydriatic. Certain disease processes start in this region, for example retinal tears and retinitis pigmentosa.

THE ABNORMAL FUNDUS

PAPILLOEDEMA (Fig. 12.4)

This is a swelling of the optic nerve head due to raised intracranial pressure. There is an absence of inflammatory changes and little or no disturbance of visual function. In severe papilloedema the patient may notice transient loss of vision for a second or two (visual obscurations). In the initial stages of papilloedema there is an increased redness of the disc with blurring of its margins; the blurring appears first at the upper and lower margins, particularly in the upper nasal quadrant. The physiological cup becomes filled in and disappears, and the retinal veins are slightly distended. Spontaneous pulsation of the retinal veins is usually absent.

As the condition progresses the disc becomes definitely swollen (Fig. 12.6). In order to measure the degree of swelling of the disc, start with a high plus lens in the ophthalmoscope and reduce the power of the lens until the centre of the disc is just in focus.

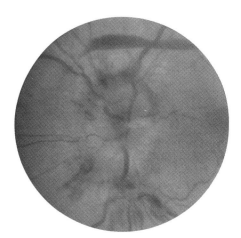

Fig. 12.6   Severe papilloedema with retinal haemorrhages.

The retina, a short distance from the disc, is then brought into focus by further reduction of the power of the lens. This further reduction indicates the degree of swelling of the disc (3 dioptres is equivalent to 1 mm of swelling).

If papilloedema develops rapidly, there will be marked engorgement of the retinal veins with haemorrhages and exudates on and around the disc, but with papilloedema of slow onset there may be little or no vascular change, even though the disc may become very swollen (Fig. 12.7). The retinal vessels will, however, bend sharply as they dip down from the swollen disc to the surrounding retina. The oedema may extend to the adjacent retina, producing greyish-white striations near the disc (Paton's lines), and a macular fan of hard exudates temporal to the fovea may develop in some cases. These appearances result from swelling of the ganglion cell axons in the nerve and retina as a result of interference with axoplasmic flow.

Papilloedema occurs in patients with space-occupying lesions, but is particularly liable to occur in children with tumours of the cerebellum and fourth ventricle. It is rare in patients with pituitary tumours. An acute form of papilloedema with haemorrhage extending into the vitreous is characteristic of sub-

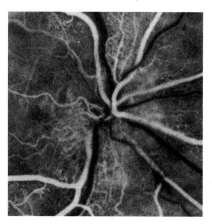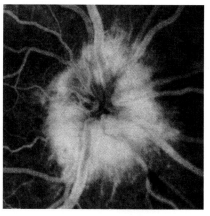

Fig. 12.7   Fluorescein retinal angiogram of fundus in papilloedema. Note the late phhase leakage of the dye.

arachnoid haemorrhage. A subdural haematoma may produce a clinical picture similar to that of a cerebral tumour. Papilloedema is uncommon in acute meningitis, but is a feature in subacute and chronic meningitis and in patients with brain abscess. It may be the only physical sign in benign (idiopathic) intracranial hypertension. Papilloedema occurring in malignant hypertension is accompanied by arterial changes characteristic of this condition and haemorrhages, exudates and cotton wool spots extending far beyond the region of the disc.

Pseudopapilloedema (Fig. 12.8) is an anomaly of development of the optic disc that produces an appearance resembling true papilloedema. However, in this condition there is no oedema of the optic disc and therefore the emerging retinal blood vessels are not obscured by swollen axons.

OPTIC NEURITIS

Inflammatory or demyelinating disease may affect any part of the optic nerve, producing an optic neuritis, the characteristic symptom of which is loss of vision. There is often pain on moving the eye, and the pupil on the affected side shows a diminished and ill-sustained contraction to a bright light (see p. 247).

When the disease affects the optic nerve head (papillitis) there is hyperaemia and some swelling of the optic disc. It must not be confused with papilloedema due to raised intracranial pressure, in spite of their similar ophthalmoscopic appearances. The two conditions can be distinguished by the severe visual impairment that occurs with optic neuritis, as compared with the minimal loss in papilloedema. In optic neuritis swelling of the optic disc is usually slight, distension of the retinal veins is less marked than in papilloedema, haemorrhages and exudates are rarely present, and there may be signs of intra-ocular inflammation, such as a hazy vitreous. Optic neuritis is usually followed by optic atrophy (Fig. 12.9), with reduced visual acuity and central or paracentral scotoma. It may occur alone, bilaterally or during the course of multiple sclerosis.

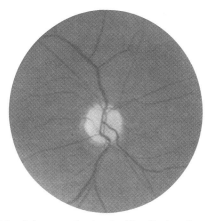

Fig. 12.9 Primary optic atrophy. The disc is pale and whiter than normal, and its edges are unusually sharply demarcated from the retina. The retinal vessels are slightly attenuated.

OPTIC ATROPHY

In optical atrophy the optic disc is paler than normal and may even be white (Fig. 12.9). Because there is wide variation in colour of the normal disc, a useful sign of optic atrophy is reduction in the number of capillaries on the disc. In optic atrophy the number of capillaries that cross the disc margin is reduced from the normal 10 to 7 or less (*Kestenbaum's sign*). From the appearance of the disc it is customary, although not always very useful, to divide optic atrophy into primary and secondary types. In the *primary* type the disc is flat and white with clearcut edges. *Secondary* optic atrophy follows swelling of the optic disc due to papilloedema. The disc is greyish-white in colour and its edges are indistinct.

Optic atrophy may occur in a number of disorders, of which the following are a few:

- Where there is interference with the blood supply to the optic nerve, as in occlusion of one of the ciliary vessels supplying the optic nerve head (*ischaemic optic neuropathy*)
- Where there is pressure on the nerve, whether in

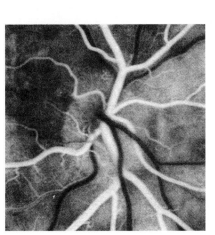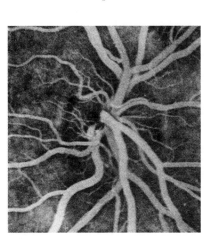

Fig. 12.8   Fluorescein retinal angiogram of fundus in pseudopapilloedema.

its intraocular, intraorbital, intracanalicular or intracranial portions

- Following optic neuritis
- Following trauma, where the optic nerve or its blood supply is involved
- In toxic poisoning due to substances such as tobacco, alcohol, lead, etc.
- In certain congenital disorders, when it is frequently associated with other neurological signs
- Following widespread chorioretinal inflammation or degeneration.

OPAQUE OR MYELINATED NERVE FIBRES

These are usually seen as one or more bright white patches radiating for a short distance from the optic disc (Fig. 12.10). The patch has a characteristic feathered edge and retinal vessels may disappear for a short distance within it. This condition is a harmless and non-progressive congenital anomaly.

MYOPIC CRESCENT

This is a crescent of white sclera, usually on the temporal side of the optic disc but in some cases extending all round it. When marked it may be associated with other degenerative changes in the fundus, which, if they involve the macula, will result in reduction of central vision.

RETINAL HAEMORRHAGES

These occur in a number of different conditions and are due to one or more of the following factors:

- Increased blood pressure within the retinal vessels, as in hypertension
- Decreased retinal arterial pressure due to proximal large vessel disease
- Abnormalities in the walls of the retinal vessels, as in diabetes mellitus or occlusion of the retinal veins
- Abnormalities in the circulating blood, as in severe anaemia, leukaemias, and bleeding diatheses.

When *superficial*, within the nerve fibre layer of the retina, the haemorrhages are elongated and flame-shaped, whereas when deep they are round blotches or spots. *Subhyaloid* haemorrhages, situated in front of the retina, are occasionally seen as very large round haemorrhages with a straight, horizontal upper border; they sometimes occur in diabetic retinopathy and after a subarachnoid haemorrhage.

RETINAL ARTERIOSCLEROSIS

This occurs either as an exaggeration of the general ageing process of the body or in association with hypertension. It is characterized by:

- Broadening of the arterial light reflex, producing a 'copper wire' or 'silver wire' appearance
- Tortuosity of the vessels
- Nipping, indentation or deflection of the veins where they are crossed by the arteries
- In hypertension, flame-shaped haemorrhages and 'cotton wool' spots in the region of the macula.

HYPERTENSIVE RETINOPATHY (Fig. 12.11)

This is characterized by a generalized narrowing of the retinal arteries, particularly in the young patient. In older patients these changes are masked by the accompanying arteriosclerosis. If the hypertension is severe, fullness of the retinal veins and flame-shaped haemorrhages occur around the optic disc, and there is disc oedema extending towards the macula, sometimes accompanied by a star-shaped collection of yellow exudates around the macula (Fig. 12.11). The retinopathy seen in some cases of acute and chronic nephritis is due to the associated hypertension.

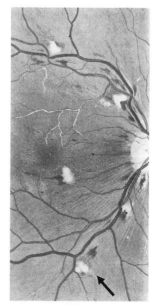

Fig. 12.11   Hypertensive retinopathy. The arteries are irregular in calibre and show 'silver wiring'. Arteriovenous nipping is present. Characteristic 'flame-shaped' haemorrhages and 'cottonwool' spots (arrow) can be seen.

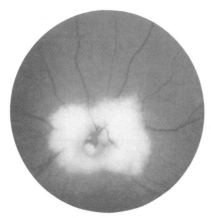

Fig. 12.10   Opaque (myelinated) nerve fibres. The white area obscures the disc, but this is a normal variant.

DIABETIC RETINOPATHY (Fig. 12.12)

The fundamental change in this condition is the formation of capillary microaneurysms, seen as tiny red spots around the macula. Microaneurysms are not seen in such abundance in any other condition. Retinal haemorrhages and exudates may occur; the haemorrhages are punctate or round, and the exudates have a waxy yellow-white appearance. In the more severe form of diabetic retinopathy—proliferative retinopathy—new vessels extend into the vitreous and bleed. The resulting glial proliferation may destroy vision by covering the macula or by producing a retinal detachment. Patients with diabetic retinopathy often have associated arteriosclerotic or hypertensive changes in their fundi.

RETINOPATHIES IN DISORDERS OF THE HAEMOPOIETIC SYSTEM

In severe anaemias the fundus may be paler than normal and a few small flame-shaped haemorrhages and cotton wool spots may be present.

In polycythaemia the retinal vessels are dark, tortuous and dilated. There may be oedema of the optic disc, and a few retinal haemorrhages may be observed.

In the leukaemias the retinal veins may be tortuous and dilated. In the later stages of these diseases the arteries and veins may be yellowish in colour, and the fundus may have a generalized pallor. Retinal haemorrhages of various types may occur, the characteristic ones in leukaemia being round with a pale centre.

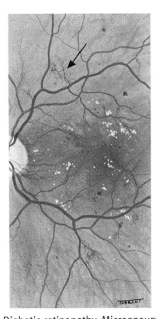

Fig. 12.12   Diabetic retinopathy. Microaneurysms (tiny red dots), blot haemorrhages, hard exudates and areas of new vessel formation (arrow) are characteristic of this condition. In many patients hypertensive retinopathy is also present.

OCCLUSION OF THE CENTRAL ARTERY OF THE RETINA

The optic disc and surrounding retina are pale, and there is a cherry-red spot at the macula which contrasts with the milky pallor of the adjacent retina. The retinal arteries are narrow or even thread-like (Fig. 12.13). Embolic occlusion of branch retinal vessels may occur from atheromatous emboli causing a zone of retinal infarction (Fig. 12.14).

OCCLUSION OF THE CENTRAL VEIN OF THE RETINA

There is intense swelling of the optic disc, gross venous dilatation and numerous retinal haemorrhages which extend in all directions. Branch retinal veins may be affected in isolation, with less resultant abnormality in the retina (Fig. 12.15).

CHOROIDITIS

In acute choroiditis there are one or more round or oval whitish patches in the fundus, lying deep to the

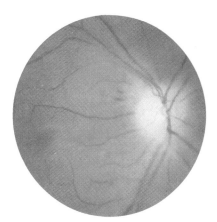

Fig. 12.13   Acute central artery occlusion. The vessels are attenuated, the retina is pale and oedematous and there are a few flame-shaped haemorrhages. the disc is slightly swollen and there is a cherry red spot at the macula indicating preserved choroidal circulation.

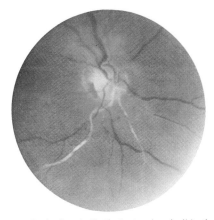

Fig. 12.14   Retinal emboli. Cholesterol emboli in the retinal arteries of a patient with atheromatous disease of the internal carotid artery in the neck.

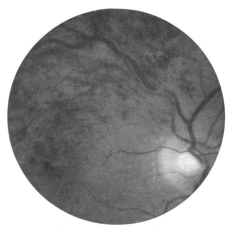

Fig. 12.15   Branch retinal vein occlusion. There are flame-shaped retinal haemorrhages. The disc is normal.

retinal vessels. These patches have ill-defined edges and the vitreous may be hazy. When the acute phase subsides, flat white scars with pigment around their edges are left. The numerous causes of choroiditis include tuberculosis, syphilis (which may cause a disseminated choroiditis), and toxoplasmosis (which characteristically produces lesions at the maculae).

EXAMINATION OF THE EYE IN CHILDREN

The points made in Chapter 18, on the examination of children in general, also apply to the examination of children's eyes. In particular, children may object strongly to lights and instruments, particularly when they are wielded by white-coated strangers. Allow the child to get used to the surroundings while taking a history from the parent. At the same time, constantly observe the child, noting the visual behaviour, the position and movements of the eyes, and the general appearance of each eye.

The assessment of visual acuity should then be made. Babies should rapidly fix a large object and follow it. The examiner's face is the best visual target. In infants, the visual acuity can be assessed by the ability to follow rolling white balls of varying sizes. From the age of $2\frac{1}{2}$ years a more accurate estimate of acuity can be made using the Sheridan–Gardiner test. In this test the child, or the child's mother, holds a card with a number of letters on it. The examiner then shows the child one of the letters on an identical card and asks the child to point to the same letter on his or her own card. When the child has understood the test the examiner moves to a distance of 6 m and shows the child a series of letters of decreasing size, until the child fails to make a match. This test is also useful for assessing visual acuity in patients with whom the examiner has no common language, in illiterate patients, and in patients with dysphasia.

Next, the position and movements of the eyes should be assessed. The least disturbing method is to observe the corneal light reflex; a light held at about 1 m should produce a reflection in the centre of the pupil of each eye. If the reflection in one eye is at a different location to that in the other, there is probably a squint. If squint is suspected, a cover test should be performed (see p. 244). The range of movement of the eyes should then be assessed and the pupillary responses to light, and to accommodation, should be observed. Finally, the media and fundi are examined with the ophthalmoscope. It is best to carry out ophthalmoscopy without touching the child as this can produce resistance and tight closure of the eye. Begin with a relatively dim light and gradually increase the brightness.

SOME CLINICAL PROBLEMS

THE RED EYE

A red eye is usually a sign of ocular inflammation. The dilated vessels giving rise to this appearance produce either *conjunctival* injection (posterior conjunctival vessels) or *ciliary* injection (anterior ciliary vessels). There are essentially four conditions which must be distinguished:

- Conjunctivitis
- Keratitis
- Iritis
- Acute glaucoma.

In assessing these conditions a history of pain and any blurring of vision are important clues to the diagnosis. Examination of the pupil is the most helpful diagnostic sign:

- In *conjunctivitis* pain is usually mild or absent and vision is unaffected. There is injection particularly involving the palpebral conjunctiva, and often also the bulbar conjunctiva, associated with a sticky discharge. The pupil is normal.
- In *keratitis* there is moderate to severe pain exacerbated by blinking, often with photophobia and loss of vision, particularly if the keratitis involves the visual axis. There may or may not be some discharge. The cornea will show signs of inflammation (uptake of fluorescein dye), but the pupil is normal.
- *Iritis* is associated with a dull, boring pain made worse by exposure to bright light (*photophobia*). Vision is reduced to varying degrees depending on the severity of the inflammation (see also p. 292). The pupil is small, and may be irregular if there have been previous attacks.
- *Acute glaucoma* presents suddenly with severe pain, marked loss of vision and often vomiting. There is ciliary injection, the cornea is cloudy and the pupil remains fixed in the mid-dilated position.

- *Subconjunctival haemorrhage*, resulting from rupture of a small conjunctival blood vessel, is an alarming but benign cause of a red eye associated with no pain, no discharge and no loss of vision.
- In *carotico-cavernous sinus fistulae* the conjunctival vessels are often dilated and arterialized and vision may be affected, but there is usually no pain.

SUDDEN LOSS OF VISION

It is important to decide whether the patient's vision was lost suddenly or whether the patient suddenly became aware of relatively long-standing or slowly progressive loss of vision in one eye, for example by inadvertently covering the other eye. Sudden visual loss is usually unilateral and often results from vascular disease. Sudden transient loss of vision, sometimes described as coming on like a curtain falling over the eye, and resolving gradually after a few minutes, is usually due to emboli in the retinal vessels. Sudden permanent loss of vision in one eye occurs from central retinal artery occlusion, or from optic nerve ischaemia, due to involvement of the ciliary circulation. The ciliary vessels are often involved in giant cell arteritis. When a retinal detachment involves the macula, it may cause sudden loss of vision.

In all cases of sudden loss of vision, it is essential to test the pupillary light response. When there is disease in the retina or in the optic nerve there will be an afferent pupillary defect (p. 247). Sudden blindness with normal pupillary responses to light strongly suggests a functional cause for the loss of vision. Bilateral sudden loss of vision may also be psychogenic in origin, but it can result from acute compression of the optic chiasm and optic nerves, for example in pituitary apoplexy (i.e. infarction of a pituitary tumour). Infarction of both occipital lobes, from vertebrobasilar disease or due to embolism from the heart, similarly may produce bilateral loss of vision and in this disorder the pupillary light responses are normal.

UNEQUAL PUPILS (ANISOCORIA)

Approximately 12% of normal individuals have a slight, but clinically evident, pupillary inequality. Such physiologically unequal pupils react normally. Pathological pupils dilate and constrict abnormally. In the absence of local disease of the eye, a small pupil may be due to paralysis of the dilator pupillae muscle, which is supplied by sympathetic nerve fibres. The sympathetic nerve fibres also supply part of levator palpebrae superioris. Damage to these sympathetic nerve fibres, derived from the stellate cervical sympathetic ganglion, produces slight drooping of the lid on the affected side (*ptosis*). The small pupil, together with slight ptosis, constitutes *Horner's syndrome* (Fig. 12.16). The easiest way to confirm a diagnosis of Horner's syndrome is to put the patient into a semi-darkened room for a minute or two. If Horner's syndrome is present, the affected pupil will dilate very poorly; the normal contralateral pupil dilates much better.

An abnormally dilated pupil suggests a defect of the parasympathetic supply to the iris sphincter muscle, which may be pre-ganglionic (*oculomotor palsy*) or post-ganglionic (*tonic pupil*). The internal ophthalmoplegia in a third nerve palsy result from damage to the parasympathetic fibres, which arise in the Edinger–Westphal nucleus of the oculomotor nerve. This is invariably associated with partial or complete weakness of the external ocular muscles supplied by the oculomotor nerve (p. 242) and the enlarged pupil reacts very poorly to both light and accommodation. A *tonic pupil* (Holmes–Adie pupil), which is initially larger than normal but becomes smaller with time, reacts very slowly and shows a greater constriction to accommodation than to light (*light-near dissociation*). In both pre- and post-ganglionic parasympathetic blockade the pupil is supersensitive to weak cholinergic drugs instilled into the conjunctival sac (e.g. pilocarpine 0.125% solution).

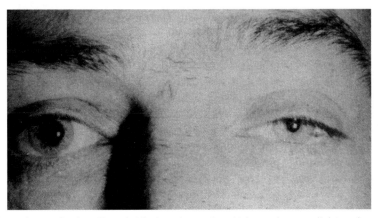

Fig. 12.16   Horner's syndrome. On the affected side there is ptosis, which may be very slight, and a small pupil (miosis) which reacts to both light and accommodation.

A common cause of an unexplained large and unreactive pupil is accidental medication with mydriatics. The pupillary changes in neurosyphilis, the Argyll Robertson phenomenon, are described in Chapter 11.

TRAUMA

FOREIGN BODIES

In all, 25% of ocular injuries are foreign bodies in the cornea. Symptoms range from mild discomfort to severe pain. Inspection of the cornea with a magnifying glass will aid identification of the foreign body. Further localization may be obtained by instilling sterile 2% fluorescein solution. It is important to search for foreign bodies elsewhere in the conjunctival sac, particularly *subtarsal* foreign bodies (see p. 291 on how to evert the upper lid).

Intraocular foreign bodies occur when small pieces of metal, glass, plastic or similar material penetrate the cornea or sclera. Any intraocular foreign body, particularly if it is of vegetable origin, may produce a severe purulent panophthalmitis. Retained iron foreign bodies cause *siderosis*, resulting in gradual loss of vision. It is imperative to X-ray all suspected intraocular and orbital foreign bodies.

Lid lacerations involving the lid margin must be recognized owing to the serious complications, such as ingrowing lashes (*trichiasis*), which may follow inadequate repair. If a laceration of the medial end of the lid also involves the lacrimal drainage system, then *epiphora* may result.

PENETRATING INJURIES

Penetrating or perforating injuries of the eye result in distortion of the ocular anatomy. There may be prolapse of iris, ciliary body, lens, vitreous or retina. An X-ray is essential to exclude a foreign body.

BLUNT INJURIES

Mild blunt trauma to the eye and orbit may produce quite marked swelling and bruising of the lids—a 'black eye'. Subconjunctival haemorrhage and corneal epithelial abrasion may also occur; the latter, although painful, heals rapidly.

More severe contusion of the globe may result in bleeding into the anterior chamber (*hyphaema*). This may vary from a small level of red cells to a large clot. Dislocation of the lens, vitreous haemorrhage and retinal detachment can also occur.

Blunt trauma to the orbit can cause fractures. In particular the orbital contents may prolapse through a fracture of the floor of the orbit producing a '*blowout fracture*'. Fracture–dislocation of the zygomatic bone and arch produces the cosmetically unsightly malar fracture.

CHEMICAL INJURIES

Acid or alkali coming into contact with the cornea and conjunctiva can cause serious complications, including loss of the eye. Severe chemical injuries cause a whitening of the conjunctiva and a marbled appearance to the cornea: there is a danger of corneal perforation in these injuries. A careful history is essential for identifying the noxious substance, and standard litmus paper should be used to test the pH of the tear film to confirm the diagnosis.

THERMAL INJURIES

The globe is usually spared because of the blink reflex. Scarring of the lids after a facial burn can result in exposure and subsequent damage to the cornea.

SPECIAL TECHNIQUES IN OPHTHALMOLOGY

A refraction test will ascertain the optical power of an eye. This is performed subjectively by placing neutralizing lenses in front of the eye and simultaneously assessing visual acuity. An objective refraction is performed using neutralizing lenses in conjunction with a *retinoscope*.

The intraocular pressure is measured by *tonometry*. It is performed by measuring the force required to flatten a given area of the cornea using an *applanation tonometer*, which is usually attached to a slit lamp.

In addition to standard direct ophthalmoscopy, *binocular indirect ophthalmoscopy*, using a light source supported on the examiner's head and a hand-held lens in front of the patient's eye, allows a much greater area of the fundus to be visualized and permits stereopsis on the part of the examiner.

A *slit lamp* consists of a binocular microscope mounted on a table with an adjustable beam of light. This can produce a fine slit of light enabling one to examine a magnified optical section of the various structures of the eye.

Fundus photography is a useful adjunct to the diagnosis and management of retinal and choroidal disorders. When used in conjunction with the intravenous injection of sodium fluorescein, detailed assessment of the retinal and choroidal vasculature (Figs. 12.7 and 12.8) may be obtained using a blue filter with the fundus camera to excite fluorescence as the dye circulates (*fluorescein angiography*).

Ultrasonography, using sound waves with frequencies of 5–20 MHz is used in the diagnosis of retinal detachments and both intraocular and orbital tumours. MRI Scanning has largely replaced this technique.

Radiopaque dye may be introduced into the lacrimal drainage system to identify sites of obstruction (*dacrocystography*).

Computed tomography (CT) and magnetic resonance imaging (MRI) are useful in the diagnosis of orbital disease (see Fig. 12.2).

VISUAL HANDICAP

The word *blindness* is emotive and for many people implies total loss of vision, but this is rarely the case. In the UK a person can be legally registered blind if they are 'unable to perform any work for which eyesight is essential' (DoH/Dept of Employment regulations). This usually implies a visual acuity less than 6/60. Alternatively, a person can be registered as partially sighted with vision between 6/60 and 6/18, particularly if there is an associated field defect.

ELECTROPHYSIOLOGICAL TESTS

Visual evoked potentials (VEP), recorded from the occipital cortex using scalp electrodes while the subject views an alternating black and white checker board stimulus, are used in the diagnosis of disease of the visual pathway. The principal waveform recorded from the scalp is a positive deflection occurring about 100 ms after the stimulus (the P100 wave). This is attenuated in amplitude and increased in latency in disease, especially disease of the optic nerve, for example optic neuritis or optic nerve compression.

Electroretinograms measure the electrical potential across the eye, recorded from a special corneal electrode, with a reference electrode placed on the forehead. Flash, flicker or pattern stimuli are used to generate electrical responses derived from activation of the retina. The waveform is useful in assessing patients with hereditary or acquired retinal degenerations.

13
THE EAR, NOSE AND THROAT

INTRODUCTION

The ear, nose and throat are functionally interrelated. For example a patient with sinus disease who has pus dripping into the back of the nose and over the opening of the eustachian tube may present either with acute suppurative otitis media or with infection in the pharynx.

In this chapter each region will, of necessity, be described as a separate entity. However in clinical practice the close associations between disease processes in the ear, nose and throat makes it important to ensure that the whole region is examined.

THE EAR

ANATOMY

The ear comprises the external, middle and inner ears. The pinna and the ear canal (external auditory meatus) form the *external ear*. The *pinna* consists of fibrocartilage covered with perichondrium and skin and is characterized by a series of folds the most important of which are the helix and antihelix.

The *meatus* has a cartilaginous (outer) and a bony (inner) component. The skin of the outer part of the meatus contains sebaceous glands and normal skin appendages such as hair, but in the deeper parts of the canal the skin is no more than a layer of epithelium. Squamous debris from the outer part of the drum and from the external ear canal migrates to the outside and becomes mixed with sebum to form wax.

The *eardrum* (the tympanic membrane) lies obliquely across the bottom of the meatus and separates the middle and external ears (Fig. 13.1). It is normally semi-translucent and grey and consists of two parts. The lower two thirds (the *pars tensa*) consists of an outer layer of squamous epithelium, a middle fibrous layer, and an inner layer of mucous membrane which is continuous with the epithelium of the middle ear cleft. By contrast the *pars flaccida*, in the upper third of the drum (the attic), lacks a middle fibrous layer and is the part of the drum that is most prone to retract in patients who have a long-standing negative middle ear pressure. A fibrous ring (the *annulus*) surrounds the whole membrane and stabilizes the drum in the surrounding bone. Within the middle ear are three small bones (the *ossicles*) which transmit sound from the drum to the *cochlea*. These are the *malleus, incus* and *stapes*. The handle of the malleus lies within the fibrous layer of the pars tensa and has a short process at its upper end and a flattened lower end (the *umbo*). These features can readily be seen on otoscopy. When examined with an auriscope there is also a 'cone of light' passing down from the umbo to the annulus antero-inferiorly (Fig. 13.2).

Within the *middle ear* the incus articulates with the malleus laterally and with the stapes medially. The articulation of the long process of the incus with the stapes (the incudostapedial joint) is the weakest link in the ossicular chain and is liable to disruption from trauma or long-standing infection. The *chorda tympani* (a branch of the seventh cranial nerve) passes horizontally, medial to the malleus and lateral

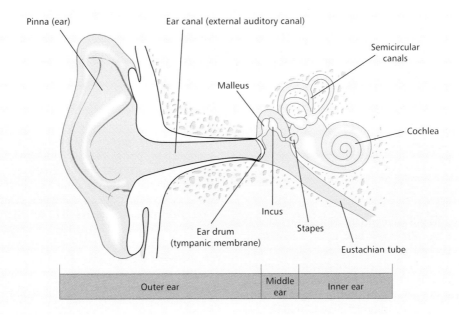

Fig. 13.1   The anatomy of the ear.

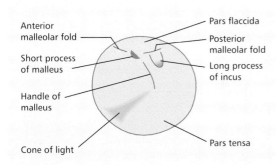

Fig. 13.2   The tympanic membrane.

to the long process of the incus, carrying taste fibres from the anterior two thirds the tongue. None of these features within the middle ear can be seen clearly unless the drum is retracted.

SYMPTOMS OF EAR DISEASE

The main symptoms of ear disease are:

- Aural pain (*otalgia*)
- Discharge (*otorrhoea*)
- Hearing loss
- A sensation of sound in the absence of an appropriate auditory stimulus (*tinnitus*)
- A sensation of abnormal movement (*vertigo*).

OTALGIA

The sensory innervation of the external ear canal, tympanic membrane and middle ear arises from the fifth, ninth and tenth cranial nerves together with branches of the great auricular nerve and the lesser occipital nerve (anterior primary rami of the second and third cervical nerves). Since divisions of the cranial nerves also supply the larynx and pharynx as well as the temporomandibular joint and teeth, primary pathology in any of these areas may give rise to referred pain in the ear. Any patient who presents with otalgia but who has normal findings on otoscopy requires examination of these other sites.

The causes of aural pain are listed in Box 13.1. Of the otological causes, acute infection (*perichondritis*) requires immediate hospitalization and treatment with intravenous antibiotics. A *subperichondrial haematoma* requires prompt drainage if deformity (a *cauliflower ear*) is to be avoided. The term malignant

---

BOX 13.1   Causes of otalgia.

Otological causes
- Acute otitis externa
- Furunculosis
- Viral infection—myringitis bullosa
- Perichondritis
- Acute otitis media
- Acute barotrauma
- Herpes zoster (Ramsay Hunt syndrome)
- Malignant otitis externa
- Neoplasia

Non-otological causes
- Tonsillitis
- Dental disease
- Temporomandibular joint pathology (Costen's syndrome)
- Cervical spine disease
- Carcinoma in the upper air and food passages

otitis externa is a misnomer. The pathology is an osteomyelitis of the skull base arising in the external meatus in immunocompromized patients—especially people with diabetes. It is due to *Pseudomonas* infection and results in granulation tissue formation and damage to the lower cranial nerves. Non-otological causes include malignancy in the larynx and hypopharynx. These conditions are discussed separately.

OTORRHOEA

A discharge from the ear may be:

- Purulent
- Serous
- Sanguineous.

The character of pus is important as it gives a clue as to the site of the pathology (Box 13.2). Intermittent, profuse, inoffensive mucoid otorrhoea suggests that there is a perforation of the pars tensa of the tympanic membrane, for only the middle ear has mucous glands. The route for this infection is from the nasopharynx and eustachian tube (tubo-tympanic middle ear disease). A chronic, offensive and scanty discharge may be the first symptom of a cholesteatoma caused by infected keratin formed in a retraction pocket or an attic perforation (attico-antral disease). This is serious since it may lead to intracerebral infection, facial nerve palsy or erosion of the inner ear with imbalance or hearing loss. In a chronically discharging ear the onset of bleeding may indicate malignant change. Severe trauma is associated with a bleeding from the meatus and, if the temporal bone is fractured, may be accompanied by leakage of cerebrospinal fluid.

HEARING LOSS

Hearing losses may be:

- Conductive
- Sensorineural
- Mixed.

Conductive hearing loss is due to a disorder in the external ear canal, tympanic membrane or middle ear. Characteristically, the patient retains normal speech discrimination and will hear well with adequate amplification.

Sensorineural hearing loss is due either to cochlear (sensory) or retrocochlear (neural) pathology and very frequently speech discrimination is markedly impaired. In particular, patients with a sensory hearing loss may find that a small increase in the intensity of the auditory stimulus above threshold leads to discomfort due to distortion. This is known as *recruitment* and is the result of damage to the hair cells in the cochlea. The patient may also notice an apparent difference in the pitch or frequency of a tone between the two ears (*diplacusis*).

Most losses are gradually progressive and are related to ageing. Some may be inherited or secondary to occupational or social *noise exposure*. Many drugs are also ototoxic and there are also associations between hearing loss and several neurological and renal disorders.

Occasionally sudden loss occurs and should be treated as an emergency with steroids and vasodilators. In the majority the aetiology remains unknown but identifiable causes include viral infections, head injuries, a perilymph fistula or, rarely, an acoustic neuroma (Box 13.3).

TINNITUS

Tinnitus is a sensation of sound in the absence of an appropriate auditory stimulus and can be caused by almost any pathology in the auditory pathways. It is

---

BOX 13.2　Characteristics of otorrhoea in relation to site and aetiology.

Watery
- Cerebrospinal fluid leak
- Eczema of the external meatus

Purulent
- Acute otitis externa
- Furunculosis

Mucoid
- Chronic tubotympanic suppurative otitis media

Mucopurulent/sangineous
- Trauma
- Acute otitis media
- Carcinoma of the middle ear

Foul smelling
- Chronic attico-antral suppurative otitis media with cholesteatoma

---

BOX 13.3　Causes of deafness.

Conductive
- Congenital atresia of the external meatus or congenital ossicular fixation
- Wax or foreign body in the external meatus
- Otitis externa
- Middle ear effusion
- Trauma to the drum or ossicular chain
- Otosclerosis
- Chronic suppuration (tubotympanic or attico-antral)
- Carcinoma of the middle ear

Sensorineural
- Genetic
- Prenatal: rubella
- Perinatal: hypoxia, jaundice
- Trauma: noise, head injury, surgery
- Infective: meningitis, measles, mumps, syphilis
- Degenerative: presbyacusis
- Ototoxicity: aminoglycosides, diuretics, cytotoxics
- Neoplastic: acoustic neurinomas
- Idiopathic: Ménières, sudden deafness

also occasionally found in patients with no discernible hearing loss.

A ringing, rushing or hissing sound in the ear characterizes most cases. It must be distinguished from *autophony*, an abnormal perception of the patient's own voice which is likened to the sensation experienced when holding a seashell to the ear. In the majority of cases cure is impossible. However, treatment with the use of a hearing aid or a tinnitus masker (an external source of continuous soft sound) may make life more tolerable.

VERTIGO

Vertigo is an hallucination of movement such that the patient either feels the world moving or has a sensation of moving in the world. It is a symptom that is characteristic of an acute labyrinthine (peripheral) or central pathology (Box 13.4).

A more persistent or slowly progressive loss of function produces vague symptoms such as dizziness, instability or a sensation of swaying or tilting. Vertigo must also be distinguished from gait abnormalities due to cerebellar disease or to disorders of proprioceptive sensory input. Occasionally such symptoms may be associated with oscillopsia—an inability to stabilize a visual image on the retina.

EXAMINATION OF THE EAR

The instruments used for examination of the ear are included in Fig. 13.3.

PINNA AND POSTAURICULAR AREA
Look first at the pinna and the surrounding skin. Congenital abnormalities may be associated with

BOX 13.4   Causes of vertigo.

Of sudden onset
- Acute viral labyrinthitis (vestibular neuronitis)

With focal features
- Brainstem ischaemia (TIA)
- Multiple sclerosis
- Migraine
- Temporal lobe epilepsy

With deafness and tinnitus
- Ménière's syndrome
- Acoustic neuroma

With particular head posture
- Benign positional vertigo

After trauma
- Post-traumatic vertigo
- Perilymph fistula

With motion
- Motion sickness

Drug induced
- Vestibulotoxic drugs, e.g. gentamicin, salicylates, quinine, antihypertensives

With aural discharge
- Middle ear disease

With systemic disorders
- Postural hypotension
- Syncope
- Cardiac dysrhythmia
- Carotid sinus hypersensitivity
- Anxiety and panic attacks
- Hyperventilation syndrome

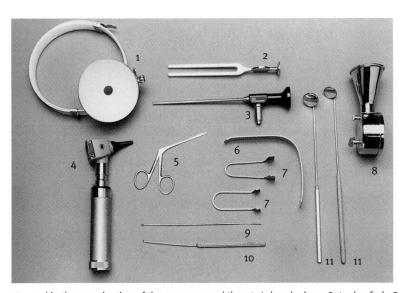

Fig. 13.3   Instruments used in the examination of the ear, nose and throat. 1, head mirror; 2, tuning fork; 3, rigid endoscope (for nose and back of nose examination) – Hopkins' rod; 4, otoscope; 5, crocodile forceps; 6, tongue depressor; 7, Thudichums' nasal specula; 8, Barony box; 9, Jobson Horne ear probe; 10, wax probe; 11, mirrors for indirect laryngoscopy.

accessory skin tags, abnormal cartilaginous fragments in the skin surrounding the ear, or small pits and sinuses. Look also for any pre- or postauricular lymphadenopathy and for abnormal protrusion of the pinna, which is commonly associated with failure of development of the antihelical fold (bat ear).

A scar or bone loss in the postauricular area indicates previous surgery and a hot, tender swelling in this region, with the pinna pushed forwards, suggests the possibility of mastoid infection.

Incomplete development (*microtia*) is commonly seen in conjunction with narrowing (atresia) of the external meatus, but the auricle can also be displaced from its normal position (*melotia*) or pathologically enlarged (*macrotia*). These abnormalities may be associated with cysts or infection in a pre-auricular sinus. Occasionally, otitis externa is associated with a tender postauricular lymph node. If the external meatus is clear the scalp should also be examined as a site of primary infection.

EXTERNAL EAR CANAL

The external auditory canal should first be examined using a hand-held auriscope (Fig. 13.4). To bring the cartilaginous meatus into line with the bony canal, retract the pinna backwards. In all cases use the largest speculum that will comfortably fit the ear canal. The auriscope should be held like a pen between thumb and index finger with the ulnar border of the hand resting gently against the side of the patient's head (Fig. 13.4). In this way head movement during examination results in synchronous movement of the speculum which limits the risk of direct trauma to the ear canal. Wax may be removed with a Jobson Horne probe or wax hook (Fig. 13.3) or by syringeing with water. Syringeing is contraindicated if there is a history of previous perforation or discharge. It is also important to ensure that the water is at body temperature lest vertigo is induced by direct stimulation of the labyrinth (a caloric effect). Keratin debris, pus or mucopus in the meatus should be removed under direct vision using an operating microscope and in cases of *purulent or mucopurulent* otorrhoea a swab should be taken for microbiology. *Foreign bodies* in the ear canal are found mainly in children. They may be difficult to remove without a general anaesthetic.

THE TYMPANIC MEMBRANE

Repeated infection or negative middle ear pressure may cause the drum to become thickened, to exhibit hyaline degeneration (seen as white plaques in the drum—tympanosclerosis) or to become thinned and atelectatic. Fluid effusions in the middle ear (serous otitis media) result in an increased vascularity and dullness of the drum. *Eustachian tube dysfunction* results in absorption of air in the middle ear with drum retraction and apparent foreshortening or undue prominence of the short process of the malleus. If the negative middle ear pressure is persistent then a *retraction pocket* may form. Perforations are either marginal or central (Fig. 13.5). Marginal defects extend to the annulus whereas with central perforations there is a rim of retained membrane between the defect and the annulus. Both are described by their position in relation to the handle of the malleus (anterior, posterior or inferior) and by their size; if the perforation involves most of the tympanic membrane it is recorded as being subtotal.

ASSESSMENT OF HEARING

It is possible to make a crude preliminary assessment of the severity of a hearing impairment from the clinical history. Ask whether the patient can hear the doorbell or telephone (sound outputs around 60 dB) and ask if conversation in a quiet environment can be heard (normal levels are at about 40 dB). If the patient prefers a raised voice in quiet surroundings this implies a degree of hearing loss. With practice, free-field tests (asking the patient to repeat words spoken at varying intensities), using phonetically balanced words (e.g. dustbin, policeman), number combinations or combinations of numbers and letters, give further information. For these tests the examiner stands to the side of the ear to be tested and masks the non-test ear using tragal movement. The test starts with a whispered voice at 6 cm (approximate intensity 15 dB) and proceeds with a whispered voice at 15 cm (35 dB). If there is no response, a conventional voice at 60 cm (50 dB) is used; this is then repeated, if necessary, at 15 cm (55–60 dB) from the test ear. Unfortunately responses in this simple test are often difficult to

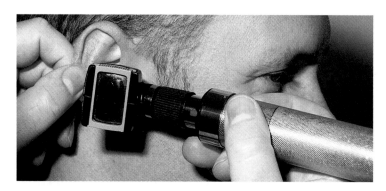

Fig. 13.4 Examination of the right ear using the auriscope. Note the left hand applying gentle traction to the pinna. The fingers of the right hand rest on the patient's cheek.

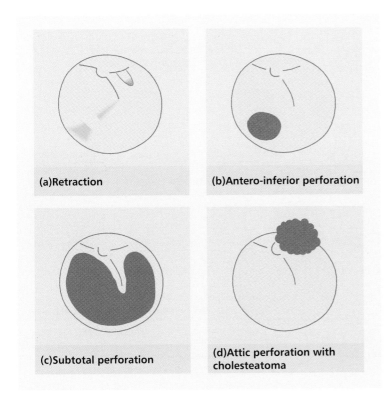

(a)Retraction

(b)Antero-inferior perforation

(c)Subtotal perforation

(d)Attic perforation with cholesteatoma

Fig. 13.5 Perforations of the tympanic membrane.

quantify and may be interpreted erroneously in those with poor English comprehension.

Further information about hearing may be obtained at the bedside by using a vibrating tuning fork. A fork of 512 Hz is normally used since higher frequencies are less accurate at identifying differences between air and bone conduction and lower frequency forks produce vibration that may be misinterpreted. In clinical practice two tests are employed.

The *Rinne test* (Fig. 13.6) compares hearing by air and bone conduction. It is performed by striking the tuning fork and holding it in line with the external ear canal (air conduction) and then against the postauricular skin (bone conduction). The patient is asked in which test position the sound is heard louder. In normal subjects air conduction is better than bone conduction (Rinne positive) and this response is also found in those patients who have a sensorineural deafness. In conductive deafness the converse is true (Rinne negative).

In the *Weber test* the base of the vibrating tuning fork is placed in the midline. The patient is then asked whether the sound is heard in the midline or whether it is lateralized. The normal response is to hear the sound in the midline; this is also true if the hearing is symmetrically reduced. However, if there is normal hearing on one side and a pure sensorineural loss on the other the tuning fork will be heard louder in the normal ear. Conversely, if there is a purely conductive hearing loss the tuning fork will

be heard louder on the side with the conductive deficit. These tests are illustrated in Fig. 13.6.

It should be borne in mind that patients with a small conductive loss (up to 30 dB) may remain Rinne positive: it is only when the difference between air and bone conduction exceeds 40 dB that the Rinne test is negative on 90% of occasions. Moreover, patients with a profound unilateral sensorineural hearing loss or a dead ear will report a Rinne negative response if the contralateral ear has normal or reasonable hearing. This is because, during this sort of clinical testing, the interposition of the mass of the head will cause sounds to be attenuated or masked in the ear furthest from the sound source. Attenuation of sound transmission for air conduction sound is marked but is much less for bone conduction. Thus a vibrating tuning fork held adjacent to the test ear will be heard only in that ear, but the same tuning fork placed on the mastoid process will also be heard in the non-test ear. For these reasons masking the non-test ear should always validate a negative response. In a clinical situation such masking can be achieved by intermittent rubbing of the tragal cartilage which produces white noise of approximately 50 dB intensity. If masking of more than 50 dB is required a Bárány box should be used to mask the contralateral ear (Fig. 13.3).

AUDIOMETRY

Formal audiometry is used to assess the degree of hearing loss and in assessing the likely site of pathol-

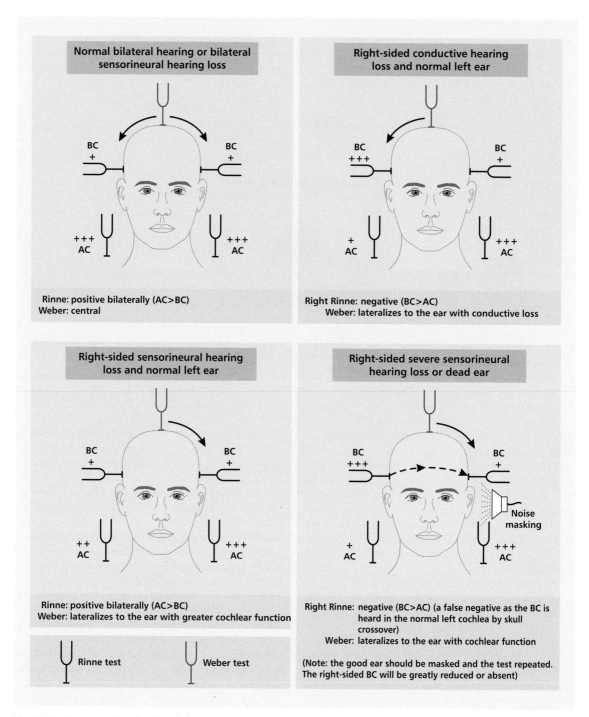

Fig. 13.6 Interpretation of tuning fork tests.

ogy in the auditory pathways. This is covered in more detail at the end of this chapter (see p. 320).

ASSESSMENT OF VESTIBULAR FUNCTION

Vestibular input is composed of information from the utricle, the saccule and the semicircular canals. These receptors respond to changes in gravity and to linear and angular acceleration and the information

that results is integrated to allow compensatory eye movements through central pathways. These include the vestibulo-ocular reflex (eye movements in response to vestibular stimulation) and postural adjustments. However, balance and orientation is not solely dependent on sensory input from the vestibular system. The eyes and muscle, joint and skin receptors also provide complex information as to body position. All this input is integrated and modulated by the cerebellum and investigation of the unsteady patient therefore requires that a full neuro-otological examination is performed. The cardiovascular system should also be examined where appropriate.

EYE MOVEMENTS

Eye movement should be observed with good illumination. Conjugacy should be tested, and any concomitant squint noted.

Following this the eyes should be observed in the primary position of gaze (looking forwards) to ensure that there is no spontaneous nystagmus. Pursuit (slow) movements, which depend on the fovea and the occipital cortex of the brain, can then be assessed by asking the patient to track an object moved horizontally and vertically slowly across the visual field at about 35 cm distance. This should be followed by asking the patient to rapidly alternate gaze between two objects held approximately 30 degrees apart; this tests saccadic (fast) movements which are driven by the frontal lobes and the pontine gaze centres.

Nystagmus is defined by the direction of the fast movement (p. 246). The characteristic saw-toothed nystagmus of vestibular disease has a slow labyrinthine and a fast central component and is enhanced by movement of the eyes in the direction of the fast phase. Such movements should also be assessed using Frenzel's glasses. These have 20 dioptre lenses that abolish visual fixation for the patient. They also contain internal illumination to facilitate observation of the eyes during testing. Eye closure or darkness can also be used to abolish fixation but measurements of the position of the eyes must then be made using *electronystagmography (ENG)*. This measures changes in electrical potentials brought about by eye movement using two electrodes placed on the adjacent skin. The velocity, amplitude and frequency of the eye movements are recorded on a paper strip.

POSITIONAL TESTING

From a seated position on an examination couch, and with the head turned 45 degrees to the right or left, the patient is rapidly lowered 30 degrees below the horizontal (*Hallpike's manoeuvre*, Fig. 13.7). The patient is instructed not to shut the eyes and to report sensations of vertigo while the examiner carefully looks for induced nystagmus. If none occurs the test is repeated with the head turned in the opposite direction.

In *benign paroxysmal positional nystagmus* there is a latent period of 5–10 seconds before the onset of vertigo and rotatory nystagmus is then seen which beats towards the lowermost ear. Fatigue of the response occurs so that immediate repetition of the test will produce little abnormality (adaptation). The pathophysiology of this disorder is not fully

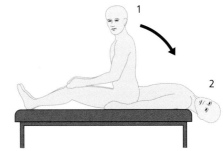

Fig. 13.7 Hallpike's manoeuvre.

understood but the symptoms tend to disappear with time. Alcohol abuse and psychotropic drugs may also cause transient positional nystagmus.

Persistent positional nystagmus implies central pathology. In this syndrome the nystagmus appears immediately, is not necessarily associated with vertiginous symptoms, and shows no adaptation. This is a feature of cerebellar brainstem disease and lesions in the region of the fourth ventricle.

FISTULA TEST

If there is evidence of middle ear disease and the patient is vertiginous then this simple test is indicated. Compression of the tragus into the external meatus or insufflating air into the ear using a speculum with a pneumatic bulb results in a sense of imbalance or vertigo and may be accompanied by nystagmus. Such a positive test implies an abnormal communication between the middle ear and the vestibular labyrinth.

ROMBERG'S TEST

The patient stands with the feet together and with the arms outstretched, initially with the eyes open and then with them closed. Patients with disorders of the posterior columns of the spinal cord will sway (or even fall) when the eyes are closed, but will stand normally with the eyes open. Patients with uncompensated unilateral labyrinthine dysfunction show instability to the side of the lesion that is more marked with their eyes closed. Patients with central dysfunction sway to both sides, whether the eyes are open or shut.

GAIT ASSESSMENT

The patient is asked to walk with the eyes open. Patients with uncompensated peripheral vestibular pathology will tend to veer towards the affected side, whereas those affected with a central pathology may stagger a few steps in one direction before veering to the other side.

CALORIC TEST, ROTATIONAL TESTING AND POSTUROGRAPHY

Caloric tests are the most commonly performed routine test for assessing the performance of the vestibular end-organ and are described on page 322.

Rotational testing assesses the response to angular acceleration but the method has the disadvantage that the ears cannot be separately tested. The same is true of the newer technique of posturography, which measures body sway using computer software. The patient stands on a specially constructed platform with a movable visual surround and is assessed under a variety of test circumstances. The advantage of this method is that all the inputs to posture can be separately tested. However, the hardware involved is expensive and, perhaps as a result of this, it has not yet been widely adopted.

RADIOLOGICAL EXAMINATION

Plain views of the temporal bone show the site of the sigmoid sinus and the tegmen tympani (the roof of the middle ear) and give an impression of the degree of mastoid aeration. However, such X-ray films only show evidence of gross disease and interpretation may be difficult. For these reasons computed tomography (CT) scanning and magnetic resonance imaging (MRI) have superseded them. Congenital abnormalities of the ossicular chain and atresia of the external ear canal can be more precisely defined by CT scanning, as can the position of the facial nerve (Fig. 13.8). Modern CT scans will also accurately show fractures or bone erosion due to cholesteatoma (Fig. 13.9) or diseases such as cancer of the middle ear. MRI is particularly useful in visualizing vascular lesions such as glomus tumours, and in assessing the internal auditory meatus to rule out acoustic neuromas.

THE NOSE AND PARANASAL SINUSES

ANATOMY

The nose is formed of two nasal bones which articulate with the nasal process of the maxilla on each side. Immediately caudal to the bones are cartilages (upper lateral cartilages) which are fused to the bones above and which form a continuum with the septal cartilage beneath. The tip of the nose is surrounded by a further set of cartilages (lower lateral cartilages) which support the nostrils and prevent collapse of the soft tissues on inspiration (Fig. 13.11).

The interior of the nose is divided into two parts by the nasal septum which is formed of cartilage anteriorly (quadrilateral cartilage) and bone posteriorly (perpendicular plate of the ethmoid; Fig. 13.12). On the lateral wall are paired turbinates (conchae) which project into the nasal cavity (Figs. 13.10 and 13.14). These structures, and the septum, are covered with mucous membrane which serves to warm and humidify the inspired air.

The paranasal sinuses are air-filled spaces which open into the nose through small openings on the

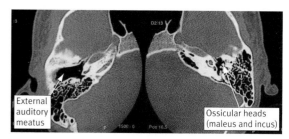

Fig. 13.8   Axial CT scans of ear showing absence of external auditory meatus on one side (right).

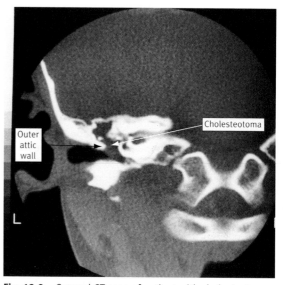

Fig. 13.9   Coronal CT scan of patient with cholesteatoma in the middle ear. Erosion of the outer attic wall is present.

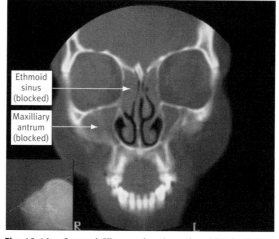

Fig. 13.10   Coronal CT scan showing ethmoid, labyrinth and maxillary antral opacification in a patient with sinusitis.

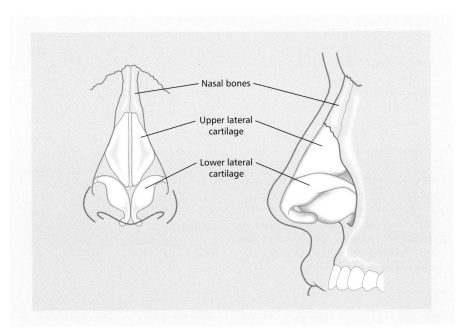

Fig. 13.11 Anatomy of the nose.

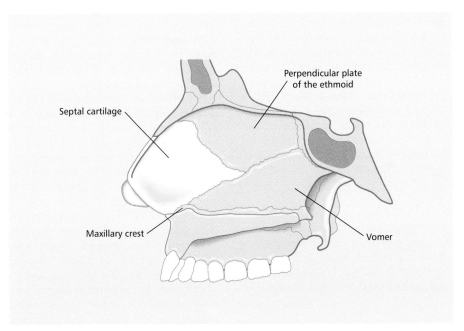

Fig. 13.12 The nasal septum.

lateral wall (ostia). They are cleansed by mucus which is secreted into the sinuses and swept by cilia through the ostia to be mixed with mucus secreted in the nose. This, in turn, is moved to the back of the nose (posterior choanae) where it is swallowed. Blockage of the ostia due to inflammation in the nose, with retention of mucus and superadded infection, is the presumed mechanism for sinus infection, Fig. 13.10 (rhinosinusitis). An apical tooth abscess of the upper jaw may also drain into the maxillary sinus causing acute sinusitis.

SYMPTOMS OF NASAL DISEASE

The important symptoms of nasal and sinus disease are:

- Nasal obstruction
- Discharge (*rhinorrhoea*)
- Sinus pain
- Sneezing and coughing
- Disturbances of smell.

Orbital pain, proptosis, diplopia, periorbital swelling and conjunctival chemosis may develop if the infection spreads to the orbit from the adjacent paranasal sinuses. Symptoms referable to the ear (otalgia or hearing loss due to serous otitis media) may also result if there is pathology in the postnasal space.

NASAL OBSTRUCTION

Obstruction of the nasal passages is one of the primary complaints of patients with nasal disease. Nasal blockage may be unilateral or bilateral. Long-standing nasal obstruction suggests structural deformity such as a deviated nasal septum or nasal polyposis. Variation between sides implies enhancement of the nasal cycle due to mucosal disease. The latter is a natural phenomenon under hypothalamic control that causes a cyclical variation in patency between the two sides of the nose. Awareness of the cycle is not normal and if the patient is conscious of it then this implies mucosal engorgement.

RHINORRHOEA

Nasal discharge (*rhinorrhoea*) may be bloody, purulent, watery or mucoid and either unilateral or bilateral.

Epistaxis (a nose bleed) varies in severity from an insignificant intermittent problem to a life-threatening major haemorrhage. The arterial supply of the nose is from branches of the sphenopalatine (external carotid), and from the anterior and posterior ethmoidal arteries (internal carotid). These vessels anastomose on the anterior nasal septum (Little's area) where they are easily traumatized. Bleeding is also associated with hypertension, nasal trauma and clotting disorders. *Watery discharge* suggests allergic rhinitis whereas *purulent discharge* may be secondary to a foreign body in the nose or may be a sign of sinus infection.

NASAL PAIN

Nasal pain *per se* is uncommon Pain centered over a sinus indicates infection or, rarely, a malignancy. However, it should be borne in mind that pain over the face is quite common and may be due to a variety of causes including trigeminal neuralgia or migraine.

SNEEZING

Sneezing is a protective expulsive reflex that helps clear the nasal airway of irritants. The most common cause is allergic rhinitis, which may provoke paroxysmal attacks associated with sneezing, rhinorrhoea, nasal obstruction and palatal and conjunctival itching.

DISTURBANCES OF SMELL

Anosmia is a total loss of smell that may accompany head injury. *Hyposmia* is a reduction in the sense of smell and is commonly found in patients who have obstruction of the olfactory cleft in the nose due, for example, to nasal polyps.

Casosmia is an unpleasant smell detected mainly by others and which is due to chronic sepsis in the nose: this is most commonly found in patients with atrophic change and secondary anaerobic infection. An even more intensely unpleasant smell is called *ozaena*; this can be found in patients with tumours or foreign bodies within the nose.

EXAMINATION OF THE NOSE

The external nose should be examined in a good light by observation and palpation. The shape of the nose should be noted. There is some reduction in the elasticity of the soft tissues of the nose with age, resulting in drooping of the nasal tip (nasal ptosis), and there may be deformities of the nasal bony and cartilaginous dorsum following a nasal fracture. Saddle deformity of the nose may follow destruction of the bony septum or cartilaginous septum from a variety of causes.

Palpation of nasal bones helps to distinguish cartilaginous from bony distortion. Also palpate the facial skeleton, paying particular attention to the orbital margins. Note any tenderness, swelling, expansion or depression of bone, for example after injury or when malignancy is suspected. Facial swelling is unusual in maxillary sinusitis but occurs with dental root infections and in carcinoma of the maxillary antrum. Finally, the palate and alveoli should be inspected and palpated from inside the mouth using a gloved finger.

A preliminary examination of the nasal vestibule and intranasal contents can usually be made by exerting gentle upward pressure on the tip of the nose with the finger and using reflected illumination from a head mirror. The nasal vestibule is lined with skin and contains vibrissae: these may become prominent in later life, particularly in men. The nasal cavity is then examined with Thudichum's nasal speculum (Fig. 13.12). The nasal septum should lie in the midline, but may be deviated or thickened. When deviated, hypertrophy of the contralateral inferior turbinate may also develop causing bilateral nasal blockage. Look for any area of granulation on the nasal septum and for a septal perforation. Perforations may be secondary to nose-picking, surgical trauma, granulomatous conditions or inhalation of industrial dusts, notably nickel and chrome.

Other than the nasal septum the most obvious intranasal structure is the inferior turbinate, situated on the lower portion of the lateral nasal wall. The submucosal vascular bed shows considerable alteration in size with changes in ambient humidity and temperature. In allergic rhinitis the inferior turbinate may be hypertrophied and its mucosa pallid and wet. In vasomotor rhinitis the mucosa is also swollen but is classically reddened.

Probing may allow distinction to be made between a nasal polyp and a hypertrophied inferior turbinate. The former will be soft and mobile and, because

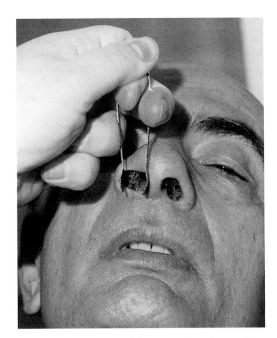

Fig. 13.13   Examination of the nose using the nasal speculum.

simple nasal polyps lack pain fibres, the patient will experience no discomfort. By contrast, probing of the inferior turbinate will cause transient mild discomfort. In a child a polyp may be seen seemingly arising from the roof of the nose. This should *not* be probed as it may be the intranasal presentation of a meningocele.

The middle turbinate is also subject to variations in size and shape. Beneath the middle turbinate lies the middle meatus. Here the maxillary, frontal and anterior ethmoidal sinuses drain into the nose. Ethmoidal nasal polyps also present in the nose at this site.

POSTNASAL SPACE (NASOPHARYNX)

The posterior choanae and the postnasal space can be inspected by means of a small mirror inserted into the mouth and oriented so that it lies just behind the soft palate. This manoeuvre is difficult and best performed with the patient leaning forward, with the mouth open and the tongue firmly depressed with a Lack's tongue depressor. A mirror is warmed with the flame of a spirit lamp and passed into the mouth over the upper surface of the tongue until it lies in the space between the uvula, the tongue and the faucial pillars. This method has now been superseded in most centres by the use of rigid telescopes (Hopkin's rods: Fig. 13.3). These can be passed with ease in the majority of patients, under local anaesthesia, and give an unparalleled view not only of the lateral wall and septum but also of the postnasal space. The opening of the Eustachian tube in the nasopharynx can be readily seen and the fossa of Rosenmuller, which is the site

of origin of postnasal space carcinomas, lies directly above and behind this opening. Hypertrophy of the posterior end of the inferior turbinate (mulberry turbinate) may also be seen in the posterior choanae and, in children and young adults, an adenoid mass may be visualized.

TESTS OF NASAL FUNCTION

NASAL PATENCY

A crude assessment of patency can be made during clinical examination. The technique differs according to age. In a neonate patency is best estimated by observing any movement of a wisp of cotton wool held in front of each nostril. In children and adults holding a Lack's tongue depressor (Fig. 13.3) at the nose causes moist expired air to mist the metal which allows a subjective assessment of airflow on each side. The patient should also be asked to inspire maximally; collapse of the rim of the nares may occur if the lower lateral cartilages are weakened or malpositioned.

More objective assessment is difficult. Rhinomanometry, which measures nasal airflow and resistance, and acoustic rhinometry, which measures nasal volume and cross-sectional area, have remained specialized research tools. Their use has not become routine because such measurements are time-consuming and seem to offer little advantage over clinical examination. There have also been difficulties in agreeing standards for these techniques.

ALLERGY TESTING

The simplest way of confirming extrinsic allergy is to undertake skin prick tests. The patient should not be taking antihistamines as this may give a false negative response.

The forearm is used and a solution containing the allergen is introduced into the superficial epidermis using a sterile lance. The common allergens (pollens, animal danders, house dust and house dust mite), together with any agents that have been suspected from the history, should be tested and compared to controls (histamine and saline). A positive response produces a wheal and flare that can be graded. However, a negative response does not definitely exclude atopy and, if clinical suspicion is strong, the radio-allergosorbent test (RAST)—which measures specific serum IgE—may be indicated. This test is, however, expensive.

MUCOCILIARY CLEARANCE

This should be assessed when impaired ciliary function is suspected, for example Kartagener's syndrome (impaired ciliary motility). The patient should taste saccharin placed on the anterior end of the inferior turbinate in approximately 20 minutes. Undue prolongation of this time suggests ciliary pathology.

MISCELLANEOUS TESTS

Nasal provocation tests have a limited place in routine investigation but may be indicated if skin tests are equivocal. They are, however, time consuming as only one allergen at a time can be tested. Eosinophil counts from smears of nasal secretion are used for research purposes only.

RADIOLOGICAL EXAMINATION

Radiological examination of the nose has little to offer in the management of nasal fractures. Manipulation of the nasal bones and septum is required if a fracture has resulted in displacement, but this is best assessed by clinical inspection.

Plain X-rays are often used in the investigation of sinus disease. In children the maxillary antra are poorly pneumatized and the frontal sinuses have not yet developed. However, the ethmoidal sinuses are well developed and are best shown on an occipito-frontal radiograph. With increasing age, the maxillary sinuses enlarge below the nasal floor and the frontal sinuses enlarge into the frontal bone. However, the latter are usually asymmetrical and sometimes fail to develop altogether. Maxillary sinusitis is best demonstrated in posteroanterior radiographs in the occipito-mental plane; with head tilt any fluid level in the antrum will be seen. In chronic infections the mucosa becomes thickened, but the X-ray appearance is indistinguishable from the mucosal thickening secondary to an allergic or vasomotor rhinitis. A lateral X-ray may demonstrate mucosal thickening or a fluid level in the sphenoid sinus. It is also useful in estimating the degree of adenoidal hypertrophy.

CT scanning of the sinuses, with sections taken in the coronal and axial planes, using bone window settings, has considerable advantages over conventional X-rays and is useful in the investigation of chronic infection, trauma and neoplasia (Figs 13.10 and 13.14). However, the radiation dose is considerable

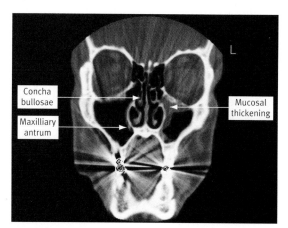

Fig. 13.14 Coronal CT scan showing hypertrophied mucosa in the left maxillary antrum and bilateral aeration of the middle turbinates (concha bullosae).

and the technique should therefore only be used when surgery seems inevitable. Magnetic resonance imaging (MRI) is also of considerable use since it readily distinguishes retained secretions from soft tissue masses.

THROAT

ANATOMY

The regions that comprise the throat include the oral cavity, the pharynx (oropharynx, nasopharynx and hypopharynx), the larynx and the major salivary glands.

The oral cavity includes the anterior two thirds of the tongue, the lips, hard palate and teeth, and the alveoli of the maxilla and mandible. The tongue is a mass of interlaced muscle covered by squamous epithelium. It contains numerous taste buds and is essential for efficient articulation, mastication and deglutition. The teeth provide the mechanics for grinding food. The primary dentition is complete by about 3 years and the secondary (permanent) dentition commences at about 6 years and is complete by the age of 18. The teeth in the maxilla are intimately related to the maxillary sinus and may be a source of infection in the maxillary antrum.

The pharynx stretches from the base of the skull to the cricopharyngeal sphincter below (Fig. 13.15). The nasopharynx has already been described. The oropharynx is bounded above by the soft palate and below by the upper surface of the epiglottis. The palatine tonsils are situated in its lateral wall between the anterior and posterior pillars of the fauces.

The hypopharynx consists of the posterior pharyngeal wall, the piriform fossae and the post-cricoid area. The piriform fossae, which comprise the lateral walls of the pharynx adjacent to the larynx, are important for they are the routes by which food is passed into the upper oesophagus.

The prime function of the larynx is to protect the upper airway. Voice production is a secondary function that has evolved with time. It has a rigid structure consisting of cartilages, the most prominent of which is the thyroid cartilage, which articulate with the cricoid cartilage below. The epiglottis is attached to the inner surface of the thyroid cartilage and helps swallowing.

The larynx consists of three compartments (Fig. 13.16):

- The glottis
- The supraglottis
- The subglottis.

The *glottis* is formed by the vocal folds. Into the posterior third of each fold is imbedded the vocal process of the arytenoid cartilage. In turn this is acted upon by many of the intrinsic muscles of the larynx which, by changing the position of the arytenoid, help to control the movements of the vocal folds.

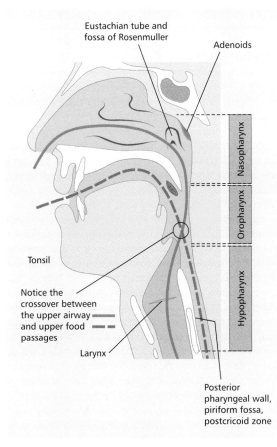

Fig. 13.15   The three regions of the pharynx.

The *supraglottis* extends from the false cords below to the hyoid bone above. The *subglottis*, which is the narrowest part of the upper respiratory tract, extends from the glottis to the lower border of the cricoid. The action of the false cords and the sphincteric action of the aryepiglottic folds and epiglottis above prevent food and liquid from entering the lower respiratory tract.

Phonation occurs with movement of the vocal folds into the midline. This produces a rise in the subglottic pressure, which, with controlled exhalation, causes the vocal cords to vibrate. Changes in volume of the voice are caused by alterations in the subglottic pressure, whereas alterations in pitch are due to modification of the length of, and tension within, the vocal folds. The quality of this basic laryngeal sound is further altered by the resonating cavities of the pharynx, mouth and nose.

The pharynx is innervated from the pharyngeal plexus (IX, X, XI cranial nerves) and all the intrinsic muscles of the larynx (except for cricothyroid) are supplied by the recurrent laryngeal nerve (X) which loops around the arch of the aorta on the left and subclavian artery on the right before entering the larynx inferiorly. The cricothyroid is supplied by the external branch of the superior laryngeal nerve (X).

The only salivary glands of clinical importance are the parotid and submandibular glands. The parotids produce a serous secretion; submandibular secretion is more seromucinous. The parotid duct opens into the mouth opposite the second upper molar tooth

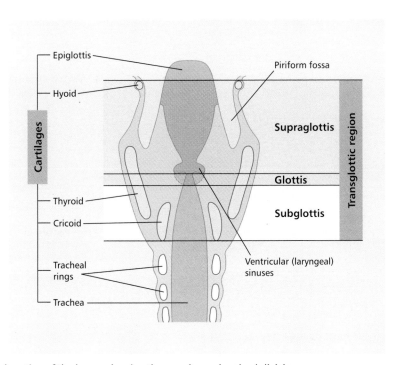

Fig. 13.16   Coronal section of the larynx showing three major regional subdivisions.

and the submandibular ducts open into the floor of the mouth adjacent to the frenulum of the tongue. Both of these areas should be inspected in any routine examination. The importance of these glands lies in the properties of the saliva produced, as this lubricates the food and facilitates articulation and mastication as well as being important in the appreciation of taste. Saliva is also essential in maintaining oral hygiene as it contains IgA and thus has a protective role.

The lymph nodes in the head and neck (Fig. 13.17) provide a barrier to the spread of disease, either inflammatory or neoplastic. Enlargement implies that there is primary disease within the nodes or that they have become involved secondary to pathology in the head and neck. Occasionally they may become involved due to pathology below the clavicle.

SYMPTOMS OF THROAT DISEASE

Patients with disease in these areas commonly present with:

- Pain
- Stridor (noisy breathing)
- Dysphonia (hoarseness)
- Dysphagia (difficulty in swallowing)
- A lump in the neck.

Occasionally lesions in the upper airway may present with symptoms such as overspill of food and ingested fluids into the upper trachea or nose, or with weight loss.

SORE THROAT

A sore throat is one of the commonest symptoms in clinical medicine. The term is often used by patients to describe any symptom felt within the mouth and throat.

The commonest causes in the oral cavity are carious teeth or periodontal disease. Ulceration associated with trauma, lichen planus, herpes or Vincent's angina may also be painful, as are aphthous ulcers. Painful vesicles, which break down to create small ulcers on the palate, occur with *herpes zoster*

Inflammatory disease in the tonsils is the most common cause of oropharyngeal pain. *Acute follicular tonsillitis* is due to *Streptococcus* infection and presents with a punctate, yellow exudate due to pus filling the tonsillar crypts. In glandular fever the tonsils are covered with a white pseudomembrane. This, and other viral infections, probably predisposes to subsequent acute attacks of inflammation. A grey membrane may be the result of infection with *Corynebacterium diphtheriae*. With these alternatives in mind, a throat swab should always be taken for culture and sensitivity in these patients. The frequency and severity of attacks of tonsillitis as estimated by the amount of time lost from schooling or work and the necessity for antibiotics should be noted: such considerations help to decide whether tonsillectomy is merited.

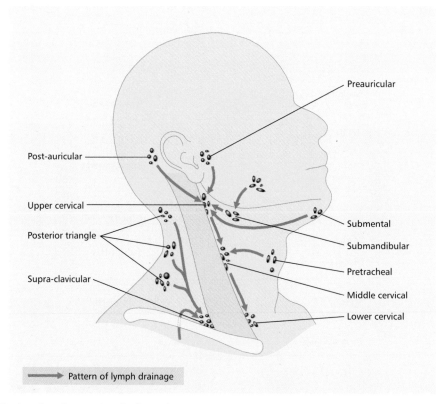

Fig. 13.17   The lymph node groupings in the neck.

An abscess adjacent to the tonsil (*quinsy*) may also be associated with painful dysphagia and trismus (spasm in the lower jaw). Drainage is often required and the tonsils should be removed to prevent recurrence. A squamous cell carcinoma of the tonsil presents as an exophytic mass or as an ulcer and is frequently associated with pain.

Ulceration in the oropharynx is also seen in glandular fever, rubella and streptococcal tonsillitis, as well as from trauma due to ill-fitting dentures or broken teeth.

STRIDOR
Stridor is noisy breathing associated with upper airway obstruction. It is associated with a variety of conditions (Box 13.5). Because of the narrowness of their airways, stridor is of particular importance in infants and children. Supraglottitis (which occurs most commonly between the ages of 3 and 7 and which is associated with infection due to *Haemophilus influenzae* type B) may present with rapidly progressive airway obstruction and dyspnoea, fever, pharyngeal pain and drooling from the corner of the mouth. Examining the throat in such a patient can induce laryngospasm and should be avoided. Blood culture and immediate treatment with antibiotics should be started and the airway secured by intubation or tracheostomy.

Acute laryngotracheobronchitis presents with a longer history (24–48 hours) and the airway obstruction tends to be less severe. The patient will have a hoarse voice and the secretions formed tend to be thick and tenacious.

Laryngeal carcinoma may also cause stridor if it is neglected, either due to direct invasion of the vocal fold with fixation, or because of recurrent laryngeal nerve involvement.

DYSPHONIA
Dysphonia may be due to organic or non organic causes (Box 13.6). Acute vocal abuse, acute inflammation, smoke inhalation or exposure to dust will all cause dysphonia. In most cases the symptoms are self-limiting. Hoarseness followed by increasing airway obstruction is the typical presentation of a laryngeal neoplasm but neurological damage to the recurrent laryngeal nerve from disease in the cervical oesophagus, the apex of the lung, the aorta or the subclavian artery may also cause disruption, as can lesions in the posterior fossa or the jugular bulb. Systemic disorders such as hypothyroidism also predispose to dysphonia. Tumours in the piriform fossa present with muffling of the voice rather than true dysphonia. The voice is said to be like someone eating a hot potato.

Non-organic causes include chronic misuse of the voice, which may result in oedema of the vocal folds (Reincke's oedema), a vocal fold nodule (hyperkeratosis), papilloma or polyp. Any laryngeal abnormality must always be biopsied as it may be due to carcinoma. If benign changes are present speech therapy is necessary.

Any patient with dysphonia which has lasted for more than 4 weeks should have a referral to exclude malignancy.

DYSPHAGIA
Any lesion that interrupts the normal sequence of coordinated muscular activity that is necessary for swallowing (Box 13.7) may cause dysphagia. Patients with persistent symptoms, especially if they are associated with regurgitation, weight loss, dysphonia, otalgia or a mass in the neck, require urgent investigation. Pooling of saliva in the piriform fossae or at the upper oesophagus seen at laryngoscopy implies obstruction in the cervical oesophagus or in the postcricoid space. Malignancy in the postcricoid area is more common in women due to the predisposition engendered by Plummer–Vinson syndrome.

BOX 13.5 Causes of stridor.

Neonatal
- Congenital tumours and cysts
- Laryngomalacia
- Subglottic stenosis

Children
- Supraglottitis (epiglottitis)
- Laryngotracheobronchitis
- Acute laryngitis
- Foreign body
- Retropharyngeal abscess
- Papillomatosis

Adults
- Acute laryngitis
- Laryngeal trauma
- Laryngeal carcinoma
- Supraglottitis (epiglottitis)

BOX 13.6 Causes of dysphonia.

Organic
- Inflammatory: infective laryngitis, inhalation of fumes
- Neoplasia: carcinoma, papillomata
- Neurological: thyroidectomy, carcinoma of lung/breast, myasthenia, spasmodic dysphonia
- Systemic: hypothyroidism, rheumatoid arthritis

Non-organic
- Habitual dysphonias: oedema, nodules, polyps or contact ulcer on vocal folds
- Psychogenic: musculoskeletal tension; ventricular dysphonia, conversion disorders, mutational falsetto

BOX 13.7   Causes of dysphagia.

- Neuromuscular: motor neurone disease, multiple sclerosis, myasthenia gravis
- Intrinsic lesions: oesophageal stricture, oesophageal web, achalasia, pharyngeal pouch, pharyngeal and oesophageal neoplasia
- Extrinsic lesions: thyroid enlargement, primary or secondary neoplasia, aortic aneurysm
- Systemic: scleroderma
- Psychosomatic: globus pharyngeus

LUMP IN THE NECK

Certain deep cervical lymph nodes are described by name. The most prominent of these is the *jugulodigastric node*, which lies anterosuperior in the jugular chain and which can be palpated just posterior to the angle of the mandible. This is the most commonly enlarged node in upper respiratory tract infections, especially following tonsillitis.

The diagnosis is suggested by the age of the patient (Box 13.8). An enlarged cervical node in an adult has an 80% chance of being malignant. Features that suggest malignancy are progressive enlargement, hardness, lack of tenderness, fixation to deep structures and size (a node greater than 2 cm in diameter is likely to be malignant). In children the likelihood of malignancy is much smaller with only 20% of cervical lumps destined to be malignant.

In all such patients the nose and throat should be examined and blood taken for a full blood count and sedimentation rate. A chest X-ray should also be performed. A fine needle aspiration biopsy of the node will diagnose more than 95% of metastatic squamous cell carcinomas and will obviate the need for an excision biopsy in many cases. However, fine needle aspiration biopsy is much less reliable for other tumour types and if fine needle biopsy produces an unsatisfactory or equivocal result an excision biopsy may be necessary.

BOX 13.8   Causes of neck lumps by age.

Less than 20 years
- Inflammatory
- Congenital: thyroglossal and branchial cysts, midline dermoid, cystic hygroma
- Lymphoma

20–40 years
- Salivary gland pathology: calculus, infection, tumour
- Thyroid pathology: goitre, inflammatory thyroiditis, lymphoma, tumour
- Chronic infection: HIV, tuberculosis, actinomycosis

Greater than 40 years
- Secondary malignancy
- Primary malignancy: lymphoma

EXAMINATION OF THE THROAT

With practice it is possible to inspect all of the oral cavity, the pharynx and the larynx. It is preferable to examine the anterior oropharynx with a headlight or with a head mirror. This ensures adequate illumination and keeps both hands free for the manipulation of instruments. First check the lips, teeth and gums, the floor of the mouth and the openings of the submandibular and parotid ducts. If salivary gland pathology is suspected, bimanual palpation, with one gloved finger in the mouth and synchronous palpation of the gland, may help to define pathology. Then tongue mobility (XII) should be assessed.

A Lack's tongue depressor (Fig. 13.3) is then introduced so that its tip lies at the junction of the posterior and middle thirds of the dorsum of the tongue. The tonsillar pillars, the palatine tonsils, soft palate and uvula can then be inspected in turn. The tonsils should be symmetrical and any gross asymmetry should be viewed with suspicion. Likewise the soft palate should be symmetrical and the gag reflex (IX) present.

The more distant portions of the pharynx can be inspected only with a laryngeal mirror or fibre-optic laryngoscope. For indirect laryngoscopy the patient is asked to remove any dentures and to protrude the tongue. A cotton swab held between the examiner's thumb and index finger grasps the latter (Fig. 13.18). The patient is then encouraged to concentrate on taking slow deep breaths and, with the mouth opened wide, a warmed laryngeal mirror is introduced gently but firmly to the soft palate just proximal to the uvula. The soft palate is displaced upwards and backwards by the mirror and, by instructing the patient to say 'aah' or 'eeee', the larynx is elevated towards the examining mirror and examined.

The *supraglottis*, the *glottis* and the *subglottis* are examined in turn. The whole length of each vocal fold should be clearly visible and the mobility of each side noted. If there is difficulty due to gagging, visualization may be improved by anaesthetizing the soft palate and posterior oropharyngeal wall with a 2% lignocaine spray to minimize palatal sensation.

If no view is obtained, then the nose should be anaesthetized and a fibre-optic rhinolaryngoscope introduced through the nose and over the back of the soft palate. This will allow a relaxed view in almost every case.

For reasons already alluded to, examination of the neck is an essential part of the routine assessment of any patient with suspected or proven disease in the throat. Examination for lymph nodes should follow a well-rehearsed routine so that no groups of nodes are missed. Such an examination starts by inspection of the neck from the front in a good light and with the area well exposed, and continues, with the examiner standing behind the patient, with systematic palpation of the principal lymph node areas.

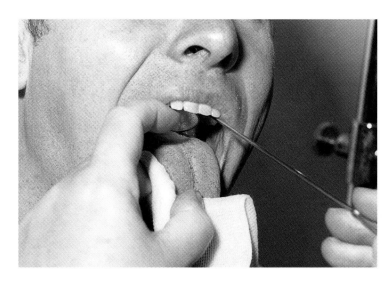

Fig. 13.18 Examination of the larynx and the laryngopharynx by indirect laryngoscopy.

Start by palpating the nodes in the *posterior auricular region* and then progressively feel for the nodes on the *anterior border of the trapezius muscle* down to the *supraclavicular fossa*. The latter area is palpated from behind forwards. The examining fingers then pass up the jugular vein, where the most important groups of nodes in the head and neck are situated, towards the ear. The *jugular, parotid* and *preauricular* areas are then examined, followed by *submandibular* and *submental* nodes. Finally the nodes associated with the *anterior jugular chain* are examined. This brings the fingers to the thyroid gland.

The position and size of the *thyroid* should be noted: since it lies deep to the small strap muscles of the neck, it is often best examined with the patient's neck partially flexed to relax the overlying structures. Consider whether the gland is enlarged and, if so, decide whether the enlargement is uniform or confined to one or other lobe. Significance also attaches to whether the gland is smooth or nodular and whether it is possible to get the fingers below the gland on palpation. Irregularity, hardness and fixation of the gland to neighbouring structures are features of neoplasia.

If there is a midline mass, observe it as the patient swallows a little water. The thyroid gland is invested with pretracheal fascia and moves as the patient swallows. Such a manoeuvre may draw a small *retrosternal thyroid goitre* above the examining fingers. Midline lumps should also be assessed with the patient protruding the tongue. Movement suggests attachment to the base of the tongue and implies the presence of a *thyroglossal cyst*.

The larynx should be mobile from side to side and, if the thyroid cartilage is held between thumb and first finger and gently moved against the cervical spine, should grate. This grating sensation (*laryngeal crepitus*) is caused by the rubbing of the cricoid and thyroid cartilages against the cervical spine and is a normal phenomenon. If hypopharyngeal pathology such as a *postcricoid neoplasm* is present, or if there is a mass in the prevertebral space displacing the larynx forward and away from the cervical spine, this crepitus cannot be demonstrated. Finally, examination of the neck should be concluded by auscultation of the carotid arteries and, if indicated, of the thyroid gland.

RADIOLOGICAL EXAMINATION

The value of a plain film of the oral cavity is confined to viewing dental disease. CT scanning is, otherwise, superior. A soft tissue lateral neck X-ray is useful in demonstrating pathology in the nasopharyx but has little value in detecting disease of the hypopharynx. Moreover it is not a sensitive investigation in the detection of foreign bodies.

A barium swallow is useful in localizing obstruction in the oesophagus, but is less helpful in evaluating the hypopharynx. Endoscopy under anaesthetic is the preferred investigation in such cases and is also essential in any patient with suspected malignancy. In any case where pathology is identified a biopsy should be obtained.

All patients with proven malignancy should also have a CT scan. This helps to stage the disease and may demonstrate metastastatic spread that has eluded palpation.

SPECIAL INVESTIGATIONS

PURE TONE AUDIOMETRY

This measures the threshold for pure tone sounds introduced into each ear at different frequencies. Standardized sound levels are used, compared to a hearing level of 0 dB. This is the threshold found when testing otologically normal adults in a sound-proofed booth using sound attenuation headphones.

The better hearing ear is tested first at frequencies from 250 to 8000 Hz to determine the threshold in decibels at each frequency. Initially an intensity well above threshold is chosen and the patient is instructed to respond when sound is heard. The sound level is then first reduced in 10-dB steps until there is no response and is then increased in 5-dB steps until the threshold is reached. Initial testing is at 1000 Hz is repeated at 2000, 4000, 8000, 500 and 250 Hz. The other ear is then tested. Bone conduction is assessed in an identical way, but using a bone vibrating headset. Different symbols are used for right and left ears and for recording responses with air and bone conduction (Fig. 13.19).

In pure sensorineural hearing loss the bone conduction thresholds mirror the air-conducted thresholds but in a conductive hearing loss, as with the Rinne test, the bone conduction thresholds exceed those for air. The *air–bone gap* (the difference between air and bone thresholds) gives a measure of the degree of conductive hearing loss. The bone conduction thresholds are also often referred to as the *cochlear reserve*. They are an indication of the best air conduction thresholds that could theoretically be obtained after surgery to correct a conductive hearing loss.

SPEECH AUDIOMETRY

A pure tone audiogram does not test speech discrimination and it is this that defines hearing disability. For this reason a speech audiogram is often required.

A speech audiogram measures the patient's ability to recognize and repeat lists of phonetically balanced words arranged in groups and delivered at different intensities to the test ear from a tape recording. The percentage of words correctly repeated by the subject is noted at each intensity. With normal hearing a score of 100% discrimination is achieved at a sound intensity of 45–55 dB. Patients with pure conductive deafness will also achieve 100% discrimination, but only at a much higher intensity. Patients with sensorineural deafness are often unable to achieve 100% discrimination due to recruitment (Fig. 13.20).

IMPEDANCE AUDIOLOGY

An impedance bridge has an earpiece that is inserted into the external meatus. Through this pass three channels. The first delivers a continuous tone into the ear canal during the test (probe tone); the second has a microphone to record the sound intensity level within the ear canal; and the third channel is connected to a manometer so that the ear canal pressure can be altered (Fig. 13.21).

The external meatus acts as a rigid tube with a compliant end (the drum). Sound introduced into the ear will be absorbed according to the compliance of the middle ear. In the normal ear the tympanic membrane is at its most compliant when the middle ear and ear canal pressures are equal. In such circumstances the majority of the sound introduced into the

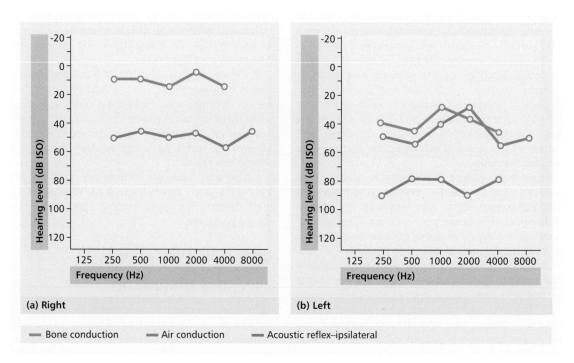

(a) Right

(b) Left

— Bone conduction   — Air conduction   — Acoustic reflex–ipsilateral

Fig. 13.19 Pure tone audiogram showing a right conductive deafness and a left sensorineural deafness with recruitment. The right ear was masked with narrow band noise while testing the left ear for both air and bone conduction.

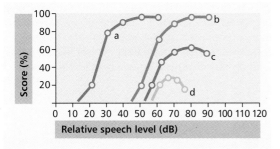

Fig. 13.20 Speech audiogram: **(a)** normal; **(b)** conductive deafness; **(c)** sensory loss; **(d)** neural lesion.

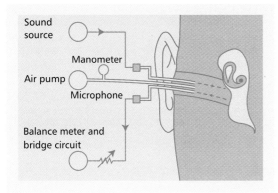

Fig. 13.21 Components of the acoustic impedance bridge. (After S.R. Mawson and H. Ludman in Diseases of the Ear, 4th edn (1979) published by Edward Arnold, London.)

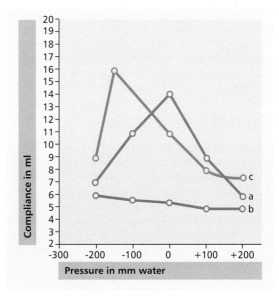

Fig. 13.22 Three types of tympanometry curve: **(a)** normal; **(b)** tympanic effusion or adhesive otitis; **(c)** negative middle ear pressure (eustachian tube dysfunction).

system is transmitted into the ear and the amount of sound energy reflected back and measured by the microphone is minimal. When the pressure difference between the external and middle ear is increased or decreased using the manometer the tympanic membrane becomes less compliant. This increases the impedance to transmitted sound and increases the sound energy reflected back to the probe.

These changes can be plotted graphically on a *tympanogram* (Fig. 13.22), which gives a measure of movement of the ear drum and the compliance of the middle ear. Impedance is increased when the tympanic membrane is thickened or when there is fluid in the middle ear and is decreased when the drum is hypermobile or atrophic.

The impedance probe can also be used to record changes in the middle ear compliance secondary to contraction of the stapedius muscle. This phenomenon, the *stapedial reflex*, can be measured on the ear that is ipsi- or contralateral to the probe. It is a bilateral reflex mediated via brainstem nuclei with input from the normal auditory pathways and output from the facial nerve—which innervates the stapedius muscle.

EVOKED RESPONSE AUDIOMETRY

This is one form of a group of tests in which evoked responses in the brain are recorded following a sound applied to the ear. As with impedance audiology these tests are objective in that they require no response from the patient. The responses are obtained using an averaging computer. When sufficient numbers of identical sound stimuli are presented, all like responses become superimposed one on another while random activity (from the background EEG) is cancelled out.

BRAINSTEM EVOKED RESPONSES (BSER)

For this test two active electrodes are used, placed on the vertex and on the mastoid. Sound is introduced through earphones and either tone pips or filtered or broad-tone clicks are used. The averaged response shows 7 peaks:

- First peak—cochlear hair cells
- Second peak—cochlear nucleus
- Third peak—superior olivary nucleus
- Fourth and fifth peak—synapses at the inferior colliculus
- Sixth peak—medial geniculate body
- Seventh peak—auditory cortex.

It is usual to measure the time taken for the impulse to travel from peaks 1 to 5 (I–V latency). Compressive lesions of the acoustic nerve will cause delay of the impulse as it travels along the nerve with increased latency. Delay also occurs in patients with brainstem tumours or with multiple sclerosis. This technique can also be used to measure hearing threshold by altering the frequency and intensity of the clicks and noting the intensity, at a given frequency, at which the brainstem auditory evoked response (BSAER) ceases to have definable peaks. This can be a useful test of hearing in the unborn and in infancy.

ELECTROCOCHLEOGRAPHY (ECOCHG)

This test requires the insertion of a needle through the tympanic membrane. It can be undertaken under local anaesthetic in adults. Most of the information comes from the basal turn of the cochlear and is therefore only related to high frequencies.

Broad-band clicks are used and the action potential from the cochlear nerve, the summating potential (related to movement of the cochlear membrane) and the cochlear microphonic recorded. This technique can also be used to assess threshold but is mostly used to assess the presence of endolymphatic hydrops such as occurs in *Ménières disease*.

CALORIC TESTING

This simple test is performed with the patient lying on a couch with the head at 30 degrees, in order to bring the lateral semicircular canals into the vertical plane. The patient is instructed to fix upon a point in central gaze and the external ear canal is irrigated with water at 30°C and then at 44°C for 30–40 seconds. This causes a thermal gradient across the temporal bone, which is thought to produce convection currents within the endolymph. Cold water induces nystagmus away from the ear being irrigated, and warm water induces nystagmus towards the ear under test (ACTH—away from cold and towards hot). Each ear is irrigated with water at both temperatures, with a suitable delay of several minutes between each test, and the induced nystagmus recorded and analysed using electronystagmography.

As with spontaneous nystagmus of peripheral origin, caloric-induced nystagmus can be significantly enhanced by the abolition of optic fixation. Peripheral lesions tend to cause a diminished response

on one side (a canal paresis), although a directional preponderance (where nystagmus in one direction is more prominent than the other) may also be observed (Fig. 13.23). This latter finding is most likely to occur with central disorders, especially in the brainstem.

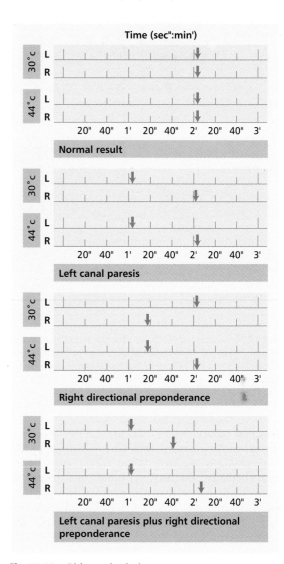

Fig. 13.23 Bithermal caloric tests.

14
GYNAECOLOGY AND OBSTETRICS

GENERAL POINTS

When a gynaecological history is taken and an examination performed, tact, discretion, consideration and the maintenance of proper confidentiality are fundamental, as some of the most intimate details of a woman's life are being elicited. Patients have complex expectations of their doctors, and it is reasonable to conform to these insofar as they allow the process of medical diagnosis to proceed smoothly. A genuine interest in the problem presented, combined with a gentleness of manner, allows both doctor and patient to feel at ease while the process of assessment continues. Adequate time should be allowed, but a sense of direction is essential as it can become difficult to separate the important from the trivial.

PRESENTING PROBLEMS AND GYNAECOLOGICAL HISTORY

General open-ended questions are better than more specific ones in the early stages of history-taking. Avoid questions which imply criticism, for example, when assessing a request for termination of pregnancy: 'How could you have forgotten to take your pill?' Such a question will probably ruin the basis for continuing a constructive interview. It is helpful to ask specifically, 'Which pill were you using?' or 'Did you have any episodes of vomiting or diarrhoea about the time you conceived?' Once the interview is progressing satisfactorily, an opportunity must be made to ask about *menstrual upset*, *post-coital bleeding* and *dyspareunia* (pain or difficulty with intercourse), as these symptoms, if present, will need further investigation. Sometimes a woman may be too apprehensive to discuss her problems freely. This should be acknowledged as soon as it is recognized; open discussion will often resolve this anxiety. If necessary, the help of a colleague with particular skills should be sought, for example for psychosexual problems.

Menstruation—the cyclical loss of sanguineous fluid from the uterus in mature women—is recorded as the days of menstrual loss and the duration of the interval from the first day of one period to the onset of the next, e.g. 5/28. An additional note is useful, giving the character of the loss and the daily variation. Specific labels such as *menorrhagia*, *metrorrhagia* or *polymenorrhoea* should only be used if the pattern conforms exactly to that definition. Where the problem is infertility, specific questions should be asked about the timing and frequency of intercourse, and whether dyspareunia or other sexual difficulties have occurred. Women with these problems will not be embarrassed by such questions, as they will be expecting them. If *prolapse* has developed (where a woman has noticed a bulge at the introitus), associated symptoms of bladder or pelvic floor disturbance and backache should be sought.

HISTORY OF CURRENT AND PREVIOUS PREGNANCIES

If a woman presents with pregnancy, ascertain as gently as possible if it is welcomed or not. Remember that although relatively few pregnancies are planned, by the time of birth most babies are genuinely wanted. In particular, ask the date of the first day of the *last menstrual period (LMP)* with a note as to its likely accuracy. Also record the previous menstrual pattern before conception and whether these were natural cycles or due to the use of the contraceptive pill. The *expected date of delivery (EDD)* of the child can be calculated providing a natural 28-day cycle has been present for some months prior to the conception cycle. The EDD is then 9 months and 7 days from the onset of the last menstrual period (i.e. 280 days or 10 lunar months; the date of delivery is 266 days from the date of conception when this is known). Clearly this is only an approximation, since calendar months are not of a standard length, and *term* is regarded as a time stretching from the end of the 37th to the start of the 42nd week from the last menstrual period. This degree of variation should be explained to the pregnant woman from the outset.

Data should be assembled chronologically in 3-monthly periods (*trimesters*) and should be related to those events which would be expected to occur at an equivalent stage of a healthy pregnancy. The course and outcome of previous pregnancies must be explored, as these are essential guides to the progress of the current pregnancy. However, the woman's age will have changed and the circumstances may also be quite different. Where early loss of pregnancy has occurred previously it must be established whether this was by *spontaneous abortion* ('miscarriage') or *therapeutic termination of pregnancy* ('abortion') and on how many occasions it occurred. The gestation, symptoms leading to miscarriage, the method of termination, complications and any treatment must be noted. Valuable additional information includes the time taken for the woman to return to a normal menstrual pattern after the event.

The outcome of previous pregnancies is recorded as a *live birth*, a *neonatal death* or a *stillbirth*. The birth of a child showing any signs of independent life is recorded as a *live birth*. This now occurs beyond 24 weeks' gestation (or 500 g weight), but with improved neonatal care, viability of a fetus may soon be obtained from an even earlier stage. If such a child dies, that event in the UK requires a death certificate. Since the Human Fertilization and Embryology Act (1990), if the child is born dead after 24 completed weeks, it is recorded as a *stillbirth*, and requires a stillbirth certificate and burial. If the child is born dead at an earlier gestation it is regarded as an *abortion* or *miscarriage* and neither stillbirth certificate nor formal burial is necessary.

The foregoing statements relate to the legal requirements, but it is important to remember that all parents who lose children under any of these circumstances will need compassionate consideration and emotional support as well as professional counselling (e.g. from SANDS, the Stillbirth and Neonatal Death Society, or similar organization). They will also need to understand the reasons for the loss. When a child is born its gestation, weight (to see if this was appropriate for gestational age), and condition at birth should be ascertained. Any complications of pregnancy, delivery or the puerperium should be enumerated, as should the developmental 'milestones' of the child. Where events are uncertain, making enquiries at the hospital where the delivery occurred is essential.

A woman's *gravidity* is described by the notation *para x + y*, where *x* is the number of babies delivered, whether live births or stillbirths, and *y* is the number of pregnancies the woman has had. The latter should include any ectopic pregnancies and abortions prior to 24 weeks' gestation, whether the fetus was born dead, or born alive but too premature to survive, including both spontaneous abortions and terminations of pregnancy. *Parity* is defined as the number of babies delivered older than 24 weeks gestation (i.e. when a baby is considered to be viable).

MEDICAL HISTORY

This should be explored generally and with particular reference to the problems under investigation, for example gangrenous appendix related to infertility, a previous blood transfusion producing antibodies related to subsequent loss of pregnancy, etc. It is essential to know of any present or previous medical disorders, such as diabetes mellitus, especially when pregnancy, further medical therapy or operative treatment is being considered. Women with complex medical conditions may have gynaecological problems and even women with renal transplants may embark on pregnancy.

MEDICATION OR TREATMENT HISTORY

Any medication taken regularly, or even occasionally, must be noted. The effects of alcohol and tobacco are aggravated by a poor diet, and when drug abuse exists (associated with an increased risk of hepatitis and HIV infection), it must be recognized and treatment offered—vertical transmission of HIV can be reduced if treatment begins early. Allergic reactions should be recorded and clearly displayed, to avoid risk, and this information may be required if the patient is unable to respond.

GENERAL AND ASSOCIATED SYSTEM ASSESSMENT

Remember that changes in appetite, bowel habit, weight and responses to normal exercise, and variations in sleep patterns are all relevant to a wide variety of obstetric and gynaecological problems. Urological function, estimated by the *frequency* and *volume* of urine passed, with a specific note about *nocturia* or *dysuria*, should be recorded. The presence of *urgency* (an overwhelming desire to micturate), which may or may not result in incontinence, or *stress incontinence* (the involuntary leakage of urine from the full bladder when the intra-abdominal pressure is raised), should be assessed. Some stress incontinence is very common, particularly after childbirth or in the menopause.

FAMILY AND SOCIAL HISTORY

Employment, home conditions and the length of relationships are all of great importance when assessing the prospects for recovery from illness or the support of a child. The ethnic origins of the family may give a clue to the presence of tuberculosis or haemoglobinopathy. The possibility of cancer is one of the underlying anxieties most frequently expressed at interviews. When a congenital abnormality is suspected in the offspring of relatives, a detailed family history is important, and increasingly, antenatal screening or diagnosis is possible, for example Tay–Sachs disease, thalassaemia and cystic fibrosis.

EXAMINATION

GENERAL

This process begins as the history is being taken. Appearance, gait, demeanour and responsiveness can all be observed, and the level of intelligence and education generally assessed. Any abnormality of affect should be noted. The presence of a female chaperone for the physical examination is important for a male doctor, but such a person may inhibit the process of history-taking and so is best used at the time when the patient needs to undress. Once this has been done, measurements of height and weight (Body Mass Index) are made, as they can be particularly difficult to assess if the patient is first seen when in bed. Note too the secondary sexual development, and hair distribution.

It is important that examination should be a non-threatening process; it should be undertaken by following a predictable sequence such as the following:

- Hands (to assess the pulse)
- Arms (blood pressure)
- Eyes (conjunctivae)
- Head, chest (heart)
- Breasts (p. 370)
- Abdomen
- Legs
- Pelvic examination (PV/PR).

ABDOMINAL EXAMINATION

The system of examination described in Chapter 20 should be followed, but in addition, the possibility of pregnancy must be considered in the age range 12–55 years, or even later with newly developed fertility techniques. When an abdominopelvic mass is present its characteristics and size, either in centimetres measured from the symphysis pubis upwards, or estimated as weeks gestation of an equivalent size pregnancy, are recorded. If ascites is suspected check the supraclavicular and inguinal lymph nodes and look for an associated hydrothorax.

ABDOMINAL EXAMINATION IN PREGNANCY

Firstly, make sure the light is good, the room comfortably warm, and that there is maximum exposure (Box 14.1). Note should be made of *striae gravidarum, linea nigra,* previous *caesarean section scars* and any visible *fetal or other movements*. Ideally the patient is examined flat but she may experience hypotension and in any case be more comfortable semi-recumbent. Ask about any tender areas before palpating the abdomen, so that, initially at least, these can be avoided. Comfort and gentleness can be enhanced by using the flat of the hand as well as the examining fingers; this assists the process of relaxation and allows the outline of a mass or pregnant uterus to be defined more readily. If there is need to undertake an uncomfortable examination, this should be explained to the patient and left to the very end. Remember too, that palpation may produce uterine contractions which can obscure the details of the uterine contents.

BOX 14.1   Abdominal examination in pregnancy.

Inspection
- Striae gravidarum
- Linea nigra
- Scars
- Fetal movements

Palpation
- Fundal height
- Fetal poles and fetal lie
- Presentation—breech, head, etc.
- Attitude
- Level of presenting part
- Fetal movements
- Liquor volume

Auscultation
- Fetal heart rate

The size of the uterus is traditionally estimated from the *fundal height*, even though this is only one dimension of a globular mass which is subject to a variety of displacements. Under normal circumstances the fundal height is just above the symphysis pubis at 12 weeks' gestation, at the umbilicus at 22 weeks and at the xiphisternum at 36 weeks. When the fundus is equidistant from the symphysis pubis and the umbilicus, the gestation is 16 weeks and when equidistant from the xiphisternum and umbilicus it is about 30 weeks. From 36 weeks the fundal height is also dependent on the level of the *presenting part*, and will reduce as the presenting part descends into the pelvis (Fig. 14.1). Comparative assessments can be made by measuring either the symphysis–fundal height or the minimal girth measured at the level of the umbilicus, as each of these measurements has a correlation with gestation.

Next, determination of the number of *fetal poles* will allow the assessment of the fetal axis and in consequence the *fetal lie* (Fig. 14.2). This is the relationship of the long axis of the fetus to the long axis of the uterus. To confirm the lie, the location of the fetal limbs and back should be identified.

The *presentation*: at term, over 95% of babies present by the head, but at 30 weeks only 70% do so because of the greater mobility of the fetus and the relatively larger volume of amniotic fluid. The breech can usually be distinguished by its size, texture and ability to change shape. However, an ultrasonic examination may be necessary for confirmation.

If the baby presents by the head, the smallest diameters which are presented to the pelvis occur when the head is well-flexed, i.e. a vertex presentation. Flexion of the head is termed the *attitude*, and decreasing amounts of flexion lead to brow or face presentations which cause difficulty in labour, often requiring delivery by Caesarean section. For a breech presentation an equivalent assessment is made to determine if the breech is *extended* (frank

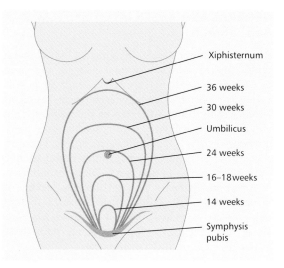

Fig. 14.01   Approximate fundal height with changing gestation.

breech), *flexed* (complete), or *footling* (incomplete) breech. Once the presenting part has a relationship to the pelvis, that relationship can be vertical (the *level* Fig. 14.3), or rotational (the *position*). When the flexed head presents, the fetal occiput is termed the *denominator*. When the face presents, the denominator is the mentum (chin) and when the breech presents it is the sacrum. Thus the position with a vertex presentation can now be defined as left occipito–lateral (LOL) or right occipito–lateral (ROL), etc. The common positions of the head before the onset of labour are LOL 50%, ROL 25%. This relationship changes during the course of labour because of internal rotation and at the end of labour the common presenting positions are left occipito-anterior (LOA) 60% and right occipito-anterior (ROA) 30%.

Engagement of the presenting part occurs when the largest diameters have passed through the pelvic brim. The number of fifths of the head palpated

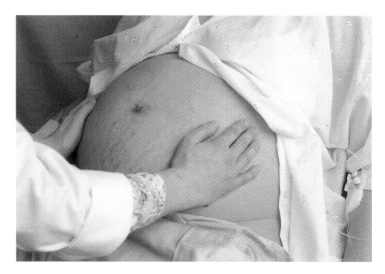

Fig. 14.02   Method of abdominal palpation to determine fetal lie and location of back.

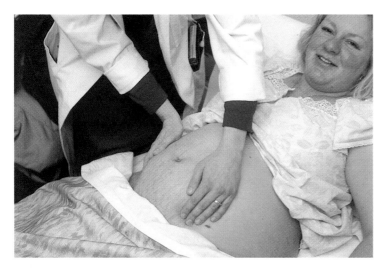

Fig. 14.03 Method of abdominal palpation to determine presenting part.

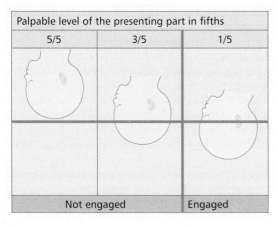

Palpable level of the presenting part in fifths		
5/5	3/5	1/5
Not engaged		Engaged

Fig. 14.04 The vertical relationship of the presenting part to the pelvic inlet (the level).

through the abdominal wall indicates its level (Fig. 14.4). Thus, if there are three or more fifths palpable, the baby's head will be unengaged. If less than three-fifths are palpable, then the baby's head is probably engaged in the pelvis, but this does depend on the overall size of the fetal head and of the pelvis. It must be remembered that the pelvic brim has an angle of approximately 45 degrees to the horizontal when the mother is lying flat. However, if the abdominal wall is reasonably thin the unengaged head can be palpated by the examiner's fingers passing round the maximum diameter and beginning to meet above the pelvic brim. When this does not occur, the widest diameter must be below the examining fingers. Fixity of the presenting part in the pelvis is also a guide.

Engagement of the baby's head in the pelvis will usually have occurred by the time the leading edge reaches the level of the ischial spines (zero station).

Fetal movements, both as recorded by the mother and observed by the examiner during the examination are noted. A record is made of the *fetal heart rate (FHR)*, normally between 115 and 160 beats/min (Fig. 14.5), and finally the *volume of liquor* is estimated. This requires considerable practice as it changes through pregnancy.

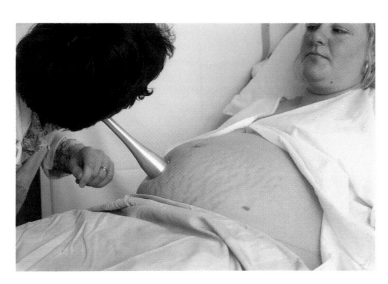

Fig. 14.05 Listening over the fetal back to the fetal heart with a Pinard stethoscope.

PELVIC EXAMINATION

The pelvic examination may be undertaken vaginally or rectally.

VAGINAL EXAMINATION

Before starting, it is most important to explain every step to the patient. Begin by inspecting the perineum in the dorsal or left lateral position (Box 14.2). A good light is required and an assistant is necessary. Women who use tampons or who have borne children should be able to tolerate a gentle vaginal examination. For those who cannot use tampons or whose hymen is intact, pelvic examination may be undertaken per rectum. Any inflammation, swelling, soreness, ulceration or neoplasia of the vulva, perineum or anus is noted (Fig. 14.6). Small warts (condylomata acuminata) appearing as papillary growths may occur

---

BOX 14.2   Vaginal examination.

Inspection of vulva

Digital palpation
- Locate cervix
- Bimanual palpation
- Pelvic tenderness
- Pelvic masses
- Assessment of uterus (position, mobility)
- Ovaries and fallopian tubes

Speculum examination
- Cervix
- Vaginal walls

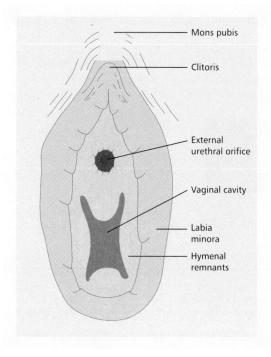

Fig. 14.06   The vulva.

Labels: Mons pubis · Clitoris · External urethral orifice · Vaginal cavity · Labia minora · Hymenal remnants

scattered over the vulva; these are due to the *human papilloma virus* (HPV). The clitoris and urethra, which may be difficult to see, are inspected, and the patient is asked to strain and then to cough to demonstrate uterovaginal prolapse or stress incontinence (Fig. 14.7). If the latter is a presenting problem it is important that the bladder is reasonably full and that more than one substantial cough is taken, as the first frequently fails to demonstrate leakage of urine.

For a digital vaginal examination, disposable gloves are used and the examining fingers are lightly lubricated with a water-based jelly. With the patient in the supine position and with her knees drawn up and separated, the labia are gently parted with the index finger and thumb of the left hand while the index finger of the right hand is inserted into the vagina, avoiding the urethral meatus and exerting a sustained pressure on the *perineal body* until relaxation of the perineal musculature occurs. Watch for any sign of discomfort. The full length of the finger is then introduced, assessing the vaginal walls in transit until the cervix is located. At this stage a second finger can be inserted to improve the quality of the digital examination, or alternatively a speculum can be used if a cervical smear is required. The examination is continued with the left hand placed on the abdomen above the symphysis pubis and below the umbilicus—the bimanual examination (Fig. 14.8). The hand provides gentle directional pressure to bring the pelvic viscera towards the examiner's fingers in the vagina and serves to assess the size, mobility and regularity of masses. The *cervix* is then identified; it is approximately 3 cm in diameter with a variably sized and shaped dimple in the middle, the *cervical os*. The os is normally directed posteriorly when the uterus is anteflexed and anteverted. The consistency of the cervix is firm and its shape is irregular when scarred. Increased hardness of the cervix may be caused by fibrosis or carcinoma. A soft cervix indicates the possibility of pregnancy; even greater caution and gentleness is then necessary. The mobility of the cervix is usually 1–2 cm in all directions and testing this movement should produce only mild discomfort. When attempts are made to move the cervix in the presence of pelvic inflammation, particularly in association with ectopic pregnancy, extreme pain (*cervical excitation*) results.

The size, shape, position, consistency and regularity of the *uterus* and the relationship of the fundus of the uterus to the cervix is estimated. Bimanual examination also enables palpation of the *ovaries* and *fallopian tubes*, although these can be difficult to feel when healthy. The pouch of Douglas is then explored through the posterior fornix via the arch formed by the uterosacral ligaments and the cervix.

SPECULUM EXAMINATION

This is an essential part of gynaecological examinations and if it is omitted then the examination must

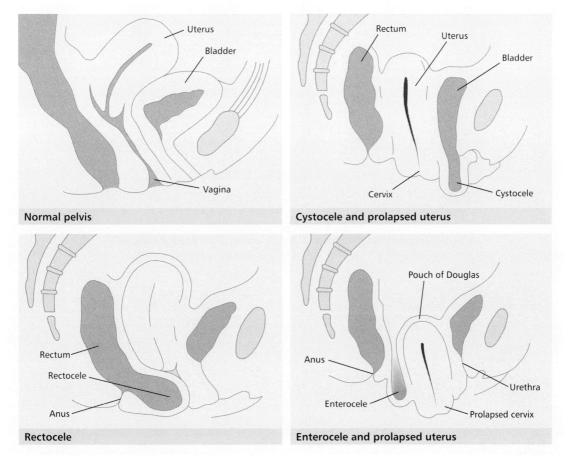

Fig. 14.07   In cystocele there is downward prolapse of the anterior part of the pelvic floor, straightening the angulation of the bladder neck and leading to urinary incontinence. In rectocele the posterior part of the pelvic floor is mostly affected, sometimes with associated faecal incontinence. In some patients the whole pelvic floor is weak with double incontinence, or with prolapse of the uterus. In enterocele there is a prolapse of viscera from the pouch of Douglas as part of severe pelvic floor weakness.

be regarded as incomplete. Several vaginal specula are available. These include the *bivalve* type (e.g. Cusco's) used for displaying the cervix (Fig. 14.9), the single or double-ended *Sims' (duckbill) speculum*, used to retract the vaginal walls, and *Ferguson's speculum*, a tube used to allow the inspection of the cervix when vaginal prolapse is so severe that a bivalve speculum fails to provide a sufficient view. Speculum examination of the vagina can be undertaken in the dorsal or left lateral position (which is used for prolapse). The speculum should be warmed to body temperature and lubricated with water or a water-based jelly. All the necessary equipment, such as spatulae, slides, forceps, culture swabs, etc., should be prepared before the examination begins (Fig. 14.10).

Technique for taking a cervical (Papanicolaou) smear

The procedure is explained to the patient and then she is asked to lie on her back. The labia are separated with the left hand as for the bimanual exam-

ination. Hold the lightly lubricated bivalve speculum in the right hand and use the index finger and thumb of the left hand to separate the introitus, then insert the speculum with the handle directly upwards, allowing it to be accommodated by the vagina (which is H-shaped in cross-section). When it has been inserted to its full length, the blades of the speculum are opened and manoeuvred so that the cervix is fully visualized. The screw adjuster or ratchet on the handle is then locked so that the speculum is maintained in place. The presence of discharge and the condition of the cervical epithelium, its colour, any ulceration, scars and retention cysts (*Nabothian follicles*) are all recorded.

In order to detect cervical pre-cancer, an Aylesbury or similar spatula is used so that the tip is appropriate for the shape of the cervix. The tip of the spatula is placed firmly in the cervical os, so as to allow the removal of surface cells from the whole of the *squamocolumnar junction* when the spatula is rotated through 360 degrees. An alternative is the brush which more effectively samples the endocervix.

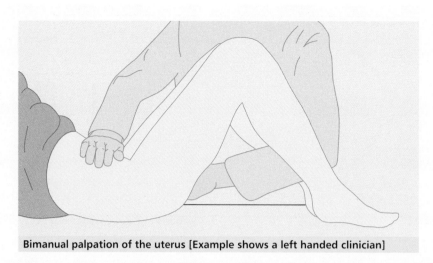

Bimanual palpation of the uterus [Example shows a left handed clinician]

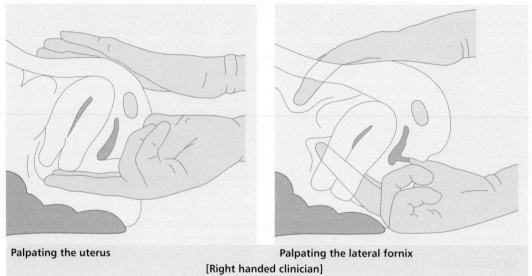

Palpating the uterus

Palpating the lateral fornix
[Right handed clinician]

Fig. 14.08   Bimanual examination of the pelvis.

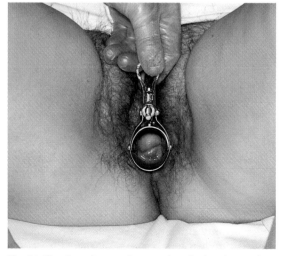

Fig. 14.09   Cusco's speculum used to display the cervix.

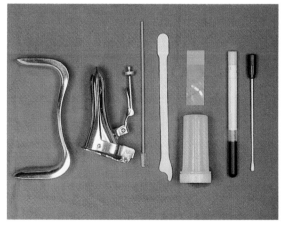

Fig. 14.10   Clinical instruments prepared for a gynaecological examination.

The material is spread thinly onto a microscope slide and immediately treated with a fixative. An example of a stained slide is shown in Fig. 14.11. At the same time a wet slide for the assessment of *monilia* (*Candida albicans*) or *Trichomonas vaginalis* can be prepared and a culture swab taken from the endocervix or vaginal vault and placed in a bacteriological transport medium. In addition a Gram-stained smear can be prepared for the detection of *Neisseria gonorrhoeae* as Gram-negative intracellular diplococci and tests for *Gardnerella*, chlamydia and herpes should be considered. (see ch. 20). An aqueous solution of iodine and potassium iodide (Lugol's iodine) can be applied to the cervix: the normal mucous membrane, which contains glycogen, stains dark brown. Those areas of abnormality which fail to take up the stain can then be identified (*Schiller's test*). The screw of the speculum is then released and the blades freed from the cervix so that it can be gently removed.

Assessment of the vaginal walls for prolapse or fistulae is done with a sims' speculum with the patient turned on her left side. The best exposure is given by Sims' position, where the pelvis is rotated by flexing the right thigh more than the left, and by hanging the right arm over the distant edge of the couch. A Sims' speculum is inserted in much the same way as above, using the left hand to elevate the right buttock (Fig. 14.12). The blade then deflects the rectum, exposing the urethral meatus, anterior vaginal wall and bladder base. The patient is then asked to strain and any vaginal wall prolapse is noted. The level of the cervix is recorded as the speculum is withdrawn. The posterior vaginal wall can then be viewed by rotating the speculum through 180 degrees. Uterine prolapse is called *first-degree* when the cervix descends but lies short of the introitus, *second-degree* when it passes to the level of the introitus, and *third-degree* (*complete procidentia*),

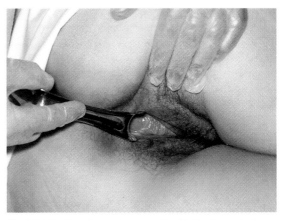

Fig. 14.12 Sims' speculum used to display the anterior vaginal wall.

when the whole of the uterus is prolapsed outside the vulva. Vaginal wall prolapse which may occur with, or be independent of, uterine prolapse consists of *urethrocele*, *cystocele*, *rectocele* or *enterocele* (prolapse of the pouch of Douglas). Several of these anatomical variations usually occur together.

VAGINAL EXAMINATION DURING LABOUR

The examination is made to determine:

- Dilatation and effacement of the cervix
- The presence or absence of amniotic membranes and the state of the liquor
- The level of the presenting part
- Absence of pulsating umbilical cord, especially if the membranes are ruptured
- The degree of moulding of the fetal head, or the presence of caput succedaneum
- The size and shape of the maternal bony pelvis.

The vulva is swabbed clean with an antiseptic such as chlorhexidine in water. Sterile surgical gloves must be worn. Initially an assessment is made of the vagina, which should normally be warm and moist. If it is dry and hot, infection should be suspected. Next the extent of *cervical dilatation* is estimated in centimetres (10 cm is equivalent to full dilatation at term) and the thinness and elasticity of the cervix, which increases with dilatation, is also assessed. The *level* of the presenting part is measured in centimetres from the ischial spines and noted as above (–), below (+) or at (0 station) that level. If caput succedaneum occurs, there may be difficulty in estimating both the exact level, and also the position of the presenting part because of the masking of the fontanelles. The *position* can then be assessed by the location and direction of a fetal ear.

The method of estimating maternal pelvic dimensions is described in textbooks of obstetrics. These measurements must be adequate in relation to the size of the baby, if a vaginal delivery is to be achieved safely.

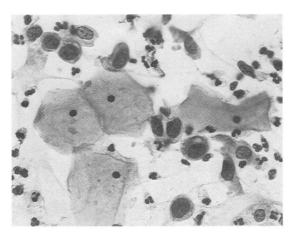

Fig. 14.11 Smear from uterine cervix. There are several abnormal squamous cells indicating in situ carcinoma of the cervix. Large pink-stained normal superficial squamous cells and many inflammatory cells are also included. (Papanicolaou stain, × 160)

RECTAL EXAMINATION   (see also p. 150)

This may be perceived by the patient as the most uncomfortable part of the whole examination. When vaginal examination is not possible or not acceptable, rectal examination permits bimanual assessment of the pelvic viscera and is particularly valuable in assessing problems which are located in the pouch of Douglas, the uterosacral ligaments, or the rectovaginal septum. Sometimes disease arising in the rectum (e.g. diverticular disease) can masquerade as a gynaecological problem.

INVESTIGATIONS

PREGNANCY TESTING

URINE

Most pregnancy tests depend on the demonstration of *human chorionic gonadotrophin (HCG)* in the urine. The sensitivity of these tests varies, but some detect as little as 50 mU/L HCG. As the developing placental tissue produces increasing amounts from about 10 days post-fertilization, very early diagnosis of pregnancy is now possible.

BLOOD

Even earlier detection of pregnancy is possible by radioimmunoassay of the beta-subunit of HCG in blood.

BACTERIOLOGICAL AND VIRUS TESTS

Bacteriological and virus tests used in gynaecology and obstetrics include the following:

- Swabs from the throat, endocervix, vagina, urethra and rectum may be needed for sexually transmitted diseases
- Bacteriological mid-stream urinalysis (MSU) is important in both obstetrics (for bacteriuria) and gynaecology (for frequency and incontinence)
- Tests for toxoplasma, rubella, cytomegalovirus and herpes simplex (TORCH) cover previous infections likely to be damaging to a pregnancy.

COLPOSCOPY

Colposcopy permits visualization of the cervix, vaginal vault (vaginoscopy) or vulva (vulvoscopy) with a low-power binocular microscope to detect pre-cancerous abnormalities of the epithelium (Fig. 14.13). Usually an abnormal cervical smear will have alerted the doctor to the need for further investigation. This can be undertaken on an out-patient basis, by exposing the cervix, treating it with acetic acid then with Lugol's iodine and viewing it through the colposcope to identify the degree, site and extent of the cervical pathology which has produced the abnormal smear. It also allows examination of the rest of the cervix, including the area most at risk (the transformation zone). Once this has been done, biopsy and appropriate treatment (e.g. laser destruction or surgical excision, by knife or large loop electrodiathermy) can be undertaken.

HYSTEROSCOPY

This is a technique for viewing the cavity of the uterus using small diameter fibre-optic telescopes and cameras (Fig. 14.14). It permits not only out-patient assessments and directed biopsies to be taken under local analgesia but also a range of other therapeutic procedures, such as endometrial ablation or resection of submuocus fibroids, which can be performed under general anaesthetic.

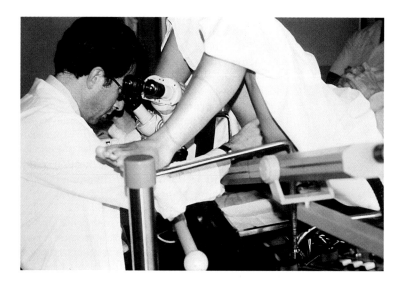

Fig. 14.13 Colposcopy.

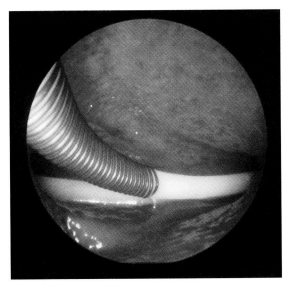

Fig. 14.14 Hysteroscopic view of an intrauterine device in situ.

ENDOMETRIAL BIOPSY (Fig. 14.15)

One of the common investigations undertaken in gynaecology is sampling of the endometrium. Formerly, this was performed by a dilatation of the cervix and curettage (D&C) to obtain histological material from the cavity of the uterus. Dilatation of the cervix is very painful and thus an anaesthetic is needed. The biopsy is not always representative and may fail to make a diagnosis in up to one-third of cases. Methods of cell sampling have been developed, including surface cytology or from larger quantities of aspirated materials, but the definitive assessment is now usually by hysteroscopy.

CYSTOSCOPY AND CYSTOMETRY

Voiding difficulties are initially investigated by checking for urinary tract infection. Assessment of post-micturition bladder volume or coincident pelvic masses by pelvic ultrasound is a useful next step.

Viewing the interior of the bladder by cystoscopy gives information of its condition and allows biopsy of the mucosa or removal of foreign bodies. The pressure/volume relationships of bladder filling, detrusor and sphincter activity and urethral flow rate can be assessed with a cystometrogram. The bladder is catheterized and filled slowly with sterile saline. The volume and pressure at which bladder filling is perceived, and at which a desire to micturate is felt, are noted. The urinary flow rate can be measured. In developments of this test electromyographic (EMG) activity in the external urethral sphincter can be measured, and the urethral pressure profile established. This is being replaced by real-time ultrasound assessment of bladder neck activity and descent. In *stress incontinence* urinary flow commences at low bladder pressure because of sphincter incompetence; in *urge incontinence* urinary flow develops at low bladder volumes because of uninhibited detrusor activity. Reflux and overflow also show as urethral leakage. Incontinence can also result from a defect in the anatomical integrity of the urinary tract, such as a congenital abnormality or fistula.

IMAGING TECHNIQUES

RADIOLOGICAL INVESTIGATIONS

HYSTEROSALPINGOGRAPHY (Fig. 14.16)

This is now used infrequently to image the uterine cavity and fallopian tubes after a radiopaque medium has been installed into the uterus. The fallopian tubal lumen and patency can also be seen. The technique is being replaced by hysterosonography.

LATERAL X-RAY PELVIMETRY

In the past, this was used to assess the diameters and shape of the pelvis when cephalopelvic disproportion was suspected. An indication for this assessment is a planned breech birth, so that the aftercoming head can be certain to pass through the pelvis without bony obstruction. Now MRI pelvimetry is usually used, in order to limit radiation exposure.

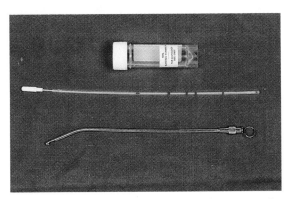

Fig. 14.15 An endometrial biopsy curette, a pipette cell sampler and fixing medium.

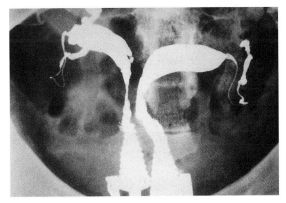

Fig. 14.16 An abnormal hysterosalpingogram: uteri didelphys (double uteri).

ULTRASOUND

Ultrasound generated from a piezo-electric crystal transducer is propagated through tissue at variable velocity depending on tissue density. The echo time and signal amplitude give an estimate of the size and consistency of the object scanned. Ultrasound scanning as used in medicine over the last 35 years appears safe. The ultrasonic assessment of gestational age, fetal normality, multiple pregnancy, placental site, blood flow and the expected changes at different gestations are all important parameters of pregnancy monitoring. Two-dimensional imaging by 'B' scanning is the primary modality, and additional information can be obtained by colour and pulsed Doppler which provide information on bloodflow. Transabdominal and transvaginal routes can be used. The former enables a wide field of view, greater depth of penetration and transducer movement; the latter, with higher frequency transducers, gives increased resolution and diagnostic power but over a more limited area.

In early pregnancy (5–7 weeks) the integrity, location and number of sacs can be viewed. At 11–13 weeks nuchal translucency, mono- or dichorionicity and gross fetal abnormality can be detected. Anomaly scanning at 18–20 weeks is performed to confirm structural normality and some functional activity. By 24 weeks uterine and placental blood flow can be assessed.

In gynaecology, apart from the assessment of masses, ultrasound is useful to acertain aspects of bladder function such as residual volumes and bladder neck activity. It is also heplful in the preoperative preparation of anal sphincter deficiency.

Hysterosonography utilizes vaginal ultrasound visualization while the uterine cavity is filled with saline or other medium to obtain views similar to that of a hysterosalpingogram without exposure to radiation.

CT SCANNING AND MRI

CT scanning has proved less useful in gynaecology than was originally anticipated and is now used mainly for staging and follow up of malignancies. MRI, however, offers an alternative to ultrasound and to X-ray imaging during pregnancy; it uses no ionizing radiation and no harmful biological effects have been detected at magnetic field strengths (0.2–2.0 tesla) in current usage. Good images are obtained with excellent differentiation of maternal and fetal tissues. Although ultrasound is much cheaper, no artefacts from bone or bowel gas occur. Echo planar imaging is useful to reduce fetal movement artefact and increases potential for the study of fetal physiology and pathology.

LAPAROSCOPY/PELVICOSCOPY

Visualization of the pelvic and abdominal viscera is valuable if it can be done without a major injury to the abdominal wall (Fig. 14.17). This is achieved by using a fibre-optic telescope illuminated by a light source remote from the patient. It is then possible to inflate the abdomen with carbon dioxide under general or local anaesthesia, so that the anterior abdominal wall is lifted away from the viscera, allowing inspection of the abdominal and pelvic contents. The main uses of laparoscopy are diagnostic (e.g. in the investigation of pelvic pain or infertility) and therapeutic (e.g. in sterilization procedures or in the treatment of a rapidly increasing number of pelvic lesions). Minimal access surgery (MAS) utilizes multiple puncture techniques with high-quality television monitors and video recorders. Treatment for ectopic pregnancy, hysterectomy, lymphadenectomy, cholecystectomy, bladder and bowel surgery are now possible in appropriate circumstances.

TESTS OF FETAL WELL-BEING

Besides those tests made to ensure the good general health of the mother, such as haemoglobin, Veneral Disease Reference Laboratories (VDRL), TPHA tests and bacteriuria screen, a number of other investigations of variable complexity can be utilized to check the fetus *in utero*. It is reasonable to use some of these tests in every pregnancy as in about 10% of mothers the outcome of apparently uncomplicated pregnancy is unpredictable. In addition, anonymous testing for asymptomatic HIV in inner London shows a number of positive results. HIV testing is offered but *not* carried out routinely.

BIOLOGICAL TESTS

Before using these tests it is important to explore the woman's attitude to the possible results. For example, would she agree to intervention if an

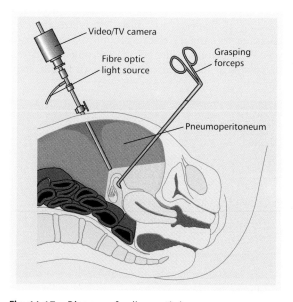

Fig. 14.17   Diagram of a diagnostic laparoscopy.

abnormality was discovered? Detailed counselling by a trained professional is essential.

Maternal blood sampling for fetal cells

It is possible to isolate from the maternal circulation fetal cells which are suitable for chromosome analysis. Trials of this promising non-invasive test are currently underway.

Chorion biopsy (chorionic villus sampling)

This is a method of obtaining chorionic material at 9–11 weeks of pregnancy, usually through the abdomen so that the genetic constitution or biochemical function of fetal cellular material can be determined. It is useful for the diagnosis of Down's syndrome, thalassaemia, and in a number of other hereditary conditions. Early and rapid diagnosis allows the therapeutic termination of an abnormal pregnancy, increasing the safety and acceptability of that procedure. There is still an increased risk of spontaneous abortion after the chorion biopsy and this technique is used only in specialized centres.

Amniocentesis

Samples of amniotic fluid can be used for:

Chromosome analysis

This is undertaken at 13–18 weeks of pregnancy and is currently much safer than chorion biopsy. The amount of desquamated fetal cells obtained is much smaller in quantity than from chorion biopsy and cell culture is necessary (which takes about 3 weeks) before a chromosomal diagnosis is made. However, rapid preliminary results can be obtained using the fluorescent immunohybridization (FISH) technique. This test is mostly used for prenatal diagnosis of Down's syndrome or when other chromosome abnormalities are suspected.

Bilirubin concentration

This is sometimes measured in amniotic fluid during the latter part of pregnancy in order to assess the health of a baby affected by maternal rhesus isoimmunization.

DNA analysis

Fetal cells obtained by amniocentesis, chorionic villus sampling or cordocentesis (see below) can be used for DNA analysis of nuclear chromatin in order to directly test for a number of genetically-determined diseases, for example Tay–Sach's disease and Duchenne muscular dystrophy, in families known to be at risk. DNA testing and chromosomal studies should both only be carried out with fully informed parental consent, and with the help of a genetic counselling service.

Cordocentesis

In this procedure a needle is inserted through the abdominal wall and into the amniotic sac to obtain fetal blood from the placental insertion of the cord. It is used when chromosomal abnormality, haemophilia, haemoglobinopathies, inborn errors of metabolism, fetal viral infections or fetal anaemia are suspected. Although the procedure carries more risk than amniocentesis, it is less traumatic than fetoscopy while permitting rapid diagnosis.

BIOCHEMICAL TESTS

Early pregnancy

Alpha fetoprotein

This is a normal fetal protein which passes from the fetus into the amniotic fluid and maternal serum. The maternal concentration of this protein varies in a predictable way with gestation. At 16 weeks' gestation increased levels suggest fetal spina bifida or anencephaly. However, similar levels can be caused by several other conditions, including threatened abortion, multiple pregnancy and exomphalos. Decreased levels are associated with the presence of an infant with Down's syndrome. A computed risk of Down's syndrome can be produced from maternal weight, gestation, parity and race, measured against alpha fetoprotein, HCG and unconjugated oestriol, and the results matched against ultrasound findings.

Labour

Fetal health in labour can be assessed by checking the liquor for the presence of meconium, by checking the responsiveness of the fetal heart rate, and by monitoring fetal movements. In addition to these simple clinical tests, *fetal pH* measured on a scalp blood sample can be used to detect acidosis. This is particularly useful if labour is prolonged, complicated or known to be high-risk, e.g. in diabetic mothers. The fetal scalp is displayed using an amnioscope and a small sample of capillary blood is obtained. If the pH of the sample is below 7.2 then delivery is an urgent priority. Continuous oximetry by near infrared reflectance although useful is not in general use.

BIOPHYSICAL TESTS

Fetal movements

In some cases of placental insufficiency fetal movements decrease or stop 12–48 hours before the fetal heart ceases to beat. In a healthy pregnancy fetal movements increase from the 32nd week of pregnancy to term, but the 12-hour daily fetal movement count falls below 10 in only 2.5% of normal pregnancies. Thus a variety of counting systems which are used by mothers for correlating fetal movement and fetal welfare have been devised. These can alert the mother that more sophisticated and detailed surveillance is required.

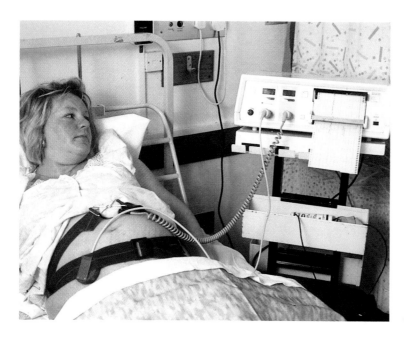

Fig. 14.18   Cardiotocography equipment.

Ultrasound

Visualization by real time

Sequential ultrasonic scanning to detect the presence of symmetrical or asymmetrical growth retardation or changes in fetal activity, breathing, movements, etc. can be used to assess placental function. If it becomes clear that fetal growth has halted or the child's survival *in utero* is in doubt, then urgent delivery should be planned with paediatric support.

Cardiotocography (CTG)

Assessment of the fetal heart rate and its variation with fetal and uterine activity can be recorded ante-natally with ultrasound using the Doppler principle (Fig. 14.18). A pressure transducer is attached to the abdominal wall so that variations in uterine activity can be matched with the ultrasound recordings. The production of an accurate recording requires patience and considerable interpretive skills.

When the membranes rupture during labour, a more accurate recording of the fetal heart rate can be produced by an electrode attached to the fetal scalp (Figs 14.19 and 14.20). The recording is triggered by the fetal ECG.

Doppler blood flow. Studies of the circulatory changes in the uterine circulation may predict fetal compromise and those in the umbilical, aortic and cerebral fetal circulation give further clues to the state of the fetus, especially in already compromised circumstances.

Placental volume. Ultrasound measurements of placental volume may also help in the prediction of fetal growth retardation.

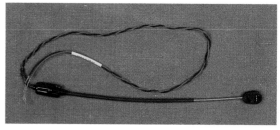

Fig. 14.19   Fetal scalp electrode.

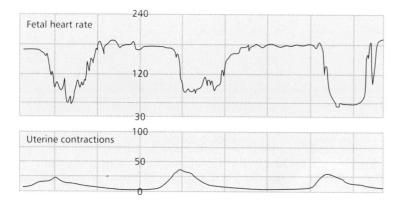

Fig. 14.20   An abnormal cardiotocograph showing late variable decelerations during uterine contractions with fetal tachycardia.

15
THE UNCONSCIOUS PATIENT

INTRODUCTION

Coma is a common medical problem. Diagnosis can usually be achieved at the bedside, provided attention is given both to the history and to the examination. In this chapter clinical methods relevant to diagnosis of the comatose patient will be described.

Consciousness is a state of normal cerebral activity in which the patient is aware of both self and environment and is able to respond to internal changes, for example hunger, and to changes in the external environment. *Sleep*, although a state of altered consciousness, is a normal variation in consciousness. The sleeping patient can be roused, both spontaneously and in response to external stimuli, to a full state of wakefulness. Altered consciousness resulting from brain disease may take the form of a *confusional state*, in which the patient's alertness is clouded; this is associated with agitation, fright and confusion, i.e. disorientation. Such patients usually show evidence of misperception of their environment, and hallucinations and delusions may occur. Confusional states must be carefully distinguished from *aphasia*, in which a specific disorder of language is the characteristic feature, and from continuous temporal lobe *epilepsy*, a form of focal status epilepticus in which the behavioural disorder is often accompanied by aphasia if the epileptic focus is left-sided. Usually this can be recognized by the occurrence of frequent but slight myoclonic jerks of facial and especially perioral muscles and by variability in the patient's confusion from moment to moment during the examination. Always pause and observe an unconscious or drowsy patient for a few moments before disturbing them.

Abnormal *drowsiness* is often found in patients with space-occupying intracranial lesions or metabolic disorders before stupor or coma supervenes. The patient appears to be in normal sleep but cannot easily be wakened and, once awake, tends to fall asleep despite verbal stimulation or clinical examina-tion. Further, while awake such patients can usually be shown to be *disorientated*. Higher intellectual function, such as the ability to perform abstract tasks or to make judgements, is disturbed. *Stupor* means a state of disturbed consciousness from which only vigorous external stimuli can produce arousal. Arousal from stupor is invariably both brief and incomplete. Stupor, and obtundation, are non-quantitative descriptions of an altered mental state that is difficult to define exactly. In *coma* the patient is less responsive: the term coma was originally used to describe a patient who is unrousable and unresponsive to all external stimuli. The *Glasgow Coma Scale* (Table 15.1) represents an attempt, now generally used, to replace these ill-defined terms with descriptions of the state of consciousness confined to three categories of performance—*eye-opening to command, verbal responses* and *motor responses*. This scale should be used to define the degree of altered consciousness (Table 15.1); non-quantitative descriptions should be avoided.

CAUSES OF COMA

The objective of clinical assessment is to achieve a diagnosis and so to plan management. Coma may be due to *metabolic* or *structural* disease of the brain: very rarely pseudocoma may occur as a psychogenic disorder. Coma results from lesions affecting the brain *widely, diffusely* or *multifocally*, or from lesions of deep, centrally placed structures in the diencephalon or brainstem (Box 15.1). For example, supratentorial mass lesions, such as tumours, may damage deep diencephalic structures, while subtentorial neoplasms may directly damage the brainstem reticular formation. Metabolic disorders, for example hypoglycaemia, hypnotic drugs or hypoxia, widely depress brain function. It is important to distinguish supratentorial (cerebral) from subtentorial (posterior fossa) space-occupying lesions. An immediate basic

TABLE 15.1   The Glasgow Coma Scale (GCS).

Eye-opening		Best verbal response		Best motor response	
Spontaneous	4	Oriented	5	Obeys commands	6
To speech	3	Confused	4	Localizes pain	5
To pain	2	Inappropriate	3	Normal withdrawal	4
None	1	Incomprehensible	2	Abnormal flexion	3
		None	1	Abnormal extension	2
				None	1

The three categories of information required in the GCS assessment require no special skills and are thus particularly suited for serial observations by relatively untrained staff. The GCS is much used in the management of head injury. This simple non-linear clinical rating scale enables relatively accurate assessment of improvement or deterioration in a patient's conscious state by physicians, nurses and ambulance staff alike. The best score is 15; the worst is 3, representing 'none' in all three categories assessed. Abnormal extension implies decerebrate posturing.

assessment will direct the subsequent series of investigations, and management (Box 15.2).

HISTORY

The history is of great importance and attempts should always be made to find witnesses of the onset of the coma. It is essential to discover whether the coma was of *gradual* or *sudden onset*. Coma occurs suddenly in vascular disorders such as *subarachnoid haemorrhage* or *stroke*, especially with cerebral or cerebellar haemorrhage. A history of trauma with concussion, followed a few days later by fluctuating drowsiness and stupor, suggests *subdural haematoma*, and should never be regarded lightly. Concussion followed by a *brief lucid interval* before rapidly deepening coma suggests *extradural haematoma*. A history of headache before coma supervenes is frequent in patients with intracranial space-occupying lesions of any cause. *Seizures* of recent onset, whether focal or generalized, strongly suggest cerebral disease, which may be due to tumour, encephalitis, abscess or trauma. Patients with *drug-induced coma* may be known by neighbours, family, medical attendants or the ambulance driver to have taken drugs by the presence of drug containers or alcohol in their homes. A history of depression may be known. A *search of the patient's clothing* may reveal hospital out-patient attendance cards, unfilled prescriptions, drugs or even syringes. Diabetic or epileptic patients often carry some form of *identification*, either in their clothing or as a wristband or necklace. If there is any suspicion that the patient might be hypoglycaemic, a blood sample should be taken for blood glucose estimation and then 20 g of 50% glucose given intravenously, before the test result is necessarily available. *Hypoglycaemia* is characterized by stupor or coma from which the patient can sometimes be roused to a resentful and aggressive state of partial awareness; there is pallor and sweati-

BOX 15.1   Outline of causes of coma.

A. Metabolic
- Hypoglycaemia
- Diabetes mellitus
- Renal failure
- Hepatic failure
- Hypothermia
- Hypothyroidism
- Cardiorespiratory failure
- Hypoxic encephalopathy

B. Drug overdosage (including alcohol)

C. Structural
Diffuse
- Meningitis
- Encephalitis
- Other infections (e.g. cerebral malaria)
- Subarachnoid haemorrhage
- Epilepsy
- Head injury
- Hypertensive encephalopathy

Focal
Supratentorial lesions
- Cerebral haemorrhage
- Cerebral infarction with oedema
- Subdural haematoma
- Extradural haematoma
- Tumour
- Cerebral abscess
- Pituitary apoplexy

Subtentorial lesions
- Cerebellar haemorrhage
- Pontine haemorrhage
- Brainstem infarction
- Tumour
- Cerebellar abscess
- Secondary effects of transtentorial herniation of brain due to cerebral mass lesions

ness, a bounding pulse, and often focal or generalized seizures.

Before beginning the examination make sure the patient is breathing adequately, that the pulse and blood pressure are satisfactory, and that there are no signs of rapid bleeding. If oxygenation is not satisfactory, whatever the breathing pattern, oxygen should be administered. If the patient is clearly in status epilepticus this must immediately be treated appropriately, and clinical examination continued afterwards (Box 15.2). Remember, also, always to consider whether there may be a fracture of the cervical spine; if this is suspected splinting of the neck and an X-ray in the AP and lateral planes is mandatory (Box 15.3). These aspects are described in Chapter 16 in relation to clinical methods in major trauma.

BOX 15.2   Immediate assessment of coma: seven questions.

Question	Check	Action
1. Airway clear?	Blood gases	Intubate, give oxygen
2. Fitting?	Blood glucose	IV glucose, IV diazepam, oxygen
3. Signs of craniofacial trauma?	CT scan	Neurosurgical opinion
4. Neck broken?	Splint neck	X-ray neck
5. Major haemorrhage?	Maintain circulation	
6. Signs of diabetes mellitus?	Check blood and urine glucose	Treat appropriately
7. Evidence of drug overdose or misuse?	Pupils/ventilation	Naloxone?

BOX 15.3   Basic neurological examination in coma.

- Assess level of consciousness (Glasgow Coma Scale, see Table 15.1)
- Signs of head injury
  — local bruising, fractures and penetrating wounds
  — bleeding from nose or ears
- Splint the neck: head injury may be associated with fracture of the cervical spine
- If no neck injury (clinically and by X-ray) check for neck stiffness
- Check resting pupillary size, and pupillary responses to light
- Ocular movements: spontaneous, following and to 'doll's head' (if no voluntary response)
- Limbs: posture, tone and movement
- Reflexes and plantar responses
- Fundi

EXAMINATION

Always proceed to examine the patient in a logical order (Box 15.3). Certain general features of the patient's clinical state are of great importance. Does the patient appear clean, well-nourished and generally cared for, or are there signs of *social decline*, such as a dishevelled appearance, lack of personal cleanliness, malnutrition or infestation? Is there evidence of trauma or exposure? A rapid search must be made for fractures and especially for signs of cranial trauma (Box 15.4). Bruising of the scalp is difficult to see but scalp oedema or haematoma can usually be palpated. Bruising of the skin behind the pinna, called a '*battle sign*', is a useful sign of basal or temporal skull fracture. Likewise, *bleeding from the external auditory meatus* is a reliable sign of a basal skull fracture. Pallor, circulatory failure and other evidence of shock must be recognized and a search made for external or internal haemorrhage, especially if trauma is suspected.

Metabolic coma is common, and has many causes (Box 15.1). It is characterized by altered consciousness without focal neurological signs or neck stiffness, and with preservation of vestibulogenic ocular movements (doll's head responses) (Box 15.5). In certain *drug-induced coma* states there may be signs of repeated intravenous injections under conditions of imperfect sterility, causing venous thrombosis in forearm or antebrachial veins. The odours of alcohol, uraemia, diabetic acidosis and hepatic coma may be recognizable in some instances. The stertorous, rapid

---

BOX 15.4   Head injury: basic management.

- Exclude intracranial haemorrhage by CT scan
- Control circulation
- Control intracranial pressure
- Control ventilation
- Obtain neurological/neurosurgical opinion

BOX 15.5   Metabolic and drug-induced coma.

- Coma without localizing signs is characteristic syndrome
- Full range of ocular movement to 'doll's head' testing
- Pupils may be small, e.g. opiate poisoning
- Altered respiratory pattern may signify metabolic acidosis (consider diabetic coma), or respiratory alkalosis (with hypercapnia)
- Decerebrate extension may occur *in extremis*
- Look for signs of metabolic disorder, e.g. jaundice, uraemia, respiratory failure, hypocalcaemia, endocrine disease (especially hypothyroidism or hypopituitarism)
- Drug-induced coma is associated with access to medication or drugs of abuse, or signs of repeated venous access

respiration of *acidotic coma* (air hunger), usually due to diabetes, can be quickly recognized (see below). The presence of jaundice, liver palms, or spider naevi, even in the absence of hepatic enlargement, raise the suspicion of hepatic coma.

Meningitis can usually be recognized by the rapid onset of drowsiness, lethargy or stupor with fever and signs of meningeal irritation (see Ch. 11). The pulse may be unexpectedly slow in relation to the fever in pyogenic meningitis, although the respirations are usually rapid. Seizures and focal neurological signs may develop and there is usually a history of headache and neck stiffness, perhaps with vomiting. In *meningococcal septicaemia* there may be a characteristic rash (Fig. 15.1). A *primary site of infection*, such as otitis media or sinusitis, may be apparent in other forms of purulent meningitis or *brain abscess*. The ocular fundi must always be examined by *ophthalmoscopy* for signs of papilloedema, retinal haemorrhages or exudates, or intra-arterial emboli, which appear as luminescent, highly refractile yellow or white plaque-like material occluding vessels (see Fig. 12.14). *Coma with neck stiffness* (Box 15.6) implies meningeal irritation and *infection* or *subarachnoid haemorrhage* must be excluded.

BOX 15.6   Causes of coma with neck stiffness (neck stiffness may be relatively inapparent in deeply comatose patients).

- Subarachnoid haemorrhage
- Meningitis
  - bacterial
  - viral (aseptic)
- Encephalitis
- Intracerebral haemorrhage
- Cerebral malaria

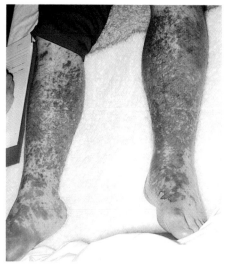

Fig. 15.1   Confluent petechial rash in an unconscious patient with overwhelming meningoccocal septicaemia and meningitis.

CONSCIOUSNESS

Define the state of consciousness by using the Glasgow Coma Scale (Box 15.1), as described above, particularly noting any variation or tendency to improve or deteriorate during the period of observation. *Change in level of consciousness* is the single most important piece of information which will indicate the need for a change of management. The scoring system applied to the Glasgow Coma Scale is useful in identifying this change. The GCS can readily be assessed by nursing staff, and is therefore a highly practical instrument. It is important to note exactly the *degree of responsiveness to external stimuli*, including conversation, calling the patient's first name, a sudden loud noise, a flash of light, contactual or painful stimulation, passive movement of the limbs and deep noxious stimuli such as squeezing the Achilles tendon, sternal pressure applied with a hard blunt object or supraorbital pressure from the examiner's thumb. Special attention must also be directed to *pupillary reactions and ocular movements*, both volitional and reflex, to the *pattern of breathing* and to *limb motor responses*, either spontaneous or reflexly evoked. Localizing responses to painful contractual stimuli are meaningful and imply preservation of sensation with associated motor responses. If localized responses are absent, there may be hemiparesis, or deep coma. Substituted flexion or extension responses of an upper limb to pain signify decortication or decerebration, respectively (see below). In the leg, extension to a painful stimulus applied to the sternum suggests decerebration or decortication.

PUPILS

Pupillary size and responsiveness to a very bright unfocused light beam (not the light of an ophthalmoscope) should be noted (Fig. 15.2). If the pupils are unequal, a decision as to which is abnormal must be made. Usually the larger pupil indicates the presence of an *oculomotor (third) nerve palsy*, whether from damage to the oculomotor nerve by pressure and displacement or from a lesion in the mesencephalon itself. Occasionally the smaller pupil may be the abnormal pupil, as in *Horner's syndrome*. If the larger pupil does not react to light it is likely that there is a *partial oculomotor nerve palsy* on that side. If the smaller pupil also fails to react to light this may be the *mid-position pupil* of complete sympathetic and parasympathetic lesions, indicating extensive brainstem damage. Pupillary dilatation in response to neck flexion or to pinching the skin of the neck is not a reliable reflex phenomenon.

In *drug-induced coma and in most patients with metabolic coma* the pupillary responses to light are normal. Exceptions to this rule are glutethimide poisoning and very deep metabolic coma, in which the pupils may become dilated and, rarely, may become

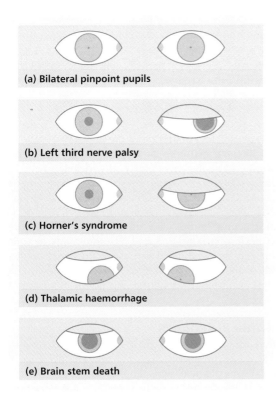

(a) Bilateral pinpoint pupils

(b) Left third nerve palsy

(c) Horner's syndrome

(d) Thalamic haemorrhage

(e) Brain stem death

Fig. 15.2 Pupillary anomalies in coma. **(a)** Bilateral pinpoint pupils occur with brain stem lesions, opiate and other drug intoxications and with pontine infarction. **(b)** Left third nerve palsy. There is ptosis, dilatation of the pupil with absence of the light reaction, and slight lateral deviation of the eye. **(c)** Horner's syndrome. There is ptosis and a small reactive pupil. **(d)** In thalamic haemorrhage the eyes tend to 'look towards the tip of the nose' and the pupils are small; later they become large and unreactive as upper brainstem involvement follows. **(e)** When brainstem death occurs the mid-brain disturbance is manifest by mid-position, fixed (unreactive) pupils with eye closure.

unreactive to light. In pontine and in thalamic haemorrhage the pupils may be very small (*pinpoint pupils*), and unreactive to light.

OCULAR MOVEMENTS

In comatose patients the eyes become slightly divergent at rest. If there is a pre-existent strabismus, deviation of the ocular axes may be pronounced, both at rest and during reflex ocular movements.

Doll's head movements

If the patient is too drowsy or stuporose to test voluntary or following eye movements, 'doll's head' movements should be tested. If possible the patient should be placed supine, although the test can be carried out in any position. The examiner grasps the patient's head with both hands, using the thumbs to hold the eyelids open gently, and firmly rocks the patient's head from side to side through about 70 degrees, and then from passive neck flexion to passive neck extension. The

patient's eyes tend to remain in the straight ahead position despite these passive movements of the head, a phenomenon like that found in some children's dolls, i.e. the patient's eyes tend to deviate in the opposite direction to the induced head movement.

This doll's head ocular movement depends on intact vestibular reflex mechanisms, and is thus a test of the peripheral sense organs involved, the labyrinths and otoliths, and their central connections in the brainstem, including the vestibular nuclei, the medial longitudinal fasciculi and the efferent pathway through oculomotor, trochlear and abducent nerves and their nuclei. Sometimes lesions in these structures can be recognized during the doll's head test by the presence of disturbances in ocular movements consistent, for example, with an abducent or oculomotor nerve palsy. Absence of the reflex on one side indicates an ipsilateral pontine lesion, but complete absence of doll's head movements may be found both in extensive structural lesions in the brainstem and in deep metabolic coma. *In most patients with drug-induced coma, however, doll's head ocular movements are intact.*

Caloric reflexes

Brainstem function can also be assessed by testing caloric reflexes. In the comatose patient, irrigation of the external auditory meatus on one side with at least 20 ml of ice-cold water induces slow conjugate deviation of the eyes towards the irrigated side after a few seconds' delay (the mnemonic COWS—cold, opposite; warm, same—is useful in remembering the direction of the ocular deviation in the comatose subject).

In the awake or drowsy patient this slow tonic deviation is masked by a fast, coarse nystagmus towards the opposite side. Normal caloric nystagmus is characteristically also found in cases of psychogenic coma. After a few minutes' delay the opposite ear should also be tested. It is important to inspect the tympanic membrane on each side *before* irrigating the external auditory meatus since it is unwise to perform this test in the presence of a large perforation, or if there is an active otitis media.

Spontaneous ocular movements

Occasionally in patients with infarction or other structural lesions in the posterior fossa *spontaneous ocular movements* may be observed. These may be accompanied by marked ocular divergence, sometimes with elevation of one eye and depression of the other. Rarely there may be a spontaneous 'see-saw' nystagmus in which one eye rotates up and the other down, the movements alternating at a very slow rate. *Rapid ocular oscillations* may occur, especially after poisoning with tricyclic antidepressant drugs, and a slow, once or twice a second, conjugate downward *bobbing* movement is sometimes a sign of cerebellar haemorrhage or tumour. In *thalamic haemorrhage* the pupils are pinpoint, and the eyes seem to be looking downwards as if at the patient's own nose. *Rapid conjugate lateral movement*, at a rhythm and rate reminiscent of cerebellar nystagmus, occurring in an unconscious patient should suggest focal motor seizures originating in the contralateral frontal lobe. Such seizures are often accompanied by deviation of the head and eyes in the direction of the 'nystagmoid movement', but not necessarily by a fully developed focal seizure involving face and limbs on the same side. *Nystagmus cannot occur in the comatose patient* because it requires ocular fixation to develop the fast, corrective phase.

PATTERN OF BREATHING
Alterations in the rhythm and pattern of breathing are an important aspect of the assessment of the unconscious patient.

Cheyne–Stokes (periodic) respiration
In Cheyne–Stokes respiration, breathing varies in regular cycles. A phase of gradually deepening respiration is followed, after a period of very deep rapid breaths, by a phase of slowly decreasing respiratory excursion and rate. Respiration gradually becomes quieter and may cease for several seconds before the cycle is repeated. Depressed, but regular breathing at a normal rate occurs in most drug-induced comas, but *Cheyne–Stokes respiration* can occur in coma of any cause, especially if there is coincidental chronic pulmonary disease. Cheyne–Stokes breathing in a comatose patient is a sign of a large unilateral space-occupying lesion with brainstem distortion, for example subdural haematoma, or of bilateral lesions from other causes, for example cerebral infarction or meningitis.

Kussmaul breathing
Deep sighing, rapid breathing at a regular rate should immediately suggest metabolic acidosis. Metabolic ketoacidosis or uraemia is the commonest cause of this acidotic (Kussmaul) breathing pattern, but a similar pattern may occur in some patients with respiratory failure, and in deep metabolic coma, especially hepatic coma.

Central pontine hyperventilation
Deep, regular breathing may also occur with rostral brainstem damage, whether due to reticular pontine infarction or to central brainstem dysfunction secondary to transtentorial herniation associated with an intra- or extracerebral space-occupying lesion. This breathing pattern is called *central neurogenic (pontine) hyperventilation*. Interspersed deep sighs or yawns may precede the development of this respiratory pattern.

Rapid shallow breathing occurs if central brainstem dysfunction extends more caudally to the lower pons. When medullary respiratory neurones are

damaged, for example by progressive transtentorial herniation, irregular, slow, deep, gasping respirations, sometimes associated with hiccups (*ataxic respiration*) may develop. In patients with raised intracranial pressure, this sequence of abnormal breathing patterns is often associated with other evidence of brainstem dysfunction, including a rising blood pressure, a slow pulse, flaccid limbs, absence of reflex ocular movements and dilatation of the pupils.

Changing patterns of respiration in an unconscious patient, particularly the development of central neurogenic hyperventilation, provide important and relatively objective evidence of deterioration. These changes in respiratory pattern may occur in structural lesions with raised intracranial pressure, in brainstem infarction and less commonly in some varieties of metabolic coma, especially hepatic coma. They are indicative of progressive and potentially fatal brainstem dysfunction, but not of its causation (Box 15.7).

MOTOR RESPONSES
It is often difficult to elicit signs of focal cerebral disease in the unconscious patient. The presence of focal neurological signs implies localized dysfunction in the central nervous system, and is important in considering the causes of altered consciousness (Box 15.8). If progressive brainstem dysfunction from raised intracranial pressure with transtentorial herniation has occurred, focal signs indicative of the causative lesion may no longer be recognizable. However, papilloedema is usually present in such cases.

In the drowsy or stuporose patient it may be possible to recognize a hemianopia by testing the

---

BOX 15.7   Coma with hyperventilation (and low *PaCO₂*).

- Metabolic acidosis
- Diabetic ketoacidosis
- Brainstem lesion, e.g. stroke
- Rising intracranial pressure
- Bacterial meningitis
- Renal failure
- Liver failure
- Pneumonia complicating brain lesion

BOX 15.8   Causes of coma with focal neurological signs.

- Epilepsy (post-ictal state)
- Stroke
- Encephalitis
- Subarachnoid haemorrhage
- Cerebral abscess
- Bacterial meningitis with cortical infarction
- Cerebral venous sinus thrombosis

response to *visual menace* or, sometimes, by testing for optokinetic nystagmus (p. 246). Visual threat, or menace, consists of threatening the patient's face, in first the left, and then the right field. Normally this threat induces rapid eye closure or a flinch. It is necessary to obtain the patient's attention transiently to assess any meaningful response and the test is, unfortunately, only rarely useful. *Hemiplegia* may be evident either from abnormal flaccidity of the arm and leg on the affected side or, in the stuporose or lightly comatose patient, by absence of spontaneous movements on that side. *Noxious stimuli*, for example pinching the skin of the forearms and thighs, deep rubbing pressure with a hard object applied to the sternum or, often most effective, lightly pricking the skin and mucous membranes near the nasal orifices on both sides, will fail to induce movement of the paralysed limbs. Sometimes in a patient with a dense hemiplegia the cheek blows flaccidly in and out with each breath on the side of hemiplegia. The *tendon reflexes* may be asymmetrical, but in most comatose patients both plantar responses are extensor (see Fig. 11.58). *Asymmetry* of these motor responses is the important feature to assess. In both structural lesions and metabolic disorders coma may be accompanied in its terminal stages by *decorticate* or *decerebrate postures*. These may occur asymmetrically and may be apparent, at first, only when induced by noxious external stimuli, such as deep sternal pressure or pinching the skin or Achilles tendon. These postural reactions are features of severe upper brainstem dysfunction and are thus usually found in association with pupillary abnormalities, absence of doll's head and caloric reflexes and a disturbed breathing pattern. Decerebrate and decorticate postures are found much more characteristically in structural coma than in metabolic coma, and thus do not usually occur in patients with drug-induced coma unless there has been additional hypoxic or ischaemic brian injury.

PERSISTENT STATES OF ALTERED CONSCIOUSNESS

Patients with extensive or diffuse injury to the brain do not always die. In some, partial recovery from coma occurs to a *persistent vegetative state (PVS)* (see Box 15.9). This term is used to describe patients who appear to be in a state of wakeful unresponsiveness, rather than in a state of unresponsive coma. Despite their apparent wakefulness, patients in a persistent vegetative state make no meaningful response to environmental stimuli.

In *PVS* the patient is immobile, with decerebrate posturing, but appears to be awake, with eyes open, but without purposeful or meaningful response to noxious stimulation.

Apparently normal sleep/wake cycles occur through the day and, when awake, the patient's eyes

---

BOX 15.9   Persistent vegetative state (PVS).

- No evidence of awareness of self or environment
- All responses are reflex in nature
- No meaningful or voluntary response to stimulation
- No evidence of language comprehension or expression
- An intermittent sleep/wake pattern
- Preserved cranial nerve responses
- Sufficiently intact hypothalamic (brainstem) autonomic function to allow prolonged survival with nursing and medical care
- Present for more than 1 month

---

may move slowly and randomly, with preserved spontaneous blinking. Reflex swallowing in response to fluid placed in the mouth, and to salivary secretion, usually occurs and there may be spontaneous chewing movements. The gag reflex is present, and the patient breathes normally. The patient is mute. Relatives often find it difficult to accept that the patient with PVS, clearly awake, is not aware. Indeed, it is not possible to assess the state of awareness in such patients, particularly if there are associated focal brain or cervical cord lesions, and it should always be assumed that some awareness may be preserved, when nursing or talking in the vicinity of a patient with PVS. In patients in PVS for longer than 6 months there is no prospect of recovery, and only few patients with PVS of any duration recover.

In *akinetic mutism*, as in PVS, the patient appears awake. The patient shows no awareness of self or environment, but may follow the examiner or a moving object with the eyes. Communication can sometimes be established, even partially, by sign language or by a code based on eye-blinking, and fragmented voluntary movements of the limbs may be possible. If the akinetic mutism is due to a localized lesion or a tumour in the third ventricular region, recovery may occur, and such patients may have excellent recall of events during the period of illness. It is wise, therefore, to remember that the apparently comatose patient may be able to hear and understand, and may later recall conversations that took place or comments made at the bedside during a phase of apparent coma.

PSYCHOLOGICAL COMA

Psychologically disturbed patients sometimes feign coma. The eyes are actually closed and the patient is usually lying in a resting position, or supine with the arms and legs extended. The eyelids resist attempts to open them and, on forced eye opening, the eyes point upwards exposing the white conjunctiva (Bell's phenomenon) as part of the patient's attempt to maintain eyelid closure. The eyelids close rapidly when released. The slow roving eye movements of organic coma cannot be simulated. Painful stimuli to the limbs may be ignored, but pin prick to the nasal mucosa or to the lips usually elicits volitional grimacing. The pupillary light responses are normal. Cold caloric testing induces nystagmus with the fast phase away from the stimulated side, rather than deviation of the eyes toward the stimulus as would occur in true coma. Examination, especially invasive tests as above, may induce return of cooperation and consciousness, or uncover a disturbed mental state.

INVESTIGATIONS

The investigation of the comatose patient is a component of the clinical management of this problem. The immediate steps to be taken are outlined in Box 15.2. Immediately treatable structural or metabolic disorders require ascertainment and management. Investigations are part of this process (Box 15.10). Several, for example blood gas determinations, electrolytes and haemoglobin, require repeated measurement during management. Others, for example X-rays of suspected fractured limbs, form part of the initial assessment (see Ch. 16).

DIAGNOSIS OF BRAIN DEATH

With the advent of improved methods of intensive care, and especially of positive pressure ventilation in

---

> **BOX 15.10   Investigations that determine management of the comatose patient.**
>
> - Cervical spine X-ray
> - CT head scan
> - Chest X-ray
> - X-ray of suspected fractures/bruised limbs
> - Blood for cross-matching
> - Check haemoglobin, haematocrit, WBC count
> - Drug screen
> - Electrolytes and liver function tests
> - Blood gases and pH

---

patients in whom spontaneous respirations have ceased, it became important to develop criteria for the diagnosis of death. This is important not only because of general recognition that brain death may have occurred in certain patients whose respiration has been maintained with a ventilator, although both the body temperature and the systemic circulation continue to be maintained spontaneously, but also because of the value of organ transplantation, for example the kidney, from such patients to others. Clearly, in both these situations the *diagnosis of brain death must be certain before any decision is made to cease attempts to keep the patient alive*. A conference of the Royal Colleges and Faculties of the United Kingdom considered this problem in 1976 in the light of previous attempts to define brain death, the changing needs of medical practice, and public concern about the issue, and agreed the guidelines in Box 15.11, which have since been validated in many clinical studies, and are accepted worldwide (Box 15.11). The criteria concentrate on the recognition of brainstem death, since independent life and consciousness is not possible without intact brainstem function.

These recommendations fall into three groups, parts A, B, and C. The patient must be deeply comatose and on a ventilator, and it must be clearly established that the patient's coma is due to *irremedial structural brain damage* (part A). Drug-induced coma, hypothermia and metabolic causes of coma and relaxant drugs must have been clearly excluded as a cause of ventilatory failure. If these conditions are fulfilled brain death may be diagnosed if no brainstem reflexes can be demonstrated (part B). Repeated tests—at least two separate evaluations should take place—are necessary, but the interval between such tests depends on the pathology and the course of the disease. Purely spinal reflexes can persist after total brainstem destruction but it must always be remembered that decorticate and decerebrate postures are far from necessarily irreversible phenomena and therefore that their presence does not inevitably indicate that brain death has occurred. Indeed some authorities would doubt a diagnosis of brain death if such reflexes persisted. All these tests should be carried out at a body temperature not less than 35°C.

BOX 15.11   Diagnostic criteria for brain death. Note that these are clinically determined criteria, and do not require special investigative techniques.
(modified from *Lancet* (1976) 2: 1069–1070)

A. Conditions in which the diagnosis of brain death should be considered
The diagnosis of a disorder that can lead to brain death must have been firmly established.

The patient is deeply comatose, being incapable of response to any stimulus, other than reflex responses.

(a) There should be no suspicion that this state is due to drugs that may depress brain function, e.g. sedatives, poisons or anaesthetic drugs. No such drugs should have been administered in the previous 24 hours.

(b) Primary hypothermia as a cause of coma must have been excluded.

(c) Metabolic and endocrine disturbances that can be responsible for or can contribute to coma must have been excluded.

The patient is being maintained on a ventilator because spontaneous respiration had previously become inadequate or had ceased altogether.

(a) Muscle relaxants and other drugs should have been excluded as a cause of respiratory failure.

(b) Blood gases, including both oxygen and carbon dioxide levels, MUST be within the normal range at the time the assessment is made; this may require the help of an anaesthetist (see below, B).

There should be no doubt that the patient's condition is due to irremediable structural brain damage.

B. Diagnostic tests for confirmation of brain death
All brain stem reflexes must be absent.

- *The pupils are fixed* in diameter and do not respond to sharp changes in the intensity of incident light.
- *There is no corneal reflex.*
- *The vestibulo-ocular reflexes are absent.*
- *No motor responses within the cranial nerve distribution* can be elicited by adequate stimulation of a somatic area.
- *There is no gag reflex response* to bronchial stimulation by a suction catheter passed down the trachea.
- *No respiratory movements* occur when the patient is disconnected from the mechanical ventilator for

BOX 15.11   (continued)

long enough to ensure that the arterial carbon dioxide tension rises above the threshold for stimulation of respiration. In practice this is best achieved by ventilating the patient with 5% CO_2 in oxygen for 5 minutes before disconnection. This ensures a $Pa\text{CO}_2$ of 8.0 kPa (60 mmHg). A period of 10 minutes' observation for respiratory movement should then be carried out.

C. Other considerations
Note the following:

- *Repetition of testing.* The interval between tests must depend upon the primary pathology and the clinical course of the disease. In some conditions the outcome is not so clearcut, and in these cases it is recommended that the tests should be repeated. The interval between tests depends upon the progress of the patient and might be as long as 24 hours.
- *Integrity of spinal reflexes.* It is well established that spinal cord function can persist after insults that irretrievably destroy brainstem functions.
- *Confirmatory investigation.* Electroencephalography is not necessary for the diagnosis of brain death. Other investigations such as cerebral angiography or cerebral bloodflow measurements are also not required for the diagnosis of brain death.
- *Body temperature.* The body temperature should not be less than 35°C before the diagnostic tests are carried out.
- *Specialist opinion and the status of the doctors concerned.* Only when the primary diagnosis is in doubt is it necessary to consult with a neurologist or neurosurgeon.
- *Decision to withdraw artificial support.* This can be considered after all the criteria presented above have been fulfilled. The decision can be made by any of the following combination of doctors:
  (a) a consultant who is in charge of the case and one other doctor
  (b) in the absence of a consultant, a deputy, who should have been registered for 5 years or more and who should have had adequate experience in the care of such cases, and one other doctor.

16
THE MANAGEMENT OF ACUTE TRAUMATIC INJURY

INTRODUCTION

Trauma is the commonest cause of death and disability in the young. Its prevention, treatment and subsequent rehabilitation are important aspects of contemporary medicine.

Major trauma is defined by an injury severity score (ISS) greater than 14. The ISS is a trauma score based on the severity of injury in the three worst injured systems. A score of 15 implies multi-system injuries. The highest possible score is 75; this is incompatible with life.

The approach to the examination of a patient with major trauma differs from that in an out-patient clinic or on the hospital ward. The trauma examination has to be rapid, and focused on the identification and correction of life-threatening injuries. No physical examination should ever be hasty, however, and thoroughness is especially important in trauma. The routine used in the trauma examination represents a departure from the 'history, examination, investigation' strategy used in ordinary clinical practice.

The process of assessment, diagnosis and management at first contact with the injured person is described as triage; where there are several injured patients, the order in which they are treated is determined by this triage.

ASSESSMENT OF MAJOR TRAUMA

The primary survey of the trauma patient, with correction of life-threatening abnormalities as they are found, is followed by essential X-rays and imaging. A slower secondary survey, comprising a complete head-to-toe examination, including examination of the back and a rectal examination, should follow. The order in which systems are examined in the primary survey is dictated by the speed with which an injury can kill the patient. Thus, airway obstruction can kill more rapidly than tension pneumothorax so it is sought and corrected first. If there is severe haemorrhage, for example from an open fracture of the femur, then the airway is still attended to first; a second person can apply pressure to the bleeding point while the airway is secured.

There is a 'Golden Hour', immediately after injury, during which the patient must be resuscitated and systematic management put in place. The Golden Hour runs from the time of injury, not from the time of arrival in hospital. In a large hospital with a well-organized accident and emergency department the management of multiple trauma is a team affair (Fig. 16.1). The team consists of a leader, an anaesthetist, a general surgeon and another specialist, such as a neurosurgeon or an orthopaedic surgeon. Each is supported by a nurse specialist. This team improves the speed and efficacy of resuscitation. If a seriously injured patient is taken to a small hospital without a trauma team, or without facilities for major surgery, the 'ABC' approach (see below), even if applied by a single doctor working with minimal nursing assistance, can save lives. This is a holding measure, useful until the patient can be transferred to a larger unit.

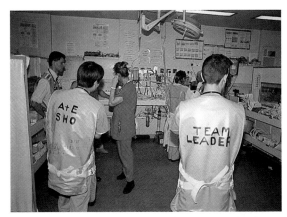

Fig. 16.1   Members of the trauma team waiting for the patient to arrive in the resuscitation room. Each member is clearly identified in order to prevent confusion during the resuscitation.

HISTORY AND MECHANISM OF INJURY

Once the initial triage is completed, it is important to get a history of the accident. The patient may be in no condition to provide this. Information from relatives, ambulance personnel, police or other eyewitnesses at the scene of the accident is essential. Much may be deduced from the mechanism of injury. In addition, enquire about any previous medical history, especially in older patients, because intercurrent illness has a bearing on survival. Search for prescription medicines, hospital appointment cards and other information in the patient's pockets and belongings.

There are three peak risk periods for death following injury (Fig. 16.2). The first, accounting for over 10% of all deaths, occurs at the scene of the accident and is due to severe injury to the central nervous system or mediastinum. The second, smaller, peak occurs about 24 hours later; it is usually due to continuing haemorrhage as a result of extensive injury. The third peak is the smallest and occurs about a week after injury; this is usually due to sepsis and multi-organ failure.

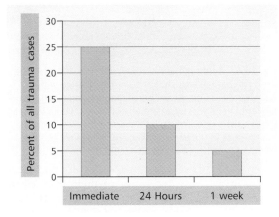

Fig. 16.2   Trimodal distribution of trauma deaths.

There are two basic mechanisms of injury: *blunt* and *penetrating*. The ratio of blunt to penetrating injury reflects the nature and degree of violence in a particular society. In the UK the ratio is 4:1. In the United States, where firearms are readily available, this ratio is reversed.

BLUNT INJURY

The most common causes of blunt injury are falls and motor vehicle accidents. The degree of injury is related to the amount of energy released in the collision between the patient and the solid object concerned. In all cases a sudden deceleration causes brain, bone and soft tissue injury; direct blows in which the velocity of injury is comparatively lower cause isolated fractures. Young people are more resistant to deceleration than older people. The speed at which a car crash will kill half of constrained car occupants is about 40 mph (65 kph) and the height from which half those falling will die is about 40 feet (12 metres). Occasionally, people survive deceleration forces much greater than this, but there are usually mitigating factors such as something to break the fall, or vehicular deceleration occurring in stages. The use of seat belts has dramatically reduced road mortality and morbidity among car occupants in traffic accidents but the use of airbags is not so obviously beneficial. Properly designed crash helmets and protective clothing similarly increase safety among motor cyclists and pedal cyclists involved in accidents.

Other causes of blunt injury include fights and, rather more rarely, blast injury from anti-personnel mines, industrial explosions and terrorist or military bombs.

PENETRATING INJURY

These are usually deliberately inflicted rather than accidental. They are classified as follows:

BLADE
Stabbing is a common injury. The overall mortality of stab wounds is about 2%. The majority of stab wounds involve the hands, arms and subcutaneous tissues of the trunk, rather than vital structures (Fig. 16.3). A deep stab wound to the chest or abdomen can cause rapid death from bleeding, due to perforation of mediastinal structures, intercostal vessels, the abdominal aorta or its main visceral branches. Bleeding from a stab wound to a small vessel, such as the facial artery in the neck, or the inferior epigastric artery inside the rectus sheath, can be life-threatening, and swift attention to such wounds is essential. The size of the entry wound is no indication of its depth, direction or severity.

BULLET
The extent of injury from a bullet wound is dependant on the energy transferred from the speeding

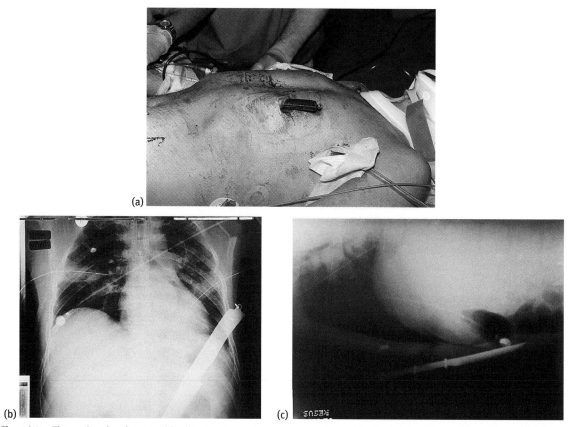

(a)

(b)   (c)

Fig. 16.3   The patient has been stabbed in the chest with a very large knife **(a)**. The AP chest X-ray **(b)** confirms this but the lateral view **(c)** shows that the blade has not penetrated the chest cavity. The knife was removed and the patient made an uneventful recovery, being discharged from hospital the next day.

bullet to the tissue. For example, a high velocity bullet from an AK47 assault rifle entering the chest between the ribs at the front of the chest, passing through the lung tissue and then leaving between the ribs at the back of the chest, causes very little damage. The same bullet, travelling much more slowly at the limits of its trajectory, may cause serious damage if it strikes mediastinal structures, the vertebral column or a solid organ such as the liver. Slower velocity bullets generally cause less damage because they possess less kinetic energy, but even a very small bullet fired from a short barrel weapon can kill instantly if it lodges in the heart or brain, or somewhat more slowly if a major artery is damaged. Survival from bullet wounds, therefore, is often a matter of luck (Fig. 16.4). Shotgun injuries are rather different. At shorter range, damage is caused by blast injury from the cartridge discharge as well as tissue destruction from a large mass of small lead pellets. At longer range the pellets travel much more slowly and tend to cause more superficial injuries but can still cause blindness at a distance of 40 metres (Fig. 16.5).

BLAST

Injuries from explosions consist of concussive blast, but there is also a risk of penetrating injury from flying fragments (Fig. 16.6). These can lodge any-

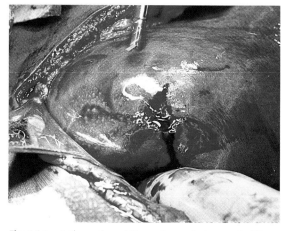

Fig. 16.4   A through-and-through gunshot wound of the liver. The patient was shot at point blank range with a long-barrelled Colt .44 calibre Magnum weapon, a powerful handgun, by an armed policeman whom he was trying to strangle. The bullet traversed the liver and was found loose in the peritoneal cavity. Only minimal bleeding from the liver wound occurred.

where in the body and cause anything from trivial superficial wounds to serious, deep wounds. Such fragments are often travelling at a high speed and their irregular shape and aerodynamic instability

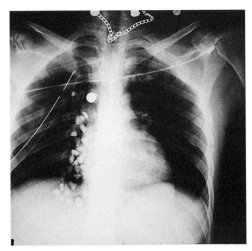

Fig. 16.5 A PA chest X-ray showing large calibre shotgun pellets in the anterior mediastinum. The weapon had been discharged at medium range and none of the pellets had punctured the myocardium.

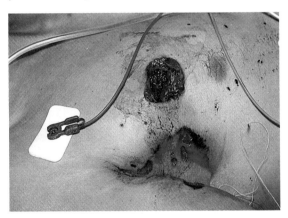

Fig. 16.6 A penetrating wound through the right anterior axillary fold caused by a bomb fragment. Note the ragged entry and exit wounds, the result of both the irregular shape of the fragment and its tumbling flight.

lead to much more energy transfer in the body than would be expected from a slower streamlined bullet following a stable trajectory.

PRIMARY SURVEY AND TRIAGE

The three principal steps in management are defined by *ABC*:

- **A** is for Airway
- **B** is for Breathing
- **C** is for Circulation

the **ABC** of resuscitation.

AIRWAY (WITH CERVICAL SPINE CONTROL)

Resuscitate the trauma patient supine. The so-called 'recovery position', with the patient lying on the left side, is not used because it makes it difficult to protect the cervical spine The airway can be managed perfectly well with the patient supine.

BASIC MANAGEMENT OF AIRWAY OBSTRUCTION

Airway obstruction, if complete, causes death within a few minutes. It must be recognized and relieved at once. Simple manoeuvres such as sweeping the index finger around the mouth to remove obstructions such as false teeth, followed by a chin lift or jaw thrust to move the tongue forwards and clear the oropharynx, can be life-saving. Once the airway has been cleared (Box 16.1), its patency can be maintained with a nasopharyngeal or oropharyngeal airway. If the patient has ceased to breathe, a cuffed orotracheal or nasotracheal tube should be inserted. This makes ventilation with a bag and oxygen easier and the inflated cuff protects the airway against vomit (Fig. 16.7). If the patient is not unconscious enough for the passage of an endotracheal tube, but requires one to maintain oxygenation or to protect the airway, then a general anaesthetic is needed.

BOX 16.1   Key points in airway management.

Basic management
- Chin lift
- Jaw thrust
- Nasopharyngeal airway
- Oropharyngeal airway

Advanced management
- Nasotracheal intubation
- Orotracheal intubation

Surgical management
- Cricothyroidotomy
- Tracheostomy

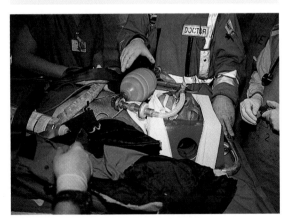

Fig. 16.7 Airway with cervical spine control. The airway has been secured with an endotracheal tube. The cervical spine is controlled by means of a hard cervical collar to prevent rotation, with wedges either side of the head to prevent lateral flexion, and a tape across the forehead to prevent flexion. All of these measures must be used to provide complete control.

It is vital to recognize the physical signs of upper airway obstruction. These are not always obvious, but should be actively sought:

- *Noisy breathing*, particularly on inspiration, should suggest partial airway obstruction.
- *Silence*. If there are a number of injured people at the scene of an accident, the silent ones should always be attended to before those crying out in pain, since there may be a simple cause for their airway obstruction which can be corrected easily. On the other hand, they may already be dead.
- *Suprasternal recession*. The inspiratory effort against a closed upper airway sucks the tissue inwards above the suprasternal notch and above the clavicles. This sign indicates the urgent need for airway relief.
- *Deepening cyanosis*. This is a sign of dangerous airway obstruction.

ADVANCED MANAGEMENT OF AIRWAY OBSTRUCTION

The airway may be blocked above the larynx by the inhalation of a foreign body or by direct trauma to the neck. In this case a surgical airway is needed. Cricothyroidotomy is the safest way to provide an airway quickly. A stab incision is made into the larynx *below* the vocal cords through the cricothyroid membrane, which lies subcutaneously between the thyroid and cricoid cartilages (Fig. 16.8). The surgical procedure should be carefully learned. Details are readily available from any operative surgery text or from the ATLS Manual of the American College of Surgeons. Cricothyroidotomy, done under a local anaesthetic, or without anaesthesia if the patient is unconscious, is much safer and faster to perform than a tracheostomy. Tracheostomy is an elective or semi-elective procedure which should be carried out by an experienced surgeon under general anaesthetic.

PROTECTING THE CERVICAL SPINE

Control of the cervical spine is essential during airway clearance, and indeed during any subsequent resuscitation. A deceleration injury may cause cervical spine fracture, which may be unstable, and it is essential to immobilize the cervical spine until its integrity has been determined by X-ray imaging. The spine is immobilized:

- In an in-line position
- Using both hands.

A *rigid* cervical collar (not a soft collar) should be applied in order to avoid spinal cord damage. Full immobilization requires:

- Sandbags on either side of the head
- A piece of wide sticky plaster across the forehead, fixed to the sides of the bed.

If the airway problem is urgent and no collar is available, then an assistant should hold the head steady while the airway is cleared (see Fig. 16.7).

BREATHING

In the absence of airway obstruction, failure of breathing is caused by:

- Severe head injury leading to cessation of central control of breathing
- Direct damage to the thoracic wall.

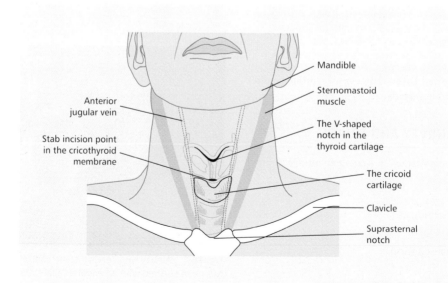

Fig. 16.8   Surface markings for cricothyroidotomy. The cricothyroid membrane is located as a depression felt between the 'V' of the thyroid cartilage and the prominent ring of the cricoid cartilage, some 2 cm below this. Caudally, the trachea can be felt disappearing into the thorax at the suprasternal notch. The transverse incision should be restricted to 2 cm in order to avoid damage to the lateral structures of the neck, the most prominent of which is the anterior jugular vein which will bleed profusely if damaged.

Thoracic injury may result in fractured ribs, a collapsed lung or bleeding into the chest, all of which restrict breathing. (see Box 16.2) The following local problems may lead to restricted breathing; all need immediate treatment from the moment they are diagnosed during the primary survey:

Tension pneumothorax

This results from the introduction of air into the pleural cavity, usually from damage to the lung surface by a fractured rib. Lung damage causes a pleural flap which allows air to enter the pleural cavity with each breath but not to leave between breaths, so that air accumulates under pressure. Left untreated, increasing intrathoracic pressure displaces the mediastinum and restricts venous return to the heart, thus eventually compromising cardiac output (Fig. 16.9(a)). The condition is exacerbated by reduced air exchange in the affected lung and there is often cyanosis. Observation of the chest wall shows that the affected side is fixed (does not move with respiration) and hyper-inflated. Palpation confirms lack of movement on the side of the lesion and deviation of the trachea away from the side of the pneumothorax. Percussion reveals hyper-resonance all over the chest wall and resonance outside the normal surface markings of the lung during inspiration. Auscultation reveals dimin-

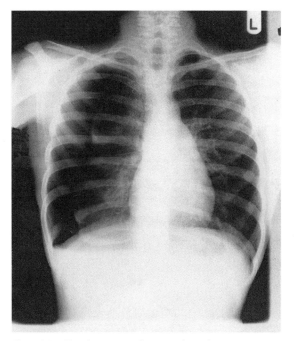

Fig. 16.9 Simple pneumothorax and tension pneumothorax.

ished or absent breath sounds. The diagnosis is made clinically and should be obvious without the use of a chest X-ray; indeed waiting for an X-ray to confirm the suspected diagnosis is a mistake that wastes precious time.

Treatment of a tension pneumothorax is by the immediate insertion of a large bore needle in the second interspace on the side of the lesion. This relieves the tension but does not treat the underlying lesion. A chest drain (Fig. 16.10) should be inserted on the side of the lesion. There is usually a brisk gush

(a)

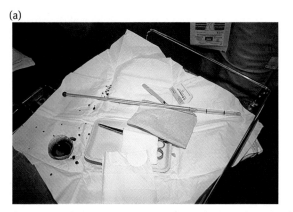

(b)

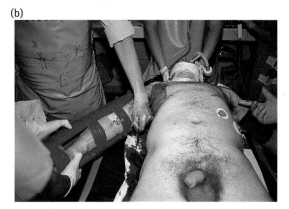

Fig. 16.10   The instrument requirements for insertion of a chest drain **(a)** are minimal. Antiseptic solution, a knife for making the incision in the chest wall, a pair of artery forceps to deepen the incision through the intercostal muscles, an intercostal tube drain with the sharp trocar removed and a stitch for securing the drain are all that are required. The drain is placed **(b)** in the fifth intercostal space in the anterior axillary line. The drain is shown pinched shut by the surgeon while the underwater seal drainage tube is prepared for connection.

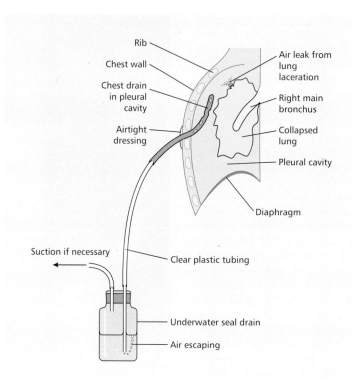

Fig. 16.11 An intercostal underwater seal tube drain. The fenestrated drain is introduced into the pleural cavity and once secured to the chest wall is connected to an underwater seal. As the pressure in the pleural cavity rises, air is forced down the tube and bubbles out through the water. This is particularly evident on coughing. Gentle breathing usually causes the water in the drainage tube to move up and down. If the patient breathes in sharply the water is drawn up the tube until the hydrostatic pressure equals the pressure inside the pleural cavity. The water thus acts as a one-way valve which prevents air entering the pleural cavity via the chest drain but allows it to escape to the atmosphere. Graduations on the side of the bottle allow the amount of any blood or other fluid leaking from the pleural cavity to be measured.

of air as the pleural cavity is opened which confirms the diagnosis and is the first step towards successful treatment. The important first step is to relieve the tension; the needle does this but converts the lesion into a simple pneumothorax. A negative pressure underwater seal drain allows the collapsed lung to reflate (Fig. 16.11).

Massive haemothorax

The signs are similar to tension pneumothorax except that the side of the lesion is dull to percussion. The patient is nearly always shocked, with a low blood pressure and elevated pulse rate, and is sweaty and short of breath (see 'Circulation' below). Insertion of a chest drain confirms the presence of blood which may be arterial or venous in origin, but which most commonly comes from a torn intercostal artery. Massive haemorrhage from the mediastinum is rarely seen in hospital as this usually causes death before a chest drain can be inserted. If more than 750 ml is drained and the bleeding continues at a rate of more than 2150 ml per hour with no signs of slowing down, then the patient needs an urgent thoracotomy in order to secure haemostasis.

Haemopneumothorax

There is both blood and air in the pleural cavity. It can occur with a simple or tension pneumothorax. Physical signs are similar to pneumothorax except that there is often a fluid level on percussion. Dullness to percussion over the lower zone gives way to a sudden increase in resonance as the pneumothorax is encountered. This sign is easier to elucidate with the patient sitting up. Treatment again is by the insertion of a chest drain. The indications for thoracotomy are the same as those for massive haemothorax, i.e. uncontrolled intrathoracic bleeding.

Simple traumatic pneumothorax

This occurs when a fixed amount of air has escaped into the pleural cavity causing partial collapse of the lung, the leak then sealing itself off (see Fig. 5.20). There is seldom any tracheal deviation and the affected side moves normally or with only slight restriction. The patient is unlikely to be short of breath, distressed or cyanosed unless there is underlying chronic obstructive pulmonary disease. Palpation may reveal some loss of movement on the affected side. The percussion note is more resonant than usual but not as resonant as that found in

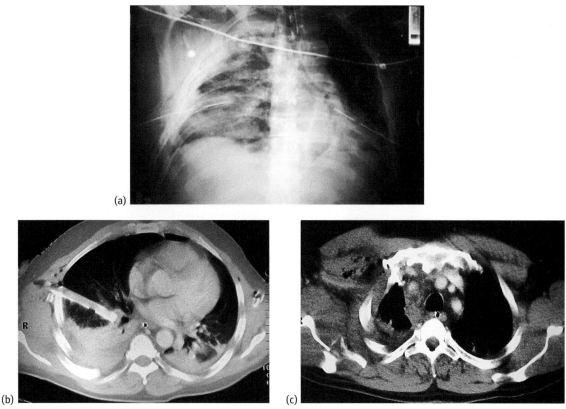

(a)

(b)   (c)

Fig. 16.12   Typical X-ray findings in a flail chest **(a)**. There are obvious multiple fractures on the right side of the chest which include the first rib. There are underlying lung contusions. Bilateral chest drains are in situ. A CT scan through the lower part of the chest **(b)** shows a collection of blood in both the pleural cavities, more on the right, with a chest drain in situ. A CT scan through the upper part of the chest **(c)** shows that the chest wall over the apex of the lung is crushed, with heavy extravasation of blood into the chest wall musculature. A ruptured right subclavian vein was subsequently repaired.

tension pneumothorax, and breath sounds may be reduced or muffled but are seldom absent. Diagnosis without chest X-ray may be difficult. The insertion of a chest drain is less urgent than with a tension pneumothorax.

Flail chest
A flail chest is present when there is more than one fracture in more than one rib (Fig. 16.12). The loose segment of the chest wall which results from this injury takes no part in breathing; it is sucked in during inspiration and bulges out during expiration. If the segment is large, gas exchange may be compromised and the patient may need to be ventilated until healing takes place—normally for about a fortnight. There is often an underlying lung injury. This may be serious, with lung contusion, ventilation/perfusion mismatch, infection and pulmonary oedema. These complications may require the use of ventilation with sedation and intubation, physiotherapy and antibiotic therapy.

Open chest wound
If there is a hole in the chest wall this should be covered with an airtight dressing, taped down on

> **BOX 16.3   Sites of haemorrhage.**
>
> - Intrathoracic
> - Intra-abdominal
> - Pelvic fracture
> - Multiple long bone fractures
> - Exsanguination

three of its four sides, or be completely sealed and a separate chest drain with a flutter valve or underwater seal inserted. Remember that an open chest wound causes collapse of the lung.

CIRCULATION

CONTROL OF HAEMORRHAGE
Circulatory collapse in the absence of airway obstruction or tension pneumothorax is due to *haemorrhage* (Box 16.3). This may be confined to the body cavities (see haemothorax above) or may be due to exsanguination from an open wound. *The lost blood is in the chest, in the abdomen, in the pelvis, in the long bones or on the floor of the resuscitation room* (Fig. 16.13).

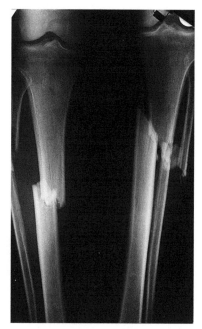

Fig. 16.13 Bilateral fractures of the tibiae and fibulae can cause three to four units blood loss into the tissues and even more than this if the fractures are open.

The diagnosis of circulatory collapse may be made by observation of the *pulse, blood pressure, urine output* and *skin temperature*. The signs of shock are:

- Elevation of pulse rate
- Fall in blood pressure
- Fall in urine output
- Central cyanosis due to circulatory failure
- Sweatiness
- Fall in peripheral temperature.

Cardiac tamponade

This is a rare cause of shock. It should be suspected in the absence of bleeding into the body cavities or externally. Accumulation of blood inside the pericardial cavity compresses the cardiac atria, impeding venous return and thus reducing cardiac output. Eventually the circulation fails. The clinical diagnosis in a shocked patient is suggested by Beck's triad, which consists of:

- Distended neck veins
- Reduced heart sounds
- Reduced blood pressure.

Pulsus paradoxus may be present. There is often a penetrating injury in the region of the mediastinum, at the front or the back of the chest. Treatment consists in removal of blood from the pericardial space, either by needle pericardiocentesis or, more reliably, by thoracotomy. Thoracotomy is preferred because the bleeding point can be secured (Fig. 16.14).

(a)

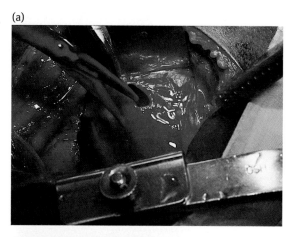

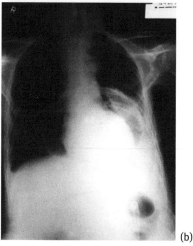

(b)

Fig. 16.14 **(a)** The surgical treatment of pericardial tamponade. The figure shows a gush of blood under pressure leaving the pericardial cavity via a stab incision which has just been made by the surgeon. **(b)** Pneumopericardium may produce similar symptoms to haemopericardium.

BOX 16.4   Signs of intra-abdominal bleeding.

- Pain
- Distension
- Guarding, rebound, rigidity
- Absent bowel sounds

Fractures of long bones

These cause major haemorrhage into soft tissues adjacent to the fractures, often without obvious external signs of bleeding. Bilateral femoral shaft fractures with a fractured pelvis can lead to haemorrhagic shock from exsanguination.

Bleeding into the abdominal cavity

Bleeding into the abdominal cavity is also often difficult to diagnose (Box 16.4). It should be suspected if the patient is obviously shocked but there is no pelvic or long bone fracture and the chest is clear. Blood in the peritoneal cavity is irritant and causes *abdominal pain, distension* and *absent bowel sounds*. If the diagnosis is unclear, then a diagnostic peritoneal lavage (DPL, see below), ultrasound scan or CT scan of the abdomen should be carried out.

Treatment of circulatory collapse

This requires administration of fluid and blood. Insert two wide-bore cannulae (16 gauge or larger) into the antecubital veins. Blood samples should be taken at this point; a full blood count, urea and electrolyte and amylase estimation and blood cross-matching should be carried out immediately on these samples (Box 16.5). Immediate resuscitation with a rapid intravenous infusion of *warm* crystalloid (low molecular weight solutions of dextrose or saline) or colloid (high molecular weight solutions of starch and other blood substitutes) solution is used to restore blood volume and blood pressure. Put in a central venous line at this time. The central venous line is used for continuous measurement of the central venous pressure (CVP), an indication of the need for blood and fluid replacement.

The trauma patient almost always needs blood, especially if arterial blood gases show a metabolic acidosis, indicating tissue hypoperfusion, and the CVP is low. If the need is clinically urgent, O Rhesus negative blood may be given until type-specific uncrossmatched or properly crossmatched blood becomes available.

External bleeding should be controlled by direct pressure on the bleeding point until surgical repair can be arranged. Most patients whose bleeding has ceased, but whose blood pressure is low, will respond to a 2-litre fluid challenge. If it proves impossible to maintain the blood pressure it must be assumed that bleeding is continuing internally. The source of the bleeding should be sought and dealt with surgically, immediately. Whole blood and crystalloid or colloid should be given in the initial stages of resuscitation. In trauma in younger, fitter patients it is probably best not to resuscitate the patient too vigorously since a restored normal blood pressure may provoke further bleeding. The CVP line should not be used for volume replacement or fluid; it is unwise to give a volume of cool fluid directly into the central circulation.

CENTRAL NERVOUS SYSTEM ASSESSMENT

The diagnosis of central nervous system (CNS) injury is made initially by a simple assessment of the level of consciousness. The patient may be alert, responsive to

voice, responsive to pain, or not responsive at all. A rudimentary assessment of limb movement may be made at the same time but it is seldom necessary to go beyond this level until later in the examination. The assessment can usefully be formalized by using the Glasgow Coma Scale (Box 16.6).

EXPOSE THE PATIENT FULLY

It is important to undress the patient *completely* in order to carry out a full examination. At the same time, it is important to keep the patient warm since trauma and blood loss invariably lead to a reduction in core temperature, even in warm climates. Once undressed, the patient should be covered with a cellular blanket, or some other warming device should be used to maintain body warmth (Fig. 16.15).

RADIOLOGY

Three X-ray examinations are of immediate use in the trauma patient:

- Cervical spine
- Chest
- Pelvis.

These augment the physical findings made during the primary survey.

(a)

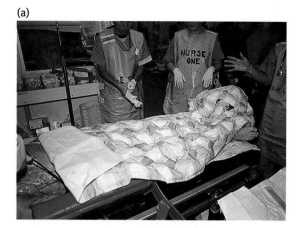

(b)

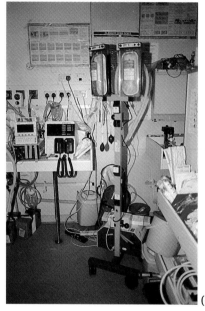

Fig. 16.15 Keeping the patient warm by means of **(a)** a warm blanket and **(b)** a blood warmer.

BOX 16.7   Criteria for low risk of cervical spine injury after trauma, such that cervical spine X-ray is unnecessary.

- No midline cervical tenderness
- No focal neurological signs
- Normal alertness
- Absence of any intoxication, especially alcohol-related
- No other painful, distracting injury

CERVICAL SPINE (Box 16.7)

A cross-table lateral view of the cervical spine is important in assessing potential spinal cord injury due to an unstable fracture of the neck. In order to be useful, the film *must show all seven cervical vertebrae* and the top half of the first thoracic vertebra. If it does not reveal these structures repeat it with traction on the patient's arms or using oblique views.

If there is doubt, and particularly if there is neck tenderness on examination, the rigid cervical collar that was fitted when the patient was first examined should be left in place. CT or MRI scans of the neck may be required to clear the cervical spine. In case of uncertainty these investigations are mandatory.

CHEST

A plain chest radiograph is useful for identifying:

- Lung contusions or mediastinal injury not suspected clinically
- Bony injury such as fractured ribs or flail chest
- Simple pneumothorax and/or haemothorax
- Diaphragmatic injury
- Correct placement of chest drains and CVP lines can be confirmed.

Interpretation is surprisingly difficult because this is an anteroposterior film taken with the patient lying flat and the normal appearances are quite different from the standard posteroanterior erect chest X-ray. The discovery of a tension pneumothorax on X-ray means that the patient has not been properly assessed clinically. The diagnosis of a ruptured diaphragm may be quite difficult to make unless a nasogastric tube has been placed and is seen inside the stomach, but within the thoracic cavity. Placing a nasogastric tube in situ before the chest X-ray is helpful since it often appears in the chest if the diaphragm is ruptured.

PELVIS

The recognition of a pelvic fracture is very important since it may be life threatening because of haemorrhage within the pelvis, and because of the risk of associated injury to pelvic organs (e.g. bladder, ureters, kidneys, uterus, rectum, iliac arteries and veins). The extent of the bony injury is generally related to the extent of the soft tissue injury.

OTHER DIAGNOSTIC X-RAYS

These are carried out as indicated when specific injuries are recognized during the secondary survey.

SECONDARY SURVEY

The secondary survey is a full physical examination, from head to toe.

FACE, HEAD AND NECK

Careful palpation of the cranium, the facial skeleton, the cervical vertebrae and associated soft tissues is important to exclude fractures. The cervical collar may be removed for this examination but in-line trac-

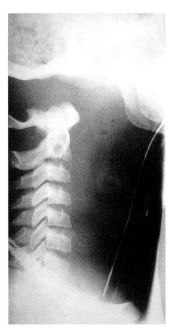

Fig. 16.16 Atlanto-occipital disruption is a rare and generally fatal injury caused by severe traction injury to the neck.

tion of the neck must be maintained by an assistant and the collar replaced afterwards unless a fracture has been clearly excluded. Be particularly alert for boggy swelling over the cranium which suggests a depressed fracture and tenderness in the neck which suggests a fractured cervical vertebra. An open wound over such an injury suggests a compound fracture. Look for penetrating injuries; a tiny stab wound to the neck may hide extensive damage to the carotid arteries, pharynx and other deep neck structures.

Facial bruising is a good clue to underlying injuries. In particular it is important to exclude any suggestion of an orbital floor blowout fracture—this is associated with periorbital haematoma and can lead to loss of sight. Serious maxillary fractures are nearly always heralded by bleeding from the nose or mouth, as is a fractured base of skull. The mouth is searched for broken teeth and a step in the mandible which suggests a fractured jaw. Finally fundoscopy can provide important information about injuries to the eye, and raised intracranial pressure, and otoscopy will reveal bleeding from the ear and blood behind the tympanic membrane. Fractured base of skull is often associated with a cerebrospinal fluid leak from the nose or ears, and the Battle sign, bruising over the mastoid bone, is another important clue to this injury.

CENTRAL NERVOUS SYSTEM

The state of the pupils is a good guide to any brain damage. A unilateral constricted pupil is caused by stretching of the optic nerve across the edge of the tentorium cerebelli as a result of early brain displacement, usually due to extradural or subdural haematoma with raised intracranial pressure; if this situation worsens the pupil becomes fixed and dilated, and the patient's conscious state deteriorates. Urgent CT assessment, followed by surgical removal of subdural or extradural haematoma and control of haemorrhage, is required. Bilateral fixed dilated pupils usually indicate brainstem contusion and a poor outcome; this pathological situation is usually associated with a Glasgow Coma Scale of 3 (Box 16.6).

The Glasgow Coma Scale (GCS) is a simple non-expert assessment of three domains of function, scored as in Box 16.6:

- Eye opening
- Best motor response
- Verbal response.

The best possible score is 15 and the worst is 3. The GCS does not give information regarding the CNS as a whole. A patient with a dense left-sided stroke may still have a GCS of 15, since the best motor response will be on the unaffected side and therefore normal. Coma is defined as a score of 8 or less; the prognosis becomes increasingly grave with lower scores and, especially, if the patient does not show progress in serial observations (see Ch. 15).

CHEST

Severe chest injuries must be recognized and corrected in the primary survey. In the secondary survey the chest is examined in more detail, together with the thoracic spine. The patient is log-rolled onto the left side by four people, maintaining in-line traction on the cervical spine and avoiding any twisting of the thoracic and lumbar spine. It is at this point that the back is searched for stab wounds or other open wounds not hitherto suspected, or tenderness associated with fractured ribs, and the thoracic and lumbar spine are gently probed for tender areas or a palpable step which might suggest a spinal fracture (Fig. 16.17).

ABDOMEN AND PELVIS

Abdominal injuries are difficult to diagnose. Abdominal symptoms are more likely to be noted in conscious patients. However, there are a number of clues. Bruising from seat-belt injuries or other direct blunt trauma should be regarded with suspicion and, or course, a penetrating abdominal injury very often means damage to internal structures. If the abdomen is soft and pain-free, major injury is unlikely (Fig. 16.18(a)). The classic signs of peritonitis, guarding, rebound tenderness and rigidity can only be elucidated in the conscious patient. A distended, rigid abdomen with absent bowel sounds

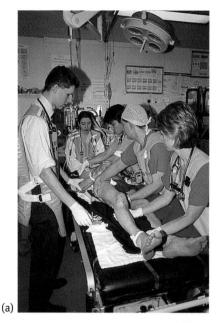

(a)

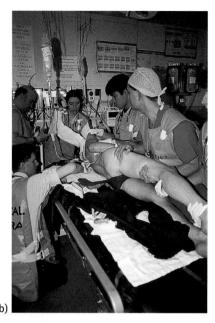

(b)

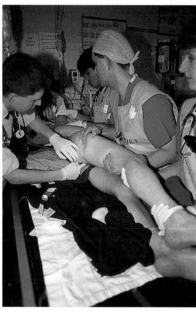

(c)

Fig. 16.17   **(a)** Preparing to log-roll a patient. Four people are needed to do this: three to roll the patient while keeping the thoracolumbar spine stable and in line, and the fourth to secure the cervical spine from the top of the table. **(b)** Once the patient is rolled the thoracolumbar spine is examined for evidence of fracture and the back of the thorax and abdomen searched for penetrating trauma. The opportunity is taken **(c)** to carry out a rectal examination.

almost certainly contains major pathology whether the patient is awake or unconscious (Box 16.8).

Haematemesis suggests upper gastrointestinal injury. Pancreatic injury is serious and a *raised amylase* alerts the surgeon to its presence in most cases. CT scanning will locate a pancreatic injury.

A *nasogastric (N-G) tube* should always be placed in the trauma patient; if there is bleeding from the nose or mouth the N-G tube is best placed orally in order to avoid the remote risk of passage of the naso-gastric tube through a fractured base of skull and into the cranial cavity.

A *rectal examination* is essential (see Fig. 16.17(c)); this should be done during the log-roll described above. Rectal wall damage should be sought, and the jagged edges of fractured pelvic bones may be felt if such injury is present. Blood on the glove is a sign of rectal or other large bowel injury. The presence of bruising in the perineum, haematuria, or a high-riding prostate, suggesting urethral injury, is a con-traindication to catheterization, and a suprapubic catheter should be placed under such circumstances. Blood coming from the urethra is usually fresh and undiluted whereas haematuria from the kidneys and

(a)   (b)

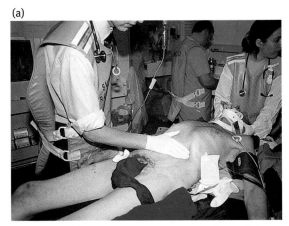 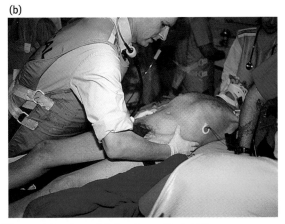

Fig. 16.18 (a) Palpating the abdomen for signs of injury and (b) examining the pelvis for signs of instability.

bladder is diluted by the urine. Renal or bladder damage should always be suspected under these circumstances. Otherwise, diagnosis in the unconscious patient relies on the special tests outlined below. Pelvic fracture can be diagnosed clinically in a conscious patient by the elucidation of pain on gentle suprapubic pressure (Fig. 16.18(b); Box 16.9).

EXTREMITIES

Fractures of the arms and legs should be carefully sought. Radiography is indicated if there is bruising or obvious deformity. Skin wounds near a fractured bone mean that the fracture is probably compound. A large haematoma, especially with a penetrating injury, suggests vascular damage and the presence of a bruit over the area found on auscultation suggests traumatic arteriovenous fistula. The peripheral pulses should be checked. An absent pulse usually means major vessel injury, unless the patient is elderly and has pre-existing vascular disease. The presence of *pain, pallor, pulselessness, coldness and poor capillary return* are diagnostic of acute ischaemia (Box 16.10). In a young fit patient pulses may still be present even if a major

---

BOX 16.8   Examination of the abdomen.

The following usually imply peritonitis due to rupture of the viscera.
- Guarding
- Rebound
- Rigidity
- Absent bowel sounds

BOX 16.9   Diagnosis of pelvic fracture.

- Unstable pelvic ring
- Perineal bruising
- Bright red blood on rectal examination
- Bony fragments on rectal examination
- Bleeding from the urethral meatus

BOX 16.10   Diagnosis of acute peripheral ischaemia.

- Pain
- Pallor
- Paraesthesia
- Pulselessness
- Paralysis
- Perishing with cold

---

blood vessel has been disrupted. An open arterial injury can be temporarily controlled by direct pressure on the wound. This is safer than application of a tourniquet which may too easily be forgotten. Venous bleeding, such as that seen after disruption of a superficial varicose vein, can be controlled either by local pressure or by elevation of the limb.

SPECIAL TESTS

Additional diagnostic tests may be carried out following the secondary survey.

The mainstay of trauma investigation is the CT scan. Highly sensitive and specific, especially with injected contrast medium, the test will identify most intrathoracic, intra-abdominal and pelvic injuries including firm and soft organ rupture, retroperitoneal injury to the urinary tract and pancreas, and ruptured thoracic aorta. A modern spiral CT scanner will perform a total body scan in less than 3 minutes. The most important thing to remember about this type of diagnostic imaging is that the patient must have a stable airway and circulation, otherwise he or she may collapse half-way through the scan.

Diagnostic ultrasound is useful in the early stages of resuscitation or if there is no access to a CT scanner. It can identify fluid in the peritoneal cavity and delineate injury to firm organs, including the kidneys, but not soft tissues, such as the gut.

Intravenous urography will help diagnose renal tract injury—this is normally done as a one-shot film procedure 1–2 minutes after intravenous injection of contrast medium, for example the same contrast used in the CT scan study. This will show whether the kidneys are working. The assessment of ureteric, bladder or urethral injury relies on more complex radiological procedures.

Finally, the diagnostic peritoneal lavage (DPL) is useful under some circumstances, usually when ultrasound or CT is unavailable. The procedure recognizes the presence of blood or bowel contents inside the peritoneal cavity but cannot indicate its source. A small incision is made below the umbilicus and a litre of warmed saline instilled, left for 15 minutes and then drained out. The procedure is positive, indicating the need for laparotomy, if the red cell count exceeds 100 000/ml, the white cell count exceeds 5000/ml, or there are bowel contents in the fluid.

MONITORING THE TRAUMA PATIENT

Finally, after these initial intensive evaluations, do not forget to continue monitoring the patient's progress. Decide what are the areas of risk, and follow them carefully. Be prepared to intervene according to a prepared plan. Do not be taken unawares by unexpected deterioration. Think ahead about what might go wrong, and how you will recognize improvement. Watch renal function, and the circulation. Check gas exchange, and assess the neurological status. Be prepared.

17
ONCOLOGY

INTRODUCTION

In its early stages, cancer is usually asymptomatic. Screening programmes, such as those for cervical and breast cancer, aim to achieve diagnosis at this pre-symptomatic stage, to enable curative treatment. However, many patients present later, for example, with a lump that has been noted for some time, or when a mass in an internal organ has caused symptomatic functional alteration, as with ovarian or renal cancers.

COMMUNICATION

People vary greatly in their knowledge and in their responses to their natural fears and anxieties about a diagnosis of cancer. For example, a person may present early or late in the course of the disease, exercise denial, demand control, desire immediate treatment, or refuse treatment altogether. The initial consultation is the best time to assess a person's knowledge and attitude to cancer and to establish rapport with both the patient and the family. This relationship is important when communicating the diagnosis and involving the patient in treatment decisions that require judgement concerning the relative costs and benefits of treatment, the expected quality and length of survival, and how to relate these elements to life priorities.

SYMPTOMS OF CANCER

There are a number of general features that suggest a diagnosis of cancer, and certain features that are specific to various cancers, mostly based on the organ involved.

GENERAL SYMPTOMS

Weight loss, fatigue, anorexia, even cachexia, are frequent early and non-specific symptoms of cancer. The serious nature of these symptoms may not be appreciated until continuing deterioration indicates a sinister underlying cause. There is no typical time course for cancer symptoms: some arise rapidly over a matter of weeks, as in acute leukaemia, lymphomas, and germ cell tumours, while others develop slowly over several years, for example, bowel and renal cancers.

Initial, non-specific symptoms later become linked to specific features indicating functional or anatomical disturbance due to the primary tumour. Sometimes, cancer may be suspected only when secondary spread causes symptoms distant from the primary neoplasm, such as the pain of bone metastases in prostate cancer, painful enlargement of the liver in colon cancer, or focal neurological disturbances (e.g. seizures) with brain metastases from lung cancer.

SITE-SPECIFIC SYMPTOMS

Specific symptoms at the primary site of origin of the cancer are usually related to:

- Pain
- Swelling
- Non-healing ulceration and bleeding
- Invasion and disruption of surrounding structures.

Usually the patient is alerted to the importance of these symptoms by their persistence and worsening. The initial symptoms of cancer are seldom specific but reflect the organ involved.

PARANEOPLASTIC SYNDROMES

The general and site-specific symptoms of cancer may be complicated by specific cancer-related syndromes due to indirect effects of the cancer. (Box 17.1).

Paraneoplastic syndromes arise in several different ways. Their importance reflects their specificity to certain types of cancer, and to their potential reversibility with treatment of the cancer, or directed to their underlying cause. Paraneoplastic disorders may arise during the course of the disease, or may be a presenting feature, sometimes evident for months or an even longer period before the cancer itself is recognized.

Autoimmune paraneoplastic syndromes occur because antibodies developing to antigens within tumour cells cross-react with antigens in other tissues causing dysfunction in these tissues. In *LEMS* antibodies to an antigen at acetylcholine release sites in motor nerve terminals lead to impaired acetylcholine release, causing muscle fatigue. This antigen is associated with small cell lung cancer but, like many of these syndromes can also occur as a spontaneous, non-cancer-related autoimmune disease.

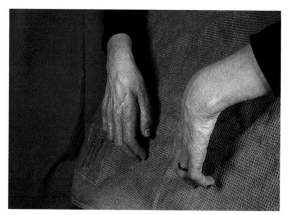

Fig. 17.1   Paraneoplastic peripheral neuropathy, associated with a thymoma.

Immunosuppression leads to *opportunistic infection* with viruses, and with other rare pathogens, such as fungi. *Coagulopathy* is particularly associated with cancers of the pancreas and stomach.

METABOLIC AND ENDOCRINE SYNDROMES

These syndromes result from the effects of specific secretions in certain cancers (Box 17.2). In all of these syndromes there are several additional possible causes, other than a remote effect of cancer. As with other paraneoplastic syndromes the cancer may present with the remote syndrome, or the paraneoplastic syndrome may develop during the course of the illness, after the diagnosis of cancer has been made and treatment commenced.

Carcinoid syndrome

This syndrome is due to the release of increased amounts of 5-hydroxy tryptamine (5-HT) and other vasoactive compounds from certain endocrine tumours, especially carcinoid tumours. It consists of:

- Episodic fever
- Flushing and facial discoloration
- Bronchospasm
- Abdominal colic and diarrhoea
- Endocardial fibrosis, with tricuspid regurgitation and right heart failure.

BOX 17.1   Paraneoplastic syndromes.

Metabolic and endocrine syndromes
- See Box 17.2

Autoimmune syndromes
- Lambert–Eaton myasthenic syndrome (LEMS)
- Cerebellar degeneration with ovarian cancer
- Peripheral neuropathy with various cancers (Fig. 17.1)

Immunosuppression
- Re-activation of *Herpes zoster* infection, especially with lymphomas

Coagulopathy
- Thrombophlebitis and pulmonary emboli associated with cancers of pancreas, stomach, breast and ovary

Pel–Ebstein fever
- An alternating daily fever associated with malignancy

BOX 17.2   Cancer-related metabolic and endocrine syndromes.

- Carcinoid syndrome
- Cushing's syndrome
- Cytokine-related hypercalcaemia
- Syndrome of inappropriate antidiuretic hormone (ADH) secretion
- Gynaecomastia

Two-thirds of carcinoid tumours arise in the mid-gut; others are found in the respiratory and genitourinary tracts. Gut carcinoids may be associated with other, hormone-producing tumours, known by their secretions as insulinoma, gastrinoma, VIPoma, and glucagonoma.

Cushing's syndrome

This syndrome is due to the uncontrolled release of corticosteroids, or of peptides with corticosteroidal effects (e.g., ectopic ACTH release) from a tumour. It usually presents with:

- Change in appearance, e.g., moon-face, hirsutism
- Altered mental state—sleeplessness and even psychotic behaviour may occur.

Uncontrolled corticosteroid secretion occurs with adrenal or pituitary tumours. Ectopic ACTH production is a feature of small cell lung cancers, and may also occur with carcinoid tumours.

Hyperuricaemia

Rapid cell turnover, especially in haematological cancers, may cause hyperuricaemia. This leads to:

- Gouty arthritis, especially affecting distal interphalangeal, knee and shoulder joints
- Renal failure.

Hypercalcaemic syndrome

Increased blood calcium levels occur with bony metastases, and with circulating humoral factors that release calcium from bone (Fig. 17.2). This causes:

- Thirst
- Drowsiness
- Bone pain
- Constipation
- Renal failure
- Ectopic calcification.

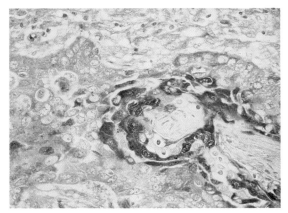

Fig. 17.2   Paraneoplastic humoral hypercalcaemia with parathyroid-related hormone protein produced by squamous carcinoma.

Syndrome of inappropriate antidiuretic hormone production (SIADH)

Water intoxication is associated with hyponatraemia and hypo-osmolality, especially with small cell lung cancer. It presents with:

- Drowsiness
- Confusion, progressing to coma.

Gynaecomastia

Inappropriate HCG production by testicular or lung cancers may cause unilateral or bilateral breast enlargement in men. Gynaecomastia also arises from liver disease, including liver cancer.

PREDISPOSING FACTORS IN CANCER

Both environmental and genetic factors are important in cancer pathogenesis.

ENVIRONMENTAL EXPOSURE TO CARCINOGENS

The social and occupational history is important in the assessment of patients with possible cancer in order to assess their likely exposure to environmental carcinogens (Box 17.3).

Exposure to infectious agents such as hepatitis virus in hepatomas, papilloma virus in cervical cancer, human immunodeficiency virus (HIV) in Kaposi's sarcoma, *Helicobacter pylori* infection in gastric cancer, and human T-cell leukaemia virus are important factors in the aetiology of cancer.

GENETIC FACTORS

It is important to consider the family history of cancer (Box 17.4). In some families Mendelian autosomal dominant predisposition to cancer occurs, involving one or a limited number of organ systems. Breast cancer, ovarian cancer and colon cancer develop in Lynch type II syndrome, renal cancer in von

---

BOX 17.3   Some environmental factors leading to cancer.

- Tobacco and lung cancer
- Alcohol and gastrointestinal cancer
- Ultraviolet light and skin cancer
- Dietary habits such as the chewing of betel nut in oral cancers
- Exposure to industrial carcinogens: asbestos exposure leads to mesothelioma, and heavy metals, leather tanning and coal tar products to bladder cancer
- Occupational hazards, e.g. radiation exposure in lung and prostate cancer
- Radon exposure in lung cancer.

Hippel–Lindau syndrome, parathyroid, adrenal, and pancreatic cancers in multiple endocrine neoplasia, and leukaemia, brain tumour and soft tissue sarcomas in the p53 deficient Li–Fraumeni syndrome. In certain other syndromes (e.g. neurofibromatosis type I of von Recklinghausen) there is particular susceptibility to CNS and peripheral nerve tumours, including vestibular schwannoma, and also to endocrine tumours (e.g. phaeochromocytoma). Other genes involved in susceptibility to specific cancers are beginning to be recognized, for example causing inherited susceptibility to breast cancer, to colon cancer associated with colonic polyposis, and to meningiomas. In the future, it is likely that testing for these susceptibility genes will be an important part of cancer screening in population-based programmes to prevent, and to offer early treatment of, cancer.

PHYSICAL EXAMINATION IN SUSPECTED CANCER

Cancer begins as a genetic change in a clone of cells or sometimes throughout a particular tissue field. At first little or no abnormality may be detected. Precursor lesions may be found on the skin, such as solar keratosis preceding squamous carcinoma, or dysplastic naevus preceding the development of melanoma.

In the mouth, lichen planus may precede oral mucosal cancer. Examination of the perineal region may reveal lichenification of the penis or vulva. Intra-epithelial neoplasia within the uterine cervix may be detected by *colposcopy*—visual inspection of the cervix and vaginal wall. Colonoscopy is used to detect dysplastic colonic polyps, and mammography to detect the microcalcification that is characteristic of ductal carcinoma in situ in the breast. In each organ system conventional physical examination is augmented by special investigative techniques, especially imaging (Box 17.5).

GENERAL ASSESSMENT

At the point of diagnosis, it is important to assess general health and fitness, and the effect that the cancer has had on the person's quality of life and functional capacity. The ECOG (Box 17.6) or

Karnovsky scales are simple Quality of Life instruments that are helpful in determining prognosis. People with low ECOG scores, about 3 or 4, have a generally poor prognosis and response to treatment. At this level the person is already severely disabled.

Recent weight loss, anaemia, and fatigue are important general features of cancer. Other non-specific features may be present, such as *finger clubbing*, *cyanosis* and *pulmonary osteoarthropathy*. Signs of metastatic or widespread disease are of especial importance in determining prognosis and the potential for therapy. For example, breathlessness

---

BOX 17.6   ECOG Performance Status Scale.

Status	Description
0.	Asymptomatic, fully active and able to carry out full predisease performance without restrictions.
1.	Symptomatic, fully ambulatory but restricted in physically strenuous activity and able to carry out performance of a light sedentary nature, e.g. light housework, office work.
2.	Symptomatic, ambulatory and capable of all self-care but unable to carry out any work activities. Up and about more than 50% of waking hours: in bed less than 50% of day.
3.	Symptomatic, capable of only limited self-care, confined to bed or chair more than 50% of waking hours, but not bedridden.
4.	Completely disabled. Cannot carry out any self-care. Totally bedridden.

may signify *pulmonary involvement*. The *painless jaundice* of pancreatic cancer and the nicotine-stained fingers of the lung cancer sufferer are important signs. Less commonly there may be roughening and thickening (*ichthyosis*), or darkening (*melanosis*) of the skin. The rash of *Herpes zoster* may be present. Leg oedema may occur due to *deep venous thrombosis*, when it is usually unilateral, or hypo-albuminaemia, or to lymphoedema, when it is usually bilateral. Symmetrical distal muscle wasting, often with painful tingling and sensory impairment may be due to *paraneoplastic peripheral neuropathy*.

In general, the presence of visible masses, distortion of the normal anatomy of an organ, enlargement of local superficial lymph nodes, or generalized lymphadenopathy, sometimes with splenomegaly, are sinister findings. In less advanced cancers a palpable mass, or a mass detectable on imaging but still localized to the tissue of origin, may be noted.

In the clinical examination, it is important to delineate the size and extent of the mass, to consider whether or not there is invasion across tissue boundaries into surrounding structures, and to detect distant, metastatic spread. Generally, the more pronounced the systemic symptoms the greater the likelihood that the disease is more extensive than it initially appears.

STAGING CANCER

Measuring the extent of the disease is termed 'staging the cancer'. A systematic approach is used, such as the *T (tumour), N (nodal), M (metastasis)* system (Box 17.7), or by site-specific conventions such as, for example, in breast cancer (Box 17.8), described as stages I, II, III, or IV. Some staging systems in use are sensitive to the tumour biology, for example those that describe the degree of infiltration of tumour in the primary tissue, as determined by

BOX 17.7   Cancer staging.

Cancers are commonly staged using the TNM (Tumour, Nodes, Metastases) system, which is a clinically-based method that can be applied to most cancers.

Clinical staging definitions

T = Size of the tumour and its spread to the skin and chest wall:
0 No primary tumour
1 Tumour no more than 2 cm
2 Tumour 2–5 cm
3 Tumour greater than 5 cm
4 Tumour with direct extension to the skin or chest wall

N = Extent of tumour spread to lymph nodes:
0 No growth present in axillary lymph nodes same side as primary tumour
1 Growth present in axillary lymph nodes same side as primary tumour, with axillary lymph nodes still moveable
2 Growth present in axillary lymph nodes same side as primary tumour, with axillary lymph nodes fixed to one another, or to other structures
3 Growth present in supraclavicular or infraclavicular nodes same side as primary tumour, or oedema of the arm

M = Metastases
0 No metastases
1 Metastases demonstrable

BOX 17.8   Breast cancer staging; how the two systems compare (the TNM system is explained in BOX 17.7).

	Clinical stage			
	1	2	3	4
T1N0M0	■			
T2N0M0	■			
T4N0M0*			■	
	1	2	3	4
T1N1M0		■		
T2N1M0		■		
T3N1M0			■	
T4N1M0			■	
	1	2	3	4
T1N2M0*			■	
T2N2M0			■	
T3N2M0*			■	
T4N2M0			■	
	1	2	3	4
T1N3M0*			■	
T2N3M0*			■	
T3N3M0*			■	
T4N3M0*			■	
T0-4, N0-3,M1				■

* Less common

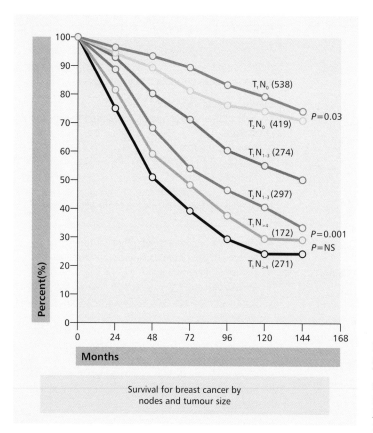

Survival for breast cancer by
nodes and tumour size

Fig. 17.3 Breast cancer; survival for operable disease, showing the relation of T and N staging to prognosis where N staging describes the number of involved nodes. From Moon T. E. et al American Journal of Clinical Oncology. 1987; 10: 396–403.

histological examination, for example, staging of cancer of the uterine cervix or of melanoma in the skin. These are important concepts, since the treatment of a tumour that has remained limited to tissue planes in its organ of origin will be different from that of a tumour that has metastasized widely throughout the body. Cancer staging provides a way of sorting patients into groups according to prognosis and so to enable the potential effect of any planned treatment to be estimated (Fig. 17.3). It is important also, therefore, in counselling the patient regarding management options.

SITE-SPECIFIC FEATURES

Cancers usually present with features suggestive of disease at their site of origin. The common presentations are noted below:

LYMPHATIC AND HAEMOPOIETIC CANCER

Lymphadenopathy occurs because there is invasion of the nodes draining the primary tumour site, or it may signify disseminated disease. When there is extensive nodal replacement by metastatic cancer in the axilla, groin or pelvis, distal lymphoedema with a woody pitting oedema involving the whole limb may occur. It is often difficult to distinguish neoplastic lymphoedema from oedema due to venous thrombosis, although cancerous lymphoedema is usually

more persistent and is not associated with venous engorgement.

Primary lymphomas cause painless, localized or generalized lymphatic enlargement, often with a smooth, rubbery texture to the enlarged glands. The haemopoietic system is often involved, leading to pallor, fever, and bruising, reflecting the anaemia, leukopenia, and thrombocytopenia of bone marrow failure (Box 17.9).

Lymphadenopathy, hepatomegaly, with fever splenomegaly and signs of weight loss are common features found on examination. Primary lymphoma sometimes commences in other organs, e.g. the lung (Fig. 17.4) or gastrointestinal tract, where it produces mass effects. Primary central nervous system lymphomas may closely resemble other neurological disorders in their clinical presentation.

RESPIRATORY SYSTEM CANCER

Primary lung cancer (Fig. 17.5) presents with symptoms and signs due to bronchial obstruction or to

BOX 17.9	Haemopoietic and lymphatic cancer.
Symptom	**Signs**
Night sweats, breathlessness	Anaemia and pallor
Fever	Leukopenia
Petechiae and bruising	Thrombocytopenia
Local pain and oedema	Lymphadenopathy

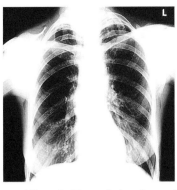
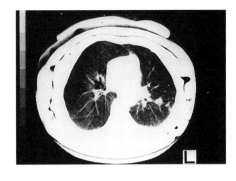

Fig. 17.4   Chest X-ray and thoracic CT scan in lymphoma. Pulmonary nodule (left lung) and hilar lymph nodes are seen in the CT image but not on the chest X-ray.

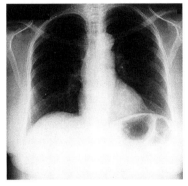
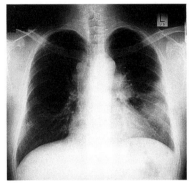

Fig. 17.5   Chest X-ray in lung cancer; left—normal chest X-ray; right—lung cancer, left lung field, with hilar lymphadenopathy.

BOX 17.10   Lung cancer.

Symptom	Signs
Cough	Clubbing
Breathlessness	Nicotine staining
Haemoptysis	Cyanosis
Pain on the medial surface the upper arm	Lower brachial root signs, Horner's syndrome

---

invasion of adjacent structures (Box 17.10). Pulmonary metastases from other primary sites, on the other hand, are frequently asymptomatic until very advanced. Common signs in primary lung cancer include those due to consolidation distal to an obstructed bronchus, to pleural or pericardial effusion, and to invasion of the chest wall. In pulmonary *lymphangitis carcinomatosa* there is extensive invasion of the pulmonary lymphatics, with or without a pulmonary mass, producing breathlessness that is disproportionately severe in comparison with the chest X-ray appearance, though not with the CT scan, which is more sensitive in revealing pulmonary infiltration and fibrosis.

Specific syndromes may occur, for example:

- Horner's syndrome (due to a malignant upper mediastinal mass), with recurrent laryngeal nerve palsy

- Brachial plexus infiltration from bronchogenic carcinoma in the apex of the lung, producing neuralgic pain along the medial surface of the upper arm near the axilla, with weakness and sensory loss in the distribution of the lower parts of the brachial plexus. This is often associated with ipsilateral Horner's syndrome (Pancoast syndrome).

CARDIOVASCULAR MALIGNANCY
The most common sign of cancer involving the vascular system is deep venous thrombosis (DVT) or thrombophlebitis in the leg (Box 17.11). There are no unique features to the DVT although sometimes there is a mass adjacent to the venous drainage. Thrombophlebitis may be associated with intravascular coagulation in small vessels, causing infarction or ulceration of the extremities (*thrombophlebitis*

BOX 17.11   Effects of venous compression by cancer.

Local venous compression by the cancer may cause:
- Superior vena caval obstruction causing cyanosis, swelling and oedema of the head and neck
- Inferior vena caval obstruction causing oedema of the lower trunk and leg
- The Budd–Chiari syndrome, consisting of hepatic venous obstruction. Thrombosis of the hepatic veins leads to portal hypertension and ascites.

obliterans) that heals only on successful treatment of the cancer. Disseminated intravascular coagulation causes generalized small vessel disease, with renal, hepatic, and cerebral failure (Fig. 17.6). Consumption coagulopathy, with a very low platelet count, may occur after severe haemorrhage.

The heart may be involved by direct extension from an adjacent malignancy (typically lung cancer), leading to arrhythmias if the atrium is invaded. Malignant invasion of the pericardium causes a blood-stained *pericardial effusion*. If cardiac tamponade develops cardiac output will be reduced, with a weak pulse, low blood pressure, and pulsus paradoxus (fall in cardiac output on inspiration). *Intracardiac thrombus*, for example, associated with renal cancer involving the inferior vena cava, can lead to a valve like obstruction to the right heart outflow with right heart failure, leading to raised jugular venous pressure and peripheral oedema, but without pulmonary oedema. *Marantic endocarditis*, a non-specific effect of generalized cancer, causes sterile vegetations on cardiac valves (Fig. 17.7), leading to systemic embolization.

Primary tumours on the left side of the heart (e.g. myxoma) are rare. They cause systemic embolism, a raised ESR and, sometimes, fever. Presentation with stroke or haematuria is typical.

BREAST CANCER

Most primary breast cancers present as a painless mass (Box 17.12) that may be associated with a discharge from the nipple. In Paget's disease of the nipple there is intra-epithelial spread of the cancer. In more advanced cases there may be tethering or dimpling of the skin of the breast, with oedema resembling an orange skin (*peau d'orange*). Sometimes the overlying skin is reddened and hot (inflammmatory breast cancer). The technique of examination of the breast is described below.

GASTROINTESTINAL CANCER

The cancer may present with an acute abdomen due to perforation, haemorrhage or obstruction of the involved organ (Box 17.13). If extensive, however, the disease causes progressive abdominal distension due to ascites and tumour mass, often with hepatomegaly or splenomegaly. If abdominal tumours present with signs of bowel obstruction; there is tympanitic distension of the abdomen, loss of normal bowel sounds, and an empty rectum. Gastric outflow obstruction may be associated with vomiting and an audible succussion splash on rocking the patient, caused by a fluid/air interface.

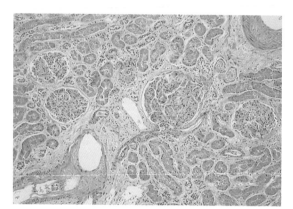

Fig. 17.6   Paraneoplastic intravascular coagulation with fibrin deposition in glomeruli of kidney.

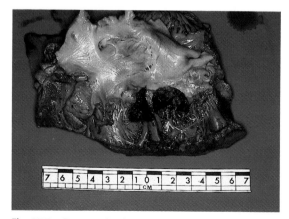

Fig. 17.7   Paraneoplastic post mortem specimen. Heart, showing marantic endocarditis and clot formation on mitral valve cusps, producing systemic emboli.

BOX 17.12   Breast cancer.

Symptom	Signs
Mass	Skin discoloration and tethering
Nipple discharge	Inflammation
Ulceration	Lymphadenopathy

BOX 17.13   Gastrointestinal malignancy.

Symptom	Signs
Dysphagia	Glossitis
Indigestion	Anaemia
Abdominal pain	Guarding
Nausea and vomiting	Jaundice and ascites
Haematemesis	Epigastric mass and tenderness
Melaena	Palpable colonic mass
Rectal bleeding	Palpable anal or retal mass
Pruritis and jaundice	Hepatomegaly and hepatic failure

BOX 17.14   Urological malignancy.

Symptom	Signs
Dysuria	Abdominal and pelvic mass
Frequency	Rectal prostatic mass
Incontinence	Penile or vulval ulceration
Haematuria	Testicular mass
Prostatism	Hard prostatic mass

GENITAL CANCER

Ulceration of the vulva or glans penis is a feature of squamous carcinoma. A genital mass (Box 17.14) is often associated with inguinal lymphadenopathy, due to secondary spread of the cancer to the regional lymphatics. Primary testicular masses are best appreciated as an irregularity in texture and shape of the testicle on bimanual palpation. The recent onset of varicocele of the testis may be a feature of primary renal malignancy. Para-aortic nodes are involved early in the disease.

PELVIC CANCER

Anal carcinoma presents with pain or haemorrhage. Routine perineal and rectal examination may reveal the cancer as a localized ulceration or mass. Rectal cancer often presents with rectal haemorrhage; an intramural mass is found by digital examination of the rectum or by proctoscopy (Box 17.15). Prostatic cancer is often palpable as enlargement of the prostate, with loss of normal consistency and of the contour of the median raphe of the gland, felt anterior to the rectum.

Pelvic cancer in women can be detected by vaginal examination. A mass may be felt within the vaginal wall or in the pelvic organs palpated through the vagina. Cancer of the cervix and uterus may be palpable or visible on speculum examination (colposcopy or hysteroscopy). Pelvic ultrasound or MRI are useful investigations (see Ch. 14).

HEAD AND NECK CANCER

Persistent ulceration of the mouth is often wrongly attributed to poorly fitting dentures. Persistent dysphagia and cough and recurrent blood-stained nasal discharge are often reported (Box 17.16). There is often pain in the mouth, tongue or face, and distortion of facial structures may develop later. Cranial nerve palsies occur, and there is lymphadenopathy or tonsillar enlargement.

MUSCULOSKELETAL CANCER

Soft tissue masses within muscular compartments, or bone masses or deformity, may develop with primary or secondary neoplasms. Primary sarcomas are sometimes necrotic, resembling soft tissue abscesses.

CENTRAL NERVOUS SYSTEM CANCER

Intrinsic brain tumours, for example gliomas, lead to progressive focal cerebral, cerebellar or spinal cord abnormalities. Seizures are common with cerebral tumours. Tumours may also arise from meninges (meningiomas), or from cranial nerves (vestibular schwannoma) or spinal nerve roots (neurofibroma). Pituitary tumours are also relatively common. Raised intracranial pressure causes early morning headache and vomiting, and papilloedema (Box 17.17). Malignant meningeal infiltration by metastatic carcinoma, lymphoma or sarcoma causes multiple cranial nerve or nerve root lesions associated with features of raised intracranial pressure, meningism, and confusion. A rapidly progressive transverse cord lesion with local pain and a spinal mass, often with evolving spinal deformity, is typical of metastatic disease involving the spine.

ENDOCRINE CANCER

The cancer presents as a localized mass in superficial endocrine glands (e.g. the thyroid gland) with features of endocrine overactivity or underactivity (Box 17.18). Neighbouring structures may be involved in contiguity, as the recurrent laryngeal nerve with thyroid cancer, and the optic nerves and chiasm with pituitary tumours. Many endocrine cancers are malignant and may metastasize to nearby lymph nodes or more widely, especially thyroid cancer.

BOX 17.17 CNS malignancy.

Symptom	Signs
Headache and vomiting	Mental function
Convulsions	Focal neurological signs
Loss of function	

BOX 17.18 Primary endocrine cancer.

Symptom	Signs
Hoarseness	Thyroid mass
Headache, sweats	Hypertension, oedema
Palpitations, nausea	Adrenal mass, pallor, hypertension, phaeochromocytoma
Hypoglycaemic coma and history of dyspepsia	Pancreatic mass, insulinoma/gastrinoma
Polyuria, polydipsia	Pituitary mass
Visual field loss	Hypopituitarism
Fatigue	Buccal pigmentation of hypoadrenalism

BOX 17.15 Gynaecological malignancy.

Symptom	Signs
Vulval pruritis	Vulval ulceration
Vaginal discharge	Cervical mass
Vaginal bleeding	Pelvic mass
Pelvic pain	Mass, discharge or bleeding

BOX 17.16 Head and neck malignancy.

Symptom	Signs
Taste, swallowing disturbed	Ulceration
Hearing, voice abnormal	Discharge and bleeding
Persistent cough	Cranial nerve palsies
Sinusitis	Lymphadenopathy

SKIN CANCER

Cancers of the skin develop in cetain predisposing conditions, for example xeroderma pigmentosa, and in light-skinned European peoples in response to excessive exposure to sunlight. Melanoma, a highly malignant tumour that metastasizes early and widely, and basal cell carcinoma, a less malignant tumour, are particularly common. Kaposi's sarcoma is a cutaneous cancer that is common in immunosuppressed persons, especially those with AIDS. The important features are a change in size, shape or in pigmentation of a pre-existing skin lesion, local irritation in the lesion, and bleeding from it. Solar keratoses are common and most do not presage malignancy. Skin cancers often develop in skin not usually exposed to the sun, except in sunbathers or outdoor workers, for example on the back or upper arm.

BREAST CANCER: THE APPROACH TO DIAGNOSIS

Cancer of the breast is a common problem in most Western countries. Considerable medical resource is expended in the early detection of breast cancer (Fig. 17.8) in order to facilitate early treatment and thus to improve the prognosis. The diagnosis may therefore be suspected from presymptomatic testing, such as mammography, or in the case of a woman who has discovered a painless mass in her breast. In both situations, careful clinical examination of the breast and its related structures is required in order to plan investigation and management and to stage the tumour.

EXAMINATION OF THE BREAST

Clinical assessment of any symptomatic mass in the breast should be completed by the performance of mammography, ultrasonography and fine needle aspiration cytology, preferably in a dedicated 'one stop' triple assessment clinic. Assessment of an asymptomatic mass, identified by mammography,

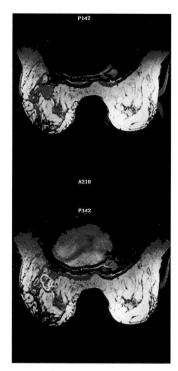

Fig. 17.9   MR scan; breast cancer. Unenhanced (upper image) and gadolinium enhanced scans of the right breast, showing a breast cancer. Arterial phase image linked to cardiac cycle.

ultrasound or MR imaging (Fig. 17.9), requires clinical examination and biopsy/excision. Examination of one breast should always be complemented by the examination of the breast on the other side, using clinical and mammographic techniques. Breast cancer occasionally occurs in men, and requires the same careful examination technique.

As for any intimate examination, the examiner should explain what is about to be done, describe the purpose of the examination, and seek verbal consent. Male doctors should ensure the presence of a female chaperone whenever possible. Cultural beliefs should be acknowledged and a request for a female examiner should be respected.

Inspection

The initial inspection of the breast should be carried out with the patient seated to assess any asymmetry, visible mass, distortion or skin tethering (Fig. 17.8). Involvement of the deeper fascia causes dimpling of the skin of the breast. Nipple discharge or ulceration, and inflammatory erythema and oedema of the dermis, termed *peau d'orange*, are all signs that suggest carcinoma of the breast. Lymphadenopathy in the axilla or supraclavicular fossa may be visible. It may cause lymphoedema of the ipsilateral arm, because the lymphatic drainage from the arm is obstructed by infiltration of the axillary nodes with cancer.

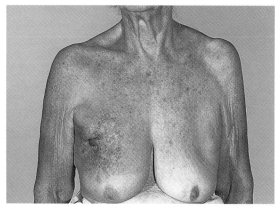

Fig. 17.8   Breast cancer: right breast mass with skin invasion causing tethering and incipient ulceration.

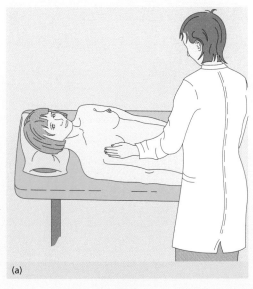

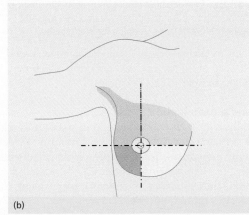

Fig. 17.10 Palpation of the breast in the supine position; the four quadrants should be carefully and systematically palpated.

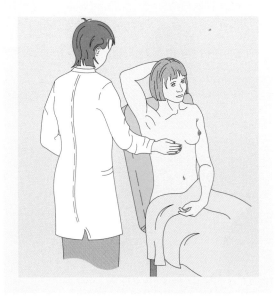

Fig. 17.11 Palpation of the breast in the semi-recumbent position; this technique may reveal additional information.

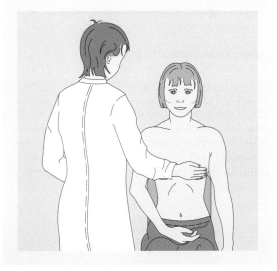

Fig. 17.12 Palpation of the axilla; it is important to ensure the patient is fully relaxed.

Palpation of the breast

At first the patient should lie in a near supine position on the examination couch so that the breast to be examined can readily be palpated between the flat of the examiner's hand and the chest wall posteriorly (Fig. 17.10). If the breasts are at all large this may best be achieved by asking the patient to lie in a semi-decubitus position with the ipsilateral arm raised, and her hand placed behind her head (Fig. 17.11). During a woman's reproductive years normal breast tissue has a lobular consistency which becomes more pronounced during the oestrogenic phase of each menstrual cycle. After the menopause, there is replacement of the breast parenchyma with adipose tissue which retains a slightly, but less marked, nodular consistency.

Gentle initial palpation of the four quadrants of the breast, including the axillary tail, is followed by more detailed palpation, using thumb and forefinger, of any suspected mass lesion(s) to define size, consistency, fixation to skin or deep fascia and relationship to nipple and areolar complex.

Palpation of the axilla

Next, examination of the axillary contents is carried out (Fig. 17.12). The examiner's right hand is placed in the patient's left axilla, and vice versa. The patient's arm is passively brought down with the examiner's other hand so as to relax the axillary tissue and allow palpation of the medial axillary wall. Sometimes it may be necessary to palpate the other three walls of the axilla.

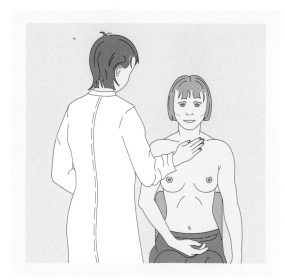

Fig. 17.13   Palpation of the anterior cervical (supraclavicular) lymph nodes from the front.

Palpation of the cervical lymph nodes

Careful palpation of the supraclavicular and infraclavicular regions, and of the anterior and posterior cervical triangles, completes the examination (Fig. 17.13).

Examination in the sitting position

Assessment of the axillary and cervical nodes should then be repeated with the patient seated to evaluate the upper axilla more closely, and to allow examination of the supraclavicular fossae from behind. This posterior approach to the supraclavicular nodes often proves to be more sensitive in the detection of minor degrees of lymph nodal enlargement (Fig. 17.14). The sitting position enables a final inspection of the

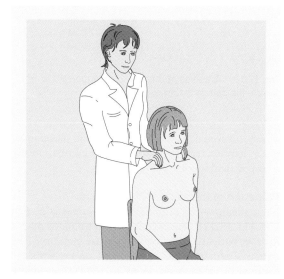

Fig. 17.14   Posterior approach to palpation of the anterior cervical nodes—often more sensitive than the anterior approach.

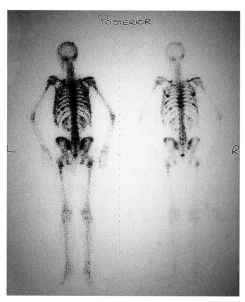

Fig. 17.15   Radionuclide whole body scan showing rib metastases in a patient with breast cancer—a useful imaging method when screening for metastases.

breasts to evaluate their shape and symmetry, and to look once more for any skin tethering which may be brought to light in this position.

General examination

Finally, a full general examination must be carried out to consider whether there are any evident distant metastases, for example, in the ribs, spine, brain or liver. Appropriate CT, ultrasound or radionuclide imaging is used to supplement this clinical examination (Fig. 17.15).

THYROID ENLARGEMENT AND THYROID CANCER

The thyroid gland is enlarged in endocrine disease (e.g. Hashimoto's thyroiditis) and in endemic iodine deficiency (endemic goitre), and also in thyroid cancer, when it may be nodular. Examination of the thyroid should be carried out systematically. The endocrine aspects of the thyroid examination are considered in Chapter 8.

IS THE THYROID ENLARGED?

The normal thyroid is impalpable, or just palpable. Enlargement may be diffuse, or nodular. The enlarged gland maybe visible in the neck, below the larynx, especially in a thin person. The gland may be enlarged below the sternum—*retrosternal goitre*—and therefore neither visible nor palpable in the neck. The latter is unusual. When assessing enlargement of the thyroid, *look at the patient in a good light*, preferably one arranged to shine across the patient from above and a little to one side. Make sure the patient's neck and shoulders are fully exposed. Ask the patient to swallow, and watch to see if you can observe the gland move up and down. *Palpate the gland* from the front, and then stand behind the seated patient and examine the gland with both hands, lightly palpating it with your fingertips on either side, as the patient swallows a few times.

Occasionally a *thyroglossal cyst*, an embryological remnant, may mimic thyroid enlargement in the neck. This can be differentiated by asking the patient to put out the tongue—the thyroglossal cyst will move up as the tongue is protruded, since it is fixed to the base of the tongue.

THYROID ENLARGEMENT

Start by considering the *size, contour and symmetry* of the thyroid. *Look* at the neck, watch the patient *swallowing*, and *protruding the tongue*. Look for signs of *overactivity or underactivity* of the thyroid gland. Then *palpate* the neck. Finally *listen for a bruit* over the gland.

In *thyrotoxicosis* the thyroid is enlarged, and has a *soft* consistency. The increased vascularity of the enlargement of Grave's disease causes a bruit that can best be heard with the bell of the stethoscope placed over the gland. Ask the patient to hold the breath briefly while you assess this. There may also be a palpable thrill. *Hard, firm, enlargement* suggests *Hashimoto's thyroiditis*, an autoimmune disease of the thyroid. This is often *multi-nodular*, and may present with *acute painful haemorrhage* into a large nodule. Haemorrhage into a thyroid nodule is always an indication for surgical assessment since it may be recurrent and cause respiratory obstruction. Hashimoto's disease is associated with *vitiligo*, and with the presence of circulating thyroid antibodies.

The thyroid gland should always be moveable during swallowing, or during palpation by the examiner. If the gland is fixed the possibility of thyroid malignancy should be considered. A single nodule also suggests thyroid cancer. Undifferentiated fast-growing tumours of the thyroid are often fixed to underlying tissues at presentation, indicating spread beyond the confines of the gland. Multiple nodules can feel firm or cystic, and may be benign, due to thyroiditis, or malignant. All thyroid nodules should be regarded with suspicion.

A retrosternal goitre, or extension of a visible goitre in the neck, can be detected by percussion over the sternum. A dull note indicates the presence of thyroid tissue in the chest.

Goitre and endocrine status

In autoimmune thyroiditis the enlarged gland may be underactive or overactive depending on the stage of the disease. In Hashimoto's disease, the disease begins with a phase of overactivity and is then followed by enlargement and underactivity as the gland is destroyed and replaced by scar tissue. Iodine-deficient goitres are often euthyroid, or mildly hypothyoid (see Fig. 8.7). In thyroid cancer the gland is usually euthyroid.

Palpating cervical nodes in thyroid disease

This is carried out as for any other clinical situation, using both anterior and posterior palpation. Nodes in the posterior triangle, the jugulo-digastric region and the supraclavicular region are particularly important when thyroid cancer is suspected.

Signs of hyperthyroidism and hypothyroism

These are described in Chapter 8.

Investigating thyroid enlargement

Ultrasound is useful in detecting cysts and nodules, especially when there is only one nodule palpable clinically. The discovery of a multi-nodular gland suggests autoimmune disease. *Needle aspiration* of nodules allows cytological analysis, an important investigation in planning further management. *CT scanning* is the definitive investigation to exclude or assess retrosternal extension of a cervical goitre. A search for thyroglobulin and cytoplasmic antibodies to thyroid cells is useful in suspected autoimmune thyroid disease. Thyroid function tests are essential in assessing management. Multiple endocrine neoplasia should be considered (see above).

PLANNING INVESTIGATION WHEN CANCER IS SUSPECTED

In general, imaging, endoscopic, biochemical and haematological investigations should be directed to suspected abnormalities, as suggested by the history and physical examination. Both functional and structural investigations, but especially imaging, are indicated (see Ch. 22).

DIAGNOSTIC IMAGING

Having identified a primary tumour, the common sites of metastatic spread should also be imaged in order to 'stage' the tumour. The different methods of imaging and assessment for each tumour site provide information for both diagnosis and staging. Not all investigations will be necessary for every patient; just those sufficient to provide the necessary information (Box 17.5).

For any potential primary tumour site investigation should start with the simplest, most informative test, and proceed to more selective tests. Frail, elderly patients do not tolerate barium enema or colonoscopy well and are better investigated first with an unprepared CT scan. Cross-sectional scanning with CT or MRI is more sensitive and more specific than plain radiology in detecting mass lesions, especially when, for example, mammography or radionuclide bone

BOX 17.19   Identifying the primary site in adenocarcinoma of unknown primary (ACUP).

Investigation	Investigational yield
CT scan	35–40%
CXR	12–24%
IVU	6–9%
Barium enema	5–9%
Barium meal	4–6%
Thyroid scan	8%

BOX 17.20   Proportion of primary sites found by CT scan (ACUP).

Site	Proportion found by CT scan
Lung	70%
Pancreas	86%
Ovary	67%
Renal	56%
Colorectal	36%
Hepatobiliary	33%
Oesophagus	20%

scanning produce equivocal results (Box 17.19 and Box 17.20).

CYTOLOGY AND HISTOLOGY

The diagnosis of cancer can only be made definitively by microscopic examination of a suitable tissue sample. After the tumour has been localized, clinically and by imaging, a biopsy taken by needle aspiration or open biopsy, or cytological study of an effusion or a bodily fluid is used for histological diagnosis (Box 17.21). Sometimes stereotaxic methods are used to localize the tumour.

In addition to classic histopathology, special immunohistochemical and molecular biological techniques, to search for particular cell-specific proteins or genes, have been applied to the diagnosis of cancers, leading to a fundamental reappraisal of many older diagnostic categories.

HAEMATOLOGY

The full blood count may reveal *anaemia*, such as microcytic hypochromic anaemia associated with gastrointestinal blood loss, or macrocytic anaemia associated with pernicious anaemia and gastric

BOX 17.21   Diagnosis of cancer.

- Cytology—effusions
  - fine needle aspirate
  - exfoliated cells (lung, cervix, bladder, pancreas)
- Histological—biopsy for pathology and immunohistochemistry

cancer, or leucoerythroblastic anaemia with bone marrow infiltration. An *elevated ESR*, though often non-specific, may be associated with rouleaux formation and hyperviscosity in myeloma. *Leucopenia and thrombocytopenia, or leucocytosis*, may be associated with leukaemia or lymphoma involving the bone marrow, often with an altered differential white blood cell count and the presence of abnormal and immature forms in the circulation.

BIOCHEMISTRY

Uraemia may complicate primary and secondary cancers of the urological tract. *Hypokalaemic alkalosis* should suggest Cushing's syndrome, which may occur as a secondary hormonal disorder (see above). *Hypotonic hyponatraemia* is a feature of inappropriate ADH secretion. In rapidly proliferating cancers, such as lymphoma or leukaemia, raised serum urate levels occur, causing acute gout. *Hypercalcaemia* follows secretion of parathyroid-related cytokines (see above), or when there is bone destruction by osteoclast activation, or by bone metastases.

Liver function is usually normal even when there is extensive metastatic involvement of the liver but there may be pronounced hypoalbuminaemia in association with cancer cachexia. Raised alkaline phosphatase is common without liver metastases. A raised lactic dehydrogenase (LDH) level may reflect released LDH directly elaborated by the tumour rather than the liver.

TUMOUR MARKERS

Tumour markers are often used in diagnosis and follow-up to ascertain tumour response (Table 17.1). For example, raised alpha fetoprotein (AFP), human chorionic gonadotrophin (hCG) and lactic dehydrogenase (LDH) levels are found in 80% of testicular

TABLE 17.1   Tumour markers commonly used in diagnosis and management.

Marker	Tumour
Alpha fetoprotein (AFP)	Gonadal germ cell tumours
Human chorionic gonadotrophin (hCG)	Hydatidiform mole
Lactate dehydrogenase (LDH)	Common but non-specific; many rapidly growing cancers
CA125	Ovarian epithelial cancers
Carcinoembryonic antigen (CEA)	Gastrointestinal cancers
CA19.9	Pancreatic cancers
CA15.3	Breast cancers
Prostate specific antigen (PSA)	Prostate cancers

germ cell tumours. However, seminomas are only associated with a raised LDH.

All tumour markers currently used in diagnosis are glycoproteins that are expressed by tumour cells and released into the circulation. They are detected by immunoassay. It is important to recognize that they are not invariably detected and that none are cancer-specific. Thus, while providing corroborative evidence, they are not in themselves sufficient for diagnosis. For example, 80% of testicular germ cell tumours produce either alpha fetoprotein or human chorionic gonadotrophin. Nonetheless, both these glycoproteins may be produced ectopically by other cancers such as small cell lung cancer.

About 80% of ovarian epithelial cancers produce CA125 but many other cancers (e.g. uterus, pancreas, lung and breast cancers, and also benign inflammatory disorders of the peritoneum) are associated with a raised CA125. Prostate specific antigen is elevated in about 80% of cancers and is also increased in the normal older male population and in benign prostatic hypertrophy, it is also found associated with some other cancers. Only 50% of bowel cancers are associated with a raised serum CEA. Thus, a normal CEA value is unhelpful and the main value of any such test is in monitoring patients once the diagnosis has been established.

NEUROPEPTIDES

Carcinoid tumours may elaborate neuropeptides. The general metabolite 5-hydroxyindole acetic acid (5HIAA) may be estimated in a 24 urine-collection, or in the serum. Substances such as insulin, gastrin, glucagon and vaso-intestinal polypeptide may also be detected in the serum. Ectopic production of ACTH, usually by lung cancers, may lead to Cushing's syndrome and elevated serum fasting cortisol with bilateral adrenal hyperplasia.

URINALYSIS

Haematuria or proteinuria should lead to investigation of the upper and lower urological tracts. Occasionally proteinuria is due to a non-local effect of cancer, such as the Bence Jones light chain proteinuria of myeloma.

CANCER OF UNKNOWN PRIMARY SITE

The patient presenting with metastatic cancer of unknown origin is a common diagnostic problem. Investigation should be determined by careful consideration of the histology followed by a thorough search for the primary. However, the investigation should be guided by pragmatism. There are few primary sites for which treatment, in the presence of metastases, will result in greatly improved survival and quality of life (Box 17.22).

With this in mind, investigations for adenocarcinoma of unknown origin should be directed at detecting cancers of the prostate, breast and ovary even though this is likely to account for only 5–10% of all cases. The two most common sites of origin are lung and pancreas, accounting for 20–30% each, but with a limited prognosis when there is metastatic disease. Routine imaging in the absence of any site-specific symptoms would therefore include nasal endoscopy (for squamous cancers), chest X-ray, mammography (in women), CT or MR scan of abdomen and pelvis, and transrectal ultrasound (in men). Apart from testicular cancer, tumour markers are not specific enough to be of diagnostic help.

Other specialized investigations should be selected by symptoms or signs suggesting particular organ system involvement. A primary site may not be found in half the patients, but most will be diagnosed by careful history and physical examination, with appropriate ancillary investigation.

BOX 17.22   Metastatic tumours for which treatment of the primary improves the prognosis.

- High grade lymphomas
- Germ cell tumours
- Squamous cancers of the oropharynx
- Adenocarcinoma of prostate, breast or ovary

18
CHILDREN AND NEONATES

INTRODUCTION

'If a child cries when you examine it, then it's probably your fault.' This rather sweeping statement was made by the late John Apley, an eminent paediatrician in Bristol. The basic philosophy is right. The examiner cannot avoid some discomfort in some parts of the physical examination, but during most of the examination the child should be contented. This is the essence of the art of examining children. A child who struggles and screams is afraid, and the examiner must spend time trying to gain their confidence. The consulting room must have a range of toys suitable for all ages, and the child should be allowed to play with whatever takes his or her fancy. If old enough, the child should be allowed to explore the room, although dissuaded from playing with expensive or potentially dangerous equipment. Younger children will be sitting on their parent's lap, and for some of the time regarding you with suspicion. Do not be afraid to stop what you are doing to pull a face or offer a toy that seems to have caught the child's attention.

As the family enter the room, they should be greeted in a friendly way, and introductions made. Ascertain who is with the child. It may not be the mother, but another family member, who, in a mixed ethnic population, may be the only one who speaks English. If you can get everyone to relax and laugh in the first few minutes, the child will relax and the subsequent history and examination will be easier. White coats have no part to play in paediatric practice as they frighten and intimidate most children. They should not be worn under any circumstances.

While talking to the mother, an essential part of the examination is to watch the child. Does the child look unwell? Is he or she interested in the surroundings and exploring them, or apathetic? Watch the child running around: are there any obvious abnormalities in the gait? Is the face normal, or are there features of abnormal development? Are there any obvious physical abnormalities? Is breathing unusually noisy? Does the child seem well-nourished, or wasted?

HISTORY

The history (Box 18.1) will normally be taken from the mother, but when you are seeing an older child, involve him or her by asking relevant points such as the site of a pain etc. Always take notice of what the mother is saying, and listen to her complaints. Do not

- Birth
- Milestones
- Mental and physical development
- School
- Specific illnesses, accidents, etc.
- Immunizations
- Contacts and travel
- Family history
- Social history
- Consanguinity and genetic risk

be tempted to interrupt a mother in full flow to try and ask what you think is a clever question. The mother will know what is worrying her about her child, and any interruptions should be to guide her rather than try and impose your diagnosis on her. Most of all, do not keep looking at your watch or the pile of notes in front of you. A mother and child must be made to feel that they have your whole attention, and that you have all the time in the world for them. Other relatives tend not to be such good historians as the parents, and if well-meaning relatives try to give you the history, make it very clear that it is the parent's view you need, even if this involves the use of an interpreter (but see above). Older children are quite capable of giving a history of their current problems and should be encouraged to do so. All the time you are talking to the parents, keep watching everything that the child is doing and their reactions.

The structure of the history is no different from that of an adult, consisting of presenting complaint, history of the present illness, and history of any previous illness. In children, enquire particularly as to the nature and severity of *previous illnesses*, the age at which they occurred, for example infectious diseases, seizures, bowel disturbances, upper respiratory tract infections, discharging ears and cough. In the case of a cough, always ask when it is worse (for example, asthma sufferers tend to cough at night and when running around), and if vomiting or a 'whoop' is present. Has the child been taking any drugs? Has he or she ever been in hospital, and if so, what was wrong? Have there been any accidents, physical injuries, burns or poisoning incidents?

Next the examiner should pay more specific attention to the *pregnancy, newborn period and developmental progress.* (Box 18.2).

At this point it is worth asking if the parents have kept any record of child health clinic attendance, such as a 'baby book', containing dates of attendance at hospital or clinic, weights, immunizations, etc.

It is important to ask about the *'milestones of development'*: When did the child first sit up, smile, crawl, walk and talk? Fuller details will be found below Table 18.2.

- Was the mother well during her pregnancy?
- Did she have any particular illnesses, or was she taking any drugs (including alcohol)?
- Was the baby born at term?
- What were the birth weight and type of delivery?
- Were there any problems in the newborn period?
  —jaundice?
  —breathing problems?
  —fits?
  —feading difficulties?
- How was the baby fed?
- If bottle-fed, which milk was used?
- When were solid foods introduced?
- Were vitamin drops given and, if so, how many?
- Was the weight gain satisfactory?

General questions are important (Box 18.3).

Ask about *routine immunizations*, and if they have all been given.

FAMILY HISTORY
- How old are the parents?
- How many children are there in the family?
- What are their ages and sex?
- Have there been any stillbirths, miscarriages or other childhood deaths in the family?
- Are there any illnesses in the siblings, parents or any near relatives?
- Is there any background of inherited disease?

SOCIAL HISTORY
Approach the social history with diplomacy; sometimes it is more prudent to leave deeper probing to a subsequent occasion. It is useful to know about living conditions, and whether either or both parents are employed. If the mother is working, there is some daily separation from the child. Ask if the child has ever been separated from her for any time in the past, as this may be the basis of a variety of behavioural difficulties. Find out if the child's parents live

- What are the child's present habits with regard to eating, sleeping, bowels and micturition?
- What sort of child is he or she?
- Is he or she robust or moody?
- Does he or she cry a lot?
- How does the child compare with siblings or friends of the same age?
- If of school age, what school does the child go to, and how is he or she getting on?
- Does the child miss much time from school and, if so, why? Ask the child if they like school, and one or two questions about it, such as who is their best friend, and the name of their teacher.

together and whether there is any difficulty in the relationship. Is there a supportive family structure involving other relatives, e.g. grandparents? If the family are immigrants, it is important to know how long they have been in their new country. The depth of enquiry in a paediatric social history must always be judged on an individual basis. If the family think that you are prying too much, you may lose the rapport that you have been building up.

Now may be the time to consider talking either to the child or to the parents without the other party being present. This may be particularly valuable in the case of adolescent children, who are often rather resentful of their parents telling you all their problems, and this is the opportunity for them to relax with you. Ask them about the illness, and also a little about themselves and their interests. Parents may also welcome an opportunity to talk in private with you, and it is often during such discussion that the real reason for the consultation emerges. This can be accomplished most easily while the child is undressing or dressing.

By this time you should already have formed an impression of the child, the family, and their relationship, and you are now ready to proceed with the examination. By now, a younger child should have found you such a fascinating person that they will be prepared to cooperate with you in most parts of the physical examination. Alternatively, the child may have become so bored that he or she is asleep. In either case physical examination should present no problems. If the child is crying loudly by now, then you are in for a difficult time, and you should be asking yourself where you went wrong.

EXAMINATION

Older children will usually cooperate sufficiently to be examined lying down, and routine physical examination is no different from an adult examination. A younger child should be examined sitting on his or her mother's lap, as any attempt to get the child to lie down will result in instant distress. Always talk to children, however young; do not be afraid of looking silly if the result is a cooperative child. Those parts of the examination which are painful or unpleasant should be left until last: if an attempt is made to examine a child's throat at the outset, the immediate response will be a crying child. Offer the child something to play with—even a stethoscope will be a source of amusement to a young infant. Children often find it amusing if you examine their toy first. Sometimes a small toy clipped onto the stethoscope is distracting enough for a young child to let you examine them without problem. Try to follow the scheme set out in Boxes 18.4 and 18.5.

Start the examination by asking the mother to undress the child. Do not make her hurry. Remember

---

> **BOX 18.4   Assessments to include in the examination of children.**
>
> - Observe
> - Listen
> - Play
> - Palpate
> - Specific clinical tests
> - Other 'background' tests

> **BOX 18.5   Schema for examination of children.**
>
> - Feet
> - Hands and pulse
> - Face
> - Head
> - Neck
> - Abdomen
> - Chest
> - Neurological
> - Eyes and fundoscopy
> - Genitalia, groins, anus
> - Other invasive clinical tests

---

that even very young children may be modest, and prefer to keep their underpants on. Wash your hands while the child is being undressed. Examination should now proceed by the usual method of inspection, palpation, percussion and auscultation; however, no set routine can be followed, and the examination is by regions rather than by systems. Each child will dictate the order of the examination by their reactions to various procedures (Box 18.5).

In general, start with the least threatening manoeuvres. Note again the state of *nutrition* now that the child is undressed. If there are bruises on young children, except on the shins, be suspicious of non-accidental injury. Are there any obvious rashes to be seen? Are there any naevi or other skin anomalies?

THE LIMBS

Often the feet are the easiest place to start. There is nothing threatening to the average child about a doctor tickling their feet. This simple trick gives you the first opportunity to touch the child, and will also allow the feet to be checked for a variety of problems such as minor varus deformities, overriding toes, or such minor plantar abnormalities as flat feet. It is then very easy to run your hands over the child's legs at the same time, noting any knee or other bony abnormalities. Note any muscle wasting or tenderness, and the movements of the knee and ankle. At the same time an assessment of the muscle tone should be made, as this seems to the child just an extension of the funny game already being played by this strange but interesting doctor. It is easy to notice at the same time whether the skin is dry or moist, and to feel any skin lesions that you may have noticed. All the time the child's reactions should be watched. Is he or she still your friend? Be prepared to stop what you are doing if the child seems to be getting upset, and spend a few minutes trying to re-establish the rapport that you have just built up.

By now there should be no major objections to the rest of the body being felt. The *arms and shoulders* should be examined next, followed by the *hands*. Do the hands have a single palmar crease, as seen in children with Down's syndrome and in a variety of other syndromes, as well as in a small proportion of normal children? Feel the *wrists* for widening of the epiphyses of the radius and ulna—a sign of rickets. Try to feel the pulse and count it, although this will be difficult in a plump, young infant; the rate is best counted at this age when auscultating the chest.

THE HEAD, FACE AND NECK

Look at the child's face and ask yourself the following questions.

- Does it look normal?
- If the baby looks odd, then do not forget to look at the parents. It may then be obvious that what you regard as abnormal may be nothing more than a family trait. If the appearance is still not too clear, ask who the baby looks like.
- Does the child have a large tongue?
- Are the ears in the normal position, or are they low-set and abnormal in any way? There are many hundreds of syndromes diagnosable by the facial appearance, and the salient features should be carefully noted.

Next note the shape of the *head*. It may be abnormally shaped, owing to premature fusion of the sutures, small if the baby is *microcephalic*, or globular if the baby is *hydrocephalic*, sometimes with dilated veins over the skin surface. It is often asymmetrical (*plagiocephalic*) in normal infants who tend to lie with their heads persistently on one side (Fig. 18.1). This shape of skull is now very much commoner because babies are placed on their backs to reduce the risk of sudden death in infancy. The parents can be reassured that the head will be normal as the baby grows up.

Assuming that you are still friends, there should be no objection to your feeling the child's head now. Leave the measurement of the head circumference to a little later in the examination, as some babies find this a little threatening, and may start crying. Feel the anterior fontanelle. It is normally small at birth, enlarges during the first 2 months, and then gradually decreases in size until final closure. It is normally closed by 18 months of age, but can close much earlier, and has been reported as staying open in a few normal girls until $4\frac{1}{2}$ years of age. Delayed closure may be seen, however, in *rickets, hypothy-*

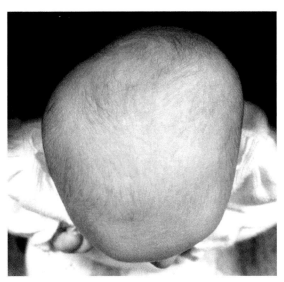

Fig. 18.1   Plagiocephalic skull.

roidism and *hydrocephalus*. An assessment of the tension of the anterior fontanelle is important. In health it pulsates and is in the same plane as the rest of the surrounding skull. A tense, bulging fontanelle indicates *raised intracranial pressure*, but it does also become tense with crying. A sunken fontanelle is a feature of dehydration. The posterior fontanelle is located by passing the finger along the sagittal suture to its junction with the lambdoid sutures. It should normally be closed after 2 months of age. Sometimes a small notch is felt over the vault of the cranium when passing the finger along the sagittal suture. This is the third fontanelle, and although it can be normal, it is seen in some chromosome abnormalities and in congenital infections such as rubella. While feeling the head, any ridging of the sutures should be noticed, suggesting premature fusion (*craniostenosis*), or overriding of the sutures if the head is small (*microcephaly*). The sutures tend to be separated in the neonatal period, and there is sometimes a continuous gap from the forehead to the posterior part of the posterior fontanelle. Sutures close rapidly, and are normally ossified by 6 months of age.

Having assessed the skull, the *neck* can be checked, paying particular attention to the presence of lymph nodes. It is common in childhood to feel small lymph nodes in the anterior and posterior triangles of the neck, as they enlarge rapidly in response to local conditions such as tonsillitis. They tend to persist for some years, but parents can generally be reassured that they are of no major significance. Examination of other lymphatic areas can be carried out at a later stage of the examination—the inguinal nodes when the napkin area is checked, and the axillary nodes when the chest is examined. In young babies the sternomastoid muscles should be checked for the thickened area known as a sternomastoid tumour.

THE ABDOMEN

The abdomen can be a little difficult to examine if the baby is crying, but most infants will be quite happy sitting on their mother's lap (Fig. 18.2). The abdomen, especially in toddlers, often gives an impression of being protuberant. Causes of true abdominal distension are shown in Box 18.6. If they are crying, it is sometimes possible to quieten them by placing them over their mother's shoulder, and examining them from behind. Small infants can be given a feed to quieten them. Look for any obvious distension or for peristaltic waves suggesting intestinal obstruction. Remember that in children up to the age of 3 years the abdomen is rather protuberant. Note the umbilicus, and whether or not there is a hernia. Palpation should be gentle and light. The liver edge can be felt in normal children up to the age of 4 years; it can be anything up to 2 cm below the costal margin. When enlarged, the spleen may be felt below the left costal margin, and in infancy it is more anterior and superficial than in the older child or adult. Slight enlargement of the spleen is common in children with many infections. Faecal masses can be felt in the left iliac fossa in constipated children, and a full or distended bladder presents as a mass arising from the pelvis. Abdominal tenderness is best detected by watching the child's facial expression during palpation. Deep palpation of the kidneys can be carried out last. Although it would be logical to examine the groin area at this time, it is often better to do this at a slightly later stage. If the child has cried persistently, it is still possible to examine the abdomen by the method of *ballottement*—as the baby breathes in, the abdominal muscles relax, and abdominal viscera and other masses, if present, can then be palpated.

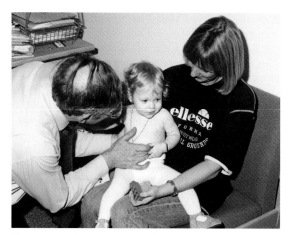

Fig. 18.2 Baby sitting on mother's lap while the abdomen is examined.

BOX 18.6   Causes of abdominal distension.

- Obese child
- Faeces (constipation, Hirschsprung's disease)
- Ascites (nephrotic syndrome, cirrhosis)
- Gas (intestinal obstruction, swallowed air)
- Pregnancy in adolescent girls
- Gastric
- Distended bladder (lower abdomen)
- Pyloric stenosis (upper abdomen)

THE CHEST

So far, nothing has been done that should cause the child any concern. Examining the chest, however, introduces the stethoscope, which sometimes worries babies. It helps to have earlier let the baby play with the stethoscope. Check for any asymmetry, and in girls for any breast development. Minor degrees of pes excavatum are a source of great anxiety to many parents, but are not usually of any importance. Indrawing of the lower ribs (*Harrison's sulcus*) may be seen in obstructive airway disease, either from asthma or a blocked nasopharynx from adenoidal hypertrophy. Note any recession when breathing, and count the respiratory rate. In a new born infant it should be 40 breaths/min, by the second year it has fallen to 30 breaths/min and by 5 years of age to 20 breaths/min. A child with pneumonia will have a grunting respiration, which is due to reversal of the normal respiratory rhythm. The grunting expiration is followed by inspiration, and then a pause. Thickening of the costochondral junction is felt in rickets (*rachitic rosary*). Palpate the anterior chest wall for the cardiac impulse and for thrills. In children under the age of 5 years the apex is normally in the fourth intercostal space just to the left of the midclavicular line. Vocal fremitus is rarely of any clinical value in children. The axillary nodes may now be felt in the same way as in adults.

Percussion of the chest is useful in older children, but in young children and infants it is only rarely of value. Percuss very lightly, and in babies directly, tapping the chest wall with the percussing finger rather than using another finger as a pleximeter. The chest is more resonant in children than in adults.

A stethoscope with a small bell chest piece is suitable for auscultation of the child's chest. Often it is less threatening to examine the back of the chest first, and much more information about the lungs can be learnt in this way. Listen for the breath sounds and adventitious sounds. Because of the thin chest wall, breath sounds are louder in children than in adults, and their character is more like the bronchial breathing of adults (*puerile breathing*). Upper respiratory tract infections in children often give rise to loud, coarse rhonchi, which are conducted down the trachea and main bronchi (Table 18.1). All is not lost if the child is crying, as this is associated with deep inspiration, and this is the time to listen for the character of the breath sounds.

TABLE 18.1   Chest signs of some common respiratory disorders of children.

Disorder	Chest movement	Percussion (if carried out)	Auscultation
Bronchiolitis	Restricted, with hyperinflation. Often tracheal tug and subcostal recession	Hyperresonant	Widespread crepitations, or wheezing
Pneumonia	Rapid, shallow respirations with audible grunt. May be reduced on affected side	Dull or normal	Localized bronchial breathing or crepitations. May have no abnormal signs
Asthma	Restricted with hyperinflation. Use of accessory muscles, and subcostal retraction	Hyperresonant	Expiratory wheeze
Croup	Inspiratory stridor, with subcostal recession	Normal	Inspiratory coarse crepitations (crackles)

When auscultating the front of the chest, the child's immediate instinct is to push the stethoscope away. Some doctors attach a small toy to the tubing to attract attention, while others prefer to distract the child with toys held in the hand (Fig. 18.3). The normal splitting of the first and second sounds is easier to hear in children than in adults. Venous hums and functional systolic flow murmurs are often heard in normal children. Count the heart rate in young children. The normal rates are as follows:

- Newborn infant 140 beats/min
- 1-year-old 110 beats/min
- 3-year-old 100 beats/min
- 8-year-old 90 beats/min
- 11-year-old 80 beats/min.

Up to this point in the examination, the baby will have been examined mainly from behind. Take the opportunity to check for spinal abnormalities such as scoliosis or kyphosis, which may otherwise be missed. If there has been no need to stand the baby up at this time, examination of the back can be deferred until the neurological examination, or when the baby is moving around when the examination has been completed.

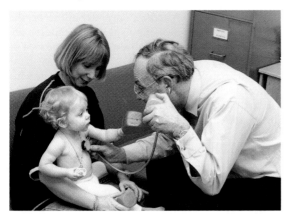

Fig. 18.3 Attracting the attention of a 10-month-old baby while examining her heart.

NEUROLOGICAL EXAMINATION

The neurological examination can usually be carried out in the normal way in older children, but in younger children the extent of the neurological examination will depend on the child's age and willingness to cooperate. Already a great deal should have been learned from initial observations. If the child is walking, the gait should have been observed and muscle tone assessed. Note any abnormal movements:

- Tics or habit spasms are repetitive but not purposeful movements, such as shrugging of the shoulders or facial grimacing
- Choreiform movements are involuntary, purposeless jerks which follow no particular pattern
- Athetoid movements are writhing and more pronounced distally.

Cooordination can best be checked by watching a child at play. It is useful to have toys available which require a degree of coordination, such as a toy farm or garage. Otherwise, a modification of the finger–nose test using a toy held in the hand can be used. If the child is old enough, watching them dressing or doing up shoelaces is a good way to assess coordination.

Check *muscle tone* if this has not already been carried out. Pick the child up if there is still a friendly relationship. This gives a good idea of the feel of a child and of the muscle tone. If the child is hypotonic, it will feel as though he or she is slipping through your hands. Muscle power is difficult to check in young children except by watching playing habits, and assessing power by ability at a variety of lifting games. Always remember to check for neck stiffness. It is detected more readily by resistance to passive flexion of the neck than by testing for Kernig's sign.

Testing of *sensation* is difficult in young children, and is probably best omitted unless there is a strong suspicion of neurological disease.

Testing the *cranial nerves* takes a little ingenuity. Eye movements are relatively easy using a toy moved in different directions in front of the baby's face; many young infants like poking out their tongue, which will check the 12th cranial nerve. If the child can be made to smile, and even if crying, any asymmetry of facial movements can be seen.

Getting a child's limbs into the correct position to test *tendon reflexes* may take some time. Often they can be elicited by using a finger rather than a patellar hammer. Tendon reflexes in young infants tend to be brisk, and the plantar responses are extensor up to 18 months of age. The persistence of an extensor response beyond the age of 2 years indicates an upper motor neurone lesion. Primitive responses should have disappeared by 3–4 months of age; their persistence indicates significant neurodevelopmental dysfunction. The primitive reflexes will be considered further in the section on examination of the newborn (see p. 393).

THE EYES

The eyes should now be checked. Inspect them for conjunctivitis, cataracts or congenital defects such as colobomata. It is very important to check for *squints*, as immediate ophthalmological referral is necessary, however young the infant. Squints are checked for by shining a light in the eyes from in front of the face; the light reflex should be at the same position in each cornea. A *cover test* should then be used (see Ch. 12), employing a doll or some other appropriate toy on which a child can focus the gaze. Pupillary accommodation and light reactions can be noted at the same time. Examination of the *fundus* is particularly difficult in infants, and forcible attempts to keep the eyes open will only make the procedure more difficult. Older children will focus on toys or distant people. In younger children only fleeting glimpses of the fundus are likely. It should be possible to see the red reflex, and sufficient of the disc to detect papilloedema.

The testing of vision, hearing, and certain motor functions in young children is included in the section on developmental screening examination (see p. 387).

With the possible exception of the eye examination, nothing so far should have upset a baby unduly. The following examinations should be carried out at the end of the consultation, as they are more likely to upset the child.

THE GENITALIA, GROINS AND ANUS

The nappy and underpants can now be removed if it is necessary to examine the groin or anus. In boys, notice the penis. This is often a source of worry to many parents, especially the lack of retraction of the foreskin. Old wives' tales abound, and few parents realize that the foreskin will only rarely retract under the age of 5 years; they should be informed that forcibly attempting retraction is not only painful but can also result in *balanitis*. Check the hernial orifices, and see if the testes have descended. To feel the testis, make sure that your hand is warm, and place a finger in the line of the inguinal canal; advance the finger towards the scrotum. This will prevent the cremasteric reflex causing the testis to disappear into the inguinal canal, which tends to happen if the scrotum is approached from below. Having located the testes in the correct place, it is important to demonstrate the normality of the boy to his parents. It is not unusual to find a testis in the inguinal canal in young babies, but it can usually be pushed into the scrotum without too much difficulty. Nothing needs to be done other than to review the boy after a few months, as the testis can be expected to descend into its normal position with increasing maturity.

In girls, check the vulva for soreness or discharge, and for abnormalities such as polyps. Fusion of the labia is not uncommon, so check that they separate normally. Enlargement of the clitoris suggests endocrine disorder.

Check for inguinal lymph nodes at this time, and palpate the femoral artery. If the femoral artery cannot be palpated, this suggests coarctation of the aorta, which requires cardiological assessment.

Examination of the anal margin can best be carried out by gently separating the buttocks with one hand on either side; the anal orifice can then be seen easily, and inspected for fissures, which are not uncommon. Rectal examination is rarely necessary in children, and if carried out should be done with a well lubricated, gloved little finger, which should be advanced very slowly. A little while spent talking and waiting will help.

THE NOSE, EARS, MOUTH AND THROAT

The worst parts of the examination as far as the child is concerned are the nose, ears, mouth and throat.

The *nose* need only be examined superficially, looking for nasal patency, any deviation of the septum, or the presence of polyps. Older children are quite good at sniffing, and this will give some idea of nasal patency.

A cooperative child will allow you to look into his or her *ears* but, if not, the child should be held by the mother, as shown in Figure 18.4. Held in such a way, the child can be kept still long enough for the eardrums to be inspected. Look carefully for the light reflex, which can be lost if the child has chronic secretory otitis media ('glue ear'). The drum may be bright red and bulging in acute suppurative otitis media.

The *mouth* and *throat* can be examined by encouraging a cooperative child to 'show me your teeth'; an open mouth will then allow a clear view of the

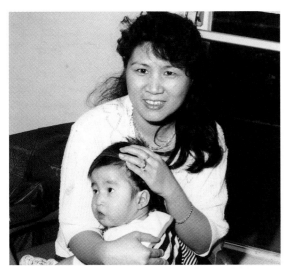

Fig. 18.4 How to hold a baby to allow the ears to be examined. The mother faces the baby to one side, and holds him firmly with one arm around the head, and the other around the upper arm and shoulder.

mouth and fauces. If uncooperative, the child will need to be held as shown in Figure 18.5. Sometimes it is not too disastrous if the child cries at this point, as this will give a very clear view of the teeth, the tonsils, and sometimes even the epiglottis. A spatula is a terrifying instrument to the average child, causing most children to clamp their teeth shut. If this happens, the spatula should be forced on to the back of the tongue to induce a gag reflex. Whatever means are used to open the mouth, the state of the teeth and mucous membranes should be noticed, as well as the tonsils and fauces. Note especially the

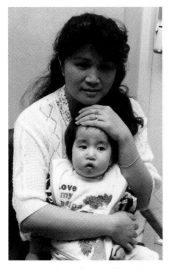

Fig. 18.5 How to hold a baby to allow the mouth and throat to be examined. The baby faces the examiner, with the mother holding him firmly with one hand on the forehead, and the other holding both arms.

white patches of *Candida* infections and Koplik's spots seen in measles.

The child should now be allowed to move freely about the room, allowing a further assessment of gait, and of any marked skeletal abnormalities.

Examination of the hips must *always* be carried out in younger children and infants (see pp. 394–395).

The general physical examination of the child, with the exception of the special examinations described in the following sections, has now been completed. It is to be hoped that you have retained the friendship of the child. Once the child is dressed, the examiner should sit quietly with the parents and explain what has been found. It is always best to have finished dressing the child before talking to the parents; they are more likely to consider what you have to say if they are not worrying about buttons or shoelaces. Always involve an older child in the discussion—he or she has every right to know what is wrong. Even young children can be told that they will be all right. Never under any circumstances deceive a child. If they find you out they will never believe you again.

SPECIAL EXAMINATIONS

The following examinations are important.

HEIGHT AND WEIGHT

Measurements of height and weight are essential in the examination of children. Height can be measured in children over the age of 2 years against a wall-mounted gauge. Younger children can be measured lying down on special measuring boards. All measurements should be made under standard conditions, and children should be weighed unclothed. If the child keeps any clothes on, this should be noted against the weight, so that subsequent weights can be taken with the child wearing the same quantity of clothing. Childhood is a period of growth, the pattern of which may be adversely affected by many disturbances of health, as well as social deprivation. Heights and weights should be compared with those of healthy children of similar sex, age and build, and for this purpose percentile charts are essential (Figs 18.6–18.9). It is also important to have some idea of the height of the parents, as it would be unrealistic to expect small parents to have large children.

Serial measurements over a period are more valuable than single measurements, and will give the growth rate—the *growth velocity*. A child who fails to grow at an appropriate velocity needs to be investigated further. However, a child presenting for the first time outside the area between the 10th and 90th percentiles should be regarded with slight suspicion, and those outside the 3rd and 97th per-

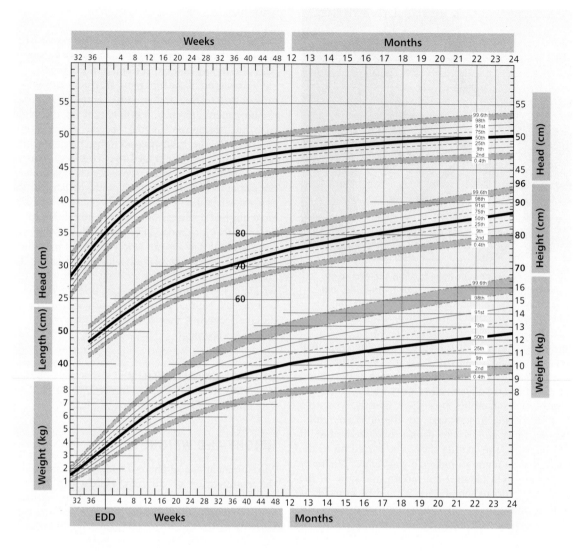

Fig. 18.6   Height, weight and head circumference: boys aged 0–2 years. © Child Growth Foundation.

centiles should be regarded as unhealthy unless proved otherwise. There are as yet no satisfactory growth charts for children of Asian origin born in the UK. As a rough guide, the mean percentile for an Asian child is the 25th percentile on the standard UK charts.

Figures 18.6–18.9 show standard height, weight, and head circumference charts for UK boys and girls from birth to 2 years, and standard height and weight charts for UK boys and girls from 0–20 years. There are special growth charts for children with Down's syndrome and Turner's syndrome. It will be seen from the percentile charts that there is a wide range above and below the mean. Each chart shows the 0.4th, 2nd, 9th, 25th, 50th, 75th, 91st, 98th and 99.6th percentiles. The meaning of the term '10th percentile' is that 10% of all normal children are lighter or shorter, respectively, at the age concerned.

Slightly different standards are applicable in different races and in different countries.

The term 'failure to thrive' is used to denote children whose weight gain is below that expected (see Figs 18.6 and 18.7).

HEAD CIRCUMFERENCE

In infants under the age of 2 years, the head circumference should be measured. The standard measurement is the occipitofrontal circumference. Hydrocephalus should be suspected when the rate of growth of the head is greater than normal for the sex, age and size of the infant. Rather than use a chart showing the head circumference alone, it is more useful to use a chart which combines head circumference, length and weight percentiles, so that the proportions of each individual child can be com-

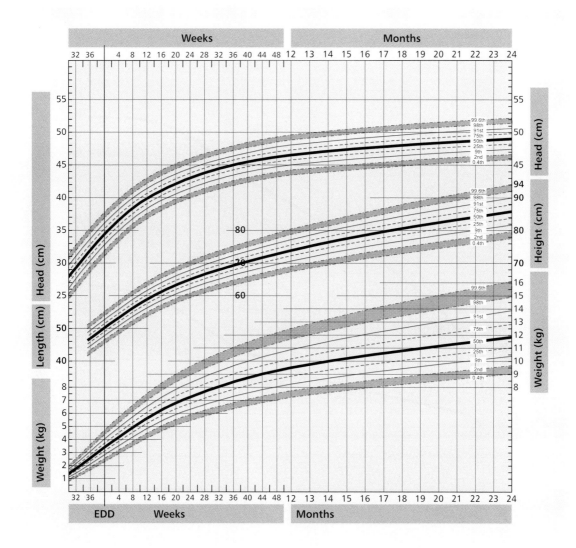

Fig. 18.7   Height, weight and head circumference: girls aged 0–2 years. © Child Growth Foundation.

pared. An additional advantage of these charts is that they allow for prematurity, and so separate charts for pre-term babies are not necessary.

BLOOD PRESSURE

Abnormalities of blood pressure are uncommon in childhood, and because the measurement of blood pressure can be frightening it need only be be measured when cardiovascular or renal disease is suspected. It should always be carried out at the end of the examination, and preferably when the child is almost dressed. Let the child play with the sphygmomanometer cuff, and talk in simple terms about what is going to happen. The size of the cuff is most important if accurate readings are to be obtained, and a variety of sizes should be available. The inflatable bag should be long enough to encircle the full circumference of the upper arm, and should be of a width roughly equal to one-third of the length of the upper arm and forearm as far as the wrist. Electronic blood pressure monitors are routinely used in most hospitals, and are more accurate than most manual methods. In small children and infants the pulse can be palpated to obtain the systolic blood pressure. In babies, the *flush method* may be used. The arm is held up and tightly bandaged to exclude the blood to the level of the cuff, which is then inflated. The bandage is then removed to reveal a white limb. The pressure in the cuff is slowly reduced; the point at which the skin flushes is an approximate indication of the systolic blood pressure. Doppler techniques more accurately measure blood pressure in children, but these are not always available. The blood pressure in the legs must be measured in all suspected cases of coarctation of the aorta.

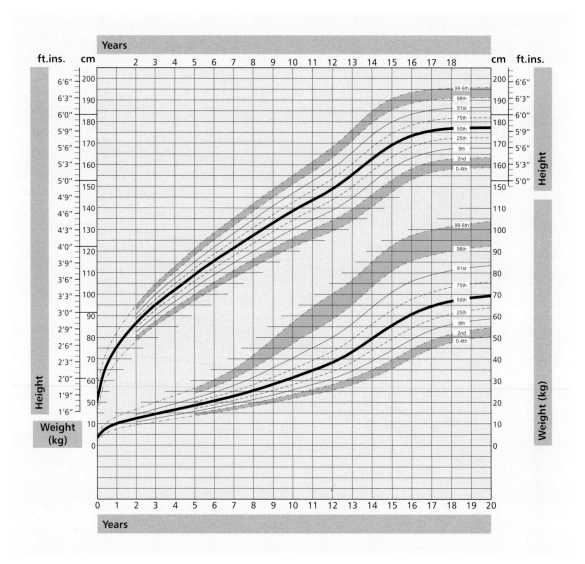

Fig. 18.8   Height and weight: boys aged 0–20 years. © Child Growth Foundation.

The blood pressure in the arms is about 65/45 in the newborn, 75/50 at 1 year, 85/60 at 4 years, 95/65 at 8 years, and 100/70 mmHg at 10 years of age.

TEMPERATURE

It is not always necessary to take the temperature as part of the routine examination of children. Fever is a very common finding in children, and may be due to excitement, exercise and minor infections, as well as to severe infections and other serious illnesses. Small infants often respond to infection with low temperatures.

Oral temperature measurements are rarely taken now, and then only in older children. Axillary temperatures are more usually taken, and are 0.5°C lower than oral temperature. Rectal temperatures are seldom if ever taken. The more usual ways of taking temperature in current use are tympanic membrane temperatures. This method is difficult in a wriggling child, and is probably best used for infants over 3 years of age. Skin temperature using chemical dot strips is widely used and easier and safer for parents to check at home than using glass thermometers. Rapid rises of temperature to 39.5 or 40°C are not uncommon in children under 5 years of age, and may be associated with a convulsion.

STOOLS

Never be afraid to see a dirty nappy, or stool. This is part of the examination of a baby, and it is important to know the normal stool appearances in childhood. The stools of a breast-fed infant may be loose and green or pasty and yellow. They have a characteristic odour. Infants fed on cows' milk preparations pass stools of a paler yellow colour and of a much firmer consistency. Babies fed on

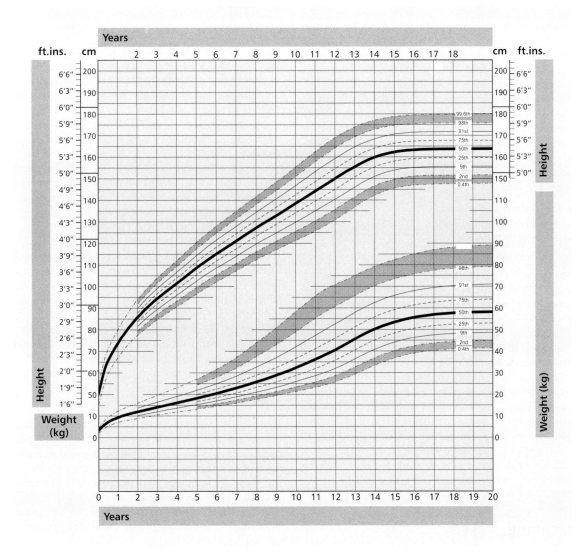

Fig. 18.9 Height and weight girls aged 0–20 years. © Child Growth Foundation.

the newer, modified cows' milk preparations have clay-coloured or greenish stools. The character of the stool in older children is more variable than in adults. Some healthy children pass frequent, loose stools containing undigested vegetable matter; 'toddler's diarrhoea'. The stools of children with coeliac disease and cystic fibrosis are bulky, odoriferous and quite characteristic.

URINE

Collection of urine specimens in infants is difficult, and special techniques are required. You may be lucky and get a 'clean catch' specimen, as many babies pass urine during examination. Alternatively, specially made sterile plastic containers with an adhesive opening can be applied to the washed genitalia. Urine can be tested immediately with reagent strips. If they are positive for leucocytes, bacteria or

nitrites the specimen should be sent immediately to the laboratory, followed as soon as possible by a second sample. Unless the child is unwell, he or she should not be treated on the strength of a positive reagent strip test, as false positives are common. Results of microscopy and culture should be awaited before treatment is commenced. Faecal contamination of urine specimens can be a problem, however the urine is collected, and it may be necessary to resort to suprapubic aspiration of bladder urine, a procedure which is not too difficult in infants.

DEVELOPMENTAL SCREENING EXAMINATION

Development is the normal process of maturation of function which takes place in the early years of life. It may be modified by emotional difficulties, environment, and physical defects and illnesses. Lack of intellectual stimulation, and of the normal experiences of childhood, may result in apparent retardation of development.

All infants should have a simple developmental screening examination at regular intervals. Table 18.2 lists the important milestones. Detailed developmental assessment is a specialist subject, but it is important for all those who examine children to be able to carry out a brief developmental screening examination, and to be aware of all the basic milestones.

It is usual to consider development under four main headings:

- Movement and posture
- Vision and manipulation
- Hearing and speech
- Social behaviour.

Screening for developmental delay involves testing the child's performance of a few skills in each of the four fields of development, and comparing the results with the average for children of the same age. The range of normal developmental progress is wide, and the milestones shown in Table 18.2 are those of an average normal baby. Delay in all fields of development is more significant than delay in one only, and severe delay is more meaningful than slight delay. There are considerable individual variations, and lateness in one particular area should not be taken as evidence of mental handicap or cerebral palsy without other corroborating features.

Allowance must always be made for those infants who were born prematurely, at least until the age of 2 years, by which time they should have caught up.

TECHNIQUES USED

The same rules apply to techniques used in developmental screening as to those of general physical examination. Time has to be spent gaining the friendship of the child. This time can be profitably utilized by offering, for example, a 10-month-old baby a small toy to see how the child grasps it and reacts to it. Let the baby play with the toys and bricks while sitting on his or her mother's lap, and if the child remains suspicious, get the mother to offer the various objects. As with all parts of the examination, much more is learned by simply watching a child play and watching his or her reactions to the surroundings.

In the UK, developmental screening is usually carried out by the health visitor. There is always an assessment at 8 months, and usually at 18 months and sometimes at 24 months but different areas have different ages of assessment, or are making 18- and 24-month tests more selective, by concentrating on 'at risk' children. The health visitor is trained in developmental skills and will refer on to a doctor babies about whom there is any suspicion.

TESTING VISION

Much will be learned about a child's vision by observation. Notice whether the child is looking around the room and at particular toys, or staring at nothing in particular, especially if there are random or nystagmoid eye movements; the latter suggests that the child is unable to see. When he or she picks toys up, is accommodation normal? The routine examination of the eye has been dealt with in the first part of this chapter.

Checks of *visual acuity* are not easy in young babies. By 6 weeks of age, infants should be following their mother with their eyes and by 6 months of age they should be able to follow a rolling ball at 3 metres. This is the basis of one method of visual testing at this age. The ability of the child to follow rolling balls of differing diameters gives an accurate assessment of visual acuity. From the age of approximately $2\frac{1}{2}$ years, the *Sheridan–Gardiner test* is used. This is a simple comparison test, with the examiner indicating letters or familiar toys on a board, and asking the child to indicate a similar object on a board held by the mother. The acuity is the ability of the child to pick out the smallest objects (Ch. 12).

TESTING HEARING

Hearing is normally checked for the first time between 6 and 8 months of age. There are special techniques (e.g. brainstem auditory evoked potential studies) for testing the hearing of newborn babies but these are indicated only in those babies at greatest risk of impaired hearing, as for example, when there is a family history of deafness, and in babies who have received ototoxic antibiotics such as aminoglycosides.

Although distraction testing, as explained below, is still carried out in some centres, this test has a large observer error and many children shown subsequently to be deaf pass the distraction test! It is more usual now to use a questionnaire, concentrating in particular on high-risk factors (see Box 18.7), and specifically on the parent's perception of the child's hearing.

To carry out the distraction test, the baby sits on the mother's lap, facing outwards. It helps if an assistant can sit facing them to distract the child with toys etc. (but not funny noises). The examiner then makes a series of soft noises to one side or the other but behind mother and child and out of the child's line of vision (Fig. 18.10). The sounds used are a special high-frequency rattle, a bell, a spoon in a cup, and the rustle of tissue paper or a whisper. At 6 months of age a baby should turn to the source of the sound when it is about 45 cm from the ear. By 9 months a baby reacts more quickly, and localizes the sound at a distance of 90 cm. If the child fails the test on the first occasion, it does not automatically mean that he

TABLE 18.2   Normal developmental milestones.

Age	Movement and posture	Vision and manipulation	Hearing and speech	Social behaviour
6 weeks	When pulled from supine to sitting, head lag is not quite complete (Fig. 18.11) When held prone, head is held in line with body When prone on couch lifts chin off couch Primitive responses persist	Looks at toy, held in mid-line Follows a moving person	Vocalizes with gurgles	Smiles briefly when talked to by mother
4 months	Holds head up in sitting position, and is steady Pulls to sitting with only minimal head lag (Fig. 18.12) When prone, with head and chest off couch, makes swimming movements Rolls from prone to supine Primitive responses gone	Watches his or her hands Pulls at his or her clothes Tries to grasp objects	Turns head to sound Vocalizes apparently appropriately Laughs	Recognizes mother Becomes excited by toys
7 months	Sits unsupported Rolls from supine to prone Can support weight when held, and bounces with pleasure When prone, bears weight on hands	Transfers objects from hand to hand Bangs toys on table Watches small moving objects	Says 'Da', 'Ba', 'Ka'	Tries to feed him- or herself Puts objects in mouth Plays with paper
10 months	Crawls Gets to sitting position without help Can pull up to standing Lifts one foot when standing	Reaches for objects with index finger Has developed a finger–thumb grasp Will place objects in the examiner's hands, but not release them	Says one word with meaning	Plays 'peep-bo' and 'pat-a-cake' Waves 'bye-bye' Deliberately drops objects so that they can be picked up Puts objects in and out of boxes
13 months	Walks unsupported May shuffle on buttocks and hands	Can hold two cubes in one hand Makes marks with pen	Says two or three words with meaning	Understands simple questions such as 'Where is your shoe?' May kiss on request Tends to be shy
15 months	Can get into standing position without support Climbs upstairs Walks with broad based gait	Builds a tower of two cubes Takes off shoes	Will say around 12 words, but mostly gobbledegook	Asks for things by pointing Kisses pictures of animals Can use a cup
18 months	Climbs stairs unaided holding rail Runs and jumps Can climb onto a chair and sit down	Builds tower of three cubes Turns pages of a book two or three at a time Scribbles Takes off gloves and socks Unzips fasteners	Is beginning to join two words together	Recognizes animals and cars in a book Points to nose, ear, etc. on request Clean and dry but with occasional accidents Carries out simple orders

BOX 18.7   Hearing questionnaire for 8-month-old babies.

CHILD'S NAME . . . .

DATE OF BIRTH . . . .

A HIGH RISK FACTORS FOR DEAFNESS

1. **FAMILY HISTORY** of deafness which required special education or hearing aid fitting in childhood or an inherited condition known to be associated with childhood deafness, even though there is no known deafness in the family.

    YES | NO

2. **CONGENITAL MALFORMATIONS** either of chromosomal, syndromic or unknown aetiology including craniofacial, branchial arch and cervical spine dysmorphologies, cleft palates, and pinna malformations even if unilateral but excluding isolated ear pits and tags.

    YES | NO

3. **CONGENITAL INFECTIONS** including clinically apparent rubella, cytomegalovirus, toxoplasmosis, herpes and syphilis and also any maternal history of possible infection in pregnancy even in the absence of neonatal stigmata.

    YES | NO

4. **PERINATAL ILLNESS** requiring admission to the Special Care Baby Unit but only to include those babies with:
    i)   Gestation of less than 32 weeks
    ii)   Birth weight of 1.25 kg or less
    iii) An Apgar score of 3 or less at 5 minutes
    iv)   Cerebral illness, e.g. intraventricular haemorrhage, convulsions, meningitis
    v)   Apnoea requiring ventilation for 4 hours or more
    vi)   Jaundice where exchange transfusion has been considered or undertaken
    vii) Administration of aminoglycosides at potentially toxic levels.

    YES | NO

5. **POSTNATAL ILLNESS** of bacterial meningitis, head injury with loss of consciousness or neurological disease.

    YES | NO

B HEARING RESPONSES

Go through parents' 'hearing' information leaflet with parents. Try to elicit from them clear examples of the baby's responses to loud and quiet sounds. Having done this

1. Do the parents have any concerns about the baby's hearing?

    YES | NO

2. Do you have any concerns about the baby's hearing?

    YES | NO

BOX 18.7   (continued)

C VOICE AND SPEECH DEVELOPMENT

The baby should enjoy using his or her voice freely with variation in pitch and tone.
The baby should have started making repetitive consonant/vowel sequences—'baba', 'mum-mum', i.e. babbling

1. Do the parents have any concerns about the baby's speech development?

    YES | NO

2. Do you have any concerns about the baby's speech development?

    YES | NO

D MIDDLE EAR PROBLEMS

1. Has the baby had recurrent ear infections requiring treatment?

    YES | NO

2. Has the baby had recurrent upper respiratory tract infections thought to be associated with hearing loss?

    YES | NO

If YES to any of the above, refer the baby to the Secondary Audiology Clinic (or to the Tertiary Clinic if suspected of having a severe loss).

E Is there parental consanguinity?

    YES | NO | UNCERTAIN

Do not make a referral on this factor alone but, if present, take particular care at this and subsequent interviews.

ACTION

F Has a referral been completed?

    YES | NO

If yes, to whom?
Signature of Interviewer . . . .
Name (Please Print) . . . .
Date of Interview . . . .

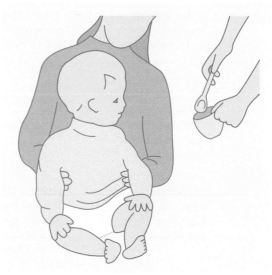

Fig. 18.10   Testing hearing at 6 months.

or she is deaf, but the test should be repeated after a further month. If the child still fails, he or she should be referred for audiological testing.

HEAD CONTROL

By 4 months babies can normally keep their head in line with the trunk when pulled from supine to sitting, and when held in the sitting position will keep their head upright. Before this age the head lags behind the trunk (Figs 18.11 and 18.12).

Table 18.2 shows the normal development milestones up to the age of 18 months, by which time obvious deviations from normal development will be apparent. Beyond this age developmental testing is more specialized, and is not the concern of this chapter. A baby who appears to have delayed development on screening will need further specialized assessment to establish causation and management.

EXAMINATION OF THE NEWBORN

The routine examination of the newborn infant (Box 18.8) is designed to assess the general state of health and to detect congenital abnormalities. It is recommended that all babies should be examined

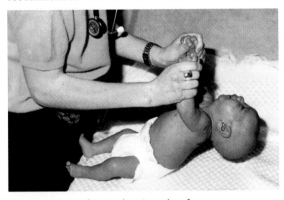

Fig. 18.11   Head control at 6 weeks of age.

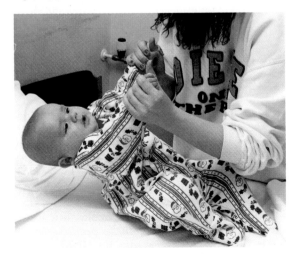

Fig. 18.12   Head control at 4 months of age.

> **BOX 18.8   Checklist for examination of the newborn.**
>
> - Apgar score 5 min after birth
> - Weight, length, head circumference
> - Passage of urine and meconium
> - Alertness and wakefulness
> - Skin colour: cyanosis, jaundice
> - Birthmarks
> - Sacral development: Down's syndrome etc.
> - Skull and fontanelles
> - Eyes
> - Mouth and tongue
> - Neck: branchial cysts
> - Limbs: digits and palmar creases, talipes
> - Chest
> - Abdomen and umbilicus
> - Perineum and genitalia
> - Neurological assessment: movements and tone, reflexes, the cry

within the first 24 hours of life, and again before the end of the first week. Many parts of the examination of the newborn infant are similar to the techniques described above for older babies and children.

The neurological status at birth has implications for the future development of the child, and has been used as an indicator of brain damage sustained during or shortly after birth. The *Apgar Score* (Box 18.9) is in general use as part of this assessment. An Apgar score of 6 or less at 5 minutes after birth is associated with neurological deficit in about 10% of cases, but a low score 1 minute after birth is less predictive of brain damage. A high Apgar score at 5 minutes, on the other hand, may not be sensitive to focal brain injury or infarction.

Weight will usually have been measured by the midwife. Length is not commonly measured now, and the head circumference (occipitofrontal) may not be done before 48 hours, to allow for moulding to subside. Note the time of passage of the first urine and meconium, which is the dark green, sticky stool of the newborn baby in the first few days of life.

Always examine a newborn baby in front of his or her mother, and involve her at all stages by explaining what you are doing. Have the baby undressed, and in a warm place. Always have warm hands, and

> **BOX 18.9   The Apgar score.**
>
> In each of the five categories a score of 0, 1 or 2 is awarded, giving a maximum score of 10. A score of 7–10 is *good*, 3–6 *moderate CNS depression*, and 0–2 *severe CNS depression*
>
> - Heart rate
> - Respiratory effort
> - Muscle tone
> - Reflex irritability
> - Colour

treat the baby gently, leaving the most unpleasant parts of the examination until last. Talk or even sing to the baby—he or she is as aware of what is going on as an older child, and should be afforded the same courtesy.

Much of the time can be spent just watching the baby, noting the state of awareness. If the baby is awake, seemingly looking around and not crying, examination of the nervous system will yield much information.

THE SKIN

Note the colour of the skin. *Peripheral cyanosis* is a common finding in the normal newborn, but *central cyanosis* indicates cardiac or respiratory disease. So-called 'traumatic cyanosis' affects the head and neck, and is produced by confluent petechial haemorrhages; it is most often seen after prolonged or obstructed labour. Jaundice is common *after* 48 hours in most pre-term and some term babies, and is considered physiological. However, jaundice *within* 48 hours of birth has to be considered pathological; the commonest cause is haemolytic disease of the newborn, but any baby jaundiced before 48 hours or after 7 days of age needs to be investigated.

Look for birthmarks, which are either pigmented lesions or haemangiomata. Most babies have a collection of dilated capillaries on the upper eyelids and nape of the neck (sometimes called 'stork bites'), which fade after a few weeks. Some babies develop a crop of small papules on the trunk during the first week (*erythema toxicum* or *urticaria neonatorum*). They are of uncertain cause, of no significance, and usually fade after a few days. Superficial peeling of the skin, especially over the periphery, is common, and is most apparent in post-term and some small-for-gestational-age babies. *Milia* are whitish, pin-head spots concentrated mainly around the nose. They are sebaceous retention cysts, and can be felt with the finger. They usually disappear within a month. *Lanugo hair* may cover the body, especially in pre-term babies and some dark-haired babies. It usually disappears over the first 2 or 3 weeks. Colour of hair at birth is no guide to subsequent hair colour. *Mongolian blue spot* is the name given to the normal dark blue areas of pigmentation commonly seen over the sacrum and buttocks or back of the legs in black or Asian babies.

THE FACE

Look at the face for obvious abnormalities such as Down's syndrome and other indications of craniofacial maldevelopment. Check the position of the ears, and whether they are normal and symmetrical. Accessory auricles are small, pedunculated skin tags, usually just in front of the ears, and can be dealt with by trying them off at the base. Make sure that the upper lip is intact.

Once superficial examination has been completed, more formal examination takes place; again, it should be regional rather than by systems, starting with the head and working down.

THE HEAD

Inspect and palpate the head. The bones of the cranial vault, being relatively soft and connected only by fibrous tissue, alter in shape readily in response to external pressure. Moulding of the skull takes place during birth, with overriding of the sutures. It usually disappears after a few days. The *caput succedaneum* is an area of oedema of the scalp over the presenting part of the head during labour. It pits on pressure and is not fluctuant. A *cephalhaematoma* is a subperiosteal haematoma which appears a few days after birth as a large, cystic swelling limited to the area of one of the skull bones. It ends to resolve relatively slowly over a few months, and may leave a calcified edge. The anterior fontanelle varies considerably at birth, but should be checked, as described above (p. 379).

THE EYES

The eyes can best be examined when the baby has his or her eyes open spontaneously. Alternatively the eyelids can be held open by an assistant, although this tends to make the baby cry. Sometimes a baby will open the eyes if given a feed. The iris gives no indication of its future colour, and is usually greyish-blue in Caucasian infants. A bluish tinge to the sclera is usual. Tears before 3–4 weeks are unusual. Even though newborn infants can see, eye movements tend to be random, often giving the impression of a transient squint. Subconjunctival haemorrhages show as a dark red patch covering the sclera, sometimes ringing the cornea. They commonly follow normal deliveries, and despite their alarming appearance are of no consequence and disappear after a few weeks. Look for evidence of conjunctivitis and check for other abnormalities as described above (p. 382).

THE MOUTH AND TONGUE

Look inside the mouth; this is easy if the baby is crying, and a spatula will not be needed. If the baby is quiet and content, this part of the examination may be left until later. Make sure that there is no cleft of the palate, and note particularly whether the uvula is normal. A bifid uvula indicates a submucous cleft of the palate which requires surgery. Rounded, thickened areas are often seen on the lips, more especially on the lower lips and are known as *suckling blisters*. This is a misnomer, as despite their name, they do not contain fluid. *Epithelial pearls* are small, white areas, best seen on the hard palate. Occasionally teeth are present at birth. They are usually incisors, and can be green in colour. If loose, they are best removed. *Macroglossia* is seen in babies with Down's syndrome, congenital hypothyroidism, Beckwith's syndrome and in some normal children.

THE NECK

The neck of a newborn baby seems rather short, and may be considered abnormal by the inexperienced. Rarely, cystic swellings are seen; *dermoid cysts* and *thyroglossal cysts* in the midline, or *branchial* cysts just in front of the upper third of the sternomastoid muscle.

THE LIMBS

Examine the limbs for abnormalities. Extra digits on the hand are not uncommon and are often familial, but are rarer on the feet. Look for a single transverse palmar crease, which is classically seen in babies with Down's syndrome, but in addition is found in a variety of dysmorphic syndromes, as well as in some normal infants. Common foot abnormalities to look for are syndactyly or talipes equinovarus; the latter requires immediate orthopaedic referral.

THE CHEST

The general appearance and shape of the chest should be noticed. Breast enlargement with exudation of a milky fluid from the nipples is sometimes seen in newborn infants of either sex. This is due to transferred maternal hormones, and disappears in a few days without causing problems. Resist the temptation to squeeze the breasts, as this may result in infection (*mastitis*). Make sure that the clavicles are intact. Note the symmetry of the chest wall, the pattern of respiration, and whether there is any indrawing on inspiration. The remainder of the chest examination is as described earlier in this chapter for older children (p. 380); percussion of the chest is of even less value at this age. Transient systolic murmurs are extremely common in the first few days, and may reflect the closing ductus arteriosus, or non-specific flow murmurs, as discussed earlier.

THE ABDOMEN

The abdomen of a newborn baby usually seems a little distended, and it moves with respiration. Slight divarication of the rectus muscles may occur, and this exaggerates this abdominal bulging. The liver edge is palpable 2–4 cm below the costal margin, and the lower poles of both kidneys can be felt easily. The bladder should not be palpable if the baby has just passed urine. Check the umbilical stump. It should contain two arteries and one vein. A single umbilical artery is associated with an increased incidence of congenital abnormalities, especially of the renal tract. The umbilical cord should become dry, and then separate between the 6th and 10th day. Some moistness of the stump then remains for a further few days. Sometimes excess granulation tissue accumulates, to form a small granuloma; this can be treated by local application of a silver nitrate stick.

THE PERINEUM AND GENITALIA

Examine the perineum for hypospadias, hydroceles, hernias or undescended testicles. Look for patency of the anus; an imperforate anus is easily overlooked unless it is specifically checked for. While looking at the buttocks and anus, see if there is a sacral dimple, which is usually a blind-ending pit and of no significance. Make sure that the back is straight and that there are no gross spinal lesions, especially spina bifida. Check female external genitalia for clitoral enlargement—which would suggest a virilizing condition such as congenital adrenal hyperplasia due to 21-hydroxylase deficiency—or labial fusion. It is not unusual for girls to have a mucous vaginal discharge, and sometimes bleeding. This is the result of transferred maternal hormones, and is usually transient. Make sure that the femoral pulses are palpable.

NEUROLOGICAL ASSESSMENT

Combine a formal neurological examination with observation of the baby's behaviour. No two babies react in the same way, but there is a broad, general pattern which applies to most. Spontaneous movement normally takes place when the baby is awake, consisting of alternating flexion and extension. Any marked difference between the two sides is abnormal. The fingers are more fully flexed than later in childhood, but spontaneous opening and closing of the hands takes place. The thumb may be tucked under the fingers.

The normal position of a newborn baby is that of flexion. When lying prone, the baby's legs are usually drawn up under the abdomen. If the baby is crying, look for any weakness or paralysis in the face suggesting injury to the facial nerve, or any deficiency of arm movements suggesting injury to the brachial plexus. Note the limb tone and, although tendon jerks are difficult to elicit at this age, they should be checked, using a finger rather than a tendon hammer.

PRIMITIVE REFLEXES

Primitive responses are present in the normal newborn infant, and disappear at variable times up to the fourth month of age. They are responses to specific stimuli, and depend to some extent on the infant's state of wakefulness. The absence of one or more of these reflexes in the newborn infant may indicate some abnormality of the brain, a local abnormality in the affected limb, or a neuromuscular abnormality. Persistence of primitive reflexes beyond the fourth month of life should alert you to the possibility of developmental delay. These reflex responses are as follows:

Rooting reflexes

In response to a touch on the cheek, a baby will turn his or her head towards the stimulus. Stimulation of the upper lip causes opening of the mouth, pouting of the lips, and tongue movements. Sucking itself is a reflex, and failure of the sucking response beyond the 36th week of gestation suggests significant neurological impairment.

Palmar and plantar grasp

A finger placed across the child's palm will cause flexion and grasping of the finger. A similar response is seen if a finger is placed on the plantar surface of the foot, but the plantar grasp is not as strong.

Stepping reflex

The baby is held upright, and the feet placed on a firm surface. As the foot presses down on the surface, the other leg flexes at the hip and knee in a stepping movement. As this response is alternated from one leg to the other, the baby makes a walking movement.

The Moro reflex

This is the best known of the primitive reflexes, but it must not be forgotten that because it is a 'startle' reaction it will make the baby cry. It should therefore be left to the end of the examination. Always be gentle in carrying out the test, and make sure that the baby is well-supported. The baby's body is supported with one arm and hand, and the head with the other hand. The hand holding the head is then lowered a few centimetres, allowing the baby's head to drop back (Fig. 18.13). In a positive response the baby abducts and extends the arms, and then flexes them. A clearly unilateral response suggests some local abnormality, such as a fracture or brachial plexus injury in the arm on the side that does not respond.

ASSESSMENT OF GESTATION

Although a full assessment of gestation is beyond the scope of this chapter, a rough approximation of the baby's gestational age should always be made, especially if the baby is small. This can be made from a combination of maternal menstrual data, and size and appearance of the baby. The flexed position of the baby at term has already been mentioned, and the more immature the baby, the less flexed he or she will be. Certain physical criteria are the basis of more formal assessments. Among these are the shape and form of the ears: is the pinna flat against the skull and unfolded, or is it folded over with a good development of cartilage? The degree of breast formation, the degree of ossification of the skull, and opacification of the skull to transillumination with a bright light are important specific features.

A neurological assessment, especially of muscle tone and movement, and the development of certain reflexes, will also give a guide to gestation. For example, by 32 weeks the baby will turn his or her head towards a diffuse light; by 34–36 weeks sucking and neck-righting reflexes will have developed.

At the end of the examination of the newborn infant, a comment should always be made of the estimated gestation.

EXAMINATION OF THE HIPS

The examination of the hips is essential but should be left to the end of the assessment because it is very uncomfortable for the baby. It is illustrated in Figures 18.14 and 18.15. It is usual to differentiate between a tendinous 'click' and the typical 'clunk' of a hip moving in and out of its socket. The latter is more a feeling than an actual noise. Skin creases on the upper posterior thigh may be asymmetrical, but this is not a reliable sign of dislocation; similarly, lim-

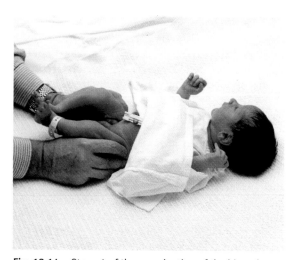

Fig. 18.14   Stage 1 of the examination of the hips: the hips are flexed, medially rotated, and pushed posteriorly. This will dislocate dislocatable hips.

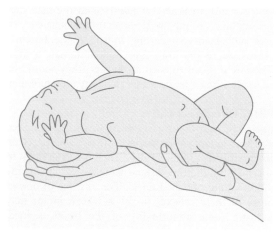

Fig. 18.13   Eliciting the Moro reflex.

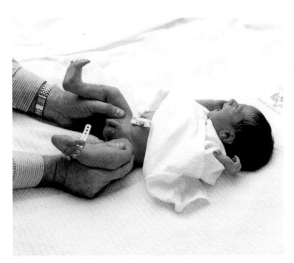

Fig. 18.15 Stage 2 of the examination of the hips: the hips are abducted, and a 'click' or a 'clunk' is felt for (see text). Note the position of the examiner's hands, with the thumbs on the medial aspect of the thigh, and the fingers over the lateral trochanters.

itation of abduction is not absolutely reliable. If there is any doubt about the hip, ultrasound examination should be carried out. Routine ultrasound examination of the hips of all newborn babies is now being carried out in some centres to screen for congenital dislocation. Some centres prefer to screen the most 'at risk' babies for congenital dislocation (see Box 18.10). If any doubt still remains, orthopaedic referral is essential.

BOX 18.10   Babies at greater risk of congenital dislocation of the hip.

- Breech extraction
- Primipara with extended breech delivery
- Females
- Family history of congenital dislocation

SCREENING FOR GENETIC DISORDERS

There are a number of disorders for which screening is available by testing at birth, and others which may be tested for by measurement of white blood cell enzymes, e.g. gangliosidosis and other lipid storage disorders. In most of these, tests are not carried out routinely except in genetically isolated populations, or in families known to be at risk. In the UK, all newborn infants are screened for phenylketonuria and hypothyroidism by a heel prick blood test at 7 days. Other conditions can be screened for in vulnerable populations (Box 18.11). Increasingly, direct DNA analysis for genetic disorders is becoming available for many inherited disorders.

Having now completed the examination, the newborn baby should be dressed and, as in every examination of children, your findings must be conveyed to the parents.

CONCLUSIONS

Throughout this chapter, emphasis has been placed on getting to know the child, and treating him or her as gently as possible. Time has to be spent getting the child's confidence and indeed building up your own confidence. This can only be acquired by examining children at each and every opportunity. One of the most rewarding parts of paediatrics is when a child sits on your lap and plays happily with you. If you can achieve this, you know how to examine children.

BOX 18.11   Inherited conditions screened for at birth.

- Phenylketonuria
- Hypothyroidism
- Haemoglobinopathies in vulnerable groups
- Cystic fibrosis in affected families
- Congenital adrenal hyperplasia

19
THE EXAMINATION OF ELDERLY PEOPLE

INTRODUCTION

It is appropriate to think of elderly people in three distinct groups: the young old (65–74), the old old (75–84), and the oldest old (85+). The social and biological characteristics of people in each of these groups is sufficiently distinct to make these categories meaningful. The emphasis in the training of health care workers, and medical students in particular, is upon disease because the detection, investigation, treatment and prevention of disease is the justification for medicine, its one specific function. However, even when detected and treated, disease often leaves disabilities. The majority of elderly, frail and disabled people, including those with severe functional impairments, live in private households. Many depend to a greater or lesser extent upon those who contribute to their social networks, whether informally or formally.

SOCIAL NETWORKS

The informal network of support consists of kin—nuclear and extended family—and friends and neighbours (Box 19.1). This network is usually not very extensive and has a long history of contact with the old person, whether rewarding, hostile or mixed. Though less skilled than a formal network, it has the great advantage of being available at all times, of being able to deal with unexpected events and emergencies, and of being flexible, familiar and continuous.

The formal network of support consists first of any basic financial entitlements, such as retirement

---

BOX 19.1 Social networks.

Informal
- Family, friends and neighbours: available, concerned and committed, familiar, flexible

Formal
- Financial entitlements: pension and other income
- Statutory services: health care and social services
- Voluntary services: church and charity

---

and supplementary pensions. The statutory agencies themselves carry out governmental economic and social policies and actually provide a service; for example, in the UK these comprise the National Health Service (including the general practitioner, district nurse and health visitor) and the local Social Services, e.g. home car, meals-on-wheels and daycare facilities. Finally, there are the voluntary organizations, and religious authorities and organizations, which are also important.

No assessment of an older person with even slight disability is complete without a description of the people who are available to help.

PRESENTATION OF DISEASE

Two major factors influence the recognition of disease processes in elderly people:

- Acceptance of ill health with a subsequent delay in seeking help
- Atypical presentation of disease processes.

Acceptance of ill health and disease as 'ageing', with its resultant disabilities, means that many elderly people *expect* to be frail, rarely complain, and often seek help late. Dramatic complaints, such as severe pain or vomiting blood, may elicit an appropriate call for help while less life-threatening episodes are accepted as part of the ageing process. Coming to terms with some disability or change is necessary at all ages and acceptance is part of survival. However, the tacit acceptance of inevitable deterioration—for example in vision, hearing, teeth and feet—may lead to treatable conditions being ignored and result in loss of independence.

The fact of atypical presentation in old age is one of the most essential elements for the student and practitioner to comprehend. The term 'geriatric giants' (Box 19.2) refers to a set of symptoms and signs that occur in old age that may have as their cause *any* disease process. Diseases as diverse in aetiology as pneumonia, myocardial infarction or drug toxicity may present *classically* or as one of the geriatric giants.

A useful analogy is a seizure occurring in a child. This is a symptom not a diagnosis. The diagnosis could be febrile illness, epilepsy, meningitis or head injury. In the same way that a fit is not a normal childhood event, falls or incontinence should not be treated as part of the normal ageing process.

There are two other important aspects concerning the unique presentation of disease in old age. One is the concept of *multiple pathology*, and the other is the recognition of the *social presentation* of disease, and the response that can subsequently occur. Multiple pathologies may be causally linked although, more typically, they are not. The art of diagnosis and management in the elderly is in identifying and treating the most important clinical problems, and utilizing a multi-disciplinary approach that compensates for as many of the other associated deficits as possible.

This holistic approach to care of the elderly recognizes that geriatric medicine has a lot to do with social problems. 'Social admission' is a pejorative term in a hospital setting. It usually indicates a lack of history-taking and examination that should have uncovered a disease process resulting in a social response (e.g. relatives leaving a person in the accident and emergency department or neighbours calling on a social worker or the police 'to do some-thing'). Recognition of this social presentation of disease allows multiple problems to be identified and treated more easily.

HISTORY

To provide adequate assessment of elderly people several aspects of the history are crucial (Box 19.3).

The first contact is extremely important (Box 19.4). It should be straightforward, relatively formal and should respect the dignity of the person. Eye contact, a greeting, an outstretched hand (expecting a returned handshake), your name and the purpose of the meeting are all that are required to begin with. These relatively simple gestures can provide a wealth of information in the first few minutes. Can the person see you? Do they smile in response to your smile? Depressed and very anxious patients may avoid eye contact. The hand contact is useful. Some patients with dementia may not respond—not recognizing the meaning of the social gesture. Frightened elderly patients may continue to clutch one's hand. An unwillingness to let go may also indicate a positive grasp reflex, a primitive reflex usually indicating frontal lobe damage and found in advanced dementia. Giving your name and purpose puts people at ease and can also be used later to assess short-term memory. Ask the person 'What is your name?'; be alert for hearing impairment. The reply indicates how a person wishes to be addressed; alternatively a person may be specifically asked.

Make sure that you are both comfortable. Sit at the same height. Ask the patient whether he or she usually wears glasses and ensure they are put on; the same applies to hearing aids and false teeth. Deafness is such a common problem that any situation where elderly people are seen regularly should have a communication aid available (from ear

---

BOX 19.2   'Geriatric giants': major clinical syndromes that may result from any disease process.

- Immobility
- Falls
- Incontinence
- Pressure sores
- Confusion

BOX 19.3   History-taking: points to note.

- The introduction
- Timing, interest
- Position and comfort
- Vision, hearing, cognition
- Environment
- Use of multiple sources of information
- Interview versus interrogation

BOX 19.4   Observations during the introduction.

- Can the patient see and hear you?
- Is behaviour normal?
- Is language normal?
- Does the patient understand your role as a doctor?
- Is the patient at ease, or in pain?
- Is there evidence of support from family or friends?

trumpet to electronic aid). If the person is deaf, note the presence of a hearing aid, sit with your face well lit (to help lip reading) and *do not shout*. Talking at the bedside in a busy environment is accepted practice. This is not privacy and is the wrong place to discuss sensitive issues such as incontinence, to test for cognitive impairment or to explore depressive symptoms. A quiet room is necessary to do the job properly.

Let the elderly patient tell the story in their own way, but help with the time sequence. Inevitably some patients will start with 'It all started when I was injured in the war'. This is really a statement about personal self-worth, and respect and politeness dictates that you should listen to a little of the story. You may use it to collect information that you were planning to ask about later.

Try to avoid interrupting a patient's story. Some patients give a rapid account of things, others are much slower. Try to adjust your pace to that of the patient, a long lifespan means a lot more potential information. However, you may need to interrupt and re-direct the conversation. Do not behave as a 'busy person', but relax and show you have time to listen, even if you are in a hurry. Give the patient your complete and undivided attention. History-taking with an elderly person can be a time-consuming but ultimately rewarding process. If you are unavoidably called away during the interview, apologize and explain what is happening. Avoid telephone interruptions; the person you are with is *always* more important.

ACTIVITIES OF DAILY LIVING (ADL)

In young patients a brief enquiry concerning all the major bodily systems can be used to rule out serious or life-threatening problems. In older patients this approach may not be appropriate; a systems enquiry can be time-consuming, producing spurious symptoms, many of which are not immediately relevant. Some sort of sifting procedure is needed. An enquiry about activities of daily living (ADL) provides a useful screen (see Table 19.1).

In general, patients who can dress, get about outdoors, are continent, can do their own housework and cooking and manage their own pension do not require much immediate enquiry other than about their presenting problem. Among the old old and the oldest old, such patients are the exception. If a daily living task cannot be carried out then it is necessary to make a detailed enquiry focusing on the reason for this.

It is useful to obtain a 'pre-morbid' ADL enabling you to describe what the patient was usually able to do before they became ill. This provides a rough goal for the outcome of treatment. A patient who was unable to get in and out of the bath, who could not dress unaided and who was incontinent prior to suf-

fering a stroke or heart attack is not likely to recover to a trouble-free life. One cannot make the assumption that an elderly person was free from disability before the onset of an acute illness.

DRUG HISTORY

Elderly people are prescribed more medication than any other age group. A treatment history checklist is useful when enquiring about current and past medications (Box 19.5).

Many patients do not take all (or even any) of their prescribed medication. Checking dates on bottles, and a tablet count, can be as a rough guide to compliance. Medicine cabinets often contain old medication kept for use in the event of future problems and many elderly people will change a new medication for an older, tested remedy without telling the doctor. Traditional treatments are also often used.

It is often necessary to be critical of the history and check key points. The simplest method of corroboration is to go over the key symptoms with the patient a few hours after the initial interview. However, it is essential to get whatever help you can from collateral sources of information. Obtain all the old case notes. Most important of all talk to a close relative or friend whenever possible. The telephone can be a vital piece of equipment for history-taking with elderly patients. A comprehensive history in an elderly person requires appropriate time and effort devoted to the process.

EXAMINATION

GENERAL

Always praise patients for their cooperation and performance. Do not complete the examination in silence—your patient may think that you have found something sinister. Explain what you are doing as you go and comment reassuringly on what you find.

Ask your patient to remove their clothes themselves. Consider whether the patient can reach their feet and manage buttons. Is their balance mechanism good? Can they get on to the examination couch unaided? Is there lateralized, proximal or distal weakness? Are there features suggesting pain? Or dyspnoea? These points may help in making a diagnosis.

Once undressed, keep the patient comfortable and use a blanket to protect their dignity. If the patient is agitated, or if you are intending a vaginal or rectal examination, a nurse should be present to assist. In the elderly the *temperature* is not always high even with obvious infection. If the temperature is low it must be measured with a low-reading rectal thermometer. Weigh the patient, record the result and *always* test the urine.

TABLE 19.1   The Barthel ADL Index (total score 20).

Item	Categories
Bowels	0 = incontinent (or needs to be given an enema)
	1 = occasional accident (once per week)
	2 = continent
Bladder	0 = incontinent/catheterized, unable to manage
	1 = occasional accident (max once every 24 h)
	2 = continent (for over 7 days)
Grooming	0 = needs help with personal care
	1 = independent face/hair/teeth/shaving (implements provided)
Toilet use	0 = dependent
	1 = needs some help but can do something alone
	2 = independent (on and off, dressing, wiping)
Feeding	0 = unable
	1 = needs help cutting, spreading butter, etc.
	2 = independent (food provided in reach)
Transfer	0 = unable — no sitting balance
	1 = major help (one or two people, physical), can sit
	2 = minor help (verbal or physical)
	3 = independent
Mobility	0 = immobile
	1 = wheelchair independent (includes corners)
	2 = walks with help of one (verbal/physical)
	3 = independent (may use any aid, e.g. stick)
Dressing	0 = dependent
	1 = needs help, does about half unaided
	2 = independent, includes buttons, zips, shoes
Stairs	0 = unable
	1 = needs help (verbal, physical), carrying aid
	2 = independent
Bathing	0 = dependent
	1 = independent (may use shower)

The Barthel Index should be used as a record of what a patient does, not as a record of what he could do. The main aim is to establish the degree of independence from any help, physical or verbal, however minor and for whatever reason. The need for supervision means the patient is not independent. Performance over the preceding 24–48 h is important but longer periods are relevant. A patient's performance should be established using the best available evidence. Ask the patient or carer but also observe what the patient can do. Direct testing is not needed. Unconscious patients score '0' throughout. Middle categories imply that the patient supplies over 50% effort. Use of aids to be independent is allowed.

BOX 19.5   Areas to cover in a treatment history.

- Current medication
- Previous hospital and family doctor medication
- Treatment from 'alternative' practitioners
- Self-medication
- Past bad experiences with medicines
- Other non-drug treatments
- Medicines kept in the home

SPECIAL CONSIDERATIONS

SKIN

Wrinkles are mainly due to past exposure to ultraviolet light and hence are not usually seen in covered areas. Elderly skin can bruise easily (*senile purpura*) and some people have skin like transparent tissue paper, especially on the backs of the hands and forearms (Figs 19.1 and 19.2). The skin around the eyes may show yellow plaques—*Dubreuilh's elastoma*. Some solar-induced changes to be aware of include keratoacanthoma, basal cell carcinoma, squamous cell carcinoma and malignant melanoma. The most common skin lesion noted is the small red Campbell de Morgan spot, a benign lesion seen most often on the trunk and abdomen.

Leg ulcers are extremely common in old age. Approximately 50% of leg ulcers are due to venous stasis (Fig. 19.3), 10% to arterial disease and 30–40% are mixed. Examination should include palpating the peripheral pulses and measurement of

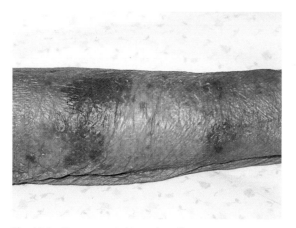

Fig. 19.1   Transparent skin and senile purpura.

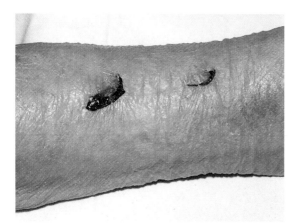

Fig. 19.2   Transparent skin.

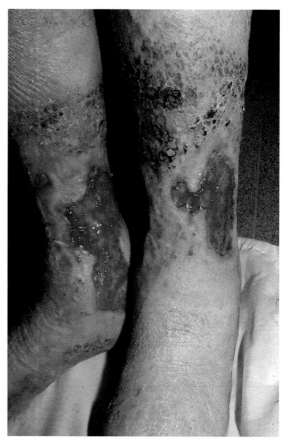

Fig. 19.3   Leg ulcers.

ankle blood pressure using a Doppler meter to determine whether the arterial circulation is adequate. The Doppler is used instead of a stethoscope in the lower limb. The resting pressure index (RPI) is calculated using the formula:

$$RPI = \frac{Brachial\ systolic\ pressure}{Pedal\ systolic\ pressure}$$

An RPI of 1.0 is normal; an RPI below 1.0 may indicate arterial disease, when the blood pressure at the ankle is less than that at the elbow.

Check cutaneous pressure areas, especially heels, hips and sacrum for signs of skin breakdown (*pressure or decubitus ulcers*).

CARDIOVASCULAR SYSTEM

Age-related structural and functional changes in the cardiovascular system account for a slight increase in mean blood pressure with increasing age. Heart valves, especially the aortic valve, can become less mobile, exacerbated by atheromatous disease and calcification. This causes an ejection systolic murmur, heard best in the aortic area, and common in older people. Degeneration and calcification of the mitral valve can result in either apical ejection murmurs or the more common pansystolic mitral regurgitant murmur (see Ch. 8). The increase in heart rate in response to stress (e.g. exercise, illness or pyrexia) is reduced in advanced old age.

A lying and standing (or sitting) blood pressure is mandatory in the examination of all elderly patients. A drop in systolic blood pressure on standing of more than 30 mmHg is defined as postural hypotension, a considerable cause of morbidity in old age.

As in younger patients, the character of the carotid pulse should be noted. All peripheral pulses should be examined and their presence or absence noted. Peripheral vascular disease is common in the aged, and palpation of vascular pulsation can be difficult due to atheroma or oedema. In the lower limbs Doppler measurement (see above) can be used to assess the peripheral circulation. The clinical signs of cardiac disease, for example valve lesions or congestive heart failure, do not alter in old age. Assessment of retinal vessels for signs of disease, such as hypertension and diabetes, can prove difficult in old people due to the frequent presence of cataracts.

RESPIRATORY SYSTEM

With ageing the elasticity of the lungs declines, so that they become more distensible. The lung fields on a chest X-ray may therefore appear overinflated. Kyphosis, due to intervertebral disc degeneration and osteoporosis, and calcification of the costal cartilages make the chest wall more rigid and less expansible. Counting the respiratory rate is one of the most useful screening examinations. At rest the normal rate will be about 15 breaths per minute. Anxiety may push this up to 20 per minute. With respiratory distress caused, for example, by heart failure or pneumonia, the respiratory rate increases in order to maintain gas transfer. It is not until rates increase to 35–40 per minute that a person looks obviously short of breath, so it is necessary to count the rate over at least half a minute. The physical signs of respiratory system disease, such as cyanosis, lip pursing and tachypnoea, are the same as in younger patients.

Coarse basal crackles caused by air-trapping due to loss of pulmonary elasticity can make interpretation of breath sounds difficult. In a sick elderly person a chest X-ray is essential, regardless of the presence or absence of signs and symptoms of pulmonary disease. Previous films, if available, help in interpretation. A major problem for ill elderly people is the position required for a good-quality posteroanterior film. A sympathetic and experienced radiographer is essential. Common changes on the X-ray include calcification from old tuberculosis, calcification in chondral cartilages and major blood vessels, pleural calcification from past pneumonia and old rib fractures.

VISION AND THE EYES

Visual acuity should be assessed and any loss of vision noted, together with a history of the development of the visual disorder. Acute and chronic causes of loss of vision should be considered during the examination (Box 19.6).

The eyes may be sunken due to loss of periorbital fat; this may be severe enough to cause drooping of the upper lid (*ptosis*) and redundant skin at the lateral borders, but may be a feature of normal ageing. The loss of fat can also cause the lower eyelid to curl in (*entropion*) and irritate the cornea, causing redness and watering (*epiphora*). The laxity also enables the eyelid to fall outwards slightly (*ectropion*) with the same results. A whitish rim around the iris (*arcus senilis*) is a zone of lipid deposition around the periphery of the cornea.

HEARING

If deafness is suspected the external ear must be inspected for wax. However, deafness is most often due to presbyacusis, an age-related degeneration of the cochlear hair cells. If a hearing aid is being worn make sure it is switched on. Communication is aided by raising your voice (but *not* by shouting), obtaining attention, sitting face to face, reducing background noise and speaking slowly and clearly.

NERVOUS SYSTEM

Consideration of higher cortical function (language, perception and memory) must not be omitted from routine testing. It is essential that the mental state be assessed early in the interview and the results recorded in the notes (see below). It is important to recognize difficulties with communication, and to consider this possibility if the history proves difficult to elicit or understand. Communication is a two-way process that involves understanding and comprehension, as well as the production of appropriate speech. Communication problems can be considered in terms of:

- Disorders of language (dysphasia)
- Disorders of articulation (dyspraxia, dysarthria)
- Disorders of voice (dysphonia) or of fluency (dysfluency).

Dysphasia is the difficulty in encoding and decoding language and hence can be *receptive*, in which the comprehension of incoming speech is lost, or *expressive*, when speech formation is impaired. Usually both these problems coexist. Dysphasia is usually associated with a left hemisphere lesion. *Dyspraxia* is difficulty initiating and carrying out voluntary movements, for example of the tongue, and hence can affect speech. *Dysarthria* has many causes, including local factors in the mouth and dentition, stroke, Parkinson's disease, motor neurone disease and other neurological disorders. *Dysphonia*, an abnormality of the voice (e.g. hoarseness), can be due to anxiety, vocal abuse, disease such as carcinoma of the larynx or hypothyroidism, and can follow surgery to the throat or even a general anaesthetic with intubation. *Dysfluency* (stammer) is found in people of all ages.

BOX 19.6   Common causes of acute and chronic loss of vision.

Acute
- Refinal detachment
- Vascular (central retinal artery/vein thrombosis)
- Angle-closure glaucoma

Chronic
- Cataract
- Macular degeneration
- Open-angle glaucoma
- Diabetic retinopathy

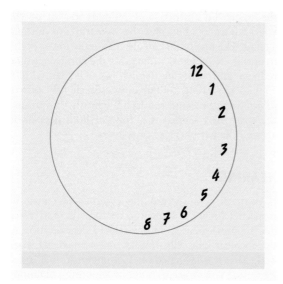

Fig. 19.4   Clock face drawing.

Pencil and paper tests can be invaluable in providing a global measure of mental competence. One test is to present a circle of about 10–15 cm diameter and ask the patient to fill in the numbers of a clock face (Fig. 19.4). This test will be abnormal in patients who have visual impairments, who have difficulty carrying out purposeful actions (*apraxia*), who have perceptual problems especially involving the right parietal lobe, or who are cognitively impaired.

In addition to the formal assessment of the peripheral nervous system by examining muscle bulk and tone, power, sensation and tendon reflexes, it is essential to observe the *walking* or gait pattern in every patient. It is common for the ankle jerks to be diminished or hard to elicit in very old people.

Examination of the gait may reveal subtle evidence of hemiparesis, poor balance (see Box 19.8), or the furniture-clutching gait of the patient with long-standing mobility problems. This assessment also provides an objective check of at least one activity of daily living. Occasionally patients report that they are capable of carrying out activities when in reality they cannot. Always check the toenails for chiropody problems (e.g. onychogryphosis) where a 'painful' gait is seen.

GASTROINTESTINAL

The majority of elderly people are edentulous. If dentures are used they should be worn during the examination so that problems with fit, for example poor speech or eating difficulties, can be corrected early. Leucoplakia appears as small white patches on the oral mucosa. It is associated with repeated mucosal trauma and may become malignant. Varicosities on the underside of the tongue are seen in about 40% of elderly people; their significance is unknown, though vitamin C deficiency has been implicated.

BOX 19.7   Faecal impaction may cause:

- Faecal incontinence (ball valve effect with spurious diarrhoea)
- Intestinal obstruction
- Restlessness and agitation in the confused (but *never itself causes confusion*)
- Retention of urine
- Rectal bleeding

Rectal examination is required as part of a full examination and especially if there are symptoms implying lower gastrointestinal, pelvic or prostatic disease. Constipation severe enough to cause faecal impaction is not uncommon and can have serious consequences (Box 19.7).

THE 'GERIATRIC GIANTS' (see Box 19.2, p397)

IMMOBILITY

Impaired mobility is one of the most common clinical presentations in geriatric practice. A careful history is invaluable in deciding the underlying problem or problems. The patient should be asked specifically what happened. In assessing this question and the answer given always try to separate cause from effect. Frequently the patient has several problems of which immobility is but one. The prognosis for recovery, however, is largely determined by the underlying cause of the patient's immobility. The crucial information is the time frame. Sudden immobility should be straightforward to diagnose, yet stroke and impacted subcapital femoral fracture can be missed. A steady deterioration in mobility over several years implies a chronic process, e.g. Parkinson's disease and osteoarthrosis. A stepwise decline indicates a disease that has periods of exacerbation and remission, for example multiple sclerosis, recurrent minor strokes or rheumatoid arthritis. Repeated rapid swings between full mobility and total immobility over a few days indicates recurrent medical problems, e.g. heart failure and urinary tract infection. The most difficult patients are those in whom the disease process caused immobility a long time ago and the picture is now clouded by the complications of immobility.

Within the bounds of common sense the patient should be asked or helped to stand up and a few steps attempted. This may reveal that a patient can walk but is immobile because he or she is unable to get out of a chair or bed unaided. Alternatively a confused patient may not have mentioned pain on standing preventing attempts to move. A chair-shaped patient indicates a long period of immobility. If the patient has no concept of walking, *apraxia*, an inability to carry out a purposeful sequence of activity despite normal power and sensation, should be suspected. This is usually due to multiple strokes, dementia or frontal lobe degenerative disease. Tentative steps with clutching of helpers may indicate loss of confidence following a fall. A dramatic staggering to the nearest bed, chair or nurse followed by an award-winning collapse suggests that a behavioral cause is possible.

Sometimes a diagnostic gait pattern is found. Typical examples are:

- The broad-based, unsteady gait of ataxia
- The apraxic gait with rapid small steps like a slipping clutch or with feet apparently glued to the floor
- The Parkinsonian gait with loss of postural reflexes, festination, a fixed posture, tremor, rigidity, hypokinesia of face and limbs, excess salivation and seborrhoea
- The gait of stroke with dragging of one leg
- The myopathic waddling gait due to weak proximal muscles, e.g. from osteomalacia.

Gait abnormality is a common problem, of course, in the presence of *osteoarthrosis* of joints, and of local problems with the feet, especially when there is *local pain*. Always remember that immobility in elderly patients is almost always a multifactorial problem.

FALLS

Falls are common in old age and are more common in women than in men, especially in the very old. Several causes may coexist (Box 19.8). The physiological changes of ageing may well be superimposed, making it a difficult task to sort out the underlying cause.

It is obvious that even a single fall should lead to a detailed history and examination. Witnesses should always be questioned too. In a patient who was previously well, a search must be made for new acute illness. If none is present the fall may be 'accidental' and due to ageing, or to environmental factors. Information about the pattern of any previous falls can be helpful; in particular their frequency, relationship with posture or time of day, any residual symptoms following the fall and any avoiding steps taken by the patient should be ascertained. Falls that occur on changing posture, particularly on standing from lying, suggest postural hypotension. A trip may occur simply as a result of poor postural reflexes associated with ageing, but may be aggravated by poor vision. Sometimes bifocal glasses can give a distorted view, leading to accidental falls. The absence of any warning implies a sudden event, usually of a neurological or circulatory nature. The most useful investigation in elderly fallers is to watch them walking.

INCONTINENCE

Incontinence is an involuntary loss of urine or faeces in an inappropriate place. Check for a past history of sphincter dysfunction. Talk to the patient and relatives. Differentiate between loss of ability to control excretion and failure to identify or get to an accept-

---

BOX 19.8   The causes of falls in elderly people.

Premonitory
- Forerunner of acute, usually infectious illness

Medication
- Multiple drug therapy
- Psychotropic drugs
- L-Dopa
- Antihypertensives

Postural hypotension
- Drugs
- Alcohol
- Cardiac disease

Neurological disease
- Multiple strokes
- Transient ischaemic attack
- Parkinson's disease
- Cerebellar disease
- Epilepsy
- Age-related loss of postural reflexes
- Spastic paraparesis (usually due to cervical spondylosis)
- Peripheral neuropathy with sensory loss

Circulatory system disease
- Silent myocardial infarction
- Vasovagal attack
- Cardiac dysrhythmias, especially Stokes–Adams disease and atrial fibrillation
- Postural

Musculoskeletal disease
- General muscle weakness (e.g. due to systemic malignancy)
- Muscular wasting due to arthritis
- Unstable knee joint
- Myopathy (e.g. osteomalacia)

Miscellaneous
- Drop attacks
- Hypoglycaemia
- Cervical spondylosis
- Alcohol
- Elder abuse (e.g. physical mistreatment)
- Poor vision
- Multisensory deprivation:
  - deafness
  - poor vision
  - labyrinthine disorder
  - peripheral neuropathy

---

able place. Clinical examination, including a rectal and a vaginal examination, evaluation of the pelvic floor muscles, and culture of a mid-stream specimen of urine are all essential (and will often give a good indication as to the cause of the problem). An incontinence chart kept for a few days may suggest a recognizable pattern of urinary and/or faecal incontinence. The specialist help of a continence adviser may be needed. Causes of urinary incontinence include infection, stress incontinence, detrusor instability, overflow, prostatism, neurogenic bladder, uterine or rectal prolapse, cystocele and atrophic vaginitis. Causes of faecal incontinence include pelvic floor weakness, carcinoma of the rectum, diverticular disease and laxative abuse. Faecal overloading with impaction and neurogenic bowel may also present with faecal incontinence.

PRESSURE ULCERS

Necrosis of skin, adipose tissue and muscle caused by pressure occurs rapidly in acutely and chronically ill elderly people. The mean capillary pressure in the skin of healthy medical students is approximately 25 mmHg. No measurements are available for normal elderly people let alone those who are ill. External pressures on the skin greater than 25 mmHg can lead to occlusion of cutaneous blood vessels; the surrounding tissues, including the skin, then become hypoxic. A bedridden patient easily generates pressures in excess of 100 mmHg, especially over the sacrum, heels and greater trochanters (96% of 'decubitus' pressure ulcers occur below the level of the waist).

About 80% of pressure ulcers are superficial (Fig. 19.5). They occur mainly in dehydrated and incontinent patients exposed to sustained pressure, especially developing postoperatively. The majority of these ulcers are preventable. Any ulcer will deepen if the pressure is not relieved. Deep ulcers (Fig. 19.6) are formed when localized high pressure applied to the skin cuts off a wedge-shaped area of tissue, usually adjacent to a bony prominence.

All at-risk patients should have anti-pressure protection started immediately a new illness or injury occurs, whether at home or in hospital. Clinical scales to determine the risk, such as the Norton scale (Table 19.2), are often used in nursing management. These scales allocate a numerical score to risk factors e.g. incontinence, immobility, sensory loss, body weight and nutrition, conscious level. All pressure area sites must be inspected at the first clinical assessment and again at regular intervals during the illness. Active management of pressure areas will help prevent ulceration. A most effective medium-priced prevention and treatment is an alternating pressure air mattress (APAM). The horizontal cells (Fig. 19.7) inflate and deflate over a short cycle, constantly supporting the patient but providing periods of low pressure at all sites.

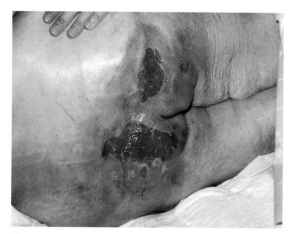

Fig. 19.5 Superficial pressure sores.

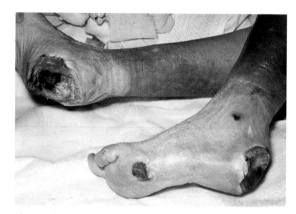

Fig. 19.6 Deep pressure sores.

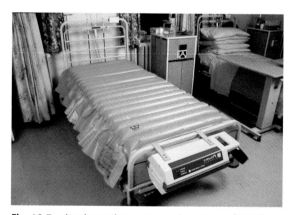

Fig. 19.7 An alternating pressure air mattress (APAM).

TABLE 19.2	Norton scale for pressure sores. Low scores carry a high risk.			
Physical	**Neural**	**Activity**	**Mobility**	**Incontinence**
4 Good	4 Alert	4 Ambulant	4 Full	4 None
3 Fair	3 Apathetic	3 Walks with help	3 Slightly limited	3 Occasional
2 Poor	2 Confused	2 Not bound	2 Very limited	2 Usually
1 Very poor	1 Stupor	1 Bedfast	1 Immobile	1 Double

CONFUSION

The term confusional state describes an abnormal mental state in which the patient is disoriented in time, place and person, often in the context of other, global disturbances of mental function. *Delirium* is an acute confusional state with global mental impairment and altered consciousness. *Dementia* is a chronic confusional state with global mental impairment in an alert patient. Delirium with increasing confusion can occur in a patient with dementia.

Acute confusional state (delirium) is one of the most common forms of *organic brain syndrome*. In most such patients there are physical and mental abnormalities that need urgent assessment. Failure to recognize it and hence to diagnose and treat the underlying condition can have fatal consequences for the patient. During hospitalization a person's level of cognitive functioning should be monitored periodically. Multiple coexisting causative factors are common. The differential diagnosis includes acute or chronic confusion, e.g. mild underlying dementia with an additional acute problem, and acute functional psychosis (*pseudodelirium*).

Chronic confusional states (dementia) must have been present for at least 3 months to be labelled as such. There is usually loss of function in multiple areas (e.g. intellectual function, memory, language). There are, however, reversible causes even of such long-lasting confusion—for example drugs, depression and endocrine abnormalities—and appropriate diagnosis and treatment may produce improvement. Chronic confusional states become increasingly common in old age (10% above age 65 years, 20% above age 80 years). Dementia is not a component of normal ageing. Regardless of age a search for the cause is warranted. The differential diagnoses include benign senescent forgetfulness, amnestic syndromes and depression (*pseudodementia*).

The two most common causes of dementia are Alzheimer's disease (AD) and multi-infarct dementia. AD is a clinical diagnosis made on the history, and by excluding other disorders. Clinical criteria for multi-infarct dementia include the presence of dementia with the history of a stepwise deteriorating course, a patchy or uneven distribution of cognitive deficits and focal neurological signs. These and other characteristic features are integrated in the *Hachinski score* (Box 19.9), used to numerically assert the likelihood of a cerebrovascular cause. Investigations in chronic confusional states are aimed at identifying potentially reversible causes. At the same time vulnerable frail patients should not be expected to undergo unpleasant tests, and scarce resources should be used appropriately.

THE CONFUSED ELDERLY PATIENT

'Patient confused, no history available' speaks volumes about the training and attitude of a doctor.

> **BOX 19.9   Hachinski scare for assessment of probability of vascular dementia.**
>
> | | |
> |---|---|
> | Abrupt onset | 2 |
> | Stepwise deterioration | 1 |
> | Fluctuating course | 2 |
> | Nocturnal confusion | 1 |
> | Relative preservation of personality | 1 |
> | Depression | 1 |
> | Somatic complaints | 1 |
> | Emotional incontinence | 1 |
> | History of hypertension | 1 |
> | History of strokes | 2 |
> | Associated atherosclerosis | 1 |
> | Focal neurological symptoms | 2 |
> | Focal neurological signs | 2 |
>
> A score of 6 or more suggests a cerebrovascular cause for the dementia

Confused patients deserve better. It is crucial to establish early on whether the patient is orientated in place, time and person. One must also decide whether the patient is alert. It is important to use a standard test of mental function (Box 19.10). Explain to the patient that you wish to test their memory. With experience, it is possible to check most of the items in the mental test score by working them into your introductory talk with the patient. Deafness and speech impairments (such as nominal dysphasia) can make people appear very cognitively impaired. Depressed patients tend to do poorly on mental test scores. If a problem is detected with a simple test proceed to a more in-depth assessment using the Mini-mental State Examination (p. 42). Assessments of mental state are most valuable when applied serially over a period of time.

ENVOI

Finally, always remember to treat an elderly patient, as any other patient, as a whole person.

> **BOX 19.10   Abbreviated mental test (AMT): total score 10 (one point for each item).**
>
> - Age
> - Time (to nearest hour)
> - Address for recall
> - Year
> - Where do you live (town or road)?
> - Recognition of two persons
> - Date of birth (day and month)
> - Year of start of First World War
> - Name of present monarch/prime minister
> - Count backwards 20–1

OTHER ISSUES

ETHNIC ELDERS

In many countries there are people from a wide range of ethnic groups, all of whom contribute to its social and economic productivity. Ethnic populations are usually derived from migrations of relatively young people, and these people age. The services provided for ethnic elders are generally inadequate. This is partly because of a desire among the host population for assimilation and acculturation to occur, partly because of an assumption that the extended family will cope with the majority of problems, and partly because of lack of understanding and awareness of the problem. The health issues experienced by ethnic elders are similar to those of the indigenous population: heart attacks, strokes, diabetes and cataracts, although they may occur with different frequency to the indigenous population. Health services would be more sensitive to the needs of ethnic minorities if emphasis were placed on the employment of staff from ethnic minorities, more widespread use of trained interpreters, better signposting and provision of health education material in appropriate languages. Always try to understand, and respect the cultural background of your patient and their family.

ELDER ABUSE/INADEQUATE CARE

There are many types of abuse. The most frequent are 'physical, psychological, financial and neglect', which in fact consist of punching, slapping, rape, bullying, intimidation, theft, over-medication and starvation—the choice of descriptive words can make a real difference. Any older person can be a victim of abuse. The most vulnerable are female partners (spouse abuse in old age), those living at home with adult children in a forced situation due to financial difficulties and unemployment, and elderly people in poorly-run institutions such as some residential and nursing homes. In the domestic setting abusers are often dependent on their victims for finance, have experienced poor long-term relationships with the victim and have health and financial problems, especially alcohol and psychological difficulties. In institutions, inadequate staff levels, poorly trained staff, repeated complaints, and poor client and environmental hygiene are all indicators of potentially abusive care.

Factors in identification can include frequent visits to doctors by carers preoccupied with their own problems, but yet often trying to indicate non-verbally their inability to cope. Marked changes in a carer's lifestyle (bereavement, unemployment, illness) can induce extra stress. There is often a poor perception of the dependency of the older person by the carer. Recognition of elder abuse is made more difficult by the physiological and the pathological changes that occur with ageing (e.g. senile purpura). The presence of some of the usual manifestations of inadequate care, especially abrasions, pressure ulcers and poor nutrition should raise the *possibility* of elder abuse. It is important to be aware of the problem, which affects up to 5% of older people. Any 4-year-old child attending accident and emergency with a broken arm will have the diagnosis of non-accidental injury within the differential diagnoses. An 84-year-old woman with a fractured neck of femur will have the cause of the fracture 'fall' either taken for granted or assumed—no one will ask, 'Was she pushed?'

Assessment includes not only a thorough physical examination (documenting positive and negative indicators of abuse) but also a sensitive history from the client including open questions about *the possibility of violent behaviour*. A full social background is necessary, including a sympathetic description of the carer's role. The person's mental state must be assessed and recorded. The diagnosis of abuse or inadequate care may not be made quickly and expert help from senior colleagues, social work, psychiatry or clinical psychology may be necessary for recognition, disclosure and management. It may be necessary to involve the police. Elder abuse is a complex phenomenon which we are only now beginning to recognize and respond to. We fail the most vulnerable people in our society, however, if we are not sufficiently aware of the problem and do not enquire *routinely* about violence within a caring setting during the history and examination.

20
THE GENITALIA AND SEXUALLY TRANSMITTED DISEASES

INTRODUCTION

There is still unwarranted stigma and shame attached to sexually transmitted diseases. Two aspects of sexually transmitted diseases are ever-present. First, an infected patient indicates that at least one other person is also infected. Thus treating a patient in isolation will not control the spread of these diseases. Second, a patient may harbour more than one sexually transmitted disease (Box 20.1). Many infections are asymptomatic and may have been acquired months or even years previously. Remember that babies, monogamous partners and victims of rape and sexual abuse can also be affected.

The interview and examination must be carried out in privacy and with confidentiality. The staff should be sympathetic, without a disapproving or moralistic attitude. As with other clinical problems, diagnosis is achieved by history (Box 20.2), examination and relevant laboratory tests. Following diagnosis, effective

---

BOX 20.1   Sexually transmitted/microbial agents in the genital tract (diseases).

Bacteria
Treponema pallidum (Syphilis)
Neisseria gonorrhoeae (Gonorrhoea)
Chlamydia trachomatis of D-K serovars (non-gonococcal urethritis)
Chlamydia trachomatis of LGV 1–3 serovars (Lymphogranuloma venereum)
Haemophilus ducreyi (Chancroid)

BOX 20.1   (continued)

Klebsiella granulomatis (Granuloma inguinale/Donovanosis)
Gardnerella vaginalis, anaerobes (Bacterial vaginosis)
Shigella species (Shigellosis)
Salmonella species (Salmonellosis)
Mycoplasma, ureaplasma (non-gonococcal urethritis)

Viruses
Herpes simplex virus types 1 and 2 (Genital herpes)
Human papilloma virus (Genital warts)
Molluscum contagiosum virus (Molluscum contagiosum)
Human immunodeficiency virus (AIDS and related diseases)
Hepatitis A, B, C and Delta viruses
Cytomegalovirus

Fungal
Candida albicans (Thrush/moniliasis/candidiasis/candidosis)

Ectoparasites
Phthirus pubis (Pediculosis pubis)
Sarcoptes scabiei (Scabies)

Protozoa
Trichomonas vaginalis (Trichomoniasis)
Entamoeba histolytica (Amoebiasis)
Giardia lambia (Giardiasis)

Nematode
Enterobius vermicularis (Enterobiasis)

---

treatment and contact tracing/partner notification should be instituted promptly. Sexually transmitted diseases in children should alert one to the possibility of sexual abuse although non-sexual transmission can occur.

HISTORY

PRESENTING SYMPTOMS

URETHRAL DISCHARGE

This is nearly always a complaint of men. Ensure that the discharge is from the urethra and not from under the foreskin. Ascertain the colour, amount and duration of the discharge. A purulent discharge suggests gonorrhoea while 'non-specific' urethritis and *Trichomonas vaginalis* are more likely to give rise to scanty mucoid or mucopurulent discharge. Sometimes the patient only notices the discharge in the morning or by the staining of his underwear. Prostatorrhoea may present as urethral discharge and is physiological.

DYSURIA

Urethral pain on passing urine may be described as burning or stinging. False dysuria may occur if urine comes into contact with inflamed areas on the prepuce or vulva (ulcerated).

URINARY FREQUENCY

Frequent passage of urine, usually in small quantity, suggests bladder infection or involvement of the trigone of the bladder from ascending urethritis. It can also indicate anxiety.

VAGINAL DISCHARGE

Ask if it is itchy or offensive. An itchy vaginal discharge is suggestive of thrush or, occasionally, trichomoniasis. Smelly discharges are usually due to trichomoniasis, bacterial vaginosis, or retained foreign bodies such as tampons. Physiological discharge can occur after sexual stimulation or during pregnancy but is not itchy or offensive. Vaginal discharge may also arise from gonococcal or chlamydial cervicitis.

DYSPAREUNIA

This is pain on sexual intercourse (see Ch. 14). In women, superficial dyspareunia is pain in the vulvo-vaginal area and can be due to vulvitis. This has to be differentiated from vulvodynia which is chronic localized burning and soreness in the vulva and may be associated with vestibulitis, vestibular papillomatosis, subclinical warts or may be idiopathic. However, the symptoms can be aggravated by intercourse or tampon insertion. Deep dyspareunia is pain deep in the vagina and may result from pelvic inflammatory disease, endometritis and other gynaecological diseases, particularly endometriosis.

GENITAL ULCER

This is described as a 'sore'. Ask if it is painful or recurrent. *Painful ulcers* are usually due to herpes, chancroid, Stevens–Johnson syndrome, Behçet's disease or trauma, whereas a *painless ulcer* may be due to syphilis or lymphogranuloma venereum. However, a painful ulcer does not exclude syphilis. The evolution of the ulcer is important. Genital herpes may start with local irritation followed by erythema, a group of papules, then blisters which ulcerate and crust before healing. If the infection was acquired in a tropical country, chancroid lymphogranuloma venereum and donovanosis should also be considered. Ask whether the patient has applied any medicament which may interfere with microbiological tests. An acute anogenital ulcer is syphilitic or herpetic unless proven otherwise, the latter if lasting more than 1 month is an AIDS defining illness.

PAINFUL SCROTAL SWELLING

This may indicate acute epididymo-orchitis which may complicate a sexually transmitted disease, or acute surgical emergencies such as torsion of the testis and strangulated inguinal hernia. It is important to remember that neoplasm of the testis may sometimes present as a painful swelling. Other causes include trauma and recent vasectomy. Acute epididymo-orchitis in sexually active men below the age of 35 is likely to result from gonococcal or chlamydial infection, and above the age of 40 from bacterial urinary tract infection such as that due to *Escherichia coli*.

PUBIC AND GENITAL ITCH

This is usually due to pediculosis pubis, scabies or other inflammatory genital conditions such as allergic dermatitis, but may be psychological. Ask if sexual or household contacts also complain of itch. In pediculosis pubis, patients may notice 'crabs' and nits on the hair shaft. Itching at night is suggestive of scabies and is likely to be generalized except for the face.

GENITAL RASH

Itchy rash on the vulva, glans penis or prepuce is seen in thrush, scabies and inflammatory dermatological conditions such as lichen sclerosis or contact dermatitis. Non-itchy rash may be seen in secondary syphilis, circinate balanitis, which is a manifestation of Reiter's disease, and in other genital dermatosis.

ANORECTAL SYMPTOMS

Anal soreness or pain, itch, rectal discharge, pain on defaecation, feeling of incomplete defaecation (*tenesmus*) and constipation may occur in infective proctitis. Anal itch (*pruritus ani*) may be secondary to rectal discharge or due to thrush, anal warts, dermatitis and poor anal hygiene. If the itch is worse at night, threadworms in particular should be considered. Pruritus ani is also commonly psychological in origin. Sexually transmitted enteric infections such as giardiasis, shigellosis and salmonellosis in homosexual and bisexual men may present with diarrhoea. Diarrhoea is also a common problem in HIV infection or may be due to HIV per se or to opportunistic infections such as cryptosporidiosis, isosporiasis and cytomegalovirus colitis

SYSTEMIC REVIEW

The skin, mouth, eyes and joints are commonly associated with sexually transmitted infections. Rash may be seen in acute HIV infection, secondary syphilis, gonococcal septicaemia and Reiter's disease. Conjunctivitis may be seen in chlamydial and gonococcal infection and is usually unilateral, while in Reiter's disease it is usually bilateral. Anterior uveitis may be seen in Reiter's disease, syphilis and HIV infection. Joints may be involved in gonococcal arthritis, Reiter's disease and late syphilis (Charcot's joints). Lower abdominal pain, may indicate pelvic inflammatory disease, while right hypochondrial pain may indicate perihepatitis or Fitz Hugh–Curtis syndrome which are all related to chlamydial or gonococcal infections.

OTHER ASPECTS OF THE HISTORY

A *past history* of genitourinary problems, sexually transmitted diseases, gynaecological diseases and obstetric problems is important. In women, the gynaecological history, e.g. dyspareunia, pelvic inflammatory disease and cervical dysplasia, and the *obstetric history*, e.g. stillbirths, miscarriages or babies with ophthalmia, may be significant. The menstrual history is vital. A delayed menstrual period with unilateral lower abdominal pain may be due to ectopic pregnancy rather than salpingitis. A change in the menstrual cycle may be due to pelvic inflammatory disease. Chlamydial cervicitis may cause postcoital bleed but other causes, including carcinoma of the cervix, must be excluded. Intrauterine contraceptive devices predispose to pelvic inflammatory disease, while the use of condoms may prevent infection. Ask whether the patient has taken any drugs, especially antibiotics, in recent months. Allergy to antimicrobials, particularly to penicillin, must be noted. Where appropriate, drug abuse and injecting drug use should be asked about. Antibiotics, diabetes mellitus, pregnancy and immunosuppression may predispose to thrush.

SEXUAL HISTORY

The patient's confidence should first be obtained by enquiring into non-threatening aspects of the medical history, then moving into more personal details such as contraception and, in the case of women, the menstrual history, before proceeding to the sexual history. Details of the sexual history should be obtained by simple questions. Ascertain the date of exposure (When did you last have intercourse/'sex'?), particulars of contacts over recent months (if married, When did you last have intercourse/'sex' with your wife/husband? followed by When did you last have intercourse/'sex' with someone else?), and whether with regular partners, casual contacts or commercial sex workers. Are sexual partners traceable, e.g. place of intercourse (which town, whether abroad)? If there are several contacts, it is useful to identify them by first names. The possibility of homosexual or bisexual contact should be ascertained (Do you have intercourse/'sex' with men, women or both?).

The incubation period of infection may be assessed from the date of exposure to the onset of symptoms, and hence the probable cause. Tropical sexually transmitted diseases should also be considered in patients presenting with genital problems acquired in the tropics. A history of intercourse with homosexual or bisexual men, injecting drug users or with persons in or from an area of high *human immunodeficiency virus* (*HIV*) endemicity may suggest acquired immune deficiency syndrome (AIDS) as the cause of multisystemic symptoms and signs in a patient.

The type of sexual practice will dictate the sites from which to take tests. It is also helpful to understand some of the common or unfamiliar terms which may be used in relation to sexual practices. 'Straight sex' indicates heterosexual (peno-vaginal) intercourse. Ask whether the person also practises insertive or receptive oro-penile intercourse (Do you have 'oral sex'?).

Certain practices in homosexual or bisexual men ('gay sex') may predispose to particular infections; for example, if there is oro-anal contact, the possibility of intestinal pathogens should be considered. Hepatitis B and HIV infection are more common in those practising receptive peno-anal intercourse. Ask whether he practises insertive ('*active*') or receptive ('*passive*') peno-anal intercourse (When did you last have 'anal sex'? or simply, Are you 'active', 'passive' or both?). Some patients practise oro-anal intercourse ('rimming'), insertive or receptive brachio-anal intercourse ('fisting'), and, rarely, urinating on to each other ('watersports') or using faeces during intercourse ('scat').

Some heterosexual couples also practise peno-anal intercourse. This should be enquired for if rectal infection is found in women, although this commonly occurs without having 'anal sex' in association with infection at other genital sites. Sex 'toys' or 'dildoes' (artificial penises) are objects inserted into the rectum or vagina. 'Fisting' and 'toys' may cause injury presenting as an acute abdomen. 'Bondage', in which the person is tied up during sex, may be associated with masochism (sexual gratification through the infliction of pain on another). This should be suspected if injury marks without an obvious cause are present on the body.

The use of condoms should be enquired into irrespective of whether the patient is using other methods of contraception. Condom usage should be advised if the person is at risk of acquiring or transmitting sexually transmitted diseases including AIDS. It is important to remember that many infections which may initially be acquired through non-sexual means, for example, hepatitis B and HIV infection among injecting drug users and haemophiliacs, may then be transmitted through sexual intercourse. Advice on non-penetrative 'safer sex' practices such as body rubbing, dry kissing and masturbating each other, can be given to infected individuals who do not wish to practise penetrative intercourse.

Psychosexual problems, including erectile dysfunction and premature ejaculation, commonly present to a sexually transmitted disease clinic. The impotence is likely to be psychogenic if it is of sudden onset, related to life events, situational or intermittent, in the presence of nocturnal emissions or early morning erectile function. Organic causes commonly have a psychogenic component.

GENITAL EXAMINATION

The patient should be examined in a well-lit room. Other non-infective genital diseases should be looked for. Gloves should be worn.

MALE GENITALIA

THE PENIS

Note the appearance and size of the penis, the presence or absence of the prepuce, and the position of the external urethral orifice. Examine the penile shaft for warts, ulcers, burrows and excoriated papules of scabies, rashes. In Peyronie's disease there may be induration or fibrotic lump inside the penile shaft. In the uncircumcised, establish that the prepuce can readily be retracted by gently withdrawing it over the glans penis. This allows inspection of the undersurface of the prepuce, the glans penis, the coronal

sulcus and the external urethral orifice (meatus) for warts (Fig. 20.1), inflammation, ulcers and other rash. Always remember to draw the prepuce forwards after examination, otherwise *paraphimosis*, painful oedema of the glans due to constriction by a retracted prepuce, may ensue.

Phimosis is narrowing of the preputial orifice, thereby preventing retraction of the foreskin. This predisposes to recurrent episodes of infection of the glans penis (*balanitis*), the prepuce (*posthitis*), or both (*balanoposthitis*). *Circinate balanitis* of Reiter's disease appears as erythematous eroded lesions which coalesce with a slightly raised and polycyclic edge. Multiple small yellow or white submucous material known as *Fordyce's spots* may be seen on the inner prepuce. These are ectopic sebaceous glands and do not require treatment. In unhygienic patients, *smegma*, which is greyish-white cheesy material arising from Tyson's glands, may accumulate under the prepuce.

Hypospadias is a congenital abnormality in which the external urethral orifice is not at the tip of the glans penis but opens at its ventral surface in the midline, anywhere from the glans to the shaft or even in the perineum. *Epispadias*, a similar opening situated on the dorsal surface of the penis, is rare.

Tiny regular papules arranged in rows around the coronal sulcus are *coronal papillae* and may be mistaken for warts. The coronal sulcus is the commonest site for a chancre. The classic Hunterian chancre, described as a single, painless, indurated ulcer with a clean base, is present in only about 40% of cases of primary syphilis. The meatus is examined for inflammation, urethral discharge, narrowing (stricture) and warts. Retract the lips of the meatus to examine for the presence of meatal chancre and intrameatal warts.

Look at the scrotal skin for any redness, swelling or ulcer. Lift the scrotum to inspect its posterior surface. Tiny dark red papules of *angiokeratoma* or round, firm, whitish nodules of *sebaceous cysts* can sometimes be seen. *Scabies* causes erythematous nodular lesions on the scrotum and glans penis. If intrascrotal swelling is present, observe whether it

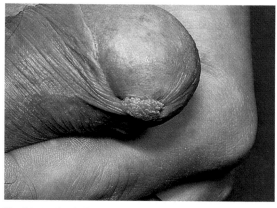

Fig. 20.1   Genital wart on the frenum of the penis.

appears to extend into the groin and note whether both testes are in the scrotum. *Ulceration* can result from a gumma, or from fungation of an underlying tumour of the testis.

THE TESTES (Fig. 20.2)

Place the right hand below the scrotum and palpate both testes. Arrange the hands and fingers as shown in Fig. 20.2; this 'fixes' the testis so that it cannot slip away from the examining fingers. The posterior aspect of the testis is supported by the middle, ring and little fingers of each hand, the right hand being inferior. This leaves the index finger and thumb free to palpate. Gently move the index finger and thumb over the anterior surface of the body of the testis and feel the lateral border with the index finger and the medial border with the pulp of each thumb. Note the size and consistency of the testis and any nodules or other irregularities. Now very gently approximate the fingers and thumb of the left hand (the effect of this is to move the testis inferiorly, which is easily and painlessly done because of its great mobility inside the tunica vaginalis). In this way the upper pole of the testis can be readily felt between the approximated index finger and thumb of the left hand. Next move the testis upwards by reversing the movements of the hands and gently approximating the index finger and thumb of the right hand, so enabling the lower pole to be palpated. The normal testes are equal in size, varying between 3.5 and 4 cm in length.

THE EPIDIDYMIS

The head is found at the upper pole of the testis on its posterior aspect and is felt between the left thumb anteriorly and the index and middle fingers posteriorly. It is a soft nodular structure about 1 cm in length. The tail lies on the posterolateral aspect of the inferior pole of the testis and is felt between the thumb and fingers of the right hand. The tail is also soft but, unlike the head, its coiled tubular structure can usually be made out. Occasionally the epididymis is situated anterior to the testis.

THE SPERMATIC CORD

Finally palpate the spermatic cord (Fig. 20.3) with the right hand. Then exert gentle downward traction on the testis, place the fingers behind the neck of the scrotum, and with the thumb placed anteriorly press forward with fingers of the right hand. The spermatic cord will be felt between the fingers and thumb; it is about 1 cm in width. The only structure that can be positively identified within it is the vas deferens, which feels like a thick piece of string.

Repeat the examination on the other side. Remember that the patient should also be examined standing up to look for *varicocele*—dilated tortuous veins in the scrotum like a bag of worms.

In the scrotum, hydrocele of the tunica vaginalis or a cyst of the epididymis are common causes of painless swelling. Hydrocele can be demonstrated by transillumination, using a bright light source held in contact with the large testicle, preferably in a darkened room. A unilateral enlarged testis must be considered malignant, particularly if painless. Other painless enlargements include testicular gumma and tuberculous involvement. Acute epididymo-orchitis, torsion of the testis, strangulated inguinal hernia and some cases of testicular neoplasm cause a painful swelling. In torsion, the epididymis cannot be differentiated from the swollen testis which lies at a higher level than the normal testis. In old age, testes may become atrophic. In younger men testicular atrophy often indicates chronic liver disease, usually alcoholic in aetiology, or it may be associated with previous torsion or varicocele. In swellings of uncertain origin ultrasound is useful.

ANORECTAL EXAMINATION

In both homosexual and bisexual men, the anorectal region should be examined. Ask the patient to lie in the standard left lateral position with the knees drawn up, or in the knee–elbow position. Examine the anal and perianal skin for *inflammation, ulceration, fissure* and *tags*. Primary syphilis and herpes

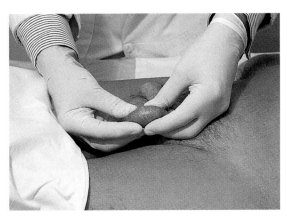

Fig. 20.2   Palpation of the testis. Gloves should be worn.

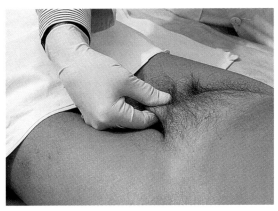

Fig. 20.3   Palpation of the spermatic cord. Gloves should be worn.

simplex virus infection can mimic an anal fissure. Anal tags should not be confused with anal warts (*condylomata acuminata*), which are sessile or pedunculated papillomata. Anal warts in turn should not be confused with the flat warty lesions of *condylomata lata*, which are the highly infectious lesions of secondary syphilis.

Gently insert a proctoscope lubricated with KY Jelly or liquid paraffin and examine the rectal mucosa for pus, inflammation, warts and threadworms. Take rectal tests. In patients who practise frequent peno-anal intercourse the anus will be lax.

FEMALE GENITALIA

Women are best examined in the lithotomy position. Examine the perineum, vulva, and labia majora and minora for discharge, redness, swelling, excoriation, ulcers, warts and other lesions. In rape and sexual abuse cases, look for evidence of trauma. Redness and swelling of the vulva with excoriations may be seen in thrush and trichomoniasis. Separate the labia and palpate Bartholin's glands; normally they are not felt. Wipe away any contaminating vaginal discharge from the vulva and urethral meatus and insert a bivalve Cusco speculum (Ch. 14) moistened with water. Note any inflammation of the vaginal wall (vaginitis) and the colour, consistency and odour of any vaginal discharge. Curdy or cheesy, white discharge suggests *thrush*, frothy greenish-yellow discharge, *trichomoniasis*, and off-white discharge, *bacterial vaginosis*. The last two conditions also have a fishy odour. Tests are taken from the posterior fornix of the vagina.

Wipe the cervix with a swab and examine it for *discharge* from the external cervical os, for *ectopy* or 'erosion' (ectopic columnar epithelium), and for *cervicitis, warts and ulcers*. Mucopurulent cervicitis may be caused by gonococcal or chlamydial infections. (Fig. 20.4). Warts on the cervix appear as either flat or papilliferous lesions. Take tests, including a smear for *cervical cytology*, to detect dysplasia

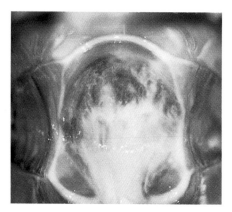

Fig. 20.4 Mucopurulent cervicitis caused by *Chlamydia trachomatis*.

and cancer of the cervix. This is particularly important because of the association of cervical cancer with genital warts. Then remove the speculum.

Next the urethral orifice is examined for discharge, inflammation and warts. If no obvious discharge is present, milk the urethra gently forward before taking specimens (see p. 416).

Examine the anal region for lesions, as in homosexual men. If indicated, insert a lubricated proctoscope and examine the rectal mucosa for discharge or inflammation, and take tests.

BIMANUAL EXAMINATION

A bimanual examination is performed to detect pelvic inflammatory disease and abnormalities of the upper genital tract. Tender uterus and fallopian tubes with positive cervical excitation test may indicate pelvic inflammatory disease.

COLPOSCOPY

In some cases, particularly in patients with cervical warts, or whose cervical cytology is dyskaryotic, the cervix should be examined under magnification using a colposcope. White areas after application of 5% acetic acid suggest cervical wart virus infection or dysplasia which can be confirmed by biopsy. Chlamydial follicular cervicitis may also be observed.

PUBIC REGIONS AND GROINS

Examine for *pediculosis pubis* ('crabs') and nits. *Molluscum contagiosum* lesions appear as pearly or pinkish umbilicated papules. Look at the groins for *tinea cruris*, *thrush* and *erythrasma*. Tinea cruris and erythrasma give rise to a rash with a well-defined border, while in thrush the border is less well-defined and erythematous papules outside the borders, known as satellite lesions, are present. Erythrasma lesions show a coral-red fluorescence under Wood's light.

Groin swelling is usually due to hernia or lymphadenopathy. Genital ulceration with tender suppurative inguinal lymph nodes (*buboes*) will suggest chancroid and lymphogranuloma venereum. In lymphogranuloma venereum, the ulcer may be transient and the buboes may have a grooved appearance resulting from lymphadenopathy above and below the inguinal ligament—'sign of the groove'. Primary syphilis gives rise to painless, mobile and rubbery lymph nodes but they can be painful if the chancre is secondarily infected. Anal, penile and vulval carcinoma may metastasize to the inguinal lymph nodes. Inguinal lymphadenopathy may be part of a generalized involvement, as in lymphoma, secondary syphilis or viral infections, e.g. infectious mononucleosis and that due to HIV infection. Donovanosis may give rise to pseudobuboes which are inguinal subcutaneous granulomata.

HUMAN IMMUNODEFICIENCY VIRUS INFECTIONS

The number of people worldwide with HIV infection has reached pandemic proportions resulting in a dramatic lowering of life expectancy in the developing world. However, the introduction of highly active antiretroviral treatment, particularly in the developed world, has delayed the onset of AIDS, with prolongation of life, but brought on accompanying problems of adverse drug reactions.

HIV infection is categorized into A, B and C (Box 20.3) broadly based on the clinical evolution of the immunodeficiency state that leads to the development of the acquired immune deficiency syndrome (AIDS), on average some 8–15 years after infection if untreated.

The first phase of HIV infection is the acute primary illness, in which fever, malaise, lymphadenopathy, muscle pain and sore throat occur, often with erythematous, maculopapular skin eruption and headache. Other features include night sweats, weight loss, diarrhoea and oral thrush. There is HIV viraemia and severe immunosuppression indicated by a high plasma HIV-RNA and a low CD4 T-lymphocyte count. Following the acute infection, the patient may be asymptomatic, or there may be persistent lymphadenopathy; the HIV-RNA decreases and the CD4 lymphocyte count increases and stabilizes (Fig. 20.5) at a baseline level: as the illness progress, patients become symptomatic (Category B) followed by the development of AIDS defining illness (Category C). These include opportunistic infections such as tuberculosis and *Pneumocystis carinii* pneumonia, and neoplasms such as Kaposi's sarcoma (Fig. 20.5) and lymphoma.

Assessment of the patient with HIV infection therefore requires a careful history and a complete examination of the body systems in order to detect the extent of the disease and its complications. It is important to remember that multi-systemic involvement is common and in each system there may be multiple causes. The mouth and the skin are important sites to examine and may provide the clue that a patient is immunosuppressed. Common chest infections include tuberculosis, *Pneumocystis carinii* and other bacterial pneumonia. Common cerebral lesions include toxoplasma and other infective abcesses and lymphoma. Diarrhoea may be caused by HIV or due to drug treatment, opportunistic infections such as isospora, cryptosporidium, cytomegalovirus and atypical mycobacterium infection, or may be sexually transmitted, for example giardiasis, shigellosis and salmonellosis in homosexual or bisexual men. The introduction of combination therapy with antiretroviral drugs which include the nucleoside reverse transcriptase inhibitors (NRTI: abacavir, didanosine, lamivudine, stavudine, zalcitabine, zidovudine), non-nucleoside reverse transcriptase inhibitors (NNRTI: delarvidine, efavirenz, nevirapine) and protease inhibitors (PI: amprenavir, indinavir, lopinavir, nelfinavir, ritonavir, saquinavir), as well as treatment for the opportunistic infections and tumours, has resulted in iatrogenic complications. NRTI may cause bone marrow suppression, peripheral neuropathy pancreatitis; the NNRTI may cause rash and hepatitis while PI may cause the lipodystrophy syndrome

---

BOX 20.3 Centre for Disease Control (CDC) HIV clinical categories.

Category A: Asymptomatic Acute infection
Persistent generalized lymphadenopathy

Category B: Symptomatic infection excluding category A and B.
Bacteria: Bacillary angiomatosis
  Listeriosis
Fungal: Candidiasis—oropharyngeal, vulvovaginal (persistent, frequent or poorly responsive to therapy)
Viral: Herpes zoster (>1 episode or >1 dermatome)
  Oral hairy leukoplakia
Constitutional symptoms: Fever (>38.5°C), diarrhoea >1 month
Other: Cervical dysplasia—moderate or severe
  Idiopathic thrombocytopenic purpura
  Pelvic inflammatory disease
  Peripheral neuropathy

Category C: AIDS defining illness
Bacteria: *Mycobacterium tuberculosis*—pulmonary, extrapulmonary
  Mycobacterium avium complex or other mycobacterial infection with disseminated disease
  Pneumonia—recurrent within 12 month period
  Salmonella septicaemia, recurrent
  Bacterial infections (multiple) in a child <13 years
Fungal: Candidiasis—oesophagus, trachea, bronchi, lungs
  Coccidioidomycosis—extrapulmonary
  Cryptococcosis—extrapulmonary
  Histoplasmosis—disseminated or extrapulmonary
  Pneumocystis carinii pneumonia
Helminth: Strongyloidosis—extraintestinal
Protozoal: Cryptosporidiosis
  Isosporiasis
  Toxoplasmosis of brain
Viral: Cytomegalovirus infection other than liver, spleen or lymph node
  HIV encephalopathy, wasting syndrome
  Herpes simplex—mucocutaneous ulcer >1 month, bronchitis, pneumonitis, oesophagitis
  Progressive multifocal leukoencephalopathy
Tumours: Cervical carcinoma, invasive
  Kaposi's sarcoma
  Lymphoma—brain, Burkitt's, immunoblastic or equivalent

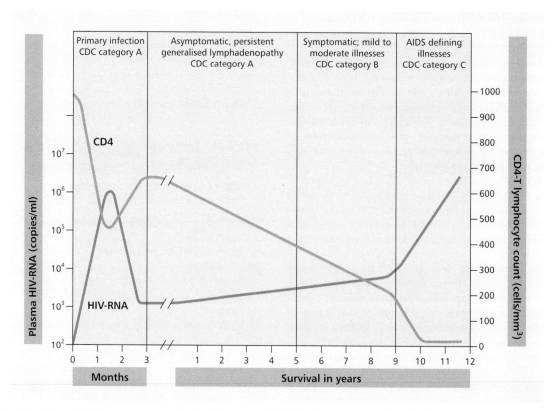

Fig. 20.5   The clinical categories associated with untreated HIV infection and survival can be loosely correlated with the plasma HIV-RNA and circulating CD4 T-lymphocyte count. Treatment with antiretrovirals and prophylaxis for opportunistic infections increases survival and can prevent or delay the progression to AIDS.

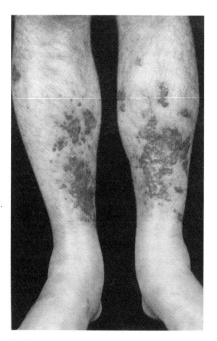

Fig. 20.6   Kaposi's sarcoma of lower legs with ankle oedema in a patient with AIDS.

(Fig. 20.7). The latter is characterized by peripheral fat wasting of the limbs and face, central adiposity resulting in a protuberant abdomen, and a buffalo

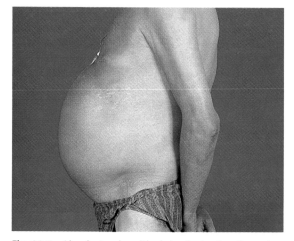

Fig. 20.7   Lipodystrophy with abdominal adiposity and thin arm resulting from protease inhibitor treatment.

hump (which has to be differentiated from Cushing's syndrome), hyperlipidaemia and insulin resistance. The thin face and limbs may be mistaken for HIV wasting syndrome and other causes of abdominal swelling should be excluded. The patient may also complain of prominent veins on the leg due to loss of fat which may be mistaken for varicose veins.

Other retroviral infections, especially with HTLV-1 virus, also cause disease in humans. HTLV-1 infection may be acquired by sexual contact. It is associated with the later development of Y cell lymphoma and leukaemia, often with hypercalcaemia, and with a slowly progressive neurological syndrome characterized by a progressive spastic paraparesis (tropical spastic paraparesis). These syndromes occur in people in regions where the infection is endemic, such as central Africa, the Caribbean, and parts of Asia.

SYSTEMIC EXAMINATION

Particular attention should be paid to the skin, mouth, eyes, joints and, in late syphilis, the cardiovascular and nervous systems.

THE SKIN

The generalized rash of secondary syphilis is usually non-itchy and commonly involves the palms and soles. Generalized rash can also be seen in drug allergy and in acute viral infections such as HIV-seroconversion illness, acute hepatitis B, acute cytomegalovirus infection and infectious mononucleosis, and acute toxoplasmosis. Gummata of the skin may be present in late syphilis. Pustular lesions of disseminated gonococcal infection are seen mainly on the limbs, particularly near joints. Excoriated papules and burrows are features of scabies. A psoriasis-like rash and keratoderma of the feet may be present in Reiter's disease. Behçet's disease causes recurrent painful oro-genital ulcers. Stevens–Johnson syndrome can also present with painful oro-genital ulceration and target lesions on the skin. In HIV infection, acute herpes zoster or scars of previous shingles, seborrhoeic dermatitis, severe fungal and bacterial infections, facial molluscum contagiosum and warts, bacillary angiomatosis and Kaposi's sarcoma may be present. The last may present with purplish nodules or plaques.

THE MOUTH

The mouth is a common site for syphilitic lesions: extragenital chancres in primary syphilis, mucous patches and snailtrack ulcers in secondary syphilis, and leucoplakia, chronic superficial glossitis and gummatous perforation of palate in late syphilis. In congenital syphilis, linear scars radiating from the mouth known as rhagades, and Hutchinson's incisors—dome-shaped incisor teeth with a central notch—may be present. Genital herpes can spread to the mouth and vice versa if the patient practises oro-genital intercourse. In HIV infection, oral hairy leucoplakia, consisting of persistent white hairy patches on the side of the tongue, and oral thrush, consisting of curdy white patches which can be removed leaving behind a raw surface (Fig. 20.8) or erythematous areas may be seen. Other oral manifestations of HIV include aphthoid ulcers, oral warts, gingivi-

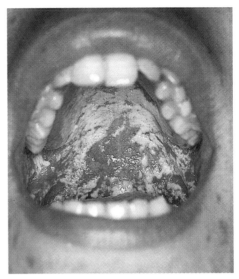

Fig. 20.8 White plaques of oral candidiasis (which can be scraped off revealing an erythematous base) in an HIV positive patient.

tis, severe peridontal disease, Kaposi's sarcoma and lymphoma.

THE EYES

Conjunctivitis can be due to direct infection by *Chlamydia*, gonococcus or herpes, or can arise indirectly, as in Reiter's disease. Iritis can be seen in Reiter's disease, secondary and late syphilis, Behçet's disease and HIV infection. Congenital syphilis can present with interstitial keratitis, iritis and choroidoretinitis. *Argyll Robertson pupils* are small irregular pupils seen in neurosyphilis, particularly tabes dorsalis. They are non-reactive to light but the *accommodation reflex* is present. In HIV infection, there may be occasional retinal exudate and haemorrhage due to retinal infarcts while cytomegalovirus infection may cause a segmental or diffuse retinitis with exudates and haemorrhage akin to a 'pizza-pie with cheese and ketchup'. Acute retinal necrosis due to other herpes viruses may also be seen.

THE JOINTS

Painful joint swelling may be present in Reiter's disease or disseminated gonococcal infection. Charcot's joints in tabes dorsalis are generally painless, deformed and hypermobile; Clutton's joints in congenital syphilis are painless bilateral joint effusions. HIV infection increases the risk of acquiring Reiter's disease.

THE ABDOMEN

Gonococcal and chlamydial infection can cause lower abdominal pain and tenderness if endometritis or salpingitis supervenes, and right hypochondrial pain and tenderness if perihepatitis (Fitz-Hugh–Curtis syndrome) is present. Sexually transmitted hepatitis includes secondary syphilis and viral hepatitis. In HIV infection, retrosternal pain (worse with food) may be due to oesphageal involvement by candida, herpes simplex virus and cytomegalovirus infection. Acute pancreatitis may complicate treatment with NRTI such as didanosine. Renal colic may result from indinavir stones.

SPECIAL INVESTIGATIONS

URETHRAL DISCHARGE

Both gonococcal and non-gonococcal urethritis may be asymptomatic and only discovered by genital tests, or when extragenital complications develop.

The urethral meatus is cleansed with a swab. If there is no visible discharge, the urethra is gently milked forward from the bulb and any discharge noted. A platinum or plastic bacteriological loop is inserted 1–2 cm into the urethra, proximal to the fossa navicularis, and the urethral material obtained is spread thinly on a glass slide for Gram-staining. Endo-urethral material for gonococcal culture is placed directly on to a suitable culture plate or sent to the laboratory in modified Stuart's transport medium. Positive cultures are tested for antimicrobial sensitivities and beta-lactamase production.

GRAM-STAINING (Box 20.4)

The presence of Gram-negative intracellular diplococci, which appear as opposing bean-shaped cocci within polymorphonuclear leucocytes under the microscope (Fig. 20.9), suggests a diagnosis of gonococcal urethritis. The presence of 5 or more polymorphonuclear leucocytes per high power field (× 1000 magnification) with a negative test for gonococci indicates non-gonococcal urethritis, the causes of which are given in Box 20.5. Exclusion of specific causes of non-gonococcal urethritis such as *Chlamydia trachomatis*, *Mycoplasma genitalium*, trichomoniasis and non-sexually transmitted diseases such as bacterial urinary tract infection leads

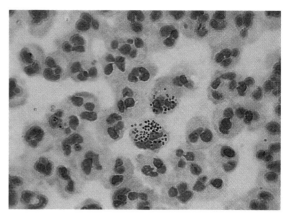

Fig. 20.9   Gram-stained smear showing Gram-negative intracellular diplococci typical of *Neisseria gonorrhoeae*.

BOX 20.5   Causes of non-gonococcal urethritis.

Sexually transmitted diseases
- *Chlamydia trachomatis* D-K serovars
- *Mycoplasma genitalium*
- Unknown/Ureaplasma?
- *Trichomonas vaginalis*
- Herpes simplex virus
- *Candida albicans*
- Intrameatal warts
- Meatal chancre

Non-sexually transmitted diseases
- Bacterial urinary tract infection
- Tuberculosis
- Urethral stricture
- Stevens–Johnson syndrome
- Benign mucous membrane pemphigoid
- Chemical
- Trauma
- Others

---

to a diagnosis of 'non-specific' urethritis. However, in the absence of adequate diagnostic facilities, urethritis due to *C. trachomatis* or *M. genitalium* is often included under 'non-specific' urethritis. If a patient has passed urine just before the test, the urethral smear may show no polymorphonuclear leucocytes because the urine will have washed out the accumulated urethral material. In such cases the patient should be asked to re-attend for an overnight or late afternoon urethral smear after holding urine for 8 or more hours.

A *wet preparation* is made by mixing urethral material obtained by scraping the urethra using a loop with a drop of normal saline on a slide. This is examined by ordinary or dark ground illumination for *Trichomonas* which appear as ovoid protozoa with beating flagellae and in jerky motion.

Direct immunofluorescent antibody (DIF) staining for chlamydial elementary bodies using monoclonal antibodies or an enzyme immunoassay (EIA) test for

---

BOX 20.4   Procedure for Gram-staining.

1   Fix the smear on the slide by passing it through a flame twice.
2   Stain with 2% crystal violet for 30 s, then wash with tap water.
3   Stain with Gram's iodine for a further 30 s and wash with water.
4   Decolorize with acetone for a few seconds.
5   Wash with water and counterstain with 1% safranin for 10 s.
6   After a final wash with water, dry by pressing between filter paper.

chlamydial antigen from genital material can be performed. Amplified DNA tests using ligase chain reaction (LCR) and polymerase chain reaction (PCR) for chlamydia are more sensitive and can use urine instead of urethral specimen. When tests for chlamydial infection are carried out, up to 40% of so-called 'non-specific' urethritis can be found to be due to *C. trachomatis*.

TWO-GLASS TEST

In the two-glass test the patient passes urine into two glasses (or clear plastic cups), approximately 100 ml in the first glass and the rest in the second. The presence of several specks or threads which sink to the bottom in the first glass, with a clear second glass, indicates *anterior urethritis*; if there are threads in both glasses, *posterior urethritis* is indicated. Hazy urine in both glasses is commonly due to phosphaturia and this clears with the addition of acetic acid. If the urine still remains hazy and there is pus in the urethral smear, this suggests either sexually transmitted 'non-specific' urethritis with ascending infection in the bladder, or bacterial urinary tract infection with descending non-sexual infection to the urethra. To obtain a presumptive diagnosis, the second glass of urine is centrifuged and the deposit Gram-stained. In 'non-specific' urethritis with ascending infection, there will be polymorphonuclear leucocytes only, whereas in bacterial urinary tract infection the smear will also show bacteria. The latter can be identified by a mid-stream urine culture. Rarely, renal tuberculosis may present with urethritis and hazy urine, which is abacterial on Gram-staining as in 'non-specific' infection. The urine must be checked for sugar, protein, blood and other abnormalities as indicated (Ch. 9).

The presence of urethritis a week or more after successful treatment for gonorrhoea indicates that the patient has post-gonococcal urethritis, a non-gonococcal urethritis unmasked following treatment for gonorrhoea.

VAGINAL DISCHARGE

A smear of the discharge can be Gram-stained to look for the spores and pseudomycelia of thrush and for '*clue cells*' indicative of bacterial vaginosis. 'Clue cells' are vaginal epithelial cells covered with *Gardnerella vaginalis*, which are Gram-variable but mainly Gram-negative coccobacilli. If after adding 10% potassium hydroxide to the discharge on the speculum, a fishy ammoniacal odour is produced, this constitutes a positive *amine* test. This, together with a vaginal pH greater than 4.5, is suggestive of bacterial vaginosis. A wet-film preparation is examined for *Trichomonas*. Cultures for *Candida* and *Trichomonas* are also performed.

Gram-stained smear and culture of cervical secretion for gonorrhoea is performed routinely. A cervical

diagnostic test for *Chlamydia trachomatis* should also be performed. If genital herpes is suspected, a cervical specimen for herpes culture should be collected.

Urethral specimens for Gram-staining and cultures for gonorrhoea should also be performed in new female patients. A Gram-stained smear, chlamydial and gonococcal cultures from the rectum may also be indicated.

In those who practise peno-oral intercourse, a pharyngeal swab should be taken for culture for gonorrhoea and chlamydia. A Gram-stained smear from the throat for gonorrhoea is useless because of the presence of other non-gonococcal *Neisseria*.

GENITAL ULCER

To investigate the cause of a genital ulcer, the base of the ulcer is first thoroughly cleansed with normal saline, then gently squeezed until a drop of serum exudates. The edge of a coverslip is applied to the drop which will adhere to it. This is put on to a glass slide and pressed down firmly between filter paper. The slide is examined under the *dark-field microscope* for the characteristic morphology and movements of *Treponema pallidum* (Fig. 20.10)—bending itself at an angle, rotating forward on its long axis or alternating between contraction and expansion of its coils. Dark-field examination should be repeated for several days if syphilis is suspected.

Sometimes dark-field microscopy may be negative from suspected syphilitic ulcers, particularly if the patient has used a topical antiseptic or antibiotic cream. If regional lymph nodes are enlarged, a *lymph node aspiration* can be performed. After infiltration of the skin with 1% lignocaine, 0.2 ml of normal saline is injected into the node, the needle moved around in the node and then aspirated. A drop is placed between a glass slide and coverslip, pressed between filter paper and examined under the dark-field microscope. In oral chancres, commensal treponemes may be confused with *Treponema pallidum*: because of this, immunofluorescent stain-

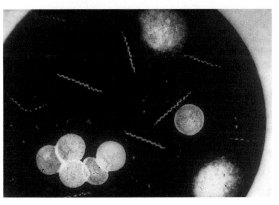

Fig. 20.10 *Treponema pallidum* seen under the dark-field microscope. The thread-like treponema can be seen, together with pus cells from a urethral discharge.

ing for pathogenic treponemes of serum from the ulcer, air-dried on a slide, is advisable.

If anogenital herpes (Fig. 20.11) is suspected, the base of the blister or ulcer is swabbed and the swab placed in a viral transport medium for herpes culture. Diagnosis of donovanosis is based upon the demonstration of Donovan bodies, which stain in bipolar fashion giving a 'safety pin' appearance within the cytoplasm of mononuclear cells in a Giesma-stained tissue smear. Tissue is obtained by infiltrating the edge of the ulcer with 1% lignocaine, and removing a small piece from the edge which is then smeared onto a glass slide or crushed between two glass slides. If chancroid or lymphogranuloma venereum is suspected, culture for *Haemophilus ducreyi* and *Chlamydia trachomatis* of the lymphogranuloma venereum serovars respectively, may be indicated using material obtained from the ulcer or bubo.

SEROLOGICAL TESTS FOR SYPHILIS

There are two groups of serological tests for syphilis: the non-specific tests for anti-cardiolipin antibody such as Venereal Disease Research Laboratories (VDRL), rapid plasma reagin (RPR), and the specific antitreponemal antibody tests such as *T. pallidum* haemagglutination (TPHA), *T. pallidum* particle agglutination (TPPA), fluorescent treponemal antibody absorption (FTA-Abs) and *T. pallidum* enzyme immunoassay (EIA) tests. The titre of the non-specific tests indicates disease activity and is useful for following-up patients, particularly those who have been treated for primary or secondary syphilis, when the test should become negative within 6–12 months. After successful treatment of all stages of syphilis, the specific tests usually remain positive while the VDRL or RPR test may slowly revert to negative but commonly remains positive in lower titre in late syphilis. A greater than twofold dilution or fourfold

increase in antibody titre following treatment indicates recrudescence or reinfection.

The presence of a positive VDRL or RPR test on two occasions with negative specific tests and the absence of any evidence of treponemal disease indicates a *biological false-positive* reaction. Acute false-positive reactions may be due to acute febrile infections such as pneumonia, malaria, HIV infection and infective endocarditis, pregnancy and vaccination; they last less than 6 months. Chronic false-positive reactions may indicate autoimmune diseases such as systemic lupus erythematosus, but can also occur in antiphospholipid syndrome, intravenous drug abusers, lepromatous leprosy and old age.

All patients should be screened for syphilis with serological tests using either the syphilis EIA, or combination of the VDRL or RPR and TPHA or TPPA. If syphilis is endemic, these tests should be repeated after 3 months if initial tests are negative. If primary syphilis is suspected, the EIA-IgM or FTA-Abs test is also performed as this is usually the first serological test to be positive. In babies with suspected congenital syphilis, the EIA-IgM or FTA-Abs tests using an IgM conjugate should be requested because of passive transfer of maternal IgG antibodies across the placenta. When treponemes cannot be demonstrated, positive results must be confirmed by a second set of tests before treatment is started.

Endemic treponematoses such as yaws, bejel and pinta, may result in positive serological tests for syphilis. It is not possible to differentiate the treponematoses by serological tests.

INVESTIGATIONS FOR HIV INFECTIONS

Screening for antibody to HIV, the causal agent for AIDS, is advisable for patients at risk of infection because of the possibility of early intervention with anti-HIV agents, preventive treatment against opportunistic infections such as *Pneumocystis carinii* pneumonia and prevention of transmission from mother to child. The latter is achieved by treating mother (antepartum, during labour and at delivery) and baby at birth with antiretrovirals, Caesarean section and avoidance of breast feeding. The test may also be indicated to confirm or exclude HIV infection as a cause of immunosuppression or problematic medical illness. Consent from the patient for the test to be carried out is desirable. Patients should be counselled as to the medical, social and emotional consequences before performing the test. The test should be repeated at 3 months to cover the 'window' period for incubating infection. HIV-RNA viral load test can also be performed for patients suspected of acute HIV infection as the HIV antibody test may initially be negative. Facilities for counselling, support and follow-up of patients with positive tests should be available. Immunological assessment must include

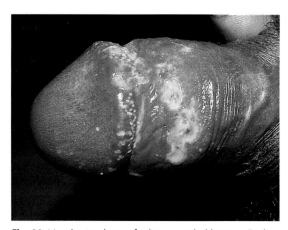

Fig. 20.11 Acute ulcers of primary genital herpes. Both herpes simplex virus types I and II can cause genital herpes.

analysis of lymphocyte subtypes, especially CD4 and CD8 counts; selective reduction in numbers of circulating CD4 cells is characteristic of the disturbed immune state. The HIV-RNA test and the CD4 T-lymphocytes count are prognostic indicators of HIV infection and can be used to monitor progression as well as treatment efficacy. Other investigations will depend on the suspected systems involved. Patients with headache or neurological signs should have a CT or MRI brain scan first to exclude intracerebral lesions before a lumbar puncture is performed.

INVESTIGATIONS IN HOMOSEXUAL AND BISEXUAL MEN

Gram-stained smears from the rectum and cultures from the rectum and throat of homosexual and bisexual men should also be obtained to exclude gonorrhoea, in addition to routine tests as for heterosexual men. In cases of proctitis, cultures for herpes simplex and *Chlamydia* may be indicated.

All homosexual and bisexual men should also be screened for hepatitis B surface antigen anti-HBc and core antibody (anti-HBc). The presence of anti-HBc indicates that the patient has been exposed to the infection. If both tests are negative vaccination against hepatitis B should be offered. If hepatitis is present, other infective causes such as secondary syphilis, hepatitis A and C as well as non-infective causes should be excluded.

Homosexual and bisexual men with diarrhoea should have their stools examined for *Giardia*, *Amoeba*, *Shigella* and *Salmonella* and if HIV infection is suspected other causes of HIV-related diarrhoea should be looked for. Threadworms may also be present.

OPHTHALMIA NEONATORUM

Ophthalmia neonatorum is defined as purulent conjunctivitis in the first 4 weeks of life. It should be differentiated from 'sticky eyes' that frequently result from blocked lacrimal ducts.

Ophthalmia neonatorum is commonly due to gonorrhoea, *Chlamydia* or non-sexually transmitted bacteria. A Gram-stained conjunctival smear can be a useful guide. The presence of polymorphonuclear leucocytes with Gram-negative intracellular diplococci is presumptive evidence of gonorrhoea but rarely may indicate *Moraxella catarrhalis* infection; culture must be carried out for full identification. The presence of pus cells with bacteria indicates bacterial ophthalmia, whereas the presence of pus alone suggests chlamydial ophthalmia. Chlamydial DIF, EIA, LCR or PCR tests, cultures for gonorrhoea and other bacteria should be performed. Mixed infections may occur.

Chest symptoms such as staccato cough and rapid breathing with poor feeding in the absence of fever may indicate chlamydial pneumonia. Auscultation of the chest may be normal but the chest X-ray may show consolidation.

If the ophthalmia is due to gonococcal or chlamydial infection, it is important to check the parents and their sexual partners.

21
ANAEMIA AND COAGULATION DISORDERS

INTRODUCTION

Blood consists of red cells, white cells, platelets and plasma. The first section of this chapter concentrates on anaemia, which results from a reduction in the number of red cells or of the haemoglobin concentration within red cells. Since the bone marrow manufactures all three cellular components of the blood, anaemia may be associated with abnormalities of white cells and platelets, for example, when there is a primary bone marrow disorder such as aplastic anaemia. However, anaemia is more commonly found as an isolated abnormality and is then usually secondary to disorders affecting the gastrointestinal tract or other organs. Thus, the clinical approach to the anaemic patient must be wide-ranging since underlying disease processes may involve any organ system. Both in the developing and developed worlds, the most important cause of anaemia is gastrointestinal (GI) blood loss. Appropriate GI investigation should be considered in all cases of unexplained anaemia.

The second section of this chapter deals with coagulation disorders, which result from abnormalities of platelet function or number, or of the plasma proteins involved in haemostasis. These abnormalities can result in either an increased risk of bleeding or, conversely, an increased risk of thrombosis.

ANAEMIA

Anaemia is present if the haemoglobin concentration is below the normal range (Box 21.1). Following acute massive blood loss the haemoglobin concentration will initially be normal. This clinical situation is dominated by hypovolaemic shock and is not further discussed here.

The causes of anaemia are numerous but can be broadly classified on the basis of the major patho-

---

BOX 21.1   Normal red cell values in adults.

	Males	Females
Hb (g/dl)	13.3–16.7	11.8–14.8
RBC ($\times 10^{12}$/l)	4.32–5.66	3.88–4.99
PCV or Hct (l/l)	0.39–0.5	0.36–0.44
MCV (fl)	80–100	

Key:

Hb	Haemoglobin
RBC	Red blood cells
PCV	Packed cell volume
Hct	Haematocrit

---

physiological mechanism. Anaemia results either from increased blood loss (bleeding or haemolysis) or from decreased red cell production. However, in the clinical situation, it is often unclear which process is dominant and a more practical classification of anaemia is based simply on red cell size (microcytic, normocytic and macrocytic) (Boxes 21.2–21.4). Although this classification is extremely valuable practically, it is not exhaustive and non-specific anaemias occur. For example, the 'anaemia of chronic disease', which can be associated with any infective, inflammatory or neoplastic process, usually results in a normocytic anaemia but in extreme cases causes a microcytic anaemia. Similarly, most haemolytic anaemias are normocytic but macrocytosis may

---

BOX 21.2   The microcytic anaemias (MCV < 80 fl).

Impaired haem synthesis
- Iron deficiency
- Anaemia of chronic disease
- Sideroblastic anaemia
- Lead poisoning

Impaired globin synthesis
- Thalassaemia

develop when haemolysis is particularly brisk, since reticulocytes are larger than mature red cells.

Certain symptoms and signs can be associated with anaemia, whatever its cause (Box 21.5). Several of these features will be strongly influenced by the coexistence of cardiovascular disease. For instance, heart failure is most likely to occur in patients with underlying coronary heart disease. Once a clinical or laboratory diagnosis of anaemia has been made, then attention should be paid to features in the history and examination that might suggest a particular underlying aetiology.

HISTORY

Patients with anaemia of any cause are likely to present with the non-specific symptoms of anaemia (Box 21.5). The age and sex of the patient are highly relevant since inherited disorders of the blood such as thalassaemia are most likely to present in childhood, while in women of child-bearing age, by far the most common cause of anaemia is iron deficiency consequent on menstrual blood loss and pregnancy.

In contrast, older women and males of any age with iron deficiency should undergo investigation aimed at detecting gastrointestinal blood loss.

The patient may describe symptoms that suggest certain underlying pathologies. For instance, drenching night sweats might indicate lymphoma whereas bone pain points towards myeloma or metastatic cancer. The past medical history may reveal important clues such as a history of peptic ulcer disease, malignancy or autoimmune disease. The use of aspirin or other non-steroidal anti-inflammatory drugs suggests that occult blood loss from gastritis is likely. Similarly, steroid therapy often results in peptic ulceration. Excess alcohol consumption is associated with gastritis, macrocytosis, folate deficiency and liver disease with consequent variceal bleeding and red cell pooling in an enlarged spleen.

The dietary history is particularly relevant in the assessment of anaemia since nutritional deficiencies of folic acid (and less frequently of iron and vitamin B_{12}) result in anaemia. Dietary folate deficiency occurs in 'skid-row' alcoholics or when the diet is deficient in green vegetables. Since there is usually adequate iron in the diet, iron deficiency is rarely due to poor diet alone. As all the vitamin B_{12} present in the human diet is ultimately of animal origin, B_{12} deficiency is only likely to occur in vegetarians and is actually inevitable in strict vegans unless appropriate supplementation is taken.

A family history of disorders of blood (e.g. sickle cell disease, thalassaemia) or autoimmune disorders is relevant, as is the ethnic origin of the patient. Sickle cell disease is found in Afro-Caribbeans whilst β-thalassaemia is commonest in the Mediterranean littoral and in the Indian subcontinent. Prolonged residence in or travel to tropical countries may suggest that malaria or other parasitic infestations are present.

Systematic questioning may reveal symptoms suggestive of an underlying disease which is causing the anaemia. Thus, a history of weight loss, dysphagia, dyspepsia, chronic diarrhoea, change in bowel habit or rectal bleeding should instigate appropriate investigations directed at the GI tract looking for GI malignancies, peptic ulcer disease, malabsorption states, colitis, haemorrhoids and other causes of GI blood loss. Similarly, a detailed genitourinary history should be taken with particular emphasis on the extent of menstrual blood loss. Many women of child-bearing age are teetering on the brink of iron deficiency and the added iron losses of menstruation or pregnancy frequently precipitate anaemia. When haematuria is heavy enough to cause anaemia, it is normally the presenting problem itself.

EXAMINATION

Certain physical signs are likely to be found in patients suffering from anaemia of any cause (Box 21.5).

Pallor is best detected by examination of the mucosae (conjunctival or intra-oral). In addition, specific causes of anaemia are often associated with characteristic physical findings (Box 21.6). Some specific points are important: B_{12} deficiency is one of the few causes of peripheral neuropathy and pyramidal tract damage and so paradoxically can present with brisk knee reflexes (pyramidal) and absent ankle jerks (neuropathy). The typical facial appearance of inadequately treated thalassaemic patients results from the massive expansion of bone marrow that occurs in an attempt to compensate for the anaemia. Expansion of the facial bones results in so-called 'chipmunk facies' and similar changes result in typical radiological features (Fig. 21.1). Leukaemia and lymphoma can result in protean physical findings. Some specific features include the florid overgrowth of gingival mucosa that occurs in monocytic leukaemias and the features of meningism (photophobia, headache, stiff neck) that result from meningeal infiltration by malignant cells.

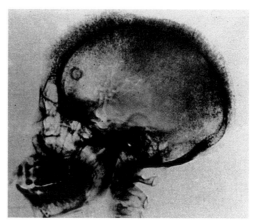

Fig. 21.1 'Hair-on-end' appearance in the calvarium in thalassaemia.

Certain other aspects of the physical examination may also be helpful. For example, anaemia associated with jaundice may well indicate haemolysis. Many haemolytic anaemias are associated with skin ulceration (Fig. 21.2). Signs of arthropathy indicate connective tissue disease. Examination of the breasts, chest or prostate may suggest carcinoma which can sometimes present with anaemia. Epigastric tenderness, abdominal masses, haemorrhoids or a rectal mucosal lesion indicate GI pathology. The presence of telangiectasias on the face, lips or within the mouth suggests a diagnosis of hereditary haemorrhagic telangiectasia which can cause iron deficiency due to chronic GI blood loss from lesions scattered throughout the length of the bowel. Enlargement of the liver, spleen and lymph nodes commonly occur in haematological diseases and they are discussed in detail below.

EXAMINATION OF THE LYMPH NODES

The distribution of the major lymph node groups that can be felt is shown in Figure 21.3. Although the

---

BOX 21.6   Specific features of different types of anaemia.

Cause of anaemia	Specific clinical findings
Iron deficiency	Angular stomatitis, painless glossitis, dysphagia due to pharyngeal web (Plummer–Vinson syndrome), koilonychia (spoon shaped nails)
Megaloblastic anaemia	Painful glossitis ('beefy' red tongue)
B_{12} deficiency	Peripheral neuropathy, subacute combined degeneration of the cord (damage to the corticospinal tracts and dorsal columns)
Haemolytic anaemias	Jaundice, gallstones, splenomegaly, skin ulceration
Sickle cell disease	Bony tenderness, osteomyelitis
Thalassaemia	'Chipmunk facies', poor growth
Malignancies	
• Leukaemia and lymphoma	Lymphadenopathy, hepatosplenomegaly, skin nodules, gum hypertrophy, meningism
• Myeloma	Bone pain and fractures
• Metastatic cancer	Bone pain and signs of primary malignancy

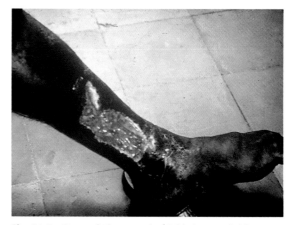

Fig. 21.2 Haemolytic anaemia (sickle haemoglobin disease); leg ulcer.

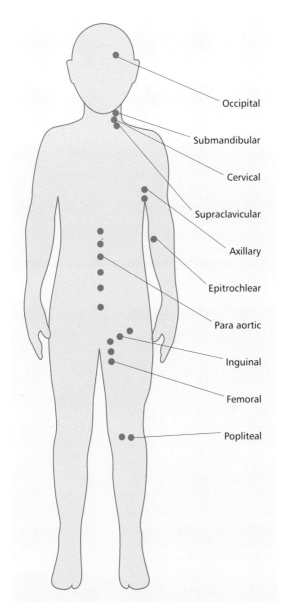

Fig. 21.3   The lymph nodes: clinical examination.

BOX 21.7   Infections that cause enlarged lymph nodes.

Site of lymph node enlargement	Infections
Submandibular	Dental infections, aphthous ulceration
Cervical	Tonsillitis (upper cervical, 'tonsillar node'), TB
Generalized lymphadenopathy (often predominantly cervical and occipital)	Epstein–Barr virus infection (glandular fever), cytomegalovirus, HIV, toxoplasmosis
Axillary	Upper limb infections (e.g. paronychia), breast infections (e.g. mastitis, abscess)
Inguinal	Lower limb infections (e.g. leg ulcers), genital infection (e.g. lymphogranuloma venereum, genital herpes)

para-aortic nodes are retroperitoneal, they can occasionally be palpated when markedly enlarged. If lymph nodes are palpated, then the following points should be considered:

- How many nodes are palpable?
- What is the diameter of the nodes?
- What is their consistency?
- Are they discrete or confluent?
- Are they mobile or fixed?
- Is the skin in the vicinity of the nodes abnormal?

Infections tend to result in tender lymphadenopathy (Box 21.7) whereas neoplastic lymph nodes are generally painless. Of course, there are exceptions to this rule and both TB and HIV infection often cause painless lymph node enlargement. Generalized lym-phadenopathy occurs in systemic infections and as a reactive process in skin diseases such as psoriasis or eczema (*dermatopathic lymphadenopathy*). Inguinal lymphadenopathy commonly occurs in normal people due to current or past infections affecting the lower limb. Marked, asymmetric or generalized enlargement of lymph nodes suggests lymphoma; this should be confirmed by excision biopsy. Lymph nodes involved by lymphoma tend to be 'rubbery' in consistency whereas nodes infiltrated by metastatic carcinoma tend to be firm or 'craggy'. The finding of regional lymphadenopathy should always prompt examination of the areas drained by those nodes (e.g. breasts, chest), searching for evidence of malignancy. Occasionally, enlargement of nodes which are impalpable themselves will result in specific clinical findings. For instance, enlargement of mediastinal nodes can cause superior vena caval obstruction manifested by venous engorgement of the neck veins, headache and papilloedema.

EXAMINATION OF THE LIVER AND SPLEEN

Haematological disorders frequently cause enlargement of liver and spleen, although the differential diagnosis is wide-ranging (Boxes 21.8 and 21.9). Palpation should begin in the iliac fossae so that massive hepatosplenomegaly is not missed. If palpable, these organs should be measured at rest in centimetres from the costal margin at the midclavicular line to the point of furthest extent. Sometimes, they are palpable only on inspiration and this should also be noted (see Ch. 7).

BOX 21.8   The common causes of hepatosplenomegaly and their associated features.

Disorder	Associated clinical findings
Myeloproliferative disorders	Usually nil
Lymphoproliferative disorders	Lymphadenopathy
Congestive cardiac failure	Tachycardia, raised JVP, displaced apex, gallop rhythm, basal crackles, dependant oedema
Chronic liver disease	Stigmata of chronic liver disease (jaundice, palmar erythema, spider naevi, ascites)

BOX 21.9   Causes of massive splenomegaly.

- Chronic myeloid leukaemia
- Myelofibrosis
- Splenic lymphoma
- Visceral leishmaniasis (kala-azar)
- Malaria (tropical splenomegaly syndrome)
- Gaucher's disease

INVESTIGATION OF THE ANAEMIC PATIENT

Investigations first should be directed at determining the type of anaemia and then at identifying an underlying pathology. A patient with significant anaemia for which the cause is not obvious should have initial investigations as in Box 21.10. Examples of normal and abnormal blood and bone marrow appearances are shown in Figures 21.4–21.15. If there is any evidence to suggest a haemolytic process (jaundice, splenomegaly, gallstones or suggestive features on the blood film), then a haemolysis screen should be included. In the majority of cases, the type of anaemia will then be apparent and further investigation can be initiated (Box 21.11). Most primary haematological disorders (e.g. leukaemia) will have an abnormal blood film and, if present, appropriate referral is indicated.

BOX 21.10   Initial investigations of anaemia.

- Full blood count
- Examination of the blood film
- Serum ferritin
- Serum B$_{12}$
- Red cell folate
- Haemolysis screen (if indicated): reticulocyte count, bilirubin, lactate dehydrogenase, haptoglobins

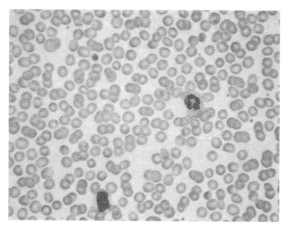

Fig. 21.4   Normal peripheral blood. The red cells show little variation in size or shape. A neutrophil granulocyte and a lymphocyte are visible and platelets are scattered through the film.

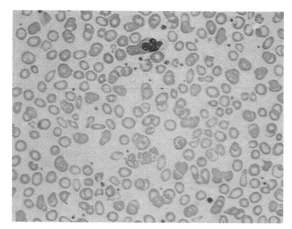

Fig. 21.5   Iron deficiency anaemia (peripheral blood). Hypochromia, microcytosis, anisocytosis and target cells are shown.

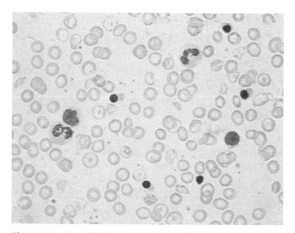

Fig. 21.6   Beta-thalassaemia major (peripheral blood). There is hypochromia, microcytosis and anisocytosis. Target cells and nucleated red cells are numerous. In beta-thalassaemia minor the peripheral blood looks like that of iron deficiency.

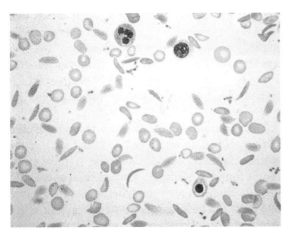

Fig. 21.7   Sickle haemoglobin disease (peripheral blood). In homozygous disease (HbSS), sickle cells and target cells are present together with occasional nucleated red cells. Heterozygotes (HbSA) have a normal peripheral blood.

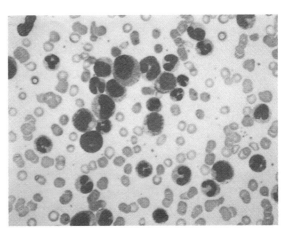

Fig. 21.10   Chronic granulocytic (myeloid) leukaemia (peripheral blood). There is an increased number of granulocytes, most of which are mature neutrophils. A few more primitive cells are also present.

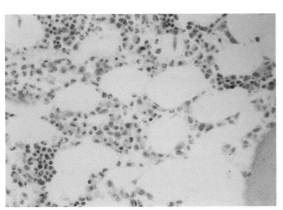

Fig. 21.8   Trephine bone marrow biopsy showing a normally cellular marrow.

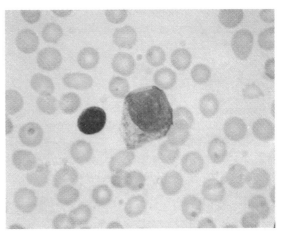

Fig. 21.11   Acute myeloblastic leukaemia (peripheral blood). The myeloblast in the centre of the field contains a cytoplasmic Auer rod.

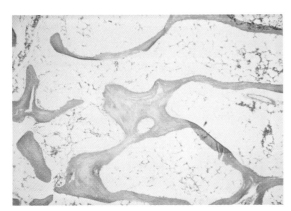

Fig. 21.9   Trephine bone marrow biopsy. The marrow is acellular and there is bone resorption in this patient with aplastic anaemia.

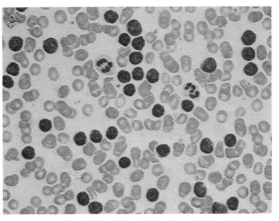

Fig. 21.12   Chronic lymphocytic leukaemia (peripheral blood). The white cell count is increased and most of the white cells are small lymphocytes.

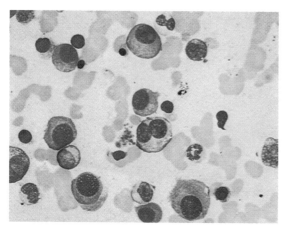

Fig. 21.13   Myelomatosis (bone marrow). The marrow is infiltrated with plasma cells and one binucleate form is present. The red cells show rouleaux formation.

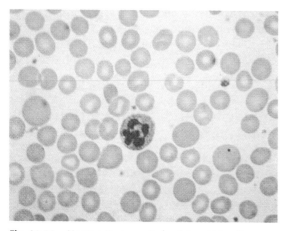

Fig. 21.14   Macrocytic anaemia (peripheral blood). Macrocytosis, anisocytosis, poikilocytosis and a hypersegmented neutrophil granulocyte are shown.

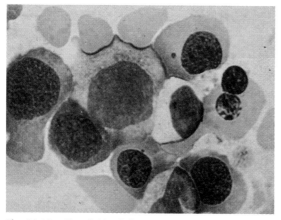

Fig. 21.15   Megaloblastic bone marrow. The majority of cells are megaloblastic erythroblasts showing failure of nuclear development and abnormal nuclear morphology.

BOX 21.11   Second line investigations of anaemia.

Cause of anaemia	Appropriate investigations
Iron deficiency	oesophagogastroduodenoscopy (OGD), colonoscopy, gynaecological examination, coeliac antibodies
Low serum B$_{12}$	Gastric parietal cell antibodies, Schilling test
Low red cell folate	Coeliac antibodies and/or duodenal biopsy—if small bowel malabsorption, refer to gastroenterologist
Evidence of haemolysis	Direct Coombs' test (DCT)—if DCT Neg: G6PD screen, refer to haematologist

If the cause of anaemia is not apparent at this stage, then proceed as in Box 21.12. Haemoglobin electrophoresis should be performed at the initial screening if the patient comes from an appropriate ethnic group. Obviously, investigation need not proceed precisely along these lines and cases should be approached on an individual basis. If the cause of the anaemia is not evident at this stage, or if a haematological disorder has been diagnosed, then referral to a haematologist is indicated.

COAGULATION DISORDERS

The term 'haemostasis' refers to the coordinated physiological processes that prevent excess blood loss following vascular injury, and that can limit and localize the thrombotic process and initiate thrombolysis. The

BOX 21.12   Third line investigations of anaemia.

Type	Investigations
Microcytic anaemias	Haemoglobin electrophoresis; search for evidence of underlying infective, inflammatory or neoplastic disorder (blood cultures, ESR, C-reactive protein, ANA, CXR, etc.)
Normocytic anaemias	Renal function; haemolysis screen (if not already performed); immunoglobulins and paraprotein screen; search for evidence of underlying infective, inflammatory or neoplastic disorder (see above)
Macrocytic anaemias	Thyroid function tests; liver function tests; haemolysis screen (if not already performed)

essential components of the haemostatic system are the integrity of the vessel wall, 'primary haemostasis' (the formation of a platelet plug) and 'secondary haemostasis' (the formation of a fibrin clot through the activation of the coagulation cascade) (Fig. 21.16). Disorders of primary haemostasis, which generally result from defects in platelet function or number, result in petechiae and bleeding from mucosal surfaces. Conversely, disorders of secondary haemostasis (as exemplified by haemophilia) usually result in haemorrhage into deeper structures such as muscles and joints (Figs 21.17 and 21.18).

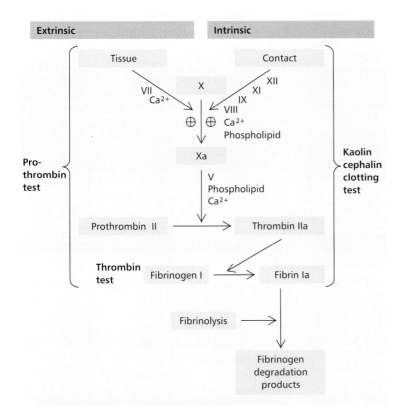

Fig. 21.16   The coagulation and fibrinolytic mechanisms.

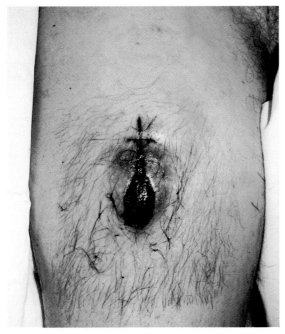

Fig. 21.17   Haematoma following an intramuscular injection in a patient with mild haemophilia.

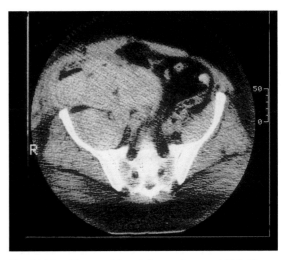

Fig. 21.18   CT scan of the abdomen (haemophilia). There is a large haematoma in the right psoas region causing right-sided abdominal pain and swelling.

HISTORY

Since bleeding after injury is a universal experience it is sometimes difficult to determine whether an individual has a significant bleeding disorder or not. Approximately 20% of the population consider themselves to be 'easy bruisers' so it is important to take a 'bleeding history' that will discriminate easy bruising from a potentially important haemorrhagic disorder. An important aspect of the history will be the duration of any bleeding tendency. A lifelong tendency suggests an inherited disorder whereas a later onset suggests an acquired disorder.

The presence of a haemostatic defect is suggested by frequent and persistent blood loss, often after minimal injury. Blood loss is often overestimated by a third party (e.g. the concerned mother of a child who has bled after dental extraction) so it is useful to try and obtain some objective evidence of excessive blood loss. Any history of prior dental extraction, surgery or vaginal delivery should be obtained since these are all significant challenges to the haemostatic system and if excess bleeding did not occur then a major haemorrhagic disorder is unlikely. Features suggestive of a haemostatic defect include the requirement for blood transfusion or for surgical intervention to stop the bleeding. Heavy menstrual blood loss is a common complaint which can result from a haemostatic defect although this is not usually the case. Certain problems are highly suggestive of specific disorders. For instance, a history of spontaneous bleeding, or of bleeding after only minimal trauma into muscles or joints is highly suggestive of haemophilia. Excessive bleeding from the umbilical stump after separation of the cord is characteristic of Factor XIII deficiency.

Certain drugs affect the haemostatic system, most obviously the anticoagulants warfarin and heparin. Sometimes patients will not spontaneously report drug ingestion because the preparation was bought 'over the counter'. Aspirin is the most important example of this; platelet function is deranged for up to 3 weeks after a single dose of the drug.

EXAMINATION

The first element of the examination is to observe the character of any bruising or haematomata. Bruising due to abnormal platelet function or number most often results in purpura—tiny pinprick bruises resulting from haemorrhage from small cutaneous vessels. When compressed, purpura do not blanch, unlike similar cutaneous lesions which result from small vessel inflammation. These latter lesions will blanch on pressure. This distinction is best made by applying pressure with a glass slide and observing whether there is any blanching or not. However, the distinction is not absolute and some types of vasculitis, such as Henoch–Schönlein purpura, also result in extravasation of blood from tiny vessels. Another common type of cutaneous bruising occurs when the supporting structures of the vessel wall are weakened by age ('senile purpura') or drug therapy (e.g. steroids). When severe, platelet abnormalities may result in retinal haemorrhage. Opthalmoscopic examination is mandatory in anyone with evidence of widespread purpura and mucosal haemorrhage.

If thrombocytopenia is suspected from the clinical findings, then consideration should be given to possible underlying causes (Box 21.13). In the paediatric setting, many of the congenital thrombocytopenic syndromes also have associated physical abnormalities, for example absent radii and radial pulses in Fanconi's anaemia. Be alert to the relevant physical findings of leukaemia and lymphoma such as lymphadenopathy and hepatosplenomegaly. Similarly, stigmata of chronic liver disease (Box 21.8) may be present. Thrombocytopenia has a wide-ranging differential diagnosis which overlaps with anaemia. A detailed general physical examination may well provide diagnostic clues.

INVESTIGATION OF THE HAEMOSTATIC SYSTEM

If a haemostatic disorder is suspected certain screening tests are essential (Box 21.14).

FULL BLOOD COUNT

A full blood count includes the platelet count (normal range $150–400 \times 10^9/1$). When abnormal this should always be correlated with examination of the blood smear. A non-exhaustive list of the potential causes of thrombocytopenia is given in Box 21.13. The clinical consequences of thrombocytopenia are detailed in Box 21.15. Myeloproliferative disorders are commonly associated with a high platelet count and, because platelet dysfunction frequently accompanies these diseases, with an increased risk of both thrombosis and bleeding.

THE PROTHROMBIN TEST (PT)

The prothrombin test measures the extrinsic coagulation pathway and final common pathway for

---

BOX 21.13   The causes of thrombocytopenia.

Mechanism	Examples
Reduced production	
• Congenital	
• Acquired	Fanconi anaemia
	Leukaemia
	Aplastic anaemia
	HIV infection
Redistribution	Chronic liver disease
Increased destruction	
• Immunological	ITP
• Non-immunological	Drugs
	Septicaemia (DIC)

BOX 21.14   Initial investigation of the haemostatic system.

Test	Purpose
Full blood count	Platelet number
Blood film	To confirm genuine thrombocytopenia; platelet cytology; other abnormalities (e.g. leukaemia)
Prothrombin test (PT)	Tests extrinsic pathway
Activated partial thromboplastin test (APTT)	Tests intrinsic pathway
Thrombin test (TT)	Tests fibrin formation

BOX 21.15   The clinical consequences of thrombocytopenia.

Platelet count ($\times 10^9$/l)	Clinical features
100–150	Nil
50–100	Possible excess bleeding after major surgery or trauma
20–50	Possible excess bleeding after minor surgery or trauma
< 20	Likelihood of spontaneous haemorrhage; purpura highly likely
< 10	Significant risk of major bleeding; cerebral haemorrhage

BOX 21.16   Tests of the coagulation system.

Test	Normal range	Comments
Prothrombin time (PT)	11–15 secs	Tests the extrinsic and final common pathway
Activated partial thromboplastin time (APTT)	33–47 secs	Tests the intrinsic and final common pathway
Thrombin time (TT)	11–15 secs	Tests the ability of exogeneous thrombin to form a clot

BOX 21.17   Causes of an abnormal PT/INR.

- Warfarin or heparin therapy
- Liver disease
- Malabsorption of vitamin K
- Haemorrhagic disease of the newborn
- Disseminated intravascular coagulation

BOX 21.18   Causes of an abnormal APTT.

- Haemophilia
- von Willebrand's disease
- Warfarin or heparin therapy
- Liver disease
- Disseminated intravascular coagulation

haemostasis (Factors VII, X, V, II and I) (Fig. 21.16 and Box 21.16). The test sample is compared with a normal control and the result expressed as a ratio. The reagents are standardized and this ratio is given as the International Normalized Ratio (INR). Common situations in which the PT/INR is abnormal are shown in Box 21.17. In practice, the test is most commonly used to monitor warfarin anticoagulant therapy and the usual therapeutic aim is an INR within the range 2–3 (normal INR = 1).

THE ACTIVATED PARTIAL THROMBOPLASTIN TEST (APTT)

The activated partial prothromboplastin test measures the intrinsic coagulation pathway and final common pathway for haemostasis (Factors XII, XI, IX, VIII, X, V, II, I) (Fig. 21.16). The result is not usually expressed as a ratio. Common causes of a prolonged APTT are given in Box 21.18. The APTT is usually used for monitoring heparin therapy.

Factor VIII and Factor IX deficiencies (Haemophilia A and B), as well as von Willebrand's disease, cause a prolonged APTT. Therefore, an isolated, prolonged, APTT should be interpreted as indicative of a significant inherited bleeding disorder until proven otherwise by specialized factor assays.

THE THROMBIN TEST (TT)

In this test, thrombin is added directly to plasma. The thrombin test therefore assesses only the very final stage of coagulation, namely the conversion of fibrinogen to fibrin. The test is abnormal when there is insufficient fibrinogen present or if there are substances present that inhibit thrombin (Box 21.19).

When there is prolongation of the PT, APTT or TT for which the cause is not apparent, then further specialized investigation is required to elucidate the cause under the direction of a haematologist.

BOX 21.19   Causes of an abnormal TT.

- Low fibrinogen levels
- Abnormal fibrinogen (dysfibrinogenaemia)
- Heparin
- Elevated fibrinogen degradation products

22
IMAGING IN MEDICINE

INTRODUCTION

The development of medical imaging began with Roentgen's demonstration in 1895 of the potential value of X-rays. Since then various other techniques for imaging the structures of the body have been introduced, but conventional X-ray images remain in common use. In general, modern methods are designed to produce good images and to minimize risk to patient and investigator. Box 22.1. lists the main imaging methods. Some modern techniques are highly specialized, as, for example, cardiac and neuroradiology. The advent of accurate and safe methods of localization in imaging and of endovascular catheterization for angiography has led to the development of interventional radiology as a sub-specialty. These methods are used to deliver therapy, to treat atheroma and to exclude aneurysms or vascular malformations from the circulation. They are also used to localize abnormalities, such as tumours, and for stereotactically directed biopsy and therapy using gamma radiation, other external irradiation methods include chemo-embolisation and thermocoagulation.

WHAT THE IMAGING DEPARTMENT NEEDS TO KNOW

The choice of investigation is based on the following:

- The clinical problem
- The degree of urgency
- The level of acceptable patient risk
- The cost.

Certain questions should always be asked before arranging an investigation (Box 22.2). The ideal, cost-effective approach is to generate a limited number of low-risk, but highly informative images. These are often of considerable technical complexity. For example, in the investigation of angina the imaging method of choice is coronary angiography,

---

BOX 22.1   Imaging methods.

- Conventional and digital radiology (X-ray imaging using photographic emulsion)
- Ultrasound imaging
- Computed tomography
- Magnetic resonance imaging
- Radioisotope imaging
- Contrast imaging of hollow structures, including barium studies, angiography, cholangiography, etc.

BOX 22.2   Considerations before arranging radiological investigation.

- Possibility of pregnancy
- History of allergy to contrast agents or iodine
- History of atopy or asthma
- Diabetes mellitus
- Previous operations, metallic implants
- Cardiac pacemakers or other electronic devices
- Drug history, especially steroids
- Mobility, e.g. walking, chair or bed-bound
- Previous imaging
- Health hazards, e.g. HIV, TB, hepatitis, MRSA

---

and this may be combined at a single session with interventional techniques to relieve partial blockage of a coronary artery by atheroma. In neuroradiology, the investigation of choice might be CT scanning in the case of suspected subarachnoid haemorrhage or acute stroke, and MR imaging in suspected tumour or multiple sclerosis. Other imaging methods in these contexts have become redundant.

LOOKING AT X-RAYS AND OTHER IMAGES

Always follow the same systematic process in inspecting any medical image (Box 22.3). Begin by checking the basic data about the patient. Check:

- Name: make sure it is the correct patient
- Hospital number: two people may have the same name—the date of birth is often used also to confirm the identity of the patient
- Date: check this carefully
- Technique: what method are you looking at?
- Check whether contrast has been used in CT or MR images
- Side marker: be sure you know which is right and left, and that the markers have been applied correctly
- Is the image oriented correctly? Or rotated?
- Are there any technical problems? Are you satisfied with the quality of the images?
- Is the whole field of interest demonstrated on the images?

- What imaging method has been used
- What organ or system has been studied.

Remember, too, that the image should be displayed so that *right-sided structures are shown to your left*, as though you were looking at the person from the front, as you would if you were in conversation with them. This convention applies to *all* medical images. If the patient has had previous imaging, be sure to sort out the various films in date order before you start to inspect them. Are there any images missing from the packet?

In studying the images, compare your findings with the radiologist's report. Your clinical knowledge of the patient will be informative in interpreting the findings, and discussion with the radiologist is always helpful, especially in deciding whether any further imaging is likely to be useful.

COMPUTED TOMOGRAPHY AND MAGNETIC RESONANCE IMAGING

CT and MR have different roles. CT imaging uses X-rays, applied in a sequence of slices, across the organ studied. Images are constructed from X-ray absorption data derived from the difference between the dose given, and the X-ray energy detected by an array of detectors opposite the source of the beam. The X-ray beam moves around the patient in a circular path. The image therefore resembles a conventional X-ray in that it is derived from the X-ray absorption (attenuation of the signal) that occurs in the tissue through which the beam passes, but the image is much more detailed. Photographic film is used to display the image, but not to produce it; the image is produced by the software in the computer and displayed on a monitor screen. CT imaging is particularly used in trauma and acute stroke, where it can readily differentiate haemorrhage from infarction. It is also important in imaging the abdominal organs, and in the investigation of parenchymal lung disease. CT is the method of choice for staging almost all solid tumours, including lymphomas. It is also the method of choice in major trauma, since spiral CT is rapid and produces high resolution images.

MR imaging uses the disturbance induced on the resonance of protons in the body tissue in a uniform magnetic field by an applied pulsed radiofrequency energy source to construct an image in any chosen plane. Conventional MR imaging is therefore especially sensitive to tissue water content, and to the presence of fat. It is possible to image certain other metabolites containing mobile protons, but such images are not yet routinely used in clinical practice. The quality of the image also depends on the software used for image construction and, especially, on the field strength of the magnet used. Most modern MR scanning equipment uses magnets with a field strength of 0.5–2 tesla. The signal to noise ratio is proportional to the square root of the field strength, so low strength magnets are less sensitive in the detection of small lesions. Most MR images are constructed with a pixel size of 1 mm × 1 mm × 5 mm slice thickness, but thinner slices are often used to accurately delineate a lesion.

MR images are produced in two basic modes:

- T_1 images are constructed from the rate of decay or relaxation of proton resonance in the plane longitudinal to the magnetic field.
- T_2 images reflect decay in the transverse plane.

The characteristics of tissue in the T_1 and T_2 images are more important than their proton density. Generally, tissue containing water is white on T_2 images ('bright lesions') and black (sometimes called 'holes') on T_1 images. Fat is white in T_1 images. Moving blood is dark, allowing blood vessels to be seen in routine images, and it is possible to reconstruct blood vessel morphology in special sequences that track a bolus of unmagnetized blood through a vessel—MR angiography. This technique is the basis of a method for non-invasive angiography. Various special methods are used to enhance the sensitivity of MR images, e.g. spin-echo sequences. In addition, contrast enhancement with gadolinium, a rare earth element, is sometimes used, particularly to differentiate solid and cystic masses, and for MR angiography (Table 22.1).

TABLE 22.1   MR imaging: recognizing structures and lesions.

	T_1	T_2
Water	Black	White
Fat	White	White
Muscle	Grey	Dark grey
Tendons/ligaments	Black	Black
Bone	Black	Black
Air	Black	Black
Tumours	Grey	White

COMMON PROBLEMS IN IMAGING

A systematic approach is used for all parts of the body, although the structures to be imaged differ.

THE CHEST

Some of the most common issues in radiology concern the chest. Common problems are shown in Figures 22.1–22.10. A systematic approach is essential (Box 22.4).

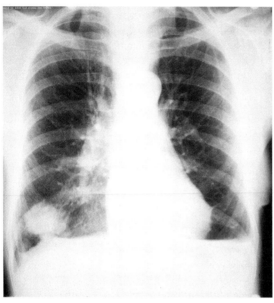

Fig. 22.1 Carcinoma of bronchus; solitary lesion in right lower lung field.

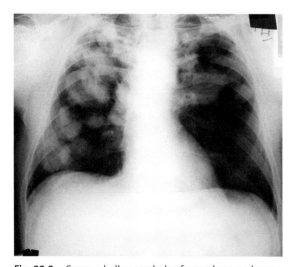

Fig. 22.2 Cannon-ball secondaries from adenocarcinoma of kidney.

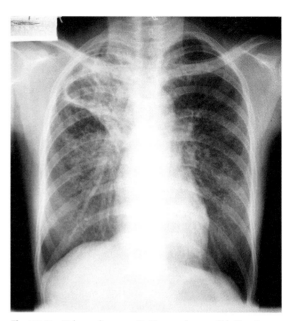

Fig. 22.3 Tuberculous cavitation and consolidation in right upper lobe.

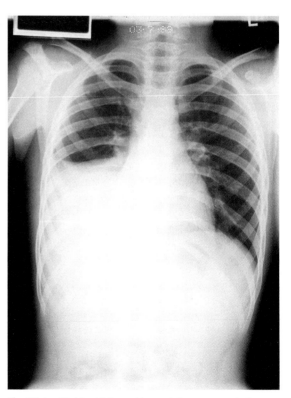

Fig. 22.4 Right middle and lower lobe pneumonia in a 14-year-old child.

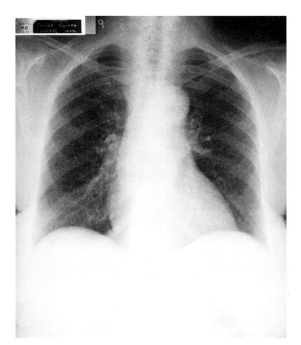

Fig. 22.5   Miliary TB; diffuse miliary tuberculosis.

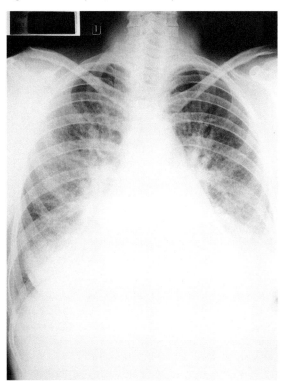

Fig. 22.6   Congestive cardiac failure; 24 hours after treatment the lungs were normal.

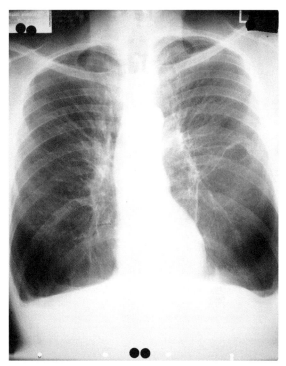

Fig. 22.7   Emphysma; large emphysematous bullae in alpha-antitrypsin deficiency.

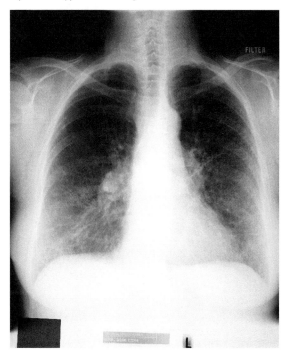

Fig. 22.8   Fibrosing alveolitis.

Measure the heart size across its widest point in the horizontal plane. Measure the pleural size across its widest point from the inner rib margins on each side. The cardiothoracic ratio (CTR) should be less than 0.5. The right hilum of the lung is lower or at the same level as the left. The mediastinum projects a little more to the left than to the right of the midline.

Evaluate the density of the lung fields on the two sides; it should be the same, allowing for the super-imposed density of breast tissue. Check the review 'areas' (Box 22.5). Try to localize the origin of any abnormalities: *lung, lymph node, pleura, heart, blood vessel or bone?* Shadowing in the lung fields has several possible causes (Table 22.2).

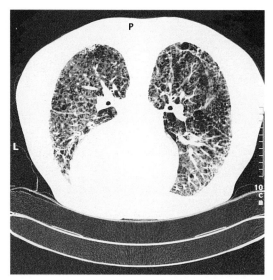

Fig. 22.9 Fibrosing alveolitis in CT scan of chest showing dilated bronchi, interstitial fibrosis and bronchiectasis.

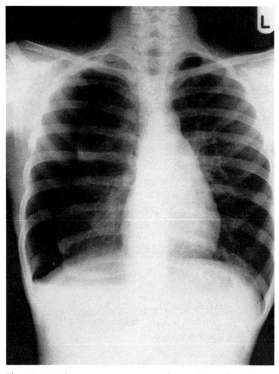

Fig. 22.10 Spontaneous pneumothorax. Note the edge of the collapsed lung visible in the right hemithorax.

BOX 22.4   Systematic evaluation of the chest X-ray.

- Heart size
- Hilar mediastinal contours
- Lungs—upper, middle and lower zones
- Review 'areas' (Box 22.5)

BOX 22.5   Areas of the chest X-ray.

A — apices
B — behind 1st rib and medial end of clavicles
C — behind the heart (cardiac)
D — below the diaphragm; pleural spaces
S — soft tissues
S — skeleton (ribs, vertebrae, sternum, clavicles)

TABLE 22.2   Diagnostic features in the chest X-ray.

Feature	Causes
Mass lesion (>3.5 cm)	Bronchogenic carcinoma
	Abscess
	Solitary metastasis
	Granuloma
	Arteriovenous malformation
	Haematoma
	Pulmonary infarct
Nodules (<1mm)	Miliary tuberculosis
(2–3 mm)	Sarcoidosis
	Metastases
	Alveolar microlithiasis
	Drug effect
(>3 mm)	Metastases and abscesses
Air/water interface	Pulmonary oedema
	Pus
	Necrotic cancer and lymphoma
	Vasculitis
Interstitial lesions	Pulmonary oedema
	Fibrosing alveolitis
	Lymphangitis carcinomatosa
	Bronchiectasis
Pulmonary collapse	Blockage of a bronchus by mucus or tumour
	Foreign body in bronchus

Solid lesions that have not changed in size over a year or more are probably benign, for example a hamartoma, an arteriovenous malformation (AVM), or a granuloma, but recent solid masses, especially if multiple, are likely to be malignant or, rarely, abscesses. A CT scan will help to differentiate these possibilities, and will aid localization for needle biopsy.

Air in the pleural space (pneumothorax) can be difficult to detect, and is easily missed. Look carefully at the apex and edges of the lung. In addition to air, the pleura may contain blood (haemothorax), inflammatory (empyema) or neoplastic effusion, or lymphatic fluid (chylothorax).

The mediastinum should be examined next. Disease in any of the tissues found in the mediastinum can cause abnormalities in this space, including thyroid, lymph nodes, thymus, aorta, heart, vertebrae and nerves. Enlargement of the heart is discussed in Chapter 6. Check each rib for fracture, texture or abnormal bone density. Look carefully at the vertebral bodies and their laminae. In women, check that both breasts are present and symetrical.

In the chest, CT imaging is useful in detecting and staging primary cancer and metastases, in the investigation of bronchiectasis and infiltrative lung disease, in the investigation of pleural lesions, and in the diagnosis of pulmonary emboli.

THE ABDOMEN AND PELVIS

Simple 'straight' X-rays of the abdomen are often used, especially in the investigation of abdominal pain or distention. Common problems are shown in Figures 22.11–22.17.

The bowel may be dilated, a feature that suggests obstruction but which also occurs in paralytic ileus. Dilated gas-filled loops of small intestine are found in small bowel obstruction, usually due to adhesions, obstructive hernias or tumours. The colon is normally less than 5 cm in diameter, and the ileum less than 3 cm in diameter. A continuous, dilated, gas-filled segment of the colon, with absence of gas more distally in the colon, suggests colonic obstruction. The colon is often enlarged in diverticular disease.

The presence of gas in the bowel is not in itself abnormal. Gas is prominent in pseudo-obstruction, a disorder of motility in which slow transit develops (see Ch. 7). Gas in the bowel wall, however, suggests that perforation may be imminent. Gas in the peritoneal cavity (pneumoperitoneum) is common after perforation or abdominal surgery, including endoscopic surgery. Pneumoperitoneum is also a feature of peritonitis, and is found with stab wounds to the abdomen. When the bowel is infarcted there may be gas in the portal vein and in the wall of the bowel. In acute necrotizing pancreatitis there may be gas in the pancreas.

Sometimes ingested foreign bodies may be seen in X-rays, including coins, dental amalgam and medicinal tablets, which often contain calcium. Glass is often radiopaque, but plastic may be radiolucent. About 10% of biliary stones and 90% of renal stones are calcified and visible on straight X-ray of the abdomen.

Calcification of blood vessels, especially the aorta, is often seen in atheromatous subjects. Remember that some objects seen on the X-ray may be outside the abdomen, in clothing or pockets, or be the result of body piercing.

Straight abdominal X-rays may be supplemented by barium contrast studies, for example barium swallow, barium meal, small bowel meal (barium follow-through), or barium enema. These techniques are less used following the advent of ultrasound, CT and, especially, flexible endoscopy (see Ch. 7).

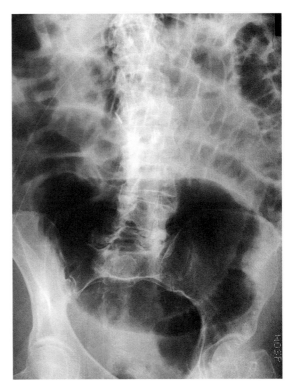

Fig. 22.11   Dilatation of small bowel due to obstruction.

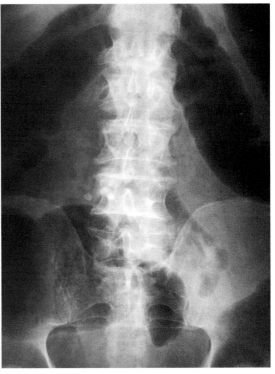

Fig. 22.12   Obstructed left inguinal hernia, with dilated colon extending into left groin.

(a)

(b)

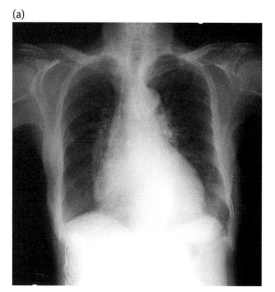
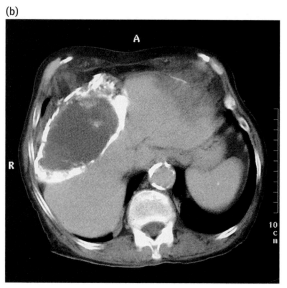

Fig. 22.13   Calcified subphrenic abscess, seen by conventional X-ray **(a)** and CT scans **(b)**.

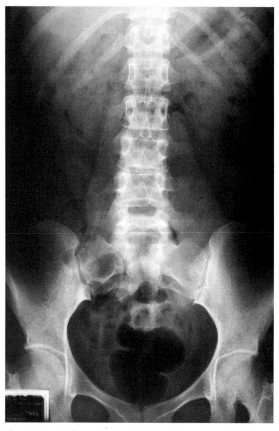

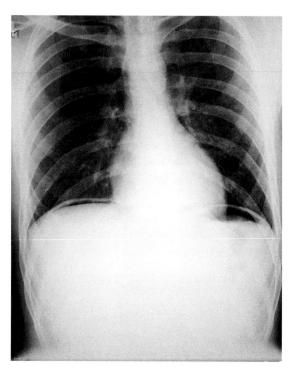

Fig. 22.15   Subdiaphragmatic air due to perforation of a viscus.

Fig. 22.14   Tuberculosis; infection of intervertebral disc at L3/4, and left psoas abscess, with enlargement of the psoas shadow.

Ultrasound is particularly valuable since it provides good images of the upper gastrointestinal tract and the pelvis. It is non-invasive, safe and portable. It can be repeated to follow progress. Its main disadvantages are that, first, it is very dependent on the skill of the operator, and, second, it is difficult to use when there is much air in the bowel. Ultrasound is much used in the investigation of solid organs, such as liver, kidneys, pancreas, gall bladder, spleen and aorta, and the pelvic organs; and it is useful in detecting tumours, granulomas, stones and abscesses and free fluid (Table 22.3).

Spiral CT has become the method of choice, after an initial ultrasound examination, in imaging abdominal organs, in particular in studying the liver

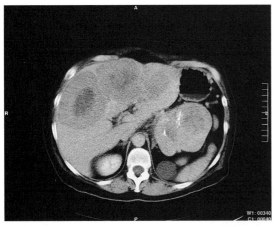

Fig. 22.16 Liver metastasis from a primary carcinoma in the tail of the pancreas.

and palpable masses, retroperitoneal structures and small or large bowel obstruction. It is also useful in evaluating and monitoring invasive procedures such as biopsies and the placement of drainage tubes.

MR imaging, because of its greater sensitivity, is used in the pelvis after an initial ultrasound has demonstrated an abnormality, and in studying the biliary tree.

Angiography is used with transvascular interventional methods in the management of arteriovenous malformations, tumours in remote locations, aneurysms and atheromatous arterial lesions, and after penetrating trauma with intra-abdominal haemorrhage.

(a)

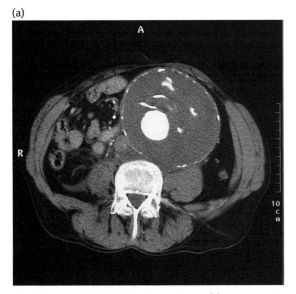

(b)

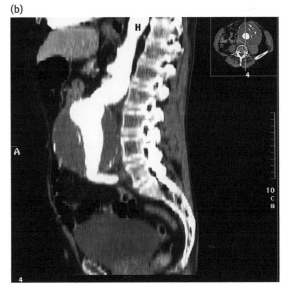

Fig. 22.17a Abdominal aortic aneurysm; **(a)** contrast enhanced axial CT image, **(b)** sagittal reconstruction.

TABLE 22.3   Ultrasound in the abdomen.

	Hyperechoic (bright)	Hypoechoic (dark)	Anechoic (black)
Liver	Haemangiomas Metastases Stones Granulomas Cirrhosis	Abscesses Metastases Hepatitis	Abscesses Cysts
Kidneys	Stones Lipoma Angioma	Carcinoma Abscesses Metastases	Cysts dilated pelvi-calyceal systems
Pancreas	Stones Chronic pancreatitis	Carcinoma Pancreatitis	Cysts and pseudocysts Abscesses
Gall bladder	Stones Polyps	Empyema Carcinoma	Abscesses Cholecystitis
Spleen	Granulomas Haemangiomas	Lymphoma Metastases Haematoma	Cysts Abscesses

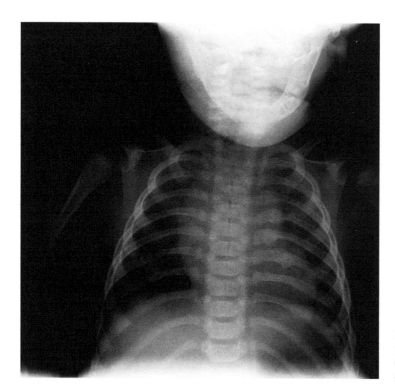

Fig. 22.18   Healed fractures of posterior left and right ribs in a 6-month-old infant, classic non-accidental injury (NAI).

Intravenous urography continues to be used in urological practice to visualize the pelvi-calyceal system, ureters and bladder, and test renal function (see Ch. 9). Radio-istope is valuable in testing renal function, and imaging liver, spleen and biliary system.

MUSCULOSKELETAL IMAGING

Certain general principles are important, particularly since all doctors are likely to be asked to give an opinion on X-rays of bones and limbs after traumatic injury, whether minor or more serious (Box 22.6). Common problems are shown in Figures 22.18–22.21. A systematic approach is essential (Box 22.7).

Bone density (Table 22.4) may be normal, reduced (osteopenia), or increased (osteosclerosis). These changes are easy to detect if focal, but difficult if diffuse. Sometimes a normal bone of standard density is placed in the field for comparison, but bone density varies with age. When a focal bone lesion (Box 22.8) is seen, it is important to look carefully at its position in the bone, and at its margins, and to note whether there is any focal matrix calcification, whether the cortex of the bone is intact and whether there is any periosteal reaction around it. Most solitary bone lesions in young people are benign, and show no periosteal reaction or swelling around them, and no associated soft tissue swelling. Aggressive (malignant) bone lesions are commoner in the elderly. Certain bone metastases have a characteristic appearance (Box 22.9). Isotope imaging is useful in detecting multiple sites of bony involvement in generalized disease and in metastatic cancer. CT

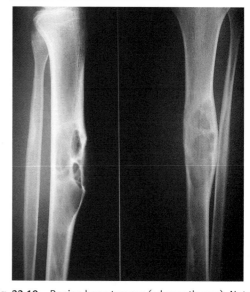

Fig. 22.19   Benign bone tumour (adamantinoma). Note the solitary, well-defined, lucent lesion with a sclerotic margin, and the absence of matrix calcification.

imaging is also sensitive in detecting and analyzing bony lesions, since it provides good images of the bony margins of the lesions, and of the associated soft tissues. MR imaging is used to assess the extent of the lesion and any local soft tissue invasion.

FRACTURES

X-rays are often the first investigation in suspected fractures and in joint disease. In traumatic fractures

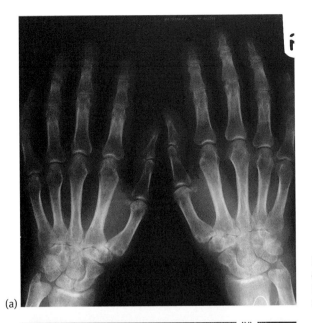

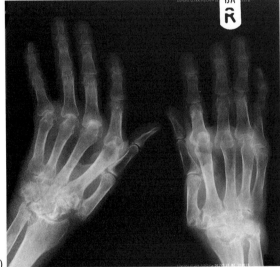

(a)

(b)

Fig. 22.20 (a) Early rheumatoid arthritis; local osteopenia, loss of joint spaces, soft tissue swelling. **(b)** Late rheumatoid arthritis: erosion of periarticular surfaces, and ulnar subluxation.

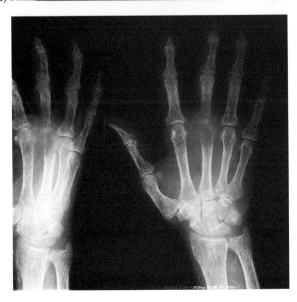

Fig. 22.21 Renal osteodystrophy; generalized demineralization, terminal phalangeal and subperiosteal bone resorption and vascular calcification.

X-rays are diagnostic and are used to check alignment of the fracture and healing. X-rays of a fracture are also important in excluding pathological fracture associated with metabolic bone disease, a focal benign bone lesion, or neoplastic invasion by metastases. In cases when there is clinical doubt after a non-diagnostic X-ray, an MR image often reveals the underlying fracture, and is the investigation of choice.

In joint disease MR imaging is now the primary imaging method because it can visualize all the soft tissue components of the joints. Osteopenia is a non-specific feature of disuse, but occurs in relation to affected joints in rheumatoid arthritis and Still's disease of children. Involvement of the distal interphalangeal joint is a feature of psoriatic arthropathy. In rheumatoid disease, involvement of joints is usually symmetrical, and the wrist is particularly susceptible.

NEUROIMAGING

Plain X-rays of the skull are now rarely performed even in casualty departments, they have been supplanted by CT imaging, which allows the whole skull to be studied in various projections on screen. If the Glasgow Coma scale score is 14/15 or less, CT scanning of the head is indicated. The skull X-ray,

TABLE 22.4   Abnormal bone density.

Generalized osteopenia	Generalized osteosclerosis	Benign focal lucent lesions	Benign focal sclerotic lesions
Osteogenesis imperfecta	Osteopetrosis (marble bone disease)	Simple bone cyst, Aneurysmal bone cyst	Bone island
Ageing	Metastatic bone disease, e.g. prostate and breast cancer	Fibrous cortical defect	Callus after fracture
Disuse, e.g. trauma and neurogenic paralysis	Dietary causes, e.g. hypervitaminosis A, fluorosis	Non-ossifying fibroma	Paget's disease of bone
Acquired metabolic bone disease, e.g. rickets, osteomalacia, hyperparathyroidism	Acquired metabolic bone disease, e.g. renal osteodystrophy	Enchondroma	Bone infarction
Myeloma	Myelofibrosis, sickle cell disease	Fibrous dysplasia Giant cell tumour of bone	Fibrous dysplasia

although simple to produce, is difficult to interpret. Only the lateral view and frontal views are likely to be available in most casualty departments. Look for the following:

- The pituitary fossa; is it expanded?
- The paranasal sinuses; is there fluid in them? (infection or CSF leak)
- Intracranial calcification; normal in the pineal gland, falx cerebri and choroid plexus of the lateral ventricles, but sometimes flecks of tumour calcification can be seen in gliomas
- Is the pineal calcification (if visible) central or displaced laterally? (subdural haematoma or other space-occupying lesion)
- skull vault; fractures, bony lesions or metastases
- skull base.

Plain films of the cervical spine are useful in assessing spondylosis (osteoarthritis) of the neck, and in recognizing narrowing of the lateral diameter of the cervical canal, leading to compressive myelopathy, especially at the C5/6 and C6/7 levels. In rheumatoid disease there may be subluxation of the upper cervical spine, especially at C1/2 when the odontoid peg is no longer securely held in place by the transverse ligament. Similarly plain films of the lumbosacral spine are also useful in spondylosis and disc disease, especially when there is chronic low back pain. Always look carefully at the alignment of the vertebral bodies in the lateral views (Box 22.10).

CT of the head is used in the management of acute head injury, suspected subarachoid haemorrhage and stroke to delineate haemorrhage and infarction. With intravenous contrast CT it is possible to show the location of the area of poor flow through the brain, even before the appearances of infarction have developed. Sometimes an intra-arterial embolus can be seen as a linear streak of high attenuation in the distribution of a vessel. Venous infarction may also be recognized acutely with this technique.

MR scanning of the brain and spine is the single most important investigation in neuroimaging, since the neural tissues themselves, together with support-

ing tissues, are well visualized. Bone is less well seen with this technique, however. As a rule of thumb, most abnormalities appear dark on T_1 weighted images, and white on T_2 weighted images.

Some common problems are shown in Figures 22.22–22.25.

RADIATION DOSAGE IN DIAGNOSTIC IMAGING

Until recently, in ordinary diagnostic practice, radiation dosage was rarely an issue of concern, since rel-

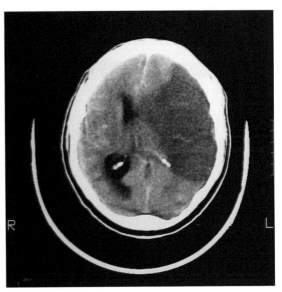

Fig. 22.22 CT head showing left middle cerebral artery (MCA) territory infarction. There is a large wedge of low attenuation extending through white and grey matter, and involving basal ganglia, indicating an infarct of at least 24–48 hours duration.

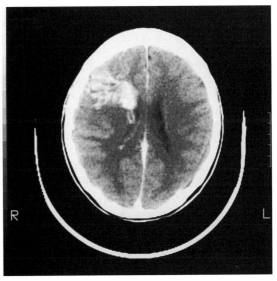

Fig. 22.23 Arteriovenous malformation (AVM) in right frontal region seen in contrast enhanced CT.

BOX 22.10   Common abnormalities of the spine.

- Degenerative disease—loss of disc height, sclerosis and osteophyte formation
- Metastatic disease—destruction of the vertebral pedicle or vertebral body
- Infection, e.g. TB—destruction of the disc and vertebral end-plate
- Arthropathy—erosion and fusion of intervertebral joints and disc spaces
- Trauma—fracture of vertebral body, transverse process and/or spinous process
- Congenital anomaly—scoliosis, hemivertebra, spina bifida, cervical ribs

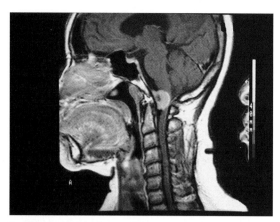

Fig. 22.24 Meningioma arising from the clivus; the lesion has a broad meningeal base.

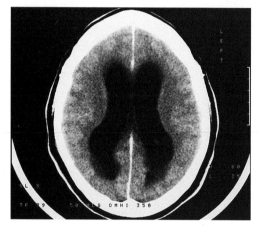

Fig. 22.25 Dilated ventricles due to obstructive hydrocephalus.

atively few X-ray images were performed and radiation exposure was low (Table 22.5). However, modern CT imaging employs relatively high dosages of X-rays, care must be exercised in not over-exposing the patient to ionizing radiation. New regulations have therefore been introduced to limit exposure.

These regulations require all those arranging an X-ray investigation to consider the hazard of exposure to radiation against the likely benefit of the test. This is a specific concern in paediatric imaging, in those with chronic conditions, and in CT imaging (Table 22.5). CT imaging accounts for about 2% of the work of an imaging department, but up to 50% of the radiation exposure. A typical CT study of the chest gives a radiation dose equivalent to 200 conventional chest X-rays (9 mSv against the conventional X-rays 0.05 mSv). Some CT studies, such as complex studies of the abdomen, will be equivalent to 1500 chest X-rays. The doses to the breast in CT examinations of the chest range from 18 to 33 mSv. In CT of the head, the

TABLE 22.5   Radiation dosage in common radiological examinations (dosage as effective dose in milliSieverts—mSv). The average dosage in CT examination is 6.6 mSv (source: National Radiological Protection Board 1993).

Examination	CT	Conventional X-ray
Head	3.5	0.2
Cervical spine	1.9	
Thoracic spine	7.8	0.9
Lumbar spine	6.0	2.2
Pelvis	9.4	1.2
Chest	9.1	0.05
Abdomen	8.8	1.14
I/V urogram	—	4.4
Barium meal	—	3.8
Barium enema	—	7.7

dose to the lens of the eye may reach 30 mSv, and as much as 130 mSv in scanning after facial trauma. Some radiation exposure can be avoided by technical modifications to the technique of CT imaging. Radionuclide imaging is also a potential source of relatively high radiation exposure (Table 22.6).

These figures suggest the need to rely on ultrasound and on MR imaging whenever possible, and to reserve CT and radionuclide functional imaging for clinical problems which cannot be resolved by any other investigation. It is always wise to consult with the radiologist in considering appropriate and cost-effective methods of investigation.

X-rays should be avoided in pregnancy, even during the first few days after conception, and adequate radio-protection should be provided during abdominal X-ray procedures in men and women of reproductive age. In any imaging department proper procedures should be observed to protect staff at all times from the possibility of accidental exposure to X-rays.

TABLE 22.6   Radiation dosage with radionuclide (isotope) imaging expressed in mSv (effective dose).

Scan type	Radionuclide	Dose
Bone scan	(^{99m}Tc phosphate)	5.0
Brain scan	(^{99m}Tc DTPA)	5.0
Liver scan	(^{99m}Tc colloid)	1.0
Thyroid	(^{99m}Tc)	0.5
	(^{123}I)	0.3
	(^{131}I)	3.0
Heart	(^{201}Tl)	25.0
	(^{99m}Tc)	7.0
Thrombus	(^{111}In)	14.0

23
BLOOD AND INTESTINAL PARASITES

INTRODUCTION

Parasitic diseases of humans are a major health problem in tropical countries, especially where clean water is in short supply; some (especially intestinal parasites) are also endemic in the West. It is important to be able to recognize parasitic infections by microscopy (see Figs 23.1 and 23.2) and, when a suitable method exists, by serological investigation. The more important of these methods are described in this chapter.

BLOOD PARASITES

The blood forms a habitat for several parasites of major importance. There are three categories: bacteria, protozoa and helminths (or worms) (Table 23.1). The main approaches to their diagnosis, often used in combination, are:

- Direct diagnosis (finding the parasite)
- Indirect diagnosis (finding antibodies to the parasite)
- Circumstantial diagnosis (by identifying the pathological changes known to be caused by this disease).

The following discussion covers these areas and is focused primarily on the major haemoparasitic diseases. The reader is recommended to consult larger works for information on other diseases not covered here but listed in Table 23.1.

MALARIA

Despite intensive worldwide attempts to contain it, malaria (caused by *Plasmodium* spp.) remains the most serious and widespread protozoan infection of humans. Current worldwide statistics suggest a prevalence of some 489 million cases of clinical malaria, of which around 2.3 million are fatal annually—especially in infancy and childhood. The disease has a wide distribution, essentially between 60°N and 40°S of the Equator. Importation of malaria into non-malaria-endemic regions is becoming an increasing problem.

Identification of the *Plasmodium* species and the percentage of red cells infected are important in subsequent management and treatment. Four species of *Plasmodium* are involved, each with characteristic morphological and staining properties.

The classic clinical feature of a malaria infection is paroxysms of fever; many patients present with fever of unknown origin. Since *P. falciparum* infection is an emergency in which any delay in diagnosis and treatment may substantially increase morbidity and mortality, it is vital to take a blood sample as soon as possible into EDTA for diagnosis. After blood collection, thin blood films stained with Giemsa should be made immediately and examined microscopically using × 600 magnification, and scanning at least 100 fields before concluding that no parasites are present. Even then, malaria cannot be excluded by a single negative film and repeat blood samples should be examined several hours later and a thick film also made.

A haematology screen using either manual techniques or automated apparatus, such as the Technicon H2, provides useful clues to the presence of *Plasmodium* spp. infection. The presence of the disease should be suspected if there is:

- A low total leucocyte count ($< 4 \times 10^9$ litre)
- Thrombocytopenia ($< 150 \times 10^9$/litre)
- Increased numbers of atypical lymphocytes ($> 4\%$).

PLASMODIUM FALCIPARUM

This species produces *falciparum*, known formerly as malignant tertian *malaria*. It is the most widespread

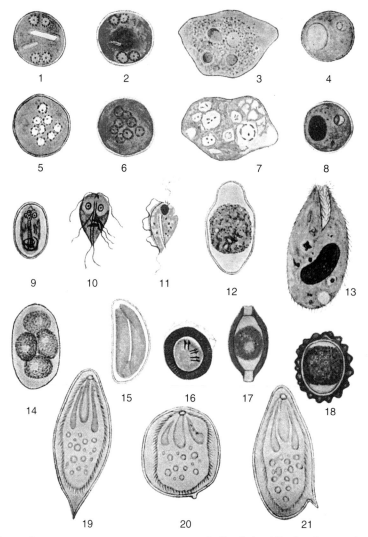

Fig. 23.1 Intestinal parasites.

1 *Entamoeba histolytica*. Fully developed four-nucleated cyst, containing chromatid bodies, as seen in a saline preparation. × 1500.

2 *Entamoeba histolytica*. Four-nucleated cyst as seen in iodine preparation. × 1500.

3 *Entamoeba histolytica*. Active form, containing ingested red blood cells, as seen in a saline preparation.
× 1500.

4 *Iodamoeba bütschlii*. Cyst, as seen in a saline preparation. Note the unstained glycogen vacuole.
× 1500.

5 *Entamoeba coli*. (Non-pathogenic) fully developed eight-nucleated cyst, as seen in a saline preparation.
× 1500.

6 *Entamoeba coli*. (Non-pathogenic) eight-nucleated cyst stained by Lugol's iodine solution. × 1500

7 *Entamoeba coli*. (Non-pathogenic) active form, as seen in a saline preparation. × 1500.

8 *Iodamoeba bütschlii* (Non-pathogenic) cyst stained by Lugol's iodine solution. × 1500.

9 *Giardia lamblia*. Cyst form, stained by Heidenhain's haematoxylin. × 1500.

10 *Giardia lamblia*. Active (trophozoite) form, stained by Heidenhain's haematoxylin. × 1500.

11 *Trichomonas hominis*. Stained by Giemsa's method.
× 1500.

12 *Isospora belli (I. Hominis)*. Undeveloped oocyst as passed in human faeces. × 500.

13 *Balantidium coli*. Active form stained by Heidenhain's haematoxylin. × 350.

14 Ovum of *Ankylostoma duodenale* (hookworm). × 500.

15 Ovum of *Enterobius vermicularis* (threadworm). × 500.

16 Ovum of *Taenia solium or T. saginata* (tapeworms).
× 500.

17 Ovum of *Trichuris trichiura* (whipworm). × 500.

18 Ovum of *Ascaris lumbricoides* (roundworm). × 500.

19 Ovum of *Schistosoma haematobium*. × 300.

20 Ovum of *Schistosoma japonicum*. × 300.

21 Ovum of *Schistosoma mansoni*. × 300.

All magnifications approximate.
Drawings by W. Cooper.

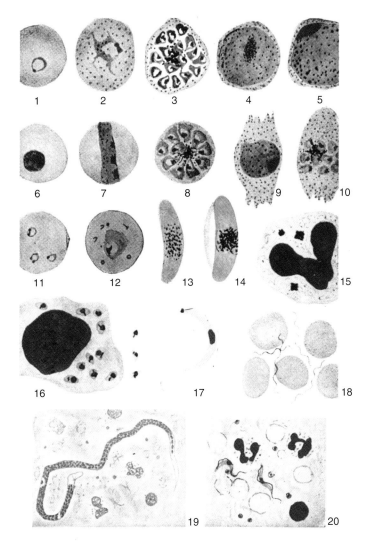

Fig. 23.2   Blood parasites.
  1 *Plasmodium vivax.* Ring stage. × 2000.
  2 *Plasmodium vivax.* Amoeboid form. × 2000.
  3 *Plasmodium vivax.* Fully developed schizont. × 2000.
  4 *Plasmodium vivax.* Male gametocyte. × 2000.
  5 *Plasmodium vivax.* Female gametocyte. × 2000.
  6 *Plasmodium malariae.* 'Compact' form. × 2000.
  7 *Plasmodium malariae.* 'Band' form. × 2000.
  8 *Plasmodium malariae.* Fully developed schizont. × 2000.
  9 *Plasmodium ovale.* Female gametocyte. × 2000.
  10 *Plasmodium ovale.* Fully developed schizont. × 2000.
  11 *Plasmodium falciparum.* Red blood corpuscle containing various types of young ring. × 2000.
  12 *Plasmodium falciparum.* 'Old' ring, showing altered staining reaction and Maurer's dots. × 2000.
  13 *Plasmodium falciparum.* Male gametocyte (or crescent). × 2000.

  14 *Plasmodium falciparum.* Female gametocyte or crescent. × 2000.
  15 *Plasmodium falciparum.* Pigment in polymorphonuclear leucocyte. × 2000.
  16 *Leishmania donovani* from a spleen smear. Some lying free, and others within the cytoplasm of an endothelial cell. × 2000.
  17 *Trypanosoma cruzi.* Adult form as seen occasionally in the blood of patients suffering from Chagas' disease (South American trypanosomiasis). × 2000.
  18 *Borrelia recurrentis.* × 2000.
  19 *Loa-loa.* × 600.
  20 *Trypanosoma rhodesiense* as seen in a thick blood film of patient suffering from African trypanosomiasis. × 1000.

Drawings by W. Cooper.

TABLE 23.1 Major blood parasites.

	Species	Vector	Reservoir host	Disease
Bacteria				
Spirochaetes	*Borrelia duttoni*	Tick	None	Tick-borne relapsing fever
	Borrelia burgdorferi	Tick	Rodent	Lyme disease
Gram-negative	*Bartonella bacilliformis*	Sandfly (*Lutzomya*)	None	Oroya fever
Protozoa				
	Plasmodium spp.	Mosquito (*Anopheles* spp.)	None	Malaria (various forms)
	Trypanosoma brucei rhodesiense and *gambiense*	Tsetse fly (*Glossina*)	Game, domestic animals	African trypanosomiasis (Sleeping sickness)
	Trypanosoma cruzi	Reduviid bugs	Dog	S. American trypanosomiasis (Chagas' disease)
	Leishmania spp.	Sandflies (*Phlebotomus*)	Dog	Leishmaniasis (visceral and cutaneous)
	Babesia spp.	Tick	Cow, rodent	Babesiosis
Helminths				
	Wuchereria bancrofti	Mosquito (*Culex, Aedes*)		Lymphatic filariasis (Elephantiasis)
	Loa loa	Horsefly (*Chrysops*)		Loaiasis
	Brugia malayi	Mosquito (*Mansonia*)	None	Lymphatic filariasis (Elephantiasis)
	Mansonella perstans (*Dipetalonema perstans*)	Mosquito (*Cullicoides*)		Covert filariasis

and causes the most serious form of malaria, accounting for 80% of malaria cases worldwide. The parasite has a high multiplication rate, infecting red cells of all ages; it therefore produces the highest parasitaemias. Incubation period is 8–15 days following the bite of an infected *Anopheles* mosquito, when the classic *ring stages* can be seen in peripheral blood. The parasite divides by binary fission within erythrocytes, a process known as *erythrocytic schizogony*, to produce infected red blood cells (*schizonts*) containing 8–32 individual *merozoites* which then invade new erythrocytes, when the schizont ruptures (schizogony). This erythrocytic cycle takes 48 hours to complete.

The ring forms consist of a rim of cytoplasm which stains blue, and a small nucleus or chromatin dot which stains purple. *P. falciparum* can be distinguished from other species in that the rings are small and delicate, with multiply invaded cells in severe infections, double chromatin dots and marginal or accole forms (Fig. 23.3(a)). Unlike the situation with other species of *Plasmodium*, the trophozoites and schizonts of *P. falciparum* 'withdraw' from the peripheral circulation and sequester in the internal organs, in particular cerebral capillaries. Thus, these two stages are not seen in the peripheral blood. Characteristic of a *P. falciparum* infection, usually of long duration (as occurs in semi-immune individuals from malaria-endemic regions), is the presence

of a few crescent-shaped male and female *gametocytes*—the sexual stage of the parasite responsible for infection of mosquitoes and transmission of the disease. The gametocytes are easily recognizable (Fig. 23.3(b)).

In many areas where *P. falciparum* occurs, other malaria species are also transmitted, and mixed infections should not be overlooked. It is important that the full number of microscope fields are examined, even when *P. falciparum* parasites are visualized in the first few fields.

A heavy parasitaemia indicates a *severe* infection (although a light parasitaemia does not exclude one) for which the patient requires urgent management. A *P. falciparum* blood film report should therefore always include an estimation of the *parasite density*. A quantitative report also allows response to treatment to be assessed where parasite resistance to chemotherapy is suspected. Parasite density can be estimated as a percentage of red cells infected, or as the number of parasites per microlitre of blood.

Calculation of the percentage of erythrocytes infected

This is performed by counting at least 1000 red cells and expressing the number of parasitized cells as a percentage of this number. Most parasitaemias range from 1 to 10%. When ≥10–20% of cells are infected

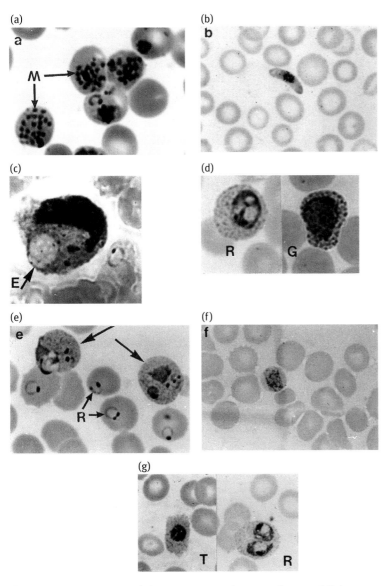

Fig. 23.3   (a) *Plasmodium falciparum* taken from *in vitro* culture showing mature erythrocytic *schizonts* containing individual *merozoites* (M). (b) Blood film from an African child with *P. falciparum* infection showing a classic sickle-shaped gametocyte. (c) Erythrophagocytosis by a peripheral blood monocyte of a non-parasitized red cell (arrow) in a *P. falciparum* infection. (d) *P. vivax* showing the large amoeboid ring (R) and gametocyte (G). The infected red cell is enlarged and the cytoplasm contains Schuffner's dots. (e) Thin blood film from a patient in Thailand showing the unusual occurrence of dual invasion of red cells by *P. vivax* and *P. falciparum*. Single invasion of *P. falciparum* is also present as indicated by the small fine rings with double chromatin dots typical of this species (photograph courtesy of M. Guy). (f) Classic 'band' trophozoite of *P. malariae* where the cytoplasm of the parasite lies diagonally across the red cell which does not contain Schuffner's dots.
(g) *P. ovale* showing the typical appearance of a trophozoite (T) within an oval-shaped red cell with fimbriated edges, and the large rings of this species in a doubly invaded erythrocyte. Like *P. vivax*, the red cells contain Schuffner's dots.

the prognosis is poor, and the patient must be treated as a medical emergency.

Measurement of the number of parasites in 1 μl of blood

Absolute numbers of parasites are estimated by counting them against the patient's leucocyte count. Malaria pigment seen within the cytoplasm of monocytes and neutrophils, and occasionally erythrophagocytosis, may be visualized in a patient who has recently recovered from an acute attack (Fig. 23.3(c)).

The World Health Organization (WHO) has suggested that the following laboratory indices should be considered as indicative of a poor prognosis in *P. falciparum* infection:

- High parasitaemia > 5% parasitized red cells (250 parasites μl/blood)
- Presence of *schizonts* in a peripheral blood film
- Peripheral leucocytosis > 12 /μl
- High serum tumour necrosis factor-alpha (TNFα)
- Haematocrit < 20% (Hb <7.1 g/dl)
- Blood glucose < 2.2 mmol/litre
- Serum creatinine > 265 μmol/litre
- Raised serum aminotransferases.

Cerebral malaria

Cerebral malaria is the most common clinical presentation of complicated *P. falciparum* infection and has an approximately 50% fatality rate despite treatment. Sequestration of *P. falciparum schizonts* from the peripheral blood and their attachment to endothelial cells, particularly cells of the post-capillary venules in the brain, causes obstruction, cerebral anoxia and associated pathological changes. The patient should be placed in intensive care.

An examination should first be carried out to establish the diagnosis (to exclude meningitis and neurotropic viruses) and to detect other parasites, hypoglycaemia, anaemia, renal failure and pulmonary oedema. Secondly, a more through examination should be performed when treatment is underway. Patients who have had an untreated *P. falciparum* infection for several weeks usually present with severe headache, drowsiness, delirium and convulsions. Examination of the fundus in such a patient is an important part of the physical examination; the presence of retinal haemorrhages in a non-comatose patient usually indicates that cerebral involvement will develop within hours. Presentation may be with unrousable coma and classic decerebrate rigidity. These features of cerebral malaria can also be caused by an associated hypoglycaemia and without blood glucose measurements the two cannot be distinguished. However, only a minority of patients respond to intravenous dextrose. In young African children living in a malaria-endemic region, the neurological signs are those of diffuse encephalopathy with symmetrical upper motor neurone signs and brainstem disturbances—including ocular palsies, stertorous breathing, hypertonicity, absent abdominal reflexes, and retinal haemorrhages.

PLASMODIUM VIVAX

Malaria caused by *Plasmodium vivax* is often referred to as *vivax* malaria; it was formerly known as benign tertian malaria. It is the main cause of malaria in temperate and subtropical regions. It is rarely encountered in West Africa where inherent immunity is present. Resistance relates to the lack of Duffy blood group antigens on the red cells of the indigenous population, which act as receptors recognized by *P. vivax* merozoites for successful invasion of the erythrocyte. It is the most common parasite in patients from the Indian subcontinent.

P. vivax preferentially invades reticulocytes, and therefore only rarely do more than 2% of the red cells become parasitized. Erythrocyte *schizogony* occurs every 48 hours within the peripheral blood and *trophozoites*, *schizonts* and *gametocytes* can be visualized in blood films. The young ring form is frequently difficult to differentiate from that of *P. falciparum*. However, the late ring form and trophozoites are large and amoeboid. The infected red cell is enlarged and if correctly stained shows well-defined Schuffner's dots (Fig. 23.3(d)). Mature schizonts contain brown pigment and between 12 and 24 *merozoites*. Mixed infections can develop and dual parasitization of a *single* cell by *P. vivax* and *P. falciparum* occasionally occurs (Fig. 23.3(e)).

P. vivax is a relapsing species with each relapse being initiated by the activation and differentiation of latent *hypnozoite* forms within hepatocytes. If treatment of *P. vivax* infection does not include concurrent treatment (with primaquine) to eliminate the hypnozoites, relapses may occur at intervals up to 3 years or more after the primary attack.

PLASMODIUM OVALE

Malaria caused by *P. ovale* is referred to as ovale malaria and was previously known as ovale tertian malaria. Like *P. vivax* it is a relapsing species, and a mixed infection with *P. falciparum* is common. It has a restricted distribution and low prevalence, mainly in West Africa.

All stages of erythrocyte *schizogony* may be present in peripheral blood and only rarely do more than 2% of red cells become parasitized. The rings are large and obvious, and multiple invasion is sometimes seen. The red cell cytoplasm contains Schuffner's dots, and 20–30% of infected cells take on an oval shape with fimbriated (ragged) ends, especially those containing late *trophozoites* and *schizonts* (Fig. 23.3(g)).

PLASMODIUM MALARIAE

Malariae malaria (formerly known as quartan malaria) is endemic in the tropics and subtropics. In Africa, it accounts for up to 25% of *Plasmodium* spp. infections and often accompanies infection with *P. falciparum*. Erythrocytic *schizogony* is slower than in falciparum and vivax malaria, taking 72 hours to complete.

Since parasite numbers are normally low (<1% of red cells are infected), laboratory confirmation requires careful examination of a thick blood film backed by a prolonged search of a thin film for identification of species. The ring forms are large ('bird's eye' rings) and the red cell cytoplasm is devoid of Schuffner's dots (unlike *P. vivax* and *P. ovale*). *Trophozoites*, *schizonts* and *gametocytes* can be seen in a blood film. Two useful features that confirm diagnosis of *P. malariae* infection are the presence of band form trophozoites (Fig 23.3(f)) and the occasional compact 'daisy head' *schizont* containing 8–12 merozoites.

There is no hypnozoite stage in *P. malariae* infection and thus no relapses.

NEW TECHNIQUES TO ASSIST CLINICAL DIAGNOSIS

During the last decade several new techniques have been developed to improve the speed and sensitivity of standard microscopy; most have limitations in developing countries for technical and financial reasons.

Species-specific *DNA probes* are available for the detection of *P. falciparum* and *P. vivax*. Probes containing repetitive sequences of *P. falciparum* DNA can detect a parasitaemia of 0.001%. This is, however, less sensitive than standard microscopy in the hands of a trained microscopist. The introduction of the polymerase chain reaction (PCR) technique has increased the sensitivity of molecular probes, which are most suited for mass screening of blood in epidemiological studies and in blood banks.

Ribosomal RNA (rRNA) probes, developed because rRNA is the most abundant cellular macromolecule and therefore an obvious target, have proved more sensitive. Using the *P. falciparum* probe, it has been possible to detect as little as 13 fg of target, representing a parasitaemia of 0.00001%.

A newly developed, commerically available diagnostic test is now available; this relies on the staining of parasite DNA and RNA by a *fluorescent probe*. The *QBC* (quantitative buffy coat) combines concentration of infected red cells by centrifugation (they have a greater density than uninfected cells) with staining of parasites with acridine orange. The manufacturers have designed simple instrumentation and tubes for the use of QBC in rural tropical environments; claims have been made that sensitivity is greater than that of a thick film.

AFRICAN TRYPANOSOMIASIS

Two organisms cause African trypanosomiasis (or sleeping sickness).

- *Trypanosoma brucei gambiense*—a chronic debilitating disease found in Central and West Africa
- *T. b. rhodesiense*, which produces a more acute disease and is found in Central and East Africa.

A related subspecies, *T. b. brucei*, with a similar East African geographical distribution, only infects animals. The different subspecies are morphologically identical and can be distinguished with certainty only by biochemical techniques, such as electrophoretic typing of their isoenzymes. The parasite is transmitted by the bite of the tsetse fly (*Glossina* spp.), a genus only found on the African continent.

Although sleeping sickness claims relatively few lives today, the risk of severe epidemics necessitates surveillance and active control measures in endemic regions. This involves the application of specific and reliable diagnostic techniques.

Demonstration of the organism itself is obviously the definitive diagnostic procedure. Trypanosomes are elongated flagellate protozoa some 14–30 μm long and 1–3 μm broad (Fig. 23.4). The flagellum arises from an organelle called the kinetoplast, which contains double-stranded DNA; this feature has been exploited for the development of molecular probes (see below). The circulating forms, termed *trypnomastigotes*, multiply by binary fission within the blood and subsequently invade a wide variety of tissues—including the brain—during the late stages of the disease.

DIAGNOSIS

Confirmation of the suspected clinical diagnosis (hepatosplenomegaly, lymphadenopathy, anaemia, thrombocytopenia, wasting and impaired mental state) is as follows:

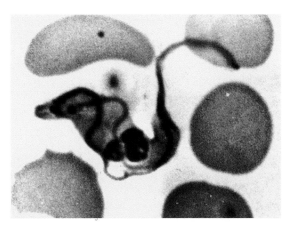

Fig. 23.4   Trypomastigote of *Trypanosoma brucei brucei* dividing by binary fission. It has two flagella, nuclei and kinetoplasts.

Examination of blood for trypnomastigotes
During early infection, actively mobile parasites may be visualized in wet blood preparations and Giemsa-stained films; this is often unsuccessful as a result of the small number of parasites present and daily fluctuations in detectable parasite numbers (*T. b. rhodesiense* is easier to find than *T. b. gambiense*). Trypanosomes must not be mistaken for microfilariae (see below) which may be present in the same blood sample.

Miniature Anion Exchange Column concentration (MAEC)
The Sephadex anion 'minicolumn' permits the detection of very small numbers of trypanosomes in specimens of blood or cerebral spinal fluid (CSF). It is an invaluable diagnostic aid in individual patients, and has also been used in field studies.

Whole blood is added to the column and washed through with an appropriate buffer. The red cells adhere to the column but the less strongly charged trypanosomes pass through in the eluate and can be concentrated by centrifugation. (Full details of this technique and availability of MAEC kits can be obtained from the WHO.)

Examination of a lymph node aspirate
Cervical lymphadenopathy, especially in the posterior triangle of the neck ('*Winterbottom's sign*'), is an important clinical diagnostic feature of *gambiense* sleeping sickness. Trypanosomes are easily identified in a wet preparation of a gland puncture and their identity confirmed by staining. This is a valuable and simple means of providing early diagnosis.

Examination of cerebral spinal fluid (CSF)
After several weeks (*T. b. rhodesiense*) or years (*T. b. gambiense*) trypanosomes invade the central nervous system, resulting in a meningoencephalitis. A lumbar puncture should, therefore, be performed in patients with confused mental status. In such instances, and in contrast with viral meningitis, tuberculous meningitis and neurosyphilis, the CSF

reveals a lymphocyte pleocytosis and an increased protein content, of which IgM represents >10%. Trypanosomes may also be seen in stained films of a centrifuged deposit, or by using CSF applied to the minicolumn described above.

Testing for anti-trypanosome antibodies
Tests used in the serological diagnosis of trypanosomiasis include an indirect fluorescent antibody test (IFA) and an enzyme-linked immunosorbent assay (ELISA) using commercially available antigens. The card agglutination test (CATT) is a recent addition to the commercial market and is widely used (particularly in field surveys) to assist in the diagnosis and control of trypanosomiasis caused by *T. b. gambiense*. Anti-trypanosomal IgM can be detected using this simple test which agglutinates freeze-dried trypanosomes fixed to the card.

DNA probes
DNA probes have yet to be completely evaluated. Analysis of trypanosome DNA reveals that in *T. b. brucei*, for example, highly repetitive sequences represent 12% of total nuclear DNA, making species-specific DNA probes a reality in diagnosis. In addition, kinetoplast DNA (kDNA) minicircles are present at approximately 5000–10 000 per genome and thus represent good candidates for use in a sensitive DNA hybridization assay.

ADDITIONAL FEATURES OF AFRICAN TRYPANOSOMIASIS
Analysis of blood and serum from an established case of trypanosomiasis reveals anaemia, thrombocytopenia, raised erythrocyte sedimentation rate (ESR), autoagglutination and rouleaux formation of red cells. The two latter features result from a very high serum IgM concentration (7–10 times the local mean).

SOUTH AMERICAN TRYPANOSOMIASIS

Trypanosoma cruzi causes South American trypanosomiasis or *Chagas' disease*. As the name implies, it occurs only in the Americas, especially in tropical and subtropical Latin American countries. It is estimated that about 16–18 million people are infected, while 65 million are at risk of infection. Chagas' disease is the main cause of chronic heart disease in endemic areas, where some 20–30% of those infected will develop Chagasic cardiomyopathy.

T. cruzi is naturally transmitted through contact with the faeces of an infected haemophagus bug of the family Reduviidae—the cone-nose or kissing bug. The faeces contain the infective *trypomastigotes* which are deposited on mucous membranes, particularly around the eye, as the bug feeds. The parasites enter through the bite wound or penetrate the membrane. Once in the bloodstream, trypomastigotes invade reticuloendothelial and other tissue cells, especially those of the heart muscle, nerves, skeletal muscle, and smooth muscle of the gastrointestinal tract. Once within the cell they lose the flagellum and become *amastigotes*, multiplying by binary fission. Parasites in the heart can cause severe myocarditis, especially in the early stages of infection. The severity of the acute myocarditis seems to seal the eventual fate of the sufferer from chronic cardiac changes which include dysrhythmias of various types, cardiomegaly and complete heart block resulting in sudden death. Muscular degeneration and denervation of segments of the alimentary tract cause mega-oesophagus, mega-stomach and mega-colon (*megasyndromes*) which can best be detected radiologically.

Chronic Chagas' disease is incurable, although two drugs (nifurtimox and benznidazole) are effective in very early infection (which is often difficult).

DIAGNOSIS
Several techniques are available for diagnosis:

Detection of trypanosomes in blood
Organisms may be detected in peripheral blood films in an early acute infection. As is the case with African trypanosomiasis, very few trypomastigotes are present. They are characteristically U- or C-shaped.

Xenodiagnosis
This is an alternative technique used in chronic cases. Uninfected, susceptible, laboratory-reared bugs are fed on the patient's blood. If trypanosomes are ingested by them they multiply, and about 25 days later trypomastigotes are found in the faeces or rectum of the bug.

Serology
The main tests are: haemagglutination and immunofluorescence. DNA probes are currently being evaluated. The incidence of transfusion-acquired Chagas' disease is high in some Latin American countries, and serological techniques for the detection of anti-*T. cruzi* antibodies have been developed for screening blood donors.

VISCERAL LEISHMANIASIS

The leishmaniases comprise several diseases caused by different species of the intracellular protozoan parasite *Leishmania*; 10 infect humans. The leishmaniases are grouped together under three headings: *visceral leishmaniasis* (VL), *cutaneous leishmaniasis*, and *mucocutaneous leishmaniasis*. This section will only deal with the life-threatening visceral disease (VL) where the parasite replicates within reticuloendothelial cells. The disease is transmitted by the bite of an infected sandfly (*Phlebotomus*). VL, or kala-azar, in the Old World is caused by *L. donovani* subspecies (*L. d. donovani* and *L. d. infantum*). It is widely distributed and not confined to the tropics; it is found in the Mediterranean basin, the Atlantic coast of Portugal, tropical Africa, parts of South America and Central and East Asia. It is currently a major problem in HIV/AIDS sufferers, for whom it is an important 'opportunist' infection.

When an infected sandfly bites man flagellate forms of the parasite (*promastigotes*) enter the blood and invade reticuloendothelial cells—notably those of the spleen and liver, where they differentiate into non-flagellate *amastigotes*. These are round oval bodies (2 to 5 μm in diameter), containing a large nucleus and rod-shaped kinetoplast (Fig. 23.5(a)). They were formerly designated Leishman–Donovan bodies (*LD bodies*) after the two researchers who initially delineated the cause of the disease. Amastigotes multiply rapidly inside the macrophages, eventually leading to rupture of the parasitized cells and dissemination throughout the body, where they are taken up by other phagocytic cells. The incubation period is very variable, but usually lies between 3 and 18 months.

DIAGNOSIS

Clinical presentation is with a high temperature and marked hepatosplenomegaly, lymphadenopathy and characteristic blood changes (see below). If untreated the infection is invariably fatal—commonly from a secondary infection. Severe immunosuppression (as in HIV infection) can make asymptomatic leishmaniasis clinically apparent. Kala-azar should therefore be suspected if the above symptoms are present in an *HIV-positive* patient. VL is often difficult to diagnose and has sometimes resulted in incorrect diagnosis such as aplastic anaemia or lymphoma. A definitive diagnosis is dependent on demonstration of the causative organism.

Demonstration of parasites in a biopsy specimen

In the human host, only intracellular amastigotes can be demonstrated. Biopsy material may be obtained from the bone marrow, lymph nodes or, preferably, the spleen. The spleen houses the greatest number of parasitized cells and will frequently give positive results even when the bone marrow proves negative. However, splenic puncture is only safe if the organ is large and firm, the platelet count is $> 50 \times 10^9$/litre and the prothrombin time normal. A film is made of the biopsied material and visualized with Romanowsky stain. Using oil immersion microscopy, amastigotes can be visualized in groups within mononuclear phagocytic cells. Because the macrophage membrane becomes fragile following parasitization of the cell, it is common for the cell to rupture when the film is being made. Thus amastigotes are frequently found lying free between cells rather than contained within them (Fig. 23.5(a)). Structurally, amastigotes of *Leishmania* species are similar and differentiation cannot be made on morphological grounds. Occasionally amastigotes can be detected in peripheral blood monocytes—especially in Indian and Kenyan VL. Blood is centrifuged, the buffy coat removed, stained and examined for amastigotes.

Culture of biopsied material

If amastigotes cannot be visualized in a film of the biopsied material, it is important to confirm the presence or absence of *Leishmania* by culturing the aspirate (which must be maintained in a sterile condition) in culture medium at room temperature (24°C) for 3–14 days. The principle is to mimic conditions within the vector gut, so encouraging any amastigotes present to differentiate and emerge from the macrophages as flagellate promastigotes (Fig. 23.5(b)).

Animal inoculation

If culture facilities are unavailable, biopsied material may be injected intraperitoneally into hamsters, which are highly susceptible to infection. After 4–6 weeks, amastigotes are usually found in large numbers in impression smears of the liver and spleen. The disadvantage of this technique is the long period of time taken for a positive result.

Serology for anti-leishmania antibodies

There are several methods, some commercially available, including IFA and ELISA employing

<table>
<tr><td>(a)</td><td>(b)</td></tr>
<tr><td>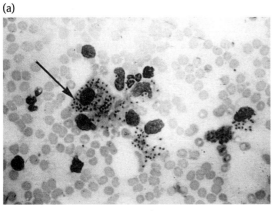</td><td>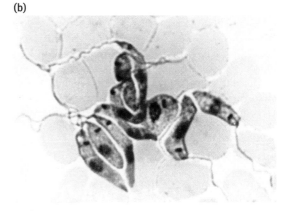</td></tr>
</table>

Fig. 23.5 *Leishmania donovani infantum* (a) amastigotes (arrowed) within macrophages in a bone marrow aspirate, and (b) culture of the same bone marrow and differentiation of amastigotes to flagellate promastigotes.

L. d. donovani promastigotes as antigen which, because of serological cross-reaction, can additionally be used to diagnose *L. d. infantum*. Cross-reactions also occur with sera from a variety of other infections, including malaria, toxoplasmosis and disseminated tuberculosis, thus limiting specificity.

Molecular probes

Because early identification of leishmaniasis can be difficult, even in a well-equipped hospital, improved methods are in demand. Present techniques use kinetoplast DNA (kDNA) probes for hybridization to parasites in tissue aspirates. Important DNA variations between different geographical isolates of *Leishmania* has resulted in the development of several thousand recombinant DNA probes which are relatively simple and cheap to prepare. Their more widespread use will open the way for earlier specific treatment; they will also assist epidemiologists concerned with more effective control interventions, and assist in determination of the link between varied clinical disease and geographical isolate.

Characteristic haematological changes

Anaemia and thrombocytopenia are typical, but not specific, features of VL. A distinctive feature is a marked granulocytopenia, sometimes amounting to an agranulocytosis. Hyper-gammaglobulinaemia often exceeds 4–5 g/dl.

FILARIASIS

This group of diseases is caused by nematodes that derive their name from a long hair-like appearance. The adults (according to species) reside in the lymphatics, connective and other tissues, whereas the larvae, or *microfilariae*, live in the blood. The larvae show what is termed *periodicity*, i.e. they are released periodically into the peripheral blood from the lungs and are therefore found in greater numbers during certain hours. Different species have characteristic periodicities. This is considered to be an adaptation by the parasite to the biting habits of their insect vectors. Being aware of the periodicity of each species is important when taking blood samples for diagnosis. Greatest numbers of microfilariae are present either during night (nocturnal periodicity, e.g. *Wuchereria bancrofti* and *Brugia* spp.) or day hours (diurnal periodicity, e.g. *Loa loa*); many patients with symptomatic infections have no demonstrable microfilariae in their blood at any time.

The most commonly encountered filarial infections which can be diagnosed from a peripheral blood film are those caused by *Wuchereria bancrofti*, *Brugia* spp., *Loa loa* and *Mansonella perstans*.

WUCHERERIA BANCROFTI

This is the most widely distributed filarial infection. The most heavily affected areas are India, South-East Asia, China, the east coast of Africa and the Pacific Islands, where the parasite causes *Bancroftian filariasis*. The number of infected individuals is estimated at 81 million worldwide. Infection occurs when larvae are deposited on the skin by an infected mosquito. The larvae enter the bite wound and make their way to the lymphatics, mature into adults and begin producing microfilariae which then enter the blood. Adults may live for up to 15 years within the same host. Diagnosis of the disease is made by detection of microfilariae in the blood (which should be collected between 22.00 and 04.00 hours). Microfilariae of *W. bancrofti* are sheathed and large (300 × 10 μm) compared with other species (Fig. 23.6) and can be identified in both wet and stained blood films.

Accompanying a *W. bancrofti* infection may be a pronounced blood eosinophilia and raised serum IgE. The adults within the lymphatics cause obstruction, especially in the leg, progressing in chronic cases to enormously enlarged limbs designated 'elephantiasis'. Lymphatic obstruction may also arise in the arm, breast or scrotum. By this stage microfilariae are rarely found in a blood film. The dilated lymph vessels occasionally rupture and discharge chyle into the urinary tract—thus producing the milky appearance known as *chyluria*; abdominal tuberculosis and malignancy are important differential diagnoses.

BRUGIA

Brugia malayi and *B. timori* also cause *lymphatic filariasis (Malayan filariasis)* and are endemic in parts of South-East Asia, India, the Philippines, Vietnam and China. The life cycle of the parasite is similar to that of *W. bancrofti*, but more frequently gives rise to a symptomless infection. Diagnosis is as for *W. bancrofti* infection.

LOA LOA

Loa loa (the 'eye worm') causes *loaisis*; as well as causing eye involvement, it can produce subcutaneous or *Calabar* swellings. The latter are recurrent large swellings—usually situated on the dorsum of the hand, wrists and forearm—which last about 3 days

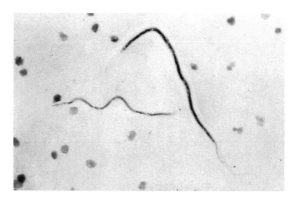

Fig. 23.6 Microfilariae in a blood film. Two species are present—the unsheathed smaller *Mansonella perstans* is readily distinguished from the larger sheathed, *Loa-loa*.

and indicate the tracks of the migrating adult worms in the connective tissue. A marked eosinophilia (60–90%) may accompany this (invasive) phase of the infection. Sometimes the worms can be seen migrating under the conjunctiva, causing considerable irritation and congestion. The adult can be extracted with fine forceps after anaesthetizing the conjunctiva.

The disease is endemic in west and central Africa. Diurnal microfilariae are best detected in peripheral blood taken between 10.00 and 15.00 hours. As with the other filarial infections, a high number of microfilariae should always be reported because serious complications can arise when treating a heavily infected individual.

MANSONELLA PERSTANS

Formerly called *Dipetalonema perstans*, this is a very common helminth found in tropical Africa and parts of South America. The microfilariae are much smaller (190 × 4 μm) than those of the other species. Although many symptoms have been attributed to this infection, none has a proven cause–effect relationship. It is often accompanied by a very marked eosinophilia.

There is considerable geographical overlap in the distribution of different species; it is therefore important to distinguish between the various microfilariae. This is usually made on differences in size, shape, presence or absence of a sheath, nuclei within the tail, and periodicity.

FAECAL PARASITES

A major reason for examination (both macroscopically and microscopically) of a faecal sample is to detect cysts and eggs, and in a minority of cases adult parasites themselves(see Fig. 23.2). Because the release of helminth (worm) eggs and protozoan cysts is irregular, three, and in some instances, six samples should be examined on separate (preferably alternate) days. In some instances (e.g. when searching for *Entamoeba histolytica* trophozoites—see below), the sample should be examined as soon as possible (preferably < 1 hour) after collection, in the *fresh* state. Although 'formed' faecal samples can be stored at 4°C overnight, examination should, when at all possible, be carried out on the same day. Samples that cannot be delivered to the laboratory promptly can be posted after emulsification in a preservative fluid (e.g. Bayer's solution or methiolate–iodine–formalin) in order to maintain parasites in a recognizable state and to allow a concentration and staining technique to be applied later.

A record of the macroscopical state of the faecal sample should always be kept, especially its composition and colour; presence of adult parasites must also be recorded.

Microscopic examination involves direct visualization of cysts, ova and parasites, and the use of a concentration technique. About 2 mg of faeces should be emulsified in a single drop (less if the sample is fluid) of warm (37°C) saline using a wooden applicator; a coverslip is then applied. When blood and/or mucus is present it should be examined separately, for it is especially likely to contain *E. histolytica* trophozoites. The presence of undigested food, bacteria, yeasts, crystals or fat globules should also be noted. The value of applying a concentration technique (to a 'formed' specimen) is that it significantly increases the likelihood of detecting ova, cysts or larvae, especially when the infective load is light. Sedimentation (e.g. modified formol–ether sedimentation) or zinc sulphate centrifugal flotation techniques can also be used; in the former, parasites are deposited at the bottom of the tube, and in the latter they float towards the surface of a liquid of high specific gravity, most debris remaining at the bottom. Although they do allow subsequent application of a staining method, concentration techniques tend to destroy trophozoites and distort the cellular exudate.

PROTOZOA

In clinical practice, the most important protozoan parasite of the gastrointestinal tract (the colorectum) is *Entamoeba histolytica*. Figure 23.7 summarizes methods used for its identification. Table 23.2 summarizes some classic differences between *E. histolytica* and *Entamoeba coli* (and other non-pathogenic amoebae); trophozoites of *E. histolytica* are invasive (and contain ingested host-erythrocytes) only if they belong to a potentially invasive zymodeme. In amoebic dysentery, direct microscopy

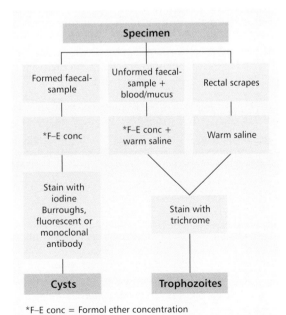

Fig. 23.7   Laboratory investigations used in the detection of *Entamoeba histolytica* in a faecal sample.

TABLE 23.2   Some differentiating features between *Entamoeba histolytica*, *Entamoeba coli* and other non-pathogenic amoebae.

	Invasive *E. histolytica*	*Entamoeba coli*	Other
Trophozoite:			
Occurrence	Present at high concentration in dysenteric stool	Never at high concentration	Variable
Size	10–60 µm	20–40 µm (often larger than *E. histolytica*)	Usually smaller, but *Balantidium coli* 50–200 µm
Mobility	Active: large pseudopodia	Sluggish, small pseudopodia	Variable
Cytoplasm	Ingested erythrocytes	Never contains erythrocytes	Variable
Cyst:			
Size	9–14.5 µm (usually nearer 10 µm)	14–30 µm (usually nearer 20 µm)	Usually smaller; but *Balantidium coli* 5–60 µm
Nucleus (fewer in young)	4 when mature	8 when mature	1–4
Cytoplasm (chromatidal bars diminish as cyst matures)	Chromatid bars present in fresh specimen. Diffuse glycogen	Chromatid bars rarely seen	*Iodamoeba* sp. has a compact glycogen vacuole
Cyst wall	Thin	Thicker than *E. histolytica*	Variable

of a fresh faecal sample (at 37°C) reveals motile trophozoites and cellular exudate. Presence of *E. histolytica* cysts in the absence of trophozoites is defined as the *cyst carrier state*. A cellular exudate may coexist with both this and *Balantidium coli*, and also with *Shigella* spp. and *Campylobacter jejuni* infection.

The presence of polymorphonuclear neutrophils, macrophages, erythrocytes and epithelial cells should be noted. Pus cells and macrophages are present in greater numbers in *Shigella* sp. compared with *E. histolytica* dysentery, whereas the pH of a faecal sample is usually more acid in *E. histolytica* compared with *Shigella* spp. infection. Table 23.3 summarizes other protozoan parasites which may be detected in a faecal sample, together with their site of origin. Some of these are depicted in Fig. 23.2.

Giardia lamblia is a small intestinal protozoan parasite that can cause small intestinal malabsorption, resulting in a faecal sample with a high fat content. While the cyst form is often detectable, albeit intermittently, in a faecal sample, jejunal fluid or biopsy is usually required to reveal the flagellated trophozoite.

Cryptosporidium parvum. and *Isospora belli* (and probably *Sarcocystis hominis*) can also be associated with malabsorption and are opportunistic in AIDS. Oocysts are easily recognizable in a faecal sample, jejunal fluid or biopsy.

DIAGNOSIS

There are several useful staining techniques for protozoa. Temporary stains include Lugol's iodine, Burrough's stain, acridine orange and eosin/saline.

TABLE 23.3   Faecal protozoa.

Usual anatomical site	Amoebae	Flagellate	Ciliate	Coccidia
Small intestine		*Giardia lamblia**		*Cryptosporidium parvum** *Isospora belli** *Sarcocystis hominis** *Blastocystis hominis**†
Colo-rectum	*Entamoeba histolytica** *Entamoeba coli* *Entamoeba hartmanni* *Iodamoeba butschlei* *Endolimax nana* *Dientamoeba fragilis*	*Chilomastix mesnili* *Trichomonas hominis* *Enteromonas* spp. *Retortomonas* spp.	*Balantidium coli**	

* Pathogenic organism in many cases—depending on the zymodeme. In the case of *E. histolyytica*.
† Classification remains undetermined.

Permanent stains include Giemsa, a modified rapid Field's stain, and a trichrome method, consisting of a modification of the Gomori technique. When *Cryptosporidium parvum* and *I. belli* oocysts are being sought, it is essential to use an acid-fast technique, e.g. a modified Ziehl–Neilsen or the phenol-auramine method, since routine stains do not allow easy identification.

Rectal scrapes often give a higher yield of positive results when an *E. histolytica* infection is suspected. Exudate should be obtained proctoscopically and immediately examined microscopically. Active trophozoites, not necessarily visualized in a fresh faecal sample, may be demonstrable.

HELMINTHS

Worms (helminths) are the commonest of all intestinal parasites.

NEMATODES (ROUNDWORMS)

Nematodes are all cylindrical, pointed at both ends, and unsegmented. The male is usually smaller than the female. They contain a tough, smooth, outer cuticle and a body cavity containing a well-developed intestinal tract. The mouth may contain rudimentary teeth or cutting plates for attachment to the mucosal surface. The largest nematode parasitic to humans, *Ascaris lumbricoides* (male 15 cm; female 25 cm), may be detected either in a faecal sample or in vomit. Differentiation from the earthworm, which is not infrequently delivered to the laboratory by an anxious patient after it has been noticed in a lavatory, is usually straightforward, the earthworm being browner in colour. The hookworms (*Ankylostoma duodenale* and *Necator americanus*) are much smaller (female approximately 8 mm) and contain two hook-like teeth at the top and two triangular cutting plates at the bottom. These are very important causes of iron-deficient microcytic anaemia in most developing countries. *A. lumbricoides* and *Necator americanus* are extremely common in most tropical countries, infecting a very high proportion of the indigenous population.

Enterobius vermicularis (threadworm)

An extremely prevalent nematode (arguably the most common intestinal helminth to afflict the human species), the threadworm is worldwide in distribution. The female is 8–12 mm and the male 2–4 mm in length; the latter dies rapidly after fertilizing the female. The major clinical manifestation is pruritus ani. Both adult worms and eggs can be recovered from perianal skin. Several methods are available. A saline-moistened swab can be gently rubbed around the perianal area and afterwards agitated in a small tube of normal saline to dislodge the eggs. After centrifugation, the supernatant is decanted and the deposit examined microscopically. Alternatively, a sellotape strip can be placed across the anus in the early morning; after removal this is applied (sticky side down) on to a microscope slide.

Trichuris trichiura (the whipworm)

This is a faecal nematode which causes symptoms only in children when present at high concentration; iron-deficiency anaemia and rectal prolapse have been recorded. Eggs are readily detectable in a faecal sample.

Strongyloides stercoralis

This is the most difficult nematode to detect. Ova are not usually detectable in a faecal sample since the eggs usually hatch to produce larvae before they reach the anus; they then undergo an 'auto-infection' cycle—which may continue for the remainder of that individual's lifespan. The larvae (200–250 μm in length) may, however, be demonstrable; a culture technique often allows identification of these even when they are too scanty for detection by a concentration technique.

CESTODES (TAPEWORMS)

Although a number of different species can parasitize humans, the two most common (and important) are *Taenia solium* and *T. saginata*. The importance of *T. solium* (the pork tapeworm) is that its larva is the causative agent in neurocysticercosis. Human infection is acquired by ingestion of *T. solium* eggs. Adult worms can reach a length of 4–8 m. Flat white segments of these worms are easily recognizable. After successful chemotherapy the entire worm (complete with head, neck and strobila) should be passed in the stool. Identification of the head (*T. solium* 1 mm and *T. saginata* 1–2 mm) is important, although this is difficult after praziquantel or niclosamide chemotherapy, both of which tend to dissolve this structure. For identification, a purged stool can be poured through a sieve of fine mesh and examined for the scolex (often broken off from the rest of the body with about 0.5 cm of the neck remaining). When detected it can be squashed in a drop of saline under a coverslip and identified microscopically. It possesses four suckers and a rostellum (a double row of alternating hooks); the fish tapeworm, *Diphyllobothrium latum* (present in Finland and Sweden), may reach a length of 3–10 m in the human intestine. A rare clinical manifestation is macrocytic (B_{12}-deficient) anaemia.

Various techniques can be used for fixation and staining of adult helminths (these can be found in specialized manuals of parasitology). They are particularly useful for establishing a permanent record.

EGGS

Methods used for the concentration of nematode, cestode or trematode eggs are the same as those used for cysts. Eggs of *Schistosoma mansoni*,

S. intercalatum, S. matthei, S. japonicum and *S. mekongi* can usually be detected in a faecal sample or rectal biopsy specimen; *S. haematobium* can also occasionally be found in the latter, but is primarily a cause of urinary tract disease. Figure 23.2 shows diagrams of eggs of human helminths as seen in a faecal sample; once detected, identification of these should be straightforward. All laboratories situated in tropical and developing countries should possess a collection of samples for use as a reference collection.

POTENTIAL DIFFICULTIES IN IDENTIFICATION OF CYSTS, EGGS AND LARVAE

The greatest problem lies in pronouncing a faecal sample 'negative'. Once evidence of a parasitosis has been established, identification is relatively straight forward. However, misidentification of some non-pathogenic objects as parasites is a major problem; some of the difficulties are as follows:

- Protozoan cysts can be confused with air bubbles, fat globules or yeasts; if iodine is added to the wet preparation the internal structure of the cyst(s) can be visualized.
- Trophozoites of pathogenic strains of *Entamoeba histolytica* must be differentiated from those of non-pathogenic amoebic trophozoites, and macrophages.
- Eggs of some helminths, especially those of *Trichuris trichiura* and *Taenia* spp., can be confused with pollen grains.

- *Ascaris lumbricoides* and *Fasciola hepatica* (the liver fluke) eggs can be mistaken for vegetable cells.
- *Strongyloides stercoralis* and hookworm larvae can be confused with hairs or vegetable fibres; the latter are usually tapered at one end, whereas the former are blunt and there is no internal structure.
- Eggs of insects and mites can occasionally be found in a faecal sample—examples of a 'spurious' infection.

Some other potential pitfalls in diagnosis are as follows:

- Charcot–Leyden crystals (breakdown products of eosinophils) are sometimes found when an immune response to a foreign substance has been initiated.
- Undigested starch granules contain concentric rings, and stain blue with iodine; when partly digested they stain red with iodine.
- A cellular exudate and/or erythrocytes may be present in, for example, invasive *E. histolytica* infection.
- Macrophages, which possess a large nucleus compared with *E. histolytica* trophozoites, may be present in colonic amoebiasis.
- Polymorphonuclear leucocytes are present in bacillary dysentery; these are scanty in *E. histolytica* dysentery.
- Epithelial cells can sometimes be visualized in a faecal sample, and frequently in material obtained at sigmoidoscopy.

24
ETHICAL ISSUES IN MEDICINE

INTRODUCTION

Successful medical practice requires a relationship of trust between doctor and patient. Although in family practice this relationship may be built up over several years, in hospital practice and in an emergency it is frequently the case that the patient and the doctor are meeting for the first time. A strict code of behaviour on the part of the doctor is therefore required in order to set the scene for a trusting relationship. The code of medical ethics provides a suitable framework defining this relationship in professional, social and legal contexts. Patients expect a high standard of care when they seek help. This includes the expectation that:

● They will be consulted about decisions bearing on their treatment
● They will be informed about their illness
● They will be informed about the likely outcome of any treatment offered
● Their right to confidentiality will be respected.

The capacity of a patient to take part in clinical decisions should never be underestimated. Always assume that a patient is able fully to understand the nature of the medical problem, and its implications, whatever their educational level. Very often, it will be up to the doctor to introduce this topic at a suit-able moment in the consultation. Some patients like to discuss the limits of what they would like to know early in a consultation, and many will define clearly the appropriate limits for dissemination of information to the family. These wishes must be respected.

Other influences in considering how and what to tell a patient are often brought to bear during diagnosis and treatment. The family may feel that the patient would not be able to comprehend medical information, or that this information will be too terrible a burden for the patient to bear. Patients may make it clear that they do not wish the family to know about their medical problems or, sometimes, that they themselves do not wish to know the diagnosis. In all such instances, the needs and rights of each individual patient should be taken as paramount. Should there be any conflict in the relationships, the patient's interests are, first and foremost, always more important than those of the family. Fortunately such conflicts of interest are very rare, and are often more apparent than real. With discussion they can usually be resolved.

HISTORICAL ASPECTS

In ancient Egypt rules of conduct for physicians included adherence to established methods of treatment. Later, the Code of Hammurabi formalized scales of payment for medical services, including penalties for negligence. In ancient Greece the Hippocratic Oath, a code of medical behaviour that underlies all modern clinical practice, required proper instruction of physicians, recognized that the physician's duty was to his patient—a duty that included an injunction to do no harm—and proscribed euthanasia and abortion, together with certain other risky or unacceptable procedures, such as lithotomy or castration. In addition, this Oath recognized the special nature of the doctor–patient relationship, and stressed that this relationship should not be abused. In both the Christian and Muslim worlds the influence of Judaism in medical ethics has been strong, particularly in clarifying the responsibilities of individuals in relation to groups, as in the case of isolation of patients with serious infective conditions. This is an example of a special policy which puts the needs of the group temporarily on a level with those of the individual patient. Similar attitudes prevail in other religious environments.

AUTONOMY

The fundamental principle underlying the concept of a medical ethic is that of the autonomy of the patient. This means that the patient has the right to decide his or her own medical destiny; the physician may advise, but the patient decides. It is unacceptable for one individual—including the physician and relatives—to attempt to exert unconstrained power over the fate of another individual. Upon this notion rests the concept of seeking consent for medical interventions, for research, and for teaching from the patient. Only in the case of a minor or a mentally disturbed person, may consent be sought from the patient's lawful parents or guardians. Assent, but not consent, may be sought from relatives, for example, in the case of an unconscious patient in an intensive care unit. The physician or surgeon, therefore, has a duty not only to advise, but also to explain.

The origin of this medical ethic antedates the Christian era, and is common to Judaism, and to the Muslim world, in addition to all countries whose governance has been influenced by Christianity. It can thus be separated from any apparent religious background, itself an important aspect of the universality of the concept of a medical ethic.

CONSENT

As a general rule the patient's consent should be sought to any treatment, however minor. In many instances consent is implied, as when a patient presents to a doctor with an injury and asks for treatment. In other circumstances, a minor symptom may lead to the discovery of a serious illness requiring complex investigation and treatment. In this example consent will be required for each stage of the investigation and treatment as part of the unfolding of the diagnosis and the management proposed.

For a patient to give consent sufficient accurate information about the illness must be given to enable the patient to decide whether the proposed treatment is, generally, both acceptable and in their own interests. There are four requirements on the doctor discussing an intervention with a patient:

1. The procedure itself must be described, including the technique and its implications.
2. Information about the risks and complications must be given.
3. Associated risks (e.g. from anaesthesia or from other drugs that may be necessary) should be described.
4. Alternative medical or surgical investigations or treatments should be discussed, so that the reasons for the specific advice given are clear. In addition, the implications of the 'do nothing' option should be discussed.

THE PROCEDURE FOR OBTAINING CONSENT

The amount of information divulged will vary according to the context of the discussion and according to the needs of the patient as they emerge in the consultation. For example, an operation on the knee of a sportsman has far greater implications than the same operation in the case of a sedentary office worker. It is not appropriate to burden the patient with a textbook approach to medical knowledge. The objective is not to place the patient in the situation of having to decide between conflicting medical data, but to explain why the advice given as to the mode of management recommended is regarded as the best in the circumstances. It may happen, of course, that during discussion other factors come to light that result in the advice being altered. Clearly, this should be accepted as a happy outcome since it implies agreement as to the best course.

SETTING THE SCENE

Discussions regarding consent for investigation and treatment are emotionally charged for the patient and often, also, for the doctor. Therefore, try to arrange a suitably quiet and pleasant environment for the discussion, one that is free of interruptions and away from unnecessary observers, such as other patients or unfamiliar nurses or students. Make time for the discussion—*never* appear rushed. Use simple language that the patient can understand. Be patient. If necessary, and with the patient's permission, involve relatives. If there is likely to be a language problem, make sure that an interpreter is available.

At the end of the discussion check that the patient has actually understood. If there is any doubt, be prepared to have a further discussion; it is often better, in the case of really serious news, to have a discussion about management on several occasions, even after the treatment schedule has commenced.

IMPLICATIONS OF CONSENT OR REFUSAL

In the event that the patient declines the investigation or treatment recommended, remember that not only is this the patient's right but also that the objective of the process of discussion is to allow the patient to understand the management proposed and to come to a decision as to whether or not to proceed with it. Therefore, refusal is *not* a signal for the doctor to disengage from management of the patient but, rather, to continue to provide care to as high a level as is possible within the limits of what has been agreed and, if necessary, to continue discussion about future management.

If explicit consent is given, the patient and doctor should both sign an appropriate Consent Form. This procedure should be followed for all serious interventions. In hospital this Consent Form will be a standardized form, and a similar form should be used in family or private practice to verify that the discussion took place. The mere act of both parties signing the form does not constitute proof that consent has been lawfully given. It simply documents that a discussion occurred without describing the context, or giving details of the information described. Generally, however, it will be taken to mean that consent was obtained. It is wise, therefore, to make a separate, contemporaneous note describing what was discussed.

LEGAL REQUIREMENTS FOR CONSENT

There are three aspects of consent that are required in law:

1. The patient must be mentally and legally competent to give consent
2. The patient must have been sufficiently well informed to be able to give consent
3. Consent must have been given voluntarily, and not under duress.

COMPETENCE FOR CONSENT

Competence is difficult to define. The patient must be able to understand the discussion. If there is doubt as to the patient's competence to give consent, consent should be obtained not only from the patient but also from a responsible relative. If necessary, enlist help from senior nursing staff, or even from a psychiatrist.

Special difficulties arise with consent and the unconscious patient. If treatment is necessary in order to save life, treatment can and must be given without waiting for consent. If relatives are available, they should be consulted, but their wishes are not necessarily paramount in the decision to initiate life-saving therapy. In the UK no adult can act as a proxy for another. The relatives may thus assent to treatment, but cannot legally consent to it. This limitation also means that relatives cannot legally refuse treatment that is medically in the best interests of the patient, although a conflict of this kind should be reason to consider, carefully and in detail with the relatives, the reasons for disagreement. In some countries relatives can be given powers of guardianship that allow them to give consent for the adult person for whom they act as guardian.

Consent for the treatment of children is a matter that must be considered with care. In the UK treatment of a minor (i.e. someone under the age of 16 years) can be given without parental consent, provided that care has been taken to make sure that the child understands the nature of the treatment proposed and its possible risks, adverse effects and consequences. However, this should be a most exceptional decision. In practice, the parents' agreement should almost always be sought. An obvious exception would be in an emergency, for example after a life-threatening head injury, or when non-accidental injury is suspected. Difficult decisions sometimes arise; for example, when the prescription of contraceptive drugs to a young girl is requested in circumstances where the young person does not wish her parents to know.

APPROPRIATELY INFORMED

The point at which a patient can be considered to be appropriately informed is a matter of judgement. Some patients make it clear that they do not wish long and involved discussion, but others are comfortable with the process only when very full explanations have been given. It is often necessary to strike a balance. It is easy to frighten a patient to such an extent by recitation of unwelcome, but rare, possible complications of a procedure that they refuse treatment. This should not be the objective of discussing treatment. If a procedure is so risky that the doctor feels it is not justified, i.e. it is futile, the patient should be advised accordingly rather than being asked to decide for themselves.

NOT UNDER DURESS

That consent was given without duress should be self-evident both to the patient and to the doctor. If necessary, the patient should be given the opportunity to consider the decision after the initial discussion. The personal, religious and social beliefs of the doctor must not be allowed to intrude. If this is likely, for example in the case of a doctor required to advise on therapeutic abortion whose religious beliefs forbid this procedure, another doctor should be asked to take over the care of the patient. Remember that duress can arise unexpectedly. A patient may feel that he or she must embark on treatment in order to prevent stress at home. The right course here is to explore the nature of this stressful situation and take steps to alleviate it, in addition to considering medical treatment. Duress may be financial. There must be no financial advantage, constituting bribery or inducement, either to the patient or to the doctor in the management proposed. Political or social duress is an issue that has confronted physicians in many parts of the world in their relations with their patients, and constitutes a particularly difficult problem for an individual to resolve. It is clearly unethical.

CONSENT FOR RESEARCH

Similar rules of conduct apply to the obtaining of consent for research as for a patient's entry into a clinical trial of a new drug and for teaching. It should be a condition of all research that the question addressed is relevant, and the protocol is capable of answering the question proposed. These are matters that are the special concern of the clinical investigators and they should have been thoroughly checked by the Research Ethics Committee (see below).

CONFIDENTIALITY

All aspects of the medical consultation are confidential. This common law duty is recognized by the public and is an essential part of the background to the consultation, since it allows the patient freedom of expression in the knowledge that disclosures made within the confines of the consulting room will not be made available to others. Indeed, in some aspects of medical practice, especially in treating sexually-transmitted diseases, and in much of psychiatric practice, confidentiality is fundamental.

The principle of confidentiality applies also to the medical records. These are held by the doctor or the group practice or, in the case of hospital records, by the hospital itself. Hospital records are not available to anyone other than the medical and nursing staff treating the patient, and are immune from police powers of search. They are made available, however, with the permission of the patient, and, once disclosed, can be used in evidence in court in both civil and criminal cases. Patients have the right to inspect their own medical records after seeking access in writing. The principle of confidentiality of medical information was recognized by Hippocrates, and has been affirmed subsequently, in modern times, for example, in the Declaration of Geneva of 1968. Although, in the modern hospital, medical information is far more widely available to a number of different health professionals and administrators, the principle of confidentiality of the record must be

strictly followed. In the UK, it is rigorously supported by the General Medical Council and its breach is regarded as a serious matter. In certain other European countries, for example in France, medical confidentiality is protected by the criminal code.

The situations in which confidentiality can be relaxed include:

- When the patient or his or her legal adviser allows it
- When it is in the patient's interests
- If there is an overriding duty to society as a whole
- In cases of statutory disclosure
- In certain situations where inspection of medical records is allowed
- Sometimes after death.

WITH PERMISSION

A common example of relaxation of confidentiality with the patient's permission is when a doctor discusses the patient's problems or takes a history with others present (e.g. medical students or a nurse). The patient should be given the opportunity to ask that others leave.

IN THE PATIENT'S INTERESTS

When it is necessary that another family member be informed about the nature of a patient's illness, for example, in order to obtain information essential for effective treatment, it may be judged in the patient's best interests to break confidentiality. Another example might arise if a patient was judged mentally incompetent and it became necessary to involve the patient's legal adviser to handle the patient's financial and legal affairs during a severe illness. This generally requires permission from a court.

AN OVERRIDING DUTY TO SOCIETY

Occasionally confidentiality may be relaxed in the context of a known or possibly pending violent crime. In the case of an illness such as epilepsy or coronary heart disease that might impair the ability to control a vehicle, the responsibility to inform the authorities rests with the patient. In this instance, it is generally thought that it is in the interests of society to encourage voluntary disclosure, thus maintaining the principle of confidentiality between doctor and patient. The clinician does have discretion, however, to break this principle of confidentiality in circumstances entailing serious public risk.

STATUTORY DISCLOSURE

Confidentiality is breached in the case of certain infectious diseases, such as tuberculosis, that are statutorily notifiable to the public health authorities.

There is also a statutory duty for a doctor to help in the identification of a driver involved in a road traffic accident who, for example, might have attended a surgery or casualty department after the accident. The doctor in the witness box is in a state of privilege, and is protected against any action for breach of confidentiality when instructed by a court to disclose potentially confidential information. Similarly, a court can ask that medical documents be released to it if they are regarded as necessary for the completion of a fair trial of an accused person.

INSPECTION OF MEDICAL RECORDS

In the UK the case notes themselves belong to the hospital or the health authority, and not to the patient or the doctor. Private patient notes belong to the doctor concerned. Patients themselves have a lawful right to inspect their own medical records, and can see any medical reports concerning their own medical condition that have been prepared before they are released to another party. Such medical reports can only be prepared with the permission of the patient or at the request of a statutory body, as in the context of an order under the Mental Health Act, or in the jurisdiction of a recognized court. Generally, persons other than the patient have no right to inspect the medical records of an individual unless permission is given in writing by the patient, or the records are subject to a subpoena from a recognized court. The inspection of medical records for epidemiological purposes and for medical audit is currently allowed, since these activities are clearly necessary, but there is a need for distinct guidelines to be established relating to these activities in order to protect confidentiality.

This right of access by the patient clearly makes it important to write in the records only statements that can later be justified or defended. Value judgements about a patient are not matters for comment in medical records.

AFTER DEATH

Generally the principle of confidentiality should extend to patients who have died. In the cases of a number of deceased public figures of recent years (e.g. Winston Churchill and John F. Kennedy) this principle was not adhered to on the grounds that there were matters of public interest involved. Whether this was really the case the reader can decide.

ORGAN DONATION

When a tissue that can be replaced by the donor's own tissues, such as blood or bone marrow, is given to another patient, no special ethical problem arises. When a living donor gives an irreplaceable organ, such as a kidney, difficulties arise. The donor must be of sound mind, not under duress, and must not be placed in a position to gain financially by the gift. In other words, the ordinary principles of consent apply. The sale of organs for transplantation is forbidden in all developed countries, and is rapidly becoming illegal in all countries. Similar considerations apply to the acquisition of donor organs from a minor, a practice about which it is particularly difficult to issue sound guidelines.

Because deceased persons have only limited rights over their organs, statutes have been introduced to regulate the practice of cadaver organ donation. This regulation is still evolving, and varies from country to country. In general, in the UK an organ can be removed from a deceased person if it is known that this was the wish of that person in life, whether for purposes of therapy, research or education, provided that the next of kin agrees. An organ can also be removed with the authorization of the next of kin, without knowledge of the deceased's wishes. However, this requirement has generally not led to the easy acquisition of organs such as kidneys for transplantation in the UK, since the next of kin are often distressed during the crucial and short period when it is possible to use cadaver organs for successful transplantation. In addition, the next of kin are often concerned to follow the supposed wishes of the deceased, or to contact other relatives for a decision and, by the time a decision is made it is too late. In some of the countries of the European Union there is a presumption that a deceased person would have wished to donate organs in the absence of any explicit statement to the contrary. However, this attitude is not general and it seems unlikely that it will become so, since clinicians are unlikely to take organs if they believe that this will cause distress among relatives. Voluntary schemes requiring a decision to consent to organ donation after death are generally preferred in most countries, even though there is a shortage of suitable organs for transplantation.

Certain religious constraints should be remembered. People of the Muslim faith are forbidden to accept organ donations from animals other than humans, and will not accept porcine products, for example pig valve grafts. However, porcine insulin is acceptable, since it consists of a product of the animal and not part of the organs of the animal. Donations of organs from a living patient, for example the gift of a kidney from a relative, may be subject to the agreement of two wise men from the community, in addition to the usual ethical procedures required by any hospital in the Western world.

ABORTION AND THE RIGHTS OF THE FETUS

The passage of the Abortion Act in the UK in 1967 marked a change in society's attitudes and, broadly, an acceptance by the medical profession of this change, illustrating that concepts of what is ethically acceptable change. Nonetheless, there are still those who for religious or other reasons find the legality of abortion unacceptable. Abortion was forbidden in the Oath of Hippocrates.

Much of the current controversy concerns definition of the age of fetal viability. This has become a particular issue since fetal tissues have begun to be used in the treatment of certain diseases, and perhaps as a source of stem cells for organ growth and the production of neural and other cells for transplantation. Fetal viability is partly determined by medical science, and medical skill in keeping small premature babies alive, and partly by biological factors. If the age of viability becomes a matter for legal definition by statute, it must be recognized that this statute will need to change with advances in medical science. There is a long-standing difficulty in resolving the logical description of the appropriate medical behaviour when the rights of an unborn fetus are seen as in conflict with those of the mother herself.

The issue of fetal viability, therefore, differs from the more philosophical issue of definition of the stage in development at which the fetus becomes a person, imbued with human characteristics and subject to the same ethical considerations as a child or an adult. This issue can be resolved on religious grounds, by defining, as does the Roman Catholic Church, the onset of human life as the moment of conception, or by recognizing the onset of fetal movement, or the external recognition of pregnancy. A simpler definition is that the fetus is invested with human status at the moment that independent existence begins, i.e. after birth. This approach, however, denies the fetus the ordinary ethical considerations of the right to life, or the protection from deliberate or negligent harm, that are accorded to persons, and therefore is likely to be rejected by many thoughtful observers. Because of the dependence of the fetus on its mother, the rights of the fetus are inevitably bound up with those of the pregnant woman.

In recent years there has been an emphasis on the rights of the fetus as a person-in-embryo. It is averred that the fetus has the same rights in common law and in society as a competent adult. In this approach the issue of medical viability becomes of less relevance, since the fetus has rights whether or not it is medically viable.

RESUSCITATION

Resuscitation is generally available in hospitals in the event that cardiopulmonary arrest occurs unexpectedly. However, this is not always successful, and many patients, recognizing the terminal nature of their illness, may request that resuscitation not be attempted. This is an entirely valid request which should be respected once it is clear that the options are clearly understood by the patient.

NOT FOR RESUSCITATION

It sometimes happens that a patient is so seriously ill that there is doubt among medical and nursing attendants that it would be appropriate to resuscitate them in the event that they suffered a cardiac arrest. It should be recognized at the outset that this implies a judgement on the part of those charged with the responsibility of caring for the patient that, in some way, the patient's life is not worth saving. It should be asked whether any physician or surgeon is ever in a position to make such a judgement. Many would think that this is not a matter that one human should decide about another.

However, the question of whether or not resuscitation is to be attempted arises in clinical practice with increasing frequency, as medical technology becomes more complex and more effective, thus prolonging life into situations that would not occur but for the efforts of medical science. The situation most frequently arises when a patient has terminal cancer, and one of the medical or nursing team asks whether the 'crash team' should be called in the event the patient undergoes circulatory or ventilatory collapse. Resuscitation for a few hours or days of further pain and discomfort might be regarded as an unnecessary prolongation of the terminal illness.

The decision to withhold resuscitation is a matter for which it is proper always to seek the patient's full, informed consent. Indeed, the patient's views are paramount, and should be respected whatever the views of the clinicians, nurses or even the relatives. Relatives have no legal rights in a decision about possible resuscitation of another individual. While they may be consulted, and their views noted, they should not be allowed to influence a decision once made by an individual patient, unless it is decided that the patient is not competent by reason of dementia, or some other impairment of judgement, to come to a decision. Overt depression, for example, might be a reason for not accepting a patient's expressed wish not to be resuscitated.

Although it might be thought not helpful to a patient to discuss this issue openly, in fact the reverse is usually the case. Most patients near to death are aware of their situation and welcome the opportunity for full discussion of the issues. Indeed, it may give them the opportunity to discuss matters with their family in a more open manner than would otherwise be possible. The agreement of the patient and medical staff should be signed in the case record; most hospitals now use a formal protocol in documenting this procedure.

As a general matter of policy it is wise to involve the most senior clinician concerned with the patient's care in discussions about 'do not resuscitate' orders. Many large hospitals have a resuscitation officer, part of whose duties it is to review clinical decisions about resuscitation, since the resuscitation resource needs to be applied uniformly across the hospital, and not be more available to some patients than to others. In many hospitals policies for resuscitation and for withholding resuscitation, in consideration of the issues outlined above, have been agreed by medical and nursing staff. These should be sufficiently flexible to allow change with evolving medical technologies, and with increasing levels of knowledge and involvement of the general public in such issues. It should always be the case, of course, that a patient should be resuscitated when cardiopulmonary collapse is unexpected and the patient's wishes are unknown.

CONSENT FOR AUTOPSY

It is nowadays necessary to be explicit in asking for consent for autopsy. As part of the autopsy, tissue samples will be taken and examined, and some may be retained for future use. If this is intended, or is likely to occur, permission to retain the samples must be obtained as part of the consent for autopsy. This process of consent implies that the family will be give some idea of what studies might be undertaken, in the future, on the retained samples. It may be considered appropriate to consider whether any circumstances might develop in which the family might reasonably expect to be informed of the results of any such studies. For example, if information of a predictive or genetic nature were to be obtained in relation to the risk of vascular disease, or of specific cancers, then the family might wish to know of this. This concept of extended consent involving future actions is as yet still developing. However, it is of considerable importance in the future of pathological research, not only on autopsies, but also in the context of biopsies and blood samples obtained during ordinary medical practice.

ETHICS COMMITTEES

There are two kinds of ethics committees—the *Clinical Ethics Comittee* and the *Research Ethics Committee*.

The Research Ethics Committee in the UK is concerned only with research. It will ascertain that proper arrangements exist for safeguarding the patient's interests at all times, especially with regard to consent and to the recognition of any possible risks associated with a research protocol. Confidentiality must be maintained, and this must include the security of any computer-held records.

Research involving human subjects, whether patients or normal subjects, generated by medical staff, medical students, nurses and other paramedical staff is all properly within the remit of the Research Ethics Committee. No research is ethical that is not scientifically valid. Particular care is required in considering research in the intensive care unit and in paediatric practice, because of the difficulties of ensuring that consent can adequately be established and the level of dependence of the patients.

It is the role of the Research Ethics Committee to be impartial and authoritative. Research Ethics Committees in the UK are locally organized and independent of local hospitals. The Research Ethics Committee functions as an autonomous committee of the health authority (the local component of the Department of Health). It consists of lay members, experienced medical and nursing researchers, and other relevant professionals who understand the wide variety of ethical and legal problems that can arise in research proposals involving human subjects. Research Ethics Committees insist that records related to research should be maintained in a state such that they are available to scrutiny by others for some years after the conclusion of the research, as part of the effort to prevent fraud in research. Adequate safeguards, and agreements for restitution for any harm inadvertently caused to a patient during participation in an approved research protocol, must be in place in the institution concerned. This will often involve an agreement with a sponsoring pharmaceutical company or other responsible organization. There are European and American guidelines and arrangements in force that cover these eventualities; these must be adhered to as appropriate for the country concerned.

Review of a research protocol by the established local Research Ethics Committee is a requirement of the process of permission to commence a research protocol in Europe, and is a federal legal requirement in the USA. Indeed, the results of any research not complying with these requirements is not acceptable to the new products licensing bodies in these two parts of the world. Similar rules pertain in many other countries.

The Clinical Ethics Committee is concerned with practical clinical matters. It may be asked to consider the ethics of the application of scarce resources, for example in the selection of people for organ transplantation, the process of consent for 'do not resuscitate' decisions, decisions related to in vitro fertilization, and other matters arising in clinical practice in a hospital. This committee is constituted to be representative of staff and of patients' interests and, like the Research Ethics Committee, will have lay membership as well as professional medical and nursing membership.

VOLUNTEERS IN RESEARCH

Particularly stringent rules relate to the selection of volunteers for research who are not themselves patients. Volunteers—like patients and the investigators themselves—should not accept inducements to take part in research. Indeed, such inducements should not in any way form part of a research protocol, except insofar as provision is made to cover incidental expenses and inconvenience. Any financial interest that the investigator or the employing department may have must be clearly acknowledged. Some agreed process of compensation for patients or volunteers in research programmes to whom harm is done, whether inadvertently or as a result of negligence, is a requirement for acceptance by the Research Ethics Committee. This usually involves the need for some form of insurance.

OTHER ETHICAL PROBLEMS

There are several other problems that arise in medical practice, several of which are likely to become more important in the coming years.

MEDICAL NEGLIGENCE

Actions against doctors in the courts alleging medical negligence have become more common in many Western countries in recent years. Medical accidents, meaning inadvertent adverse events, are frequent in clinical practice, perhaps occurring in as many as 4% of all medical interventions. Few of these result in any legal action. An accusation of negligence often implies that a doctor–patient relationship has broken down. For the doctor such an action is distressing and sometimes professionally damaging even when shown to be unjustified.

In considering whether there has been negligence it is necessary to establish *causation, harm and breach of professional duty*. Breach of the responsibility of professional duty or care is addressed by asking whether the standard of care afforded the patient fell below that expected. The standard of care expected is that of the ordinary skilled practitioner in the field of expertise in question, practising in the circumstances pertaining. It is not that of the greatest expert in the land. Thus, in assessing possible negligence a court will need to establish:

- What the ordinary practice is
- That the doctor did not follow this practice
- That the doctor undertook a course of clinical management that no ordinarily skilled doctor in that specialty would have undertaken if acting with ordinary care.

A mistake in diagnosis is not necessarily negligent, and the test of the standard of care applicable to the ordinary practitioner in the specialty will be applied by the court in considering this. In the UK this is termed the Bolam test, after a particular case that led to the enunciation of the principle.

Doctors are expected to keep up to date in their expertise, and this is an aspect that is relevant to this judgement. Doctors in training are expected, by and large, to exercise an appropriate standard of care, and no patient should expect a lower standard of care simply because they are cared for by a junior doctor of less experience. This would clearly be wrong. It is imperative, therefore, that in treating a patient advice and help should be sought at all relevant times from senior colleagues.

RESOURCE ALLOCATION

In every country, even the richest, there is a limitation on the availability of medical resources. The distribution of this resource is decided in different ways. In some countries it is decided by the capacity of any individual to pay for private medical care. In others it is made available more generally but to a level decided by the limits of the resource devoted to it by a benevolent, or otherwise, government. The doctor, therefore, is often confronted by a limitation on the capacity to offer a treatment, for one or other of a number of possible reasons.

Since the doctor's responsibility is always first to his or her patient, as an individual, and not to that group of potential patients in the general population who have not yet presented for treatment, this potential limitation of resource is relevant only in the general context of the politics of resource allocation for medicine. The individual patient's rights and the doctor's responsibilities in this matter are clear. The duty to the individual must always take precedence, and every effort must always be made to treat each patient to the best of the doctor's ability and in the best interests of the patient, utilizing such resources as are available, from whatever source.

Notwithstanding this duty of care to the individual patient, the doctor does have a duty to society to improve treatments whenever possible, and to make as widely available as possible treatments to those that will benefit from them. Currently, much effort is being expended in trying to establish methods for measurement of benefit in relation to treatments, in order that resource allocation decisions, themselves a problem in medical economics rather than in medical ethics, can more rationally be formulated.

HIV

Testing for HIV requires the consent of the patient or individual. It is usual to counsel the individual before testing, since there are implications for lifestyle, future health, and even employment hinging on the result of the test. Life insurance companies usually require HIV testing only for large insured liabilities.

GENETICS

The rapidly evolving availability of relatively accurate genetic testing for susceptibility to inherited diseases, based on the modern understanding of DNA and the genetic code, has raised a number of ethical problems for which most societies are not well prepared. For example:

- Who should have genetic tests done?
- What should be done with the results?
- Who—if anyone—should have access to the information, other than the patient?
- How should expensive treatments that may be possible for genetically determined disorders be made available?
- Is it socially and economically appropriate to prevent these disorders?

The application of genetic information to medical practice is the major area of change at present. It can be expected to have profound implications for the management of most aspects of disease, and for the ways in which all societies view the acquisition and availability of medical information.

GENETIC COUNSELLING

Genetic counselling is relatively long-established. The clinical geneticist will usually be asked to assess the risks of genetically determined disease in the context of a known familial occurrence of a disease, for example Down's syndrome, Duchenne muscular dystrophy or cystic fibrosis. There is knowledge about the genetic causation of each of these conditions, and certain tests with probabilities of accuracy are available in assessing the risk for individuals in a family, and for the risk that a planned pregnancy might result in an affected offspring. Major difficulties arise in deciding whether to inform someone who has been shown by genetic testing to be certain to develop a disease in later life, for example Huntington's disease. Such decisions should ideally be made before testing is undertaken at all. Even when offering counselling about the risks for planned pregnancies similar difficulties arise. The social costs in terms of unresolved problems to individuals and their families of offering treatment or prevention for genetic disorders are largely undetermined at this time. Practice in this context will change as knowledge and experience accumulate.

LIFE INSURANCE AND GENETIC INFORMATION

There has been concern about the implications of genetic knowledge for life insurance, a problem that is similar to that related to occult HIV infection. The knowledgeable, affected person might obtain insurance knowing of their own risk, thus selecting against the insurance company. Life insurance is a business, and not a form of social security. Clearly it is in the best interests of the insurance company, which has a responsibility towards all its insured clients, to have knowledge of all relevant medical problems affecting a client in order that an appropriate risk can be assigned to an individual policy. However, this concept may need adjustment in the light of the new genetics. It remains the case, of course, that information about an individual should never be divulged to an insurance company, or to any other organization, without the written permission of the individual, and only after the implications have been discussed with the person.

PRINCIPLES OF MEDICAL ETHICS

Several modern attempts have been made to encapsulate the principles of ethical medical behaviour in a series of simple statements. The *Declaration of Geneva* (Box 24.1) represents a modern attempt to restate the Hippocratic Oath in terms acceptable to contemporary students and medical practitioners. *The International Code of Medical Ethics* (Box 24.2) was derived from these principles, and restates them in more direct terms. The *Declaration of Helsinki* (1975) sets out recommendations for the guidance of doctors wishing to undertake biomedical research involving human subjects. The recommendations of the Declaration of Helsinki are generally recognized as relevant to the design of research protocols.

BOX 24.1   Declaration of Geneva propounded by the World Medical Association, in Sydney (1968).

On admittance to the medical profession:

1. I will solemnly pledge myself to consecrate my life to the service of humanity
2. I will give my teachers the respect and gratitude which is their due
3. I will practise my profession with conscience and dignity
4. The health of my patients will be my first consideration
5. I will respect secrets that have been confided in me, even after the patient has died
6. I will maintain by all the means in my power the honour and noble traditions of the medical profession
7. My colleagues will be my brothers
8. I will not permit considerations of religion, nationality, race, party politics or social standing to intervene between my duty and my patient
9. I will maintain the utmost respect for human life from the time of conception. Even under threat I will not use my medical knowledge contrary to the laws of humanity
10. I make these promises solemnly, freely and upon my honour.

The problems raised by the interaction of modern medical practice with government and with society as a whole are important, and will require much thought and analysis in the future. This chapter cannot pretend to raise all the issues, but should be taken as an introduction to what should be a daily consideration, both in learning about, and in practising, medicine.

BOX 24.2   International Code of Medical Ethics.

Duties of doctors in general
- To maintain the highest standards of professional conduct
- To practise uninfluenced by motives of profit
- To use caution in divulging discoveries or new techniques of treatment
- To certify or testify only those matters with which the doctor has personal experience
- To ensure that any act or advice that could weaken physical or mental resistance of an individual must be used only in the interest of that individual.

The following are unethical practices
- Any self-advertisement except as expressly authorized in a national code of ethics

---

BOX 24.2   (contd)

- Collaboration in any form of medical service in which the doctor does not have professional independence
- Receipt of any money in connection with services rendered to a patient other than a proper professional fee, even if the patient is aware of it.

Duties of doctors to the sick
- There is an obligation to preserve life
- The patient is owed complete loyalty, and all the resources of medical science. Whenever a treatment or examination is beyond the capacity of the doctor, the advice of another doctor should be sought
- A doctor must always preserve absolute secrecy concerning all he knows about a patient, because of the confidence trusted in him
- Emergency care is a humanitarian duty which must be given, unless it is clear that there are others better able to give it.

Duties of doctors to each other
- A doctor must behave to his colleagues as he would have them behave toward him
- A doctor must not entice patients from his colleagues
- A doctor must observe the principles of the Declaration of Geneva.

I
A GUIDE TO REFERENCE RANGES USED IN PATHOLOGY

The term 'normal ranges', which has frequently been used in the past, is roughly equivalent in meaning to 'reference values obtained from healthy individuals'. The concept of reference ranges was introduced to avoid the ambiguities inherent in the term 'normal values'. It was purposely introduced as a vague term to force us to define in each case what is actually meant. Reference values are results of a certain type of quantity obtained from a single individual, or group of individuals, corresponding to a stated description. A reference individual is defined as 'an individual selected for comparison using defined criteria', and a reference value as 'a value obtained by observation or measurement of a particular type of quantity on a reference individual'.

The values given in Tables 1 and 2 relate (unless otherwise stated) to the adult ranges used by the laboratories in the Royal London Hospital and St Bartholomew's Hospital. Values obtained in infants and children often differ greatly from those seen in adults; additionally, a number of results are gender specific, and in each case the local laboratory should publish relevant information. If in doubt, advice should be sought from the laboratory.

It is also important to recognize that different laboratories may quote markedly different reference ranges, depending on the method they use. The main differences in results will generally be seen with enzyme and hormone assays; interpretation of results must always be performed using the local reference ranges. Staff in the local laboratory are always available to give information and advice on the tests offered by their own laboratory. It is also useful to ask for assay imprecisions as these are important in assessing a true change in the results for a particular patient.

The ranges given in the tables are expressed in the *Système International d'Unités* (SI units), a system which has been accepted internationally since 1960. SI units are used in most recent publications, although you may also find values in older works in 'traditional units'. For this reason some of the analytes in the tables are also expressed in traditional units.

Reference ranges in clinical biochemistry

APPENDIX I, TABLE 1.1   Clinical biochemistry adult reference ranges.

Tests	Reference range	SI units	Reference range	Traditional units
Serum				
Adrenocorticotrophic hormone (ACTH)—09.00hrs	10–50	ng/L	10–50	pg/mL
Adrenocorticotrophic hormone (ACTH)—24.00hrs	<10	ng/L	<10	pg/mL
Alanine aminotransferase (ALT)	<40	U/L		
Albumin	35–50	g/L	3.5–5.0	g/dL
Aldosterone—lying	135–400	pmol/L	4.9–14.4	ng/dL
Aldosterone—standing	330–830	pmol/L		ng/dL
Alkaline phosphatase (ALP)	39–117	U/L		
Alpha-1-antitrypsin	1.1–2.1	g/L	110–410	mg/dL
Alpha fetoprotein—non-pregnant	<10	U/L		
Aluminium	<0.4	μmol/L	<11	μg/L
Ammonia	<45	μmol/L	<77	μg/dL
Amylase	25–125	U/L		
Androstenedione	3–8	nmol/L	0.9–2.3	μg/L
Androstenedione—pre-pubertal	<1.0	nmol/L	<0.3	μg/L
Angiotensin converting enzyme (ACE)	10–70	U/L		
Aspartate aminotransferase (AST)	12–39	U/L		
Beta-2-microglobulin—<60 years	<2.4	mg/L		
Beta-2-microglobulin—>60 years	<3.0	mg/L		

Tests	Reference range	SI units	Reference range	Traditional units
Serum (contd)				
Bicarbonate	22–29	mmol/L	22–29	mEq/L
Bilirubin—total	<17	µmol/L	<1.0	mg/dL
Bilirubin—direct	<4	µmol/L	<0.2	mg/dL
C1 esterase inhibitor	0.15–0.35	g/L	15–35	mg/dL
C1 esterase inhibitor—functional	40–150	U/mL		
C3	0.75–1.65	g/L	75–165	mg/dL
C4	0.20–0.50	g/L	20–50	mg/dL
C reactive protein	<10	mg/L		
CA 125	<37	µ/mL		
CA 15-3	<30	kU/L		
CA 19-9	<37	kU/L		
Caeruloplasmin	0.20–0.45	g/L	20–45	mg/dL
Calcitonin	<0.08	µg/L	<80	pg/mL
Calcium	2.15–2.65	mmol/L		mg/dL
Carbamazepine	4–12	mg/L		
Carcinoembrionic antigen (CEA)	<5	µg/L	<5	ng/mL
Catecholamines—noradrenaline	<4.14	nmol/L		
Catecholamines—adrenaline	<1.31	nmol/L		
Chloride	98–106	mmol/L	98–106	mEq/L
Cholesterol—recommended	<5.2	mmol/L	<200	mg/dL
Cholesterol—population range	3.5–6.7	mmol/L	135–259	mg/dL
Cholesterol (HDL)—male	0.8–1.8	mmol/L	3.0–70	mg/dL
Cholesterol (HDL)—female	1.0–2.3	mmol/L	39–90	mg/dL
Copper	11–20	µmol/L	70–127	ug/dL
Cortisol—midnight	<50	nmol/L	<18	ug/dL
Cortisol—09.00hrs	200–650	nmol/L	7–24	ug/dL
Creatine kinase (CK)—male	<195	U/L		
Creatine kinase (CK)—female	<170	U/L		
CK MB	<25	U/L		
Creatinine—male	79–118	µmol/L	0.9–1.3	mg/dL
Creatinine—female	58–93	µmol/L	0.7–1.1	mg/dL
Creatinine clearance—male	95–140	mL/min		
Creatinine clearance—female	85–125	mL/min		
Dehydroepiandrosterone (DHEAS)—male	2.8–12.0	µmol/L	1031–4422	ng/mL
Dehydroepiandrosterone (DHEAS)—female	1.9–9.4	µmol/L	700–3464	ng/mL
Dehydroepiandrosterone (DHEAS)—pre-pubertal	<0.5	µmol/L	<184	ng/mL
11 Deoxycortisol—09.00hrs	26–46	nmol/L	0.9–1.6	ng/mL
Digoxin	1.0–2.0	µg/L		
Dihydrotestosterone (DHT)—male	1.0–2.6	nmol/L		
Dihydrotestosterone (DHT)—female	0.3–0.93	nmol/L		
Ethanol	None detectable	mg/dL		
Ferritin—male	20–260	µg/L	20–260	ng/mL
Ferritin—female	6–110	µg/L	6–110	ng/mL
Follicle stimulating hormone—male	1–10	U/L	1–10	mIU/mL
Follicle stimulating hormone—follicular	1–10	U/L	1–10	mIU/mL
Follicle stimulating hormone—mid-cycle	<50	U/L	<50	mIU/mL
Follicle stimulating hormone—luteal	1–8	U/L	1–8	mIU/mL
Follicle stimulating hormone—post-menopausal	>25	U/L	>25	mIU/mL
Fructosamine	205–285	µmol/L		
Gamma glutamyltransferase (GGT)—male	<58	U/L		
Gamma glutamyltransferase (GGT)—female	<31	U/L		
Gastrin—fasting	<40	pmol/L	<180	pg/mL
Glucose—fasting	3.9–6.1	mmol/L	70–110	mg/dL
Glycated Haemoglobin (HbA1c) (target)	<7	%		

Tests	Reference range	SI units	Reference range	Traditional units
Serum (contd)				
Human chorionic gonadotrophin (HCG)— non-pregnant	<3	IU/L	<3	mIU/mL
Hydroxybutyrate dehydrogenase (HBD)	72–182	U/L		
17-Hydroxyprogesterone—follicular	1.0–10.0	nmol/L	0.3–3.3	µg/L
17-Hydroxyprogesterone—luteal	1.0–20.0	nmol/L	0.3–6.6	µg/L
17-Hydroxyprogesterone—neonatal	<80	nmol/L	<26	µg/L
IGF-1—0–3 years	7–100	µg/L		
IGF-1—4–6 years	14–175	µg/L		
IGF-1—7–9 years	42–210	µg/L		
IGF-1—10–12 years	50–280	µg/L		
IGF-1—13–19 years	70–420	µg/L		
IGF-1—19–49 years	90–310	µg/L		
IGF-1—>50 years	80–220	µg/L		
IGFBP 3—adult	1.0–4.0	mg/L		
Immunoglobulin A	0.8–4.0	g/L	80–400	mg/dL
Immunoglobulin G	5.5–16.5	g/L	550–1650	mg/dL
Immunoglobulin M	0.4–2.0	g/L	40–200	mg/dL
Immunoglobulin E	<110	KU/L	<11	IU/mL
Insulin—fasting	<20	mU/L	<20	µU/mL
Iron—male	11–32	µmol/L	60–180	µg/dL
Iron—female	7–30	µmol/L	40–170	µg/dL
Lactate	0.5–1.3	mmol/L	0.5–1.3	mEq/L
Lactate dehydrogenase	240–480	U/L		
Lithium	0.5–1.0	mmol/L	0.5–1.0	mEq/L
Luteinizing hormone—males	1.0–8.0	U/L	1.0–8.0	mIU/mL
Luteinizing hormone—follicular	1.0–10.0	U/L	1.0–10.0	mIU/mL
Luteinizing hormone—mid-cycle	<75	U/L	<75	mIU/mL
Luteinizing hormone—luteal	1–13	U/L	1–13	mIU/mL
Luteinizing hormone—post-menopausal	>16	U/L	>16	mIU/mL
Magnesium	0.70–1.00	mmol/L	1.4–2.0	mEq/L
Oestradiol—male	<165	pmol/L	<45	pg/mL
Oestradiol—follicular	175–400	pmol/L	50–110	pg/mL
Oestradiol—mid-cycle	400–1200	pmol/L	110–330	pg/mL
Oestradiol—luteal	400–1000	pmol/L	110–272	pg/mL
Oestradiol—post-menopausal	<100	pmol/L	<30	pg/mL
Oestradiol—pre-pubertal	<37	pmol/L	<10	pg/mL
Osmolality	275–295	mOsmol/Kg		
Paracetamol	None detectable	mg/L		
Parathyroid hormone—adult	1.1–6.8	pmol/L		
Parathyroid hormone—2–15 years	1.1–3.6	pmol/L		
Phenobarbitone—adult	15–40	mg/L		
Phenobarbitone—paediatrics	10–25	mg/L		
Phenytoin	5–20	mg/L		
Phosphate	0.8–1.5	mmol/L	2.5–4.6	mg/dL
Potassium	3.5–5.1	mmol/L	3.5–5.1	mEq/L
Progesterone—follicular	>8	nmol/L	<2.5	ng/mL
Progesterone—luteal	>30	nmol/L	>10	ng/mL
Prolactin	<400	mU/L		
Prostatic specific antigen	<2.1	µg/L		
Prostatic specific antigen—>50 years	<4.0	µg/L		
Protein—total	62–77	g/L	6.2–7.7	g/dL
Pyruvate	0.03–0.08	mmol/L	0:26–0.70	mg/dL
Renin—lying	230–1000	pmol/L/hr		
Renin—standing	460–1550	pmol/L/hr		

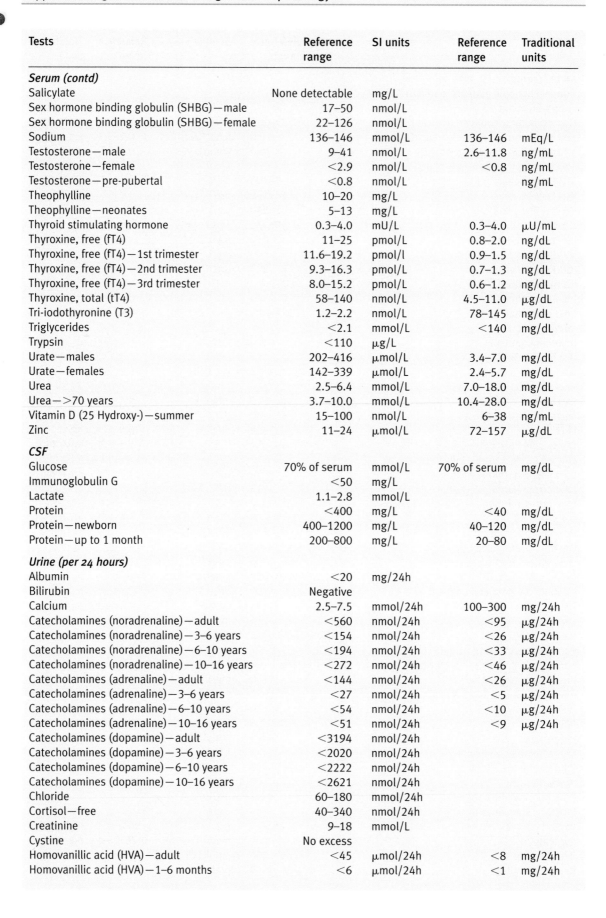

Tests	Reference range	SI units	Reference range	Traditional units
Serum (contd)				
Salicylate	None detectable	mg/L		
Sex hormone binding globulin (SHBG)—male	17–50	nmol/L		
Sex hormone binding globulin (SHBG)—female	22–126	nmol/L		
Sodium	136–146	mmol/L	136–146	mEq/L
Testosterone—male	9–41	nmol/L	2.6–11.8	ng/mL
Testosterone—female	<2.9	nmol/L	<0.8	ng/mL
Testosterone—pre-pubertal	<0.8	nmol/L		ng/mL
Theophylline	10–20	mg/L		
Theophylline—neonates	5–13	mg/L		
Thyroid stimulating hormone	0.3–4.0	mU/L	0.3–4.0	µU/mL
Thyroxine, free (fT4)	11–25	pmol/L	0.8–2.0	ng/dL
Thyroxine, free (fT4)—1st trimester	11.6–19.2	pmol/l	0.9–1.5	ng/dL
Thyroxine, free (fT4)—2nd trimester	9.3–16.3	pmol/L	0.7–1.3	ng/dL
Thyroxine, free (fT4)—3rd trimester	8.0–15.2	pmol/L	0.6–1.2	ng/dL
Thyroxine, total (tT4)	58–140	nmol/L	4.5–11.0	µg/dL
Tri-iodothyronine (T3)	1.2–2.2	nmol/L	78–145	ng/dL
Triglycerides	<2.1	mmol/L	<140	mg/dL
Trypsin	<110	µg/L		
Urate—males	202–416	µmol/L	3.4–7.0	mg/dL
Urate—females	142–339	µmol/L	2.4–5.7	mg/dL
Urea	2.5–6.4	mmol/L	7.0–18.0	mg/dL
Urea—>70 years	3.7–10.0	mmol/L	10.4–28.0	mg/dL
Vitamin D (25 Hydroxy-)—summer	15–100	nmol/L	6–38	ng/mL
Zinc	11–24	µmol/L	72–157	µg/dL
CSF				
Glucose	70% of serum	mmol/L	70% of serum	mg/dL
Immunoglobulin G	<50	mg/L		
Lactate	1.1–2.8	mmol/L		
Protein	<400	mg/L	<40	mg/dL
Protein—newborn	400–1200	mg/L	40–120	mg/dL
Protein—up to 1 month	200–800	mg/L	20–80	mg/dL
Urine (per 24 hours)				
Albumin	<20	mg/24h		
Bilirubin	Negative			
Calcium	2.5–7.5	mmol/24h	100–300	mg/24h
Catecholamines (noradrenaline)—adult	<560	nmol/24h	<95	µg/24h
Catecholamines (noradrenaline)—3–6 years	<154	nmol/24h	<26	µg/24h
Catecholamines (noradrenaline)—6–10 years	<194	nmol/24h	<33	µg/24h
Catecholamines (noradrenaline)—10–16 years	<272	nmol/24h	<46	µg/24h
Catecholamines (adrenaline)—adult	<144	nmol/24h	<26	µg/24h
Catecholamines (adrenaline)—3–6 years	<27	nmol/24h	<5	µg/24h
Catecholamines (adrenaline)—6–10 years	<54	nmol/24h	<10	µg/24h
Catecholamines (adrenaline)—10–16 years	<51	nmol/24h	<9	µg/24h
Catecholamines (dopamine)—adult	<3194	nmol/24h		
Catecholamines (dopamine)—3–6 years	<2020	nmol/24h		
Catecholamines (dopamine)—6–10 years	<2222	nmol/24h		
Catecholamines (dopamine)—10–16 years	<2621	nmol/24h		
Chloride	60–180	mmol/24h		
Cortisol—free	40–340	nmol/24h		
Creatinine	9–18	mmol/L		
Cystine	No excess			
Homovanillic acid (HVA)—adult	<45	µmol/24h	<8	mg/24h
Homovanillic acid (HVA)—1–6 months	<6	µmol/24h	<1	mg/24h

Tests	Reference range	SI units	Reference range	Traditional units
Urine (per 24 hours) (contd)				
Homovanillic acid (HVA) — 6–12 months	<8	μmol/24h	<1.5	mg/24h
Homovanillic acid (HVA) — 1–5 years	<14	μmol/24h	<2.5	mg/24h
Homovanillic acid (HVA) — 5–10 years	<33	μmol/24h	<6	mg/24h
Homovanillic acid (HVA) — 10–15 years	<39	μmol/24h	<7	mg/24h
5-Hydroxyindoleacetic acid (5HIAA)	<50	μmol/24h	<10	mg/24h
Magnesium	3.0–5.0	mmol/24h		
Melanogens	No excess			
Osmolality	50–1200	mOsm/kg		
Oxalate — male	0.08–0.49	mmol/24h	7–44	mg/24h
Oxalate — female	0.04–0.32	mmol/24h	4–30	mg/24h
Oxalate — children	0.14–0.42	mmol/24h	12–38	mg/24h
Phosphate — diet dependent	13–42	mmol/24h	0.5–1.3	g/24h
Porphobilinogen	No excess			
Porphyrins	No excess			
Potassium — diet dependent	35–90	mmol/24h	35–90	mEq/24h
Protein — total	<0.15	g/24hr	<150	mg/24h
Purgative screen	None detectable			
Sodium — diet dependent	60–180	mmol/24h	60–180	mEq/24h
Urate — diet dependent	3.5–4.2	mmol/24h	0.6–0.7	g/24h
Urea — diet dependent	166–581	mmol/24h	4.6–16.5	g/24h
Urobilinogen	No excess			
Zinc	4.5–9.0	μmol/24h	294–588	μg/24
Faeces				
Laxative screen	None detectable			
Occult blood	None detectable			
Porphyrins	No excess			
Reducing substances	None detectable			
Total fat	<18.0	mmol/24h	<5	g/24h
Weight	<200	g/24h		
Sweat				
Sodium	<60	mmol/L	<60	mEq/L
Chloride	<70	mmol/L	<70	mEq/L

Reference ranges in haematology

APPENDIX TABLE 1.2   Haematology adult reference ranges.

Tests	Reference range	Units
Blood		
Activated partial thromboplastin time (KPTT)	27–38	s
Basophils	$0.01–0.10 \times 10^9$	cells/L
Bleeding time	3–9	min
Eosinophils	$0.04–0.40 \times 19^9$	cells/L
Erythrocyte sedimentation rate (ESR)—male	1–10	mm/h
Erythrocyte sedimentation rate (ESR)—female	3–15	mm/h
Factor VIII:C	0.51–1.25	IU/mL
Factor IX	0.57–1.29	IU/mL
Fibrinogen	1.5–4.5	g/L
Folate—serum	4–18	ug/L
Folate—red cell	160–640	ug/L
G6PD	10.1–18.5	IU/gHb
Haematocrit—males	0.400–0.540	
Haematocrit—females	0.370–0.470	
Hamoglobin—male	13.5–17.5	g/dL
Haemoglobin—female	11.5–16.5	g/dL
Haemoglobin A2	1.5–3.5	%
Haemoglobin F	0.2–0.8	%
Haptoglobins	90–38	mg/dL
Lymphocytes	$1.50–4.00 \times 10^9$	cells/L
Mean cell haemoglobin (MCH)	27.0–32.0	pg
Mean cell haemoglobin concentration (MCHC)	32.0–36.0	g/dL
Mean cell volume (MCV)	80–96	fL
Methaemoglobin	<1	%
Monocytes	$0.20–0.80 \times 10^9$	cells/L
Neutrophils	$2.00–7.50 \times 10^9$	cells/L
6PGD	5.6–11.6	IU/gHb
Platelets	$150–400 \times 10^9$	cells/L
Prothrombin time (INR, PTR)	1.00–1.30	ratio
Pyruvate kinase	11–21	IU/gHb
Red blood cell count (RBC)—male	$4.5–6.5 \times 10^{12}$	cells/L
Red blood cell count (RBC)—female	$3.8–5.8 \times 10^{12}$	cells/L
Reticulocytes	0.2–2.0	%
Thrombin time	13–16	s
Viscosity (plasma)	1.50–1.72	mPa.s
Vitamin B_{12}	160–900	ng/L
White blood cell count (WBC)	$4.0–11.0 \times 10^9$	cells/L

II
COLLECTING SPECIMENS FOR LABORATORY ANALYSIS

VENEPUNCTURE

Apply a tourniquet and applied round the upper arm over the middle of the biceps so as to impede the venous but not the arterial flow. The skin at the bend of the elbow is 'painted' with 0.5% chlorhexidine in 70% alcohol or simply 70% spirit (iodine is expensive and can give rise to severe skin reactions). The skin is rendered tense by the operator's left hand; the syringe with the needle attached is held in the right hand and almost parallel with the patient's arm; the patient is asked to 'make a fist' and then the needle with the bevel upwards is inserted into a prominent vein—the median basilic vein is usually convenient—and the needle is pointed in the direction of the blood flow. The required amount of blood is then drawn up into the syringe and the tourniquet is removed before the needle is withdrawn, as otherwise a haematoma may form. For some purposes it is necessary to remove the tourniquet as soon as the needle enters the vein, so that free-flowing blood is withdrawn. As soon as the needle is withdrawn a swab is placed on the puncture site and the patient is asked to hold the forearm firmly flexed against the upper arm for a minute or so. Occasionally a vein in the forearm or wrist may prove more convenient than one at the elbow, but the procedure is then usually more painful. A vein which can be felt is generally easier to enter than one which can only be seen.

Blood obtained by venepuncture should be placed immediately in the appropriate container for the test requested. The needle must first be removed from the syringe, since forcing the blood through the needle may cause haemolysis. Appropriate containers for particular investigations should be obtained from the laboratory. Most biochemical and immunological tests require serum samples. Blood can be collected for these in tubes that do not contain anticoagulant. If plasma samples whole blood is required *Heparin and sequestrene (EDTA)* are the most generally useful anticoagulants. Sequestrene can be used for most haematological investigations and heparin for most simple chemical tests, with the exception of blood glucose, for which bottles containing sodium fluoride are necessary. For blood group and serological investigations blood should be taken into a dry sterile bottle or tube. If the specimen has to be sent to the laboratory by post, it is best to wait till the blood has clotted. Some serum should then be removed with a sterile needle and syringe; this serum is sent separately, together with the blood clot.

OTHER SPECIMENS

Urine, faeces, peritoneal fluid, pleural fluid, gastric and pancreatic juice, bile, arterial blood samples, semen, nasal secretions, cerebrospinal fluid, fluid aspirated from cysts, epididymal cysts, cutaneous cysts, etc. and pus may also be collected and sent to the laboratory for examination. Methods for the collection of these samples are discussed elsewhere in this book.

MICROBIOLOGICAL INVESTIGATIONS

Special care is necessary both in the collection and in the transport of specimens for microbiological examination to the laboratory because:

- Successful culture depends on the viability of the organisms
- Overgrowth of the normal flora present in the specimen can hinder detection of the pathogen, which is often present only in small numbers
- Careless collection techniques can lead to cross-contamination with organisms present on the patient's or operator's skin, or in the environment.

The organism can be visualized directly in the specimen, or an antibody response to the infecting organism can be demonstrated in the blood. Direct detection requires the presence of a relatively large number of organisms in the specimen, for example in pus. Organisms can also be detected by culture techniques, that is, by allowing the organism to multiply.

Genes or gene products specific to the organism can also be detected, even when only small numbers of the organism are present. These methods use immunological principles to detect antigens by complement fixing antibodies, or the *polymerase chain reaction (PCR)* to detect organism-specific proteins. Although these methods are very sensitive, unless meticulous care is taken both during collection of the specimen and during performance of the test, contamination with other antigens or proteins is a problem that reduces the specificity of the result. In addition, specificity may not be as great as expected when antigens are shared by the organism and by the patient's tissues.

SEROLOGICAL RESPONSE TO INFECTION

Traditionally, antibodies have been detected and assayed in serum. Antibody responses can also be detected in other body fluids, including CSF and saliva. The *total antibody response* and the *IgG response* are useful in measuring the incidence of disease in a community. To identify active current infection it is necessary, in general, either to demonstrate the presence of *IgM*, or a fourfold increase in titre of total antibody, during the course of the illness.

TISSUE DISCHARGES, PUS, CSF AND OTHER FLUIDS

It is important always to send a sufficient quantity of material to the laboratory. Generally, about 10–15 g of tissue or discharge and up to 25 ml of fluid are necessary. These are substantial amounts. If only very small amounts of material are available (e.g. less than an apple pip in size), it should be sent in a sterile container containing isotonic saline (never in formol saline). When only small amounts of material are available, the best results will be obtained by asking the laboratory personnel to come to the patient's bedside to make the cultures there (Figs 1–3). If it is not possible to submit material for culture in sufficient bulk then a swab may be taken. Ensure that the correct swab, supplied by the laboratory, is used. Swabs will vary according to which pathogen is sought (Box 1).

BLOOD CULTURE

Blood cultures may be set up for bacteria or viruses. Blood culture for *bacterial pathogens* is useful in the investigation of almost all infections, although it is necessary for diagnosis in only a few clinical situa-

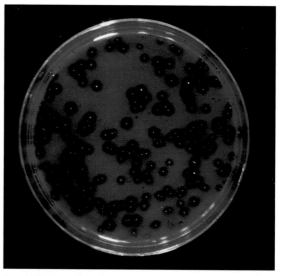

Appendix 2.2 Beta-haemolytic streptococci cultured from a throat swab on a blood agar medium.

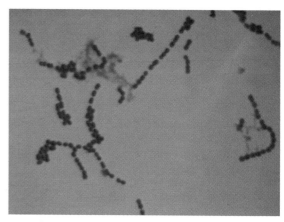

Appendix 2.3 Gram smear of culture of pus showing a growth of streptococci.

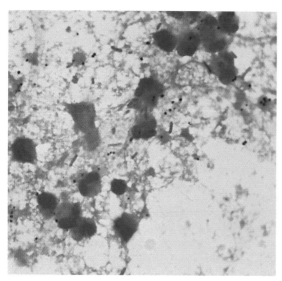

Appendix 2.1 Pus from abscess, containing Gram-positive cocci and Gram-negative rods.

BOX APPENDIX 2.1   Swabs.

- Plain swab *without* transport medium: used for hardy microorganisms only; rarely the swab of choice
- Plain swab *with* transport medium: for general bacteriology
- Swab *with* charcoal (black) transport: for *Neisseria gonorrhoeae*, and other delicate bacteria
- Plain swab *with* virus transport medium: essential to gently squeeze swab in transport medium. Virus transport medium contains antibiotics and is *not* suitable for bacterial culture
- Chlamydial swab *with* transport medium: for detection of *Chlamydia trachomatis* antigen by immunoassay. Designed for use with urogenital and ophthalmic specimens only
- Wire swab *with* transport medium: for isolation of nasal pertussis infection

tions. Bacteria are often present in blood in only very low concentrations, and their viability and growth potential may be inhibited by antibiotic treatment. Since so many different infections may be accompanied by *septicaemia* it is important to inoculate a variety of different culture media. The media used should be suitable for aerobic pathogens, anaerobic pathogens, and for fastidious species such as *Brucella* spp., *Mycobacteria* spp., *Leptospira* spp., and for non-bacterial pathogens such as fungi. Antibacterial substances present in the patient's blood can be inactivated by dilution (at least 1 : 10), by the addition of specific enzymes (e.g. penicillinase) or by absorption by resins.

Before you withdraw blood, the patient's skin and the bottle cap should be cleaned with 70% alcohol or alcohol chlorhexidine, and allowed to dry. At least three sets of blood cultures should be taken, preferably before antibiotic therapy is begun. Occasionally, particularly if endocarditis is suspected, it may be necessary to take up to six sets of cultures before a negative result can be accepted.

For the detection of *viral pathogens* sterile heparinized blood should be sent to the virus laboratory. For serological investigations clotted blood in a sterile container, without additives, is required.

URINE CULTURE

Urine specimens (Box 2) should be transferred to the laboratory within one hour of voiding, unless specific precautions are taken to prevent bacterial multiplication before cultures are set up. Urine specimens may be stored overnight at 4°C. If this is not possible, then a commercial kit for culture of the specimen at the bedside should be used. Several commercial 'chemical' kits are available, but experience in their sensitivity and specificity is limited at present.

BOX APPENDIX 2.2   Urine collections for microbiological examination.

Catheter specimen of urine (CSU)
Aspirate the urine, via a 21-gauge needle and syringe, from the rubberized part of the tubing connecting the catheter to the collection bag. *Do not collect urine from the tap outlet to the bag.*

Early morning urine (EMU)
Send the entire first-voided specimen, usually about 250 ml, to the laboratory in the large sterile container provided. Three consecutive morning specimens should be taken.

Mid-stream urine (MSU)
A urine specimen is taken during mid-micturition by the patient, after instruction, or with the assistance of a nurse, after the labia or penile orifice has been cleaned with chlorhexidine.

Mid-stream (MSU) or suprapubic aspiration techniques are suitable for general bacterial and viral culture of urine, but are unsuitable for typhoid or tuberculosis. In the diagnosis of the latter infection three early morning urine (EMU) specimens should be submitted to the laboratory. For the diagnosis of schistosomiasis the terminal 5 ml of a freshly voided specimen is required.

EXAMINATION OF FAECES

Human faeces contain approximately 10^{11} organisms/g wet weight as normal flora, whereas gut bacterial pathogens rarely exceed 10^5 organisms/g. Because of the relative scarcity of pathogens in faecal specimens, examination of a Gram-stained smear of faeces is not usually performed. However, occasionally in infections caused by *Campylobacter* spp. the typical seagull-shaped Gram-negative bacteria are present in sufficient numbers to be identifiable in a directly stained smear of a faecal specimen. The mainstay of diagnosis of bacterial infections of the gut is by culture. Correct collection and transportation of the specimen to the laboratory is particularly important, since incorrect technique can lead to the death of the pathogen or to overgrowth by normal gut flora.

COLLECTION OF THE SPECIMEN

Approximately 20 ml of stool should be collected on three separate occasions as early as possible in the illness and placed in three separate, sterile containers. For immediate transfer to the laboratory dry sterile containers are suitable but, if there is a delay in transportation to the laboratory, the faecal specimen should be placed in a suitable preservative, for example in 0.0033 M phosphate buffer mixed with an equal volume of glycerol, at pH 7.0. If possible, include any mucus or blood in the faeces in the specimen submitted.

As there are a large number of bacterial species that can cause diarrhoea, the laboratory will use many different selective culture media in order to increase the isolation rate. It is essential to note on the accompanying request form any relevant clinical details to enable the laboratory staff to seek the most likely pathogens. Important information includes a history of travel to potentially endemic areas, prior antibiotic therapy, any known outbreak of sporadic disease, possible contamination of food, and any associated immunosuppressive disease.

Many of the viruses which cause diarrhoea cannot be cultured. Diagnosis is therefore often made by immunological techniques, or by electron microscopic identification of the virus. When viral pathogens are suspected, chemical preservatives should not be used in the collection containers. Specimens should be taken into a dry sterile container and sent to the laboratory promptly, or frozen at −20°C (−70°C is optimal but rarely available). For direct detection of viral particles by electron micro-copy many particles must be present. Electron microscopy is a specific but not very sensitive technique.

Parasitic infections are discussed in Chapter 23. For detection of *Entamoeba histolytica* infestation the faecal specimen must be kept at body tempera-ture until it can be examined. Other cysts and ova can be detected by examination of stool sent in a plain sterile container.

THE RESPIRATORY TRACT

Material may be taken for detection of bacterial or viral infections. Specimens can be taken from the throat, the nasopharynx, sputum or by broncho-alveolar lavage, as appropriate.

THROAT SWABS

Vigorously swab the tonsillar areas, the posterior pharynx, and any areas of visible inflammation, exu-dation, ulceration or membrane formation. For bac-terial cultures, use a plain swab with transport medium. For viral detection, use a plain swab with virus transport medium. The specimen should be sent immediately to the laboratory, or stored at 4°C; it should not be frozen.

NASOPHARYNX

Specimens of nasopharyngeal secretions are used prin-cipally for diagnosis of *Pertussis* infection, an uncom-mon disorder in developed countries, in which immunization programmes have been largely effective in preventing whooping cough. The specimen is obtained using a wire per nasal swab. The swab is passed gently along the base of the nostril into the nasopharynx, rotated, removed and placed into trans-port medium. The laboratory may need prior warning of the arrival of the specimen so that appropriate culture media can be prepared.

For detection of viral pathogens from the nasopharynx an aspirated specimen is obtained using a suction catheter.

SPUTUM

For best results an early morning freshly expecto-rated sputum specimen should be collected in a dry, sterile bottle, preferably with the help of a physio-therapist. For isolation of mycobacteria three con-secutive morning specimens should be obtained.

BRONCHO-ALVEOLAR LAVAGE

This technique may be helpful when lower respira-tory tract infection is suspected, e.g. *Legionella* spp., *Nocardia* spp., *Pneumocystis carinii*, *Mycobacterium* spp. and *Cytomegalovirus* infections.

THE GENITAL TRACT

Different methods are used for particular clinical problems (Box 3).

THE SKIN

Dermatophytes and *Candida albicans* can be detected in keratinized specimens (e.g. hair, skin scrapings or nail cuttings), sent enclosed in black paper, for ease of recognition. Do not use sticky tape.

THE EYES

There are methods for detection of bacterial and viral pathogens. *Bacterial conjunctival infection* can be assessed in conjunctival swabs. Using a firm action, thoroughly swab the inner surface of the lower and then the upper eyelid, using a separate swab for each eye. Use a plain swab and a transport medium. For gonorrhoeal infection use a charcoal transport medium. *Intraocular infection*, assessed by bedside inoculation of tiny quantities of aspirated material, can be performed by the ophthalmologist. Viral pathogens can be detected using a swab moistened with sterile saline to collect secretions from the palpe-bral conjunctiva; this is inserted into a transport medium. Scrapings from cornea or conjunctiva can be collected by the ophthalmologist. *Chlamydia* infection can be detected in specimens of many epithelial cells, but the specimens should not consist of pus.

BOX APPENDIX 2.3   Microbiological investigation of the genital tract.

Neisseria gonorrhoeae infection
- Urethral and/or endocervical (not high vagina), rectal or throat swabs
- Use charcoal transport medium

Chlamydia trachomatis
- Endocervical (not high vaginal) or urethral specimen
- Inoculate in transport medium
- Abnormal specimens will contain pus cells
- Specimen can be stored at 2–8°C

Candida spp. and *Trichomonas* spp.
- High vaginal swab in plain transport medium

Herpes simplex virus (HSV)
- Most successful in first 3 days of infection
- Use plain sterile swab to collect vesicular fluid into viral transport medium
- Air-dried smears of scrapings from base of vesicles can be used for direct examination by immunofluorescence

Pelvic inflammatory disease
- Send endocervical swabs of pus in charcoal transport medium

III
CHEMICAL TESTS USED IN URINALYSIS

The classic tests for urinary protein, sugar, ketones and urobilinogen have largely been replaced by commercial reagent strip tests. Commercial tests incorporate modifications of the reagents used in the classic tests into convenient standardized procedures. However, traditional chemical urine tests are reliable and use commonly available reagents; it is therefore still useful to have access to them should reagent strip tests not be available.

PROTEINURIA

THE SALICYLSULPHONIC ACID TEST

To 5 ml urine in a test tube add 20% salicylsulphonic acid, drop by drop. The presence of protein is indicated by a cloudy precipitate, best seen against a black background, but up to 25 drops may be required before this forms. Continue to add salicylsulphonic acid until no more precipitate is formed. For ordinary purposes it is sufficient to express the amount present as a haze, cloud or granular precipitate, a haze representing about 20 mg protein per 100 ml; a heavier deposit should be allowed to settle (which may take an hour or so) and the quantity expressed as the proportion of the urine volume occupied by the deposit. If this proportion is one-half, the urine contains about 10 g protein/litre. False-positive results may be due to the presence of radiographic contrast medium; they may also occur in patients treated with sulphonamides, tolbutamide, para-aminosalicylic acid or large doses of penicillin, or if the urine contains a lot of uric acid.

THE BOILING TEST

Fill a small test tube two-thirds full of urine. If this is alkaline, add 10% acetic acid, drop by drop, mixing thoroughly after each drop, until pH 5 is reached as shown by pH indicator paper. Boil the top 2 cm over a flame while holding the bottom of the tube and examine against a dark background. A cloudiness indicates the presence of protein, or of phosphates which have precipitated because loss of carbon dioxide on boiling has made the urine more alkaline. If the precipitate disappears on adding more acid it was due to phosphates; if not, it is precipitated protein. If more than a light cloud persists, boil all the urine, acidifying until no more protein is deposited. Allow to settle and express semiquantitatively as described for the salicylsulphonic acid test. The two tests are comparable in sensitivity.

Treatment with tolbutamide or large doses of penicillin, or the presence of radiographic contrast medium, may cause false-positive results.

URINARY SUGAR

BENEDICT'S TEST

This is not specific for glucose and a positive reaction is given by any reducing substance present in the urine. To 5 ml of Benedict's reagent add 8 drops of urine, boil for 2 minutes and allow to cool. If a reducing substance is present, a precipitate will appear, varying from a light green turbidity to a red precipitate (see Table 1). If the reduction is due to glucose, the test gives approximately quantitative results.

URINARY KETONES

ROTHERA'S TEST

A volume of 10 ml of urine is saturated with an excess of ammonium sulphate crystals; 3 drops of a strong, freshly prepared solution of sodium nitroprusside and 2 ml of strong ammonia solution are then added. A deep permanganate colour is produced by acetone and acetoacetic acid. If Rothera's test is negative, ketones are absent.

APPENDIX TABLE 3.1	Benedict's test.
Precipitate	Sugar (g/dl)
Light green turbidity	0.1–0.5
Green precipitate	0.5–1.0
Yellow precipitate	1.0–2.0
Red precipitate	2.0 or more

GERHARDT'S TEST

Drop by drop, 10% ferric chloride solution is added to 5 ml of urine in a test tube. A precipitate of ferric phosphate usually forms, but disappears again when more ferric chloride is added. The solution becomes brownish-red if acetoacetic acid is present.

Aspirin and other salicylates, phenothiazines, phenol and some other drugs give a similar colour with ferric chloride. Boiling the urine for 5 minutes before adding the ferric chloride destroys aceto acetic acid, but the other substances which react with it are unaffected. If, therefore, urine which has been boiled still gives a positive reaction, it may be inferred that this is not due to acetoacetic acid or to other substances.

A positive ferric chloride reaction is obtained only if acetoacetic acid is present in considerable amount. If the urine reacts to Rothera's test but not to ferric chloride, it may be deduced that only a small amount is present. If both are positive, the patient is severely ketotic and requires urgent treatment.

UROBILINOGEN AND PORPHOBILINOGEN

EHRLICH'S ALDEHYDE TEST

At room temperature, 1 ml of fresh urine is mixed with 1 ml of Ehrlich's aldehyde reagent (2 g paradi-methylaminobenzaldehyde, dissolved in 100 ml of 5% hydrochloric acid). After 1.5 minutes 2 ml saturated aqueous sodium acetate is added and mixed, followed by 2 ml of a 3 : 1 (v/v) mixture of amyl alcohol and benzyl alcohol. The test tube is stoppered and its contents are shaken gently for 1 minute. After the phases have separated, a red colour in the upper (alcohol) phase indicates that urobilinogen is present, while a similar colour in the lower (aqueous) phase denotes porphobilinogen. Chloroform may be used in the test as an alternative to amyl and benzyl alcohols. It separates more quickly, into the *lower* layer, where the red colour due to urobilinogen may be seen. Normal fresh urine contains enough urobilinogen to produce a weakly positive reaction.

INDEX